The
Pot Book

"*The Pot Book* traces the secret history of marijuana, examines the disconnect between seventy years of prohibition and the American public's personal attitudes toward pot, and offers a clear-eyed look at all the uses of cannabis, including the growing list of its widespread medicinal benefits. Consulting with the top experts in the field, Dr. Julie Holland presents the current science and makes a compelling case for the need for further research, unencumbered by anti-drug hysteria, as well as an immediate change to our nation's puritanical drug laws."

JOHN DIOSO, DEPUTY MANAGING EDITOR OF *ROLLING STONE*

"The most-up-to-date and reliable source of information on the exploding frontiers of cannabis science written by the top experts in the field. I highly recommend this book."

STEVEN HAGER, *HIGH TIMES* CREATIVE DIRECTOR

"Dr. Julie Holland has assembled a virtual dream team of cannabis experts for this marijuana magnum opus."

STEVE BLOOM, PUBLISHER OF CELEBSTONER.COM, COAUTHOR OF *POT CULTURE* AND *REEFER MOVIE MADNESS,* AND FORMER EDITOR OF *HIGH TIMES*

"Dr. Holland's brilliant compendium of marijuana facts and cultural insights from the best medical minds and scientific researchers, while acknowledging the potential for abuse, makes a compelling case for cannabis as the most ancient, benign, and uplifting inebriant/sacrament/medicine humanity has ever known. Just say Know."

ALEX AND ALLYSON GREY, ARTISTS AND COFOUNDERS
OF THE CHAPEL OF SACRED MIRRORS (CoSM)

The Pot Book reveals the truth about cannabis in one timely, even-handed volume. Dr. Julie Holland has brought together the top experts discussing every aspect of this persistently misunderstood plant. *The Pot Book* is now the best single source for information and insights on marijuana."

NEAL M. GOLDSMITH, PH.D.,
AUTHOR OF *PSYCHEDELIC HEALING*

"Are you a lover or hater of the pot world? In either case this book is for you, if you want to be enlightened. I knew the book was a winner as soon as I held it and felt the good vibrations. Read it and tell your friends."

TOMMY CHONG, COMEDIAN, ACTOR,
AND CANNABIS ACTIVIST

The
Pot Book

A Complete Guide
to Cannabis

Its Role in Medicine, Politics,
Science, and Culture

Edited by Julie Holland, M.D.

Park Street Press
Rochester, Vermont • Toronto, Canada

Park Street Press
One Park Street
Rochester, Vermont 05767
www.ParkStPress.com

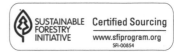

Text stock is SFI certified

Park Street Press is a division of Inner Traditions International

Note to the reader: This book is intended as an informational guide. The approaches and techniques described herein should not be seen as an endorsement to use marijuana. They also should not be used to treat a serious ailment without prior consultation with a qualified healthcare professional.

Library of Congress Cataloging-in-Publication Data

The pot book : a complete guide to cannabis : its role in medicine, politics, science, and culture / edited by Julie Holland.
    p. ; cm.
  Includes bibliographical references and index.
  Summary: "Leading experts on the science, history, politics, medicine, and potential of America's most popular recreational drug"—Provided by publisher.
  ISBN 978-1-59477-368-6
  1. Cannabis. 2. Marijuana. I. Holland, Julie, 1965–
  [DNLM: 1. Cannabis. 2. Marijuana Smoking—therapy. 3. Marijuana Abuse. 4. Marijuana Smoking—adverse effects. 5. Phytotherapy. WB 925 P859 2010]
  HV5822.C3P68 2010
  362.29'5—dc22

2010023186

Printed and bound in the United States by Lake Book Manufacturing
The text paper is 100% SFI certified. The Sustainable Forestry Initiative® program promotes sustainable forest management.

10 9 8 7

Text design by Jon Desautels and layout by Priscilla Baker
This book was typeset in Garamond Premier Pro with Helvetica Neue used as a display typeface

To send correspondence to the author of this book, mail a first-class letter to the author c/o Inner Traditions • Bear & Company, One Park Street, Rochester, VT 05767, and we will forward the communication, or contact the author at **www.ThePotBook.com**.

Dedication

To the late John Paul Morgan, M.D., chemist, genius, New Yorker, musician, scientist, professor, and friend, who passed away on February 15, 2008. His book Marijuana Myths/Marijuana Facts: A Review of the Scientific Evidence, *coauthored with Lynn Zimmer, Ph.D., and published by the Lindesmith Center in 1997, helped debunk the following myths:*

Marijuana's harms have been proven scientifically.

Marijuana has no medicinal value.

Marijuana is highly addictive.

Marijuana is a gateway drug.

Marijuana offenses are not severely punished.

Marijuana policy in the Netherlands is a failure.

Marijuana kills brain cells.

Marijuana causes an amotivational syndrome.

Marijuana impairs memory and cognition.

Marijuana can cause permanent mental illness.

Marijuana causes crime.

Marijuana interferes with male and female sex hormones.

Marijuana use during pregnancy damages the fetus.

Marijuana use impairs the immune system.

Marijuana is more damaging to the lungs than tobacco.

Marijuana's active ingredient, THC, gets trapped in body fat.

Marijuana use is a major cause of highway accidents.

Marijuana-related hospital emergencies are increasing, particularly among youth.

Marijuana is more potent today than in the past.

Marijuana use can be prevented.

Contents

Foreword by Lester Grinspoon, M.D.   xi

Introduction   1

PART ONE
An Overview of Cannabis

Introduction to Part One   6

1   The Subjective Effects of Cannabis   9
      Matthew G. Kirkpatrick and Carl L. Hart, Ph.D.

2   Early/Ancient History   17
      Chris Bennett

3   Recent History   27
      David Malmo-Levine

4   The Botany of *Cannabis*   35
      Lyle E. Craker, Ph.D., and Zoë Gardner

5   Cannabis Grow Revolution   44
      Danny Danko

6   The Endocannabinoid System   52
      *Gregory L. Gerdeman, Ph.D., and
      Jason B. Schechter, Ph.D.*

7   Anandamide and More   63
      Raphael Mechoulam, Ph.D., and Lumír Hanuš

8   Cannabis Laws in the United States   73
      Allen St. Pierre

9   On Ending Prohibition   130
      Ethan Nadelmann, J.D., Ph.D.

PART TWO
Risks of Use and Harm Reduction

Introduction to Part Two   136

10   Medical Risks and Toxicology   141
William Holubek, M.D.

11   Pulmonary Harm and Vaporizers   153
Mitch Earleywine, Ph.D.

12   Cannabis and Cognition   161
Caroline B. Marvin and Carl L. Hart, Ph.D.

13   Mental Health Risks Associated with Cannabis Use   178
Cheryl Corcoran, M.D.

14   How Real Is the Risk of Addiction?   187
Ryan Vandrey, Ph.D., and Margaret Haney, Ph.D.

15   Driving Under the Influence   196
Paul Armentano

16   Arrest Statistics and Racism   202
Harry G. Levine, Ph.D.

17   Getting Busted Is Not So Funny   207
An Interview with Tommy Chong
Julie Holland, M.D.

18   The Collateral Consequences of Cannabis Convictions   219
Richard Glen Boire, J.D.

19   Harm Reduction Psychotherapy   223
Andrew Tatarsky, Ph.D.

PART THREE
The Clinical Use of Cannabis

Introduction to Part Three   242

20   The Clinical Applications of Medical Marijuana   247
An Interview with Andrew Weil, M.D.
Julie Holland, M.D.

21   Medical Marijuana Research   252
An Interview with Donald Abrams, M.D.
Julie Holland, M.D.

22   MAPS and the Federal Obstruction of
Medical Marijuana Research   261
Rick Doblin, Ph.D.

23   The Government's Pot Farm   266
An Interview with Mahmoud A. ElSohly, Ph.D.
Julie Holland, M.D.

24   Cannabinoids and Psychiatry   282
Julie Holland, M.D.

25   Cannabinoids and Neuroprotection   295
*Sunil K. Aggarwal, M.D., Ph.D., and
Gregory T. Carter, M.D.*

26   Cannabis and HIV/AIDS   311
Mark A. Ware, M.D., and Lynne Belle-Isle

27   Multiple Sclerosis and Spasticity   318
Denis J. Petro, M.D.

28   Pain Management   328
Mark S. Wallace, M.D., and Ben Platt, M.D.

29   Sativex   336
William Notcutt, M.D., F.R.C.A., F.F.P.M.R.C.A.

PART FOUR

Cannabis Culture

Introduction to Part Four   344

30   What to Tell the Children   349
Marsha Rosenbaum, Ph.D.

31   Pot, Parenting, and Outing Myself   361
Neal Pollack

32   Cannabis: Stealth Goddess   366
Doug Rushkoff

33 Gardener's Rights, Forgetting, and Co-Evolution   373
    An Interview with Michael Pollan
    Julie Holland, M.D.

34 Cannabis, Business, and Philanthropy   383
    An Interview with Peter Lewis
    Julie Holland, M.D.

35 Thots on Pot   387
    Jeremy Wolff

PART FIVE

Steps in the Right Direction

Introduction to Part Five   396

36 Patients Out of Time   399
    An Interview with Al Byrne, L.CDR. (retired), and
    Mary Lynn Mathre, R.N., C.A.R.N.
    Julie Holland, M.D.

37 Prescribing Cannabis in California   416
    Jeffrey Hergenrather, M.D.

38 Canadian Compassion Clubs   432
    N. Rielle Capler, M.H.A.

39 Dutch Drug Policy   441
    Mario Lap

40 A Cost-Benefit Analysis of Legalizing Marijuana   447
    Jeffrey Miron, Ph.D.

41 The Marijuana Policy Project   454
    Bruce Mirken

42 The ACLU and Cannabis Drug Policy   462
    An Interview with Graham Boyd, J.D.
    Julie Holland, M.D.

    Resources   473
    References   483
    Contributors   534
    Index   544

Foreword

Lester Grinspoon, M.D.

Every age has its peculiar folly; and if Charles Mackay, the author of the mid-nineteenth-century classic *Extraordinary Popular Delusions and the Madness of Crowds,* were alive today, he would surely see "cannabinophobia" as a popular delusion along with the "tulipmania" and "witch hunts" of earlier ages. I believe that we are now at the cusp of this particular popular delusion, which to date has been responsible for the arrest of over 20 million U.S. citizens. Future historians will likely look at this epoch and recognize it as another instance of the "madness of crowds." Millions of marijuana users have already arrived at this understanding.

For a short period in the '70s, it was possible to believe that this popular delusion was beginning to lose its deeply embedded grip. Whatever the cultural conditions that made it possible, there was no doubt that the discussion about marijuana was becoming more sensible as we became conscious of the irrationality of classifying this drug as one with a high abuse potential and no medical value. If that trend had continued, it was likely that within another decade marijuana would have been sold and regulated in the United States in much the same way as alcohol.

At that time, we had reason to be optimistic. In 1971 the National Commission on Marijuana and Drug Abuse, appointed by President Nixon, had recommended the elimination of penalties for possession of marijuana for personal use and casual nonprofit transfers of small amounts. In 1973 Oregon had become the first state to decriminalize marijuana, making possession of less than an ounce a civil offense penalized by a small fine. In 1975 Alaska had eliminated all penalties for private possession and cultivation of less than four ounces. President Carter had endorsed decriminalization, as had the American Medical Association, the American Psychiatric Association, the American Bar Association, and the National Council of Churches. By 1977 most states had reduced simple possession to a misdemeanor, and by 1980 eleven states had actually decriminalized possession.

Unfortunately, this trend did not continue. The marijuana reform movement peaked in the late 1970s. In 1978 Dr. Peter Bourne, the White House drug advisor who had helped President Carter move toward reform, resigned and was replaced by Lee Dogoloff, a hardliner. In that same year the proportion of the population favoring marijuana legalization began to fall from its 1977 high of 28 percent. Under President Reagan the government instituted a program of "zero tolerance." By 1983 it was spraying the dangerous insecticide Paraquat on domestic marijuana crops and using military methods to uproot cannabis plants and arrest growers in northern California.

In 1987 Supreme Court nominee Douglas Ginsberg had to withdraw under pressure because he had smoked marijuana as a law professor. In 1989, under President George H. W. Bush, the federal government began Operation Green Merchant, which confiscated lists of people who had ordered indoor plant-growing equipment and raided their homes. The first Bush administration also worked hard to persuade Alaska to recriminalize marijuana possession and succeeded in 1990. That same year Congress passed a bill calling for federal transportation funds to be withheld from states refusing to enact a six-month suspension of the automobile licenses of people convicted of marijuana possession.

These increasingly harsh government measures (and the growing hysteria of antimarijuana citizens' groups) did not reflect any new knowledge about the dangers of this drug. The more than a third of a century since the publication of the first edition of *Marihuana Reconsidered* has produced remarkably little laboratory, sociological, or epidemiological evidence of serious health or social problems caused by marijuana. The present attitude of the government and antimarijuana crusaders bears the same relationship to reality that the film *Reefer Madness* bore in 1936. But the dissonance is even more striking now, because we know so much more.

Since 1971 millions of dollars have been spent by the National Institute of Drug Abuse to study the dangers of cannabis. This vast research enterprise has completely failed to provide a scientific basis for prohibition. Although evidence against toxicity continues to accumulate, the government persists in escalating its war on marijuana users, most cruelly on those who use it for medicinal purposes. To justify this policy—usually with the Drug Enforcement Administration (DEA) as its voice—it distorts, stretches, truncates, or simply ignores research findings.

The U.S. government's commitment to gross exaggeration of the harmfulness of cannabis has made it necessary for it to deny the drug's medical usefulness in the face of overwhelming evidence. In 1991 the DEA was inundated with requests for marijuana from people with AIDS. In response, James O. Mason, head of the Public Health Service, announced that the Compassionate IND Program, which had helped a handful of patients use marijuana legally as a medicine, would be suspended. He explained that this program undercut the administration's opposition to the use of illegal drugs: "If it is perceived that the Public Health Service is going around giving marijuana to folks, there would be a perception that this stuff can't be so bad," Mason said. "It gives a bad signal. I don't mind doing that if there is no other way of helping these people. . . . But there is not a shred of evidence that smoking marijuana assists a person with AIDS."

In 1971, I pointed out in *Marihuana Reconsidered* that since cannabis had been used by so many people all over the world for thousands of years with so little evidence of significant toxic effects, the discovery of some previously unknown serious health hazard was unlikely. I suggested that the emphasis in cannabis research should be shifted to its potential both as a medicine and as a tool to advance our understanding of brain function. Although few government resources have been committed to either of these fields, there have been compelling developments in both.

In 1990 researchers discovered the first of two receptors in the brain stimulated by THC. This exciting discovery implied that the body produces its own version of cannabinoids for one or more useful purposes. The first of these cannabinoid-like neurotransmitters was identified in 1992 and named anandamide (*ananda* is the Sanskrit word for bliss). Cannabinoid receptor sites occur not only in the lower brain but also in the cerebral cortex, which governs higher thinking, and in the hippocampus, which is a locus of memory.

These discoveries raise some interesting questions. Could the distribution of anandamide receptor sites in the higher brain explain why so many marijuana users claim that the drug enhances some mental activities, including creativity and fluidity of associations? Do these receptor sites play a role in marijuana's capacity to alter the subjective experience of time? What about the subtle enhancement of perception and the capacity to experience the physical world with some of the freshness and excitement of childhood?

Today there is a large research enterprise focusing on what is now called the endocannabinoid system, promoting a better understanding of the remarkably diverse versatility of cannabis as a medicine, a recreational drug, and an enhancer.

Despite conditions that deter medical researchers, medical applications of cannabis have seen considerable progress since 1971 under the most unusual and difficult of circumstances. New drugs are generally shepherded through the complicated federal regulatory obstacle course by pharmaceutical companies that devote vast resources to the task of taking a chemical with putative therapeutic potential and transforming it into a marketable property. For many reasons, including the fact that patent protection is impossible for a plant, no drug company is ever likely to undertake this effort on behalf of herbal marijuana. Although the U.S. government has been steadfast in its opposition to recognizing the medical utility of cannabis, ever-larger numbers of people are using marijuana medically.

Several developments have piqued interest in cannabis as a medicine. In the early 1970s many people noticed that cannabis could relieve the intense nausea and vomiting induced by cancer chemotherapeutic substances, which were then new. Marijuana often proved more effective than legal, more toxic and expensive conventional antinauseants. At about the same time, it was discovered that marijuana reliably lowered the pressure on the optic nerve in people suffering from open-angle glaucoma; many patients learned, mostly from one another, that cannabis was more effective than conventional medications in retarding the progressive loss of vision caused by this disorder.

In the mid-1980s people with AIDS discovered that cannabis relieved the nausea caused by their illness or by the medications taken to combat it. In addition, cannabis often improved their appetite and enabled them to stop losing or even to gain weight. Like most medical users of cannabis, AIDS patients have found that smoked marijuana is more effective than Marinol (dronabinol), a synthetic THC developed by a small pharmaceutical company, Unimed, with considerable financial support from the government. The federal authorities had come to believe that its availability would quell demands for herbal marijuana as a medicine. Marinol was made legally available as a prescription drug in 1985, and the government immediately placed it in Schedule II (even though it is precisely the same 21 carbon molecule that is the basis for placing marijuana in Schedule I).

DEFINITIONS OF SCHEDULED DRUGS

Schedule I

- The drug or other substance has a high potential for abuse.

- The drug or other substance has no currently accepted medical use in treatment in the United States.

- There is a lack of accepted safety for use of the drug or other substance under medical supervision.

- Examples of Schedule I substances include heroin, lysergic acid diethylamide (LSD), marijuana, and methaqualone.

Schedule II

- The drug or other substance has a high potential for abuse.

- The drug or other substance has a currently accepted medical use in treatment in the United States or a currently accepted medical use with severe restrictions.

- Abuse of the drug or other substance may lead to severe psychological or physical dependence.

- Examples of Schedule II substances include morphine, phencyclidine (PCP), cocaine, methadone, and methamphetamine.

Schedule III

- The drug or other substance has less potential for abuse than the drugs or other substances in Schedules I and II.

- The drug or other substance has a currently accepted medical use in treatment in the United States.

- Abuse of the drug or other substance may lead to moderate or low physical dependence or high psychological dependence.

- Anabolic steroids, codeine, and hydrocodone with aspirin or Tylenol (Vicodin), and some barbiturates are examples of Schedule III substances.

Schedule IV

- The drug or other substance has a low potential for abuse relative to the drugs or other substances in Schedule III.

- The drug or other substance has a currently accepted medical use in treatment in the United States.

- Abuse of the drug or other substance may lead to limited physical dependence or psychological dependence relative to the drugs or other substances in Schedule III.

- Examples of drugs included in Schedule IV are Darvon, Talwin, Ambien, Valium, and Xanax.

Schedule V

- The drug or other substance has a low potential for abuse relative to the drugs or other substances in Schedule IV.

- The drug or other substance has a currently accepted medical use in treatment in the United States.

- Abuse of the drug or other substances may lead to limited physical dependence or psychological dependence relative to the drugs or other substances in Schedule IV.

- Cough medicines with codeine are examples of Schedule V drugs.

The effort to make herbal marijuana available as a prescription drug was initiated in 1972 by the National Organization for the Reform of Marijuana Laws (NORML) and worked its way through the legal system with excruciating slowness. In 1986 John Lawn, the administrator of the DEA, finally announced that he would hold the public hearings ordered by the courts seven years before. Those hearings, which began in 1986 and lasted two years, involved many witnesses, including both patients and doctors, and thousands of pages of documentation.

The DEA's own administrative law judge, Francis L. Young, reviewed the evidence and rendered his decision in 1988. Young said that approval by a "significant minority" of physicians was enough to meet the standard of "currently accepted medical use in treatment in the United States" established by the Controlled Substances Act* for a Schedule II (prescription) drug. He added that "marijuana, in its natural form, is one of the safest therapeutically active substances known to man. . . . One must reasonably conclude that there is accepted safety for use of marijuana under medical supervision. To conclude otherwise, on the record, would be unreasonable, arbitrary, and capricious."

Young went on to recommend "that the Administrator [of the DEA] conclude that the marijuana plant considered as a whole has a currently

---

*The Controlled Substances Act (CSA), Title II and Title III of the Comprehensive Drug Abuse Prevention and Control Act of 1970, is the legal foundation of the U.S. Government's fight against the abuse of drugs and other substances. This law is a consolidation of numerous laws regulating the manufacture and distribution of narcotics, stimulants, depressants, hallucinogens, anabolic steroids, and chemicals used in the illicit production of controlled substances. The Controlled Substances Act (CSA) places all substances that were in some manner regulated under existing federal law into one of five schedules (see Definitions of Scheduled Drugs table on page xv).

accepted medical use in treatment in the United States, that there is no lack of accepted safety for use of it under medical supervision, and that it may be lawfully transmitted from Schedule I to Schedule II."

The DEA disregarded the opinion of its own administrative law judge and refused to reschedule marijuana. As the agency's lawyer remarked, "The judge seems to hang his hat on what he calls a respectable minority of physicians. What percent are you talking about? One-half of one percent?" DEA Administrator John Lawn went further, calling claims for the medical utility of marijuana a "dangerous and cruel hoax."

In the past twenty-five years, as the medical potential of cannabis has become increasingly clear, I have witnessed the growing frustration of patients who cannot obtain it legally. The U.S. government must accept responsibility for the unnecessary suffering produced by a policy that can only be described as ignorant and cruel, and for forcing its citizens to engage in criminal activity. Despite government obstructionism, many patients have learned to use marijuana therapeutically, and many more are discovering its benefits. Unfortunately, they have to endure the anxiety imposed by the threat of arrest and their feelings about breaking the law, and they are compelled to pay exorbitant street prices for a medicine that should be quite inexpensive.

When I first considered this issue in the early 1970s, I assumed that cannabis as medicine would be identical to the marijuana that is used for other purposes (the dried flowering tops of female *Cannabis indica* plants); toxicity is minimal, dosage is easily titrated, and, once freed of the prohibition tariff, it would be inexpensive. I thought the main problem was its classification in Schedule I of the Comprehensive Drug Abuse and Control Act of 1970, which describes it as having a high potential for abuse, no accepted medical use in the United States, and lack of accepted safety for use under medical supervision.

At that time I naively believed that a change to Schedule II would overcome a major obstacle to its legal availability as a medicine. I had already come to believe that the greatest harm in recreational use of marijuana came not from the drug itself but from the effects of prohibition. But I saw that as a separate issue; I believed that, like opiates and cocaine, cannabis could be used medically while remaining outlawed for other purposes.

I thought that once it was transferred to Schedule II, clinical research on marijuana would be pursued eagerly. A quarter of a century later, I have begun to doubt this. It would be highly desirable if marijuana could be approved as a legitimate medicine within the present federal regulatory system, but it now seems to me unlikely.

Today, transferring marijuana to Schedule II would not be enough to make it available as a prescription drug. Such drugs must undergo rigorous, expensive, and time-consuming tests before they are approved by the FDA. This system is designed to regulate the commercial distribution of drug company products and protect the public against false or misleading claims about their efficacy and safety. The drug is generally a single synthetic chemical that a pharmaceutical company has developed and patented. The company submits an application to the FDA and tests it first for safety in animals and then for clinical safety and efficacy. The company must present evidence from double-blind, controlled studies showing that the drug is more effective than a placebo and at least as effective as available drugs. The cost of this evaluation exceeds $200 million per drug. Case reports, expert opinion, and clinical experience are not considered sufficient. I now have doubts that it is possible to develop herbal marijuana as an officially recognized medicine via this route.

The extensive government-supported effort of the last three decades to claim a sufficient level of toxicity to justify the harsh prohibition has instead provided a record of marijuana's safety that is more compelling than that of many, if not most, approved medicines, while thousands of years of medical use have demonstrated its value. The modern FDA protocol is not the only way to establish a risk-benefit estimate for a drug with such a long history. To impose this protocol on cannabis would be like making the same demand of aspirin, which was accepted as a medicine more than sixty years before the advent of the double-blind, controlled study. Many years of experience have shown us that aspirin has many uses and limited toxicity. Even if we thought that this experience was insufficient to establish its credentials by modern standards, it would not be possible to marshal it through the FDA approval process. The patent has long since expired, and with it the enormous economic incentive to underwrite the cost of this modern seal of approval.

The plant cannabis also cannot be patented, so the only source of funding for a start-from-scratch approval would be the government, which is, to put it mildly, unlikely to be helpful. Other reasons for doubting that herbal marijuana would ever be officially approved are today's antismoking climate and, most important, the widespread use of cannabis for purposes disapproved by the government.

To see the importance of this obstacle, consider the effects of granting marijuana legitimacy as a medicine while prohibiting it for any other use. How would the appropriate "labeled" uses be determined, and how would "off-label" uses* be proscribed? And who would provide the cannabis? The federal government still provides marijuana from its farm in Oxford, Mississippi, to the four surviving patients under the now-discontinued Compassionate IND program. But surely the government could not or would not produce marijuana for many thousands of patients receiving prescriptions, any more than it does for other prescription drugs.

If production is contracted out, will the farmers have to enclose their fields with security fences? How would the marijuana be distributed? If distributed through pharmacies, how would they provide secure facilities capable of keeping fresh supplies? Would the price of pharmaceutical marijuana have to be controlled—not too high, lest patients be tempted to buy it on the street or grow their own; not too low, lest people with marginal or fictitious "medical" conditions besiege their doctors for prescriptions. What about the parallel problems with potency? When urine tests are demanded for workers, how would those who use marijuana legally as a medicine be distinguished from those who use it for other purposes?

If the full potential of marijuana as a medicine were to be achieved in the setting of the present prohibition system, all these problems and more would have to be addressed. A delivery system that successfully navigated this minefield would be cumbersome, inefficient, and bureaucratically top-heavy. Government and medical licensing boards would insist on tight restrictions, challenging physicians as though cannabis were a dangerous drug every time it was used for any new patient or purpose. There would be constant conflict with one of two outcomes: patients would not get all the benefits they should, or they would get the benefits by abandoning the legal system for the black market or their own gardens and closets.

A solution now being proposed, notably in the 1999 Institute of Medicine (IOM) Report, is what might be called the "pharmaceuticalization" of cannabis: prescription of isolated individual cannabinoids, synthetic cannabinoids, and cannabinoid analogs. The IOM Report states, "If there is any future for marijuana as a medicine, it lies in its isolated components, the cannabinoids, and their synthetic derivatives."

It goes on: "Therefore, the purpose of clinical trials of smoked marijuana would not be to develop marijuana as a licensed drug, but such trials could

---

*A labeled drug means that it has been approved by the FDA to treat a specific concern or indication. Off-label drug use means that the same drug is used to treat a different condition, one that the FDA has not approved it for.

be a first step towards the development of rapid-onset, non-smoked cannabinoid delivery systems." Some cannabinoids and analogs may have advantages over whole smoked or ingested marijuana in certain circumstances. For example, cannabidiol (CBD) may be more effective as an antianxiety drug when it is not taken along with THC, which sometimes generates anxiety. Other cannabinoids and analogs may occasionally prove more useful than marijuana because they can be administered intravenously.

Some of these commercial products may also lack the psychoactive effects, which make marijuana useful to some for nonmedical purposes, and therefore will not be defined as "abusable" drugs subject to the constraints of the Comprehensive Drug Abuse and Control Act. Nasal sprays, nebulizers, skin patches, pills, and suppositories can be used to avoid exposure of the pulmonary system to the particulate matter in marijuana smoke.

The question is whether these developments will make marijuana itself medically obsolete. Surely many of these substances will be useful and safe enough for commercial development. The question is whether pharmaceutical companies will find them worth the enormous cost of development. Some may; for example, a specific inverse cannabinoid agonist that reduces appetite might be singularly useful and highly lucrative, but for most specific symptoms, analogs or combinations of analogs are unlikely to be more useful than natural cannabis. Nor are they likely to have a significantly wider spectrum of therapeutic uses, since the natural product contains the compounds (and synergistic combinations of compounds) from which they are derived. Synthetic tetrahydrocannabinol (Marinol) has been available for years, but patients generally find whole smoked marijuana to be more effective.

The cannabinoids in whole marijuana can be separated from the burned plant products by vaporization devices that will be inexpensive when manufactured in large numbers. Inhalation is a highly effective means of delivery, and faster means will not be available for analogs (except in a few situations such as parenteral injection in an unconscious patient or one with pulmonary impairment). Furthermore, any new analog will need to have an acceptable therapeutic ratio.* The therapeutic ratio of marijuana is not known because

---

*The therapeutic ratio (also known as the therapeutic index) is a comparison of the amount of a therapeutic agent that causes the therapeutic effect to the amount that causes death. Quantitatively, it is the ratio given by the lethal dose divided by the therapeutic dose.

it has never caused an overdose death, but it is estimated on the basis of extrapolation from animal data to be 20,000 to 40,000.*

The therapeutic ratio of a new analog is unlikely to be higher than that; in fact, it may be less safe because it will be physically possible to ingest large doses. Given its remarkably limited toxicity, its medical versatility, and its potential to be considerably less expensive than any pharmaceutical-company cannabinoid-based medicine, smoked or vaporized herbal marijuana will likely long remain the gold standard for medicinal use.

There is also the matter of an analog's classification under the Comprehensive Drug Abuse and Control Act.† It is a rule of thumb that the more restrictive the classification of a drug, the less likely physicians are to prescribe it. That is why the government rescheduled Marinol from Schedule II to Schedule III in 1992. As with Marinol and Sativex (the British pharmaceutical product that has been likened to "liquid marijuana"), the commercial success of new cannabinoid products will depend to a considerable extent on how vigorously the prohibition against marijuana is enforced. While the pharmaceutical companies are less likely to be interested in developing medicines that are restrictively scheduled or even scheduled at all, one wonders how motivated they would be to develop cannabinoid products if they had to compete with natural marijuana on a level playing field—that is, if marijuana were legally available as a medicine.

I have yet to examine a patient who has used both smoked marijuana and Marinol or Sativex who finds either of the pharmaceuticals more useful; the most common reason for using one of them is the illegality of marijuana, and many patients choose to ignore the law when they believe that the difference between the two puts their health, comfort, or economic well-being at risk. If patients were legally allowed to use herbal marijuana, relatively few would choose one of these pharmaceutical products. With the present prohibition in place, the economic viability of pharmaceutical-industry-generated cannabinoid products and the motivation to develop them will be directly proportional to the vigor with which the marijuana prohibition is enforced. One of the prices of the present level of enforcement is the growing number of annual marijuana arrests (872,000 in 2007); the collateral costs are enormous. And

---

*Compare this to the therapeutic index of commonly prescribed drugs like lithium and digoxin, which is 2 to 3.

†The Comprehensive Drug Abuse Prevention and Control Act of 1970 is a U.S. federal law that, with subsequent modifications, requires the pharmaceutical industry to maintain physical security and strict record keeping for certain types of drugs.

still most patients who find cannabis useful medicinally choose illegal marijuana over presently available prescribable cannabinoids for reasons of efficacy and cost.

One has to ask whether there is any level of enforcement that would compel enough compliance to embolden drug companies to commit the many millions of dollars it will take to develop new cannabinoid products. Unimed's developmental cost for dronabinol was relatively small because the U.S. government, apparently seeking a controllable substitute for marijuana, underwrote much of it. We can safely predict that new pharmaceutical cannabinoid products will be at least as expensive as the exorbitantly priced Marinol and Sativex.

It appears, then, that in the United States two powerful forces are colliding over the issue of medicinal cannabis. On the one hand, there is a growing interest in and acceptance of the medicinal importance of cannabis, and there is every reason to believe that this development will continue to gain momentum. As it does so, it increasingly confronts the proscription against any use of marijuana. At the same time, there does not appear to be widespread interest in moving from an absolute prohibition against cannabis to a regulatory system that would allow for the responsible use of this drug. The federal government denies any medical utility to marijuana, and it appears to be vehemently opposed to any relaxation of the prohibition.

There is little doubt that pharmaceutical companies will develop some cannabinoid products that will be at least as useful as herbal marijuana, and some will be uniquely so. Also, some may be expected to be free—or nearly so—of psychoactivity; this will allow them to be placed outside of the constraints of the Comprehensive Drug Abuse Act classification, or (at most) assigned to Categories IV or V. They will require prescription and be expensive, but there will be a market. What is uncertain, and of course critical to a decision to develop new cannabinoid products, is the anticipated size of the market.

The "pharmaceuticalization" of marijuana will be economically successful only if the pharmaceutical products displace marijuana as a medicine. This seems unlikely in view of the latter's limited toxicity, easy availability, low cost relative to pharmaceuticals, ease with which it can be self-titrated, and its remarkable medical versatility. And if the legal costs of using marijuana don't stop people from choosing it over Marinol or Sativex, it is difficult to imagine a level of enforcement that would eliminate use of the plant material.

It seems inevitable that at least for some time, two distribution pathways for this medicine will coexist:

1. The conventional model of modern allopathic medicine through pharmacy-filled prescriptions for FDA-approved medicines.
2. A model closer to the distribution of alternative and herbal medicines, where there is little if any quality or quantity control.

Either way, growing numbers of people will become familiar with cannabis and its derivative products. They will learn that its harmfulness has been greatly exaggerated and its usefulness underestimated. We can expect that with this growing sophistication about cannabis, there is likely to be mounting pressure to change the way we as a society deal with people who use this drug for any reason.

Perhaps in part because so many Americans have discovered for themselves that marijuana is both relatively benign and remarkably useful, moral consensus about the evils of cannabis is uncertain and shallow. The authorities pretend that eliminating cannabis traffic is like eliminating slavery or piracy, or eradicating smallpox or malaria. The official view is that everything possible has to be done to prevent anyone from ever using marijuana, even as a medicine. But there is also an informal lore of marijuana use that is far more tolerant.

Many of the millions of cannabis users in this country not only disobey the drug laws, but feel a principled lack of respect for them. They do not conceal their bitter resentment of laws that render them criminals. They believe that many people have been deceived by their government, and they have come to doubt that the "authorities" understand much about either the deleterious or the useful properties of the drug. This undercurrent of ambivalence and resistance in public attitudes toward marijuana laws leaves room for the possibility of change, especially since the costs of prohibition are all so high and rising. Given the decades-long annual incremental increase in the number of arrests for marijuana possession, within a few years we will reach a million arrests per year.

Besides the measurable arrests and billions of dollars wasted on prohibition, there are costs more difficult to quantify. One is the lost credibility of our government. Young people who discover that the authorities have been lying about cannabis become cynical about their pronouncements on other drugs and disdainful of their commitment to justice. Another frightful cost of prohibition is the erosion of civil liberties. The use of informers and entrapment, mandatory urine testing, unwarranted searches and seizures, and violations of the Posse Comitatus Act (which outlaws the use of military forces for civilian law enforcement) are becoming more common. It is increasingly clear that our society cannot be both drug-free and free.

It is also clear that the realities of human need are incompatible with the demand for a legally enforceable distinction between medicinal and all other uses of cannabis. Marijuana simply does not conform to the conceptual boundaries established by twentieth-century institutions. It enhances many pleasures, and it has many potential medical uses, but even these two categories are not the only relevant ones. The kind of therapy often used to ease everyday discomforts does not fit any such scheme. In many cases what lay people do in prescribing marijuana for themselves is not very different from what physicians do when they provide prescriptions for psychoactive or other drugs.

The only workable way of realizing the full potential of this remarkable substance, including its full medical potential, is to free it from the present dual set of regulations—those that control prescription drugs in general and the special criminal laws that control psychoactive substances. These mutually reinforcing laws establish a set of social categories that strangle marijuana's uniquely multifaceted potential. The only way out is to cut the knot by giving marijuana the same status as alcohol—legalizing it for adults for all uses and removing it entirely from the medical and criminal control systems.

Lester Grinspoon, M.D., is professor emeritus of psychiatry at the Harvard Medical School and a well-published author in the field of drugs and drug policy. He is the author of *Marihuana Reconsidered* (Cambridge, MA: Harvard University Press, 1971, 1977; American Archives press classic edition, 1994) and *Marijuana, The Forbidden Medicine* (Princeton, NJ: Yale University Press, 1993, 1997), which is now translated into fourteen languages. Dr. Grinspoon currently maintains two medical marijuana websites (www.rxmarijuana.com and www.marijuana-uses.com) that chronicle real-life stories of people who have had positive "non-medical" experiences with marijuana. He can be contacted at lester_grinspoon@hms.harvard .edu.

Introduction

I didn't start out editing this book as an expert on cannabis. I felt more comfortable editing my last book, on MDMA (Ecstasy), because I had been studying its potential use in psychiatry for fifteen years prior to its publication. This time, I knew very little going in. And so, feeling a bit over my head, I amassed a group of experts on cannabis to help explain what I could not. Both books are nonprofit ventures; proceeds from sales of the books will fund clinical research on their respective drugs. Please see ThePotBook .com to learn more as well as to find other articles on cannabis.

I am editing this book for many of the same reasons that inspired my last book. Cannabis, like MDMA, is considered both a drug and a medicine. Both drugs are widely used recreationally but also have therapeutic potential.

As most people know, the status of medical cannabis at the federal level is different from its status at the state level. With the introduction of the Controlled Substances Act of 1970, marijuana was classified as a Schedule I drug, the strictest classification, on par with heroin, LSD, and Ecstasy; and as such, it was outlawed. However, cannabis is deemed a prescription medication in nearly a third of the United States, where it is recommended for the treatment of nausea, pain, diminished appetite, muscle spasms, insomnia . . . the list goes on. Fourteen states and the District of Columbia have legalized medical marijuana: Alaska, California, Colorado, Hawaii, Maine, Michigan, Montana, Nevada, New Jersey, New Mexico, Oregon, Rhode Island, Vermont, Washington, and Washington, D.C. In Maryland, if it can be proven that cannabis is a medical necessity, reduced penalties apply. California, Colorado, New Mexico, Maine, Rhode Island, and Montana are currently the only states to utilize dispensaries to sell medical cannabis.

With regard to drug use around the globe, when nations are compared, the World Health Organization finds clear differences across different regions of the world, with the United States having among the highest levels of legal and illegal drug use of all the countries surveyed. Drug use does not appear to be related to drug policy, however, as countries with more stringent policies (e.g., the United States) do not have lower levels of illegal drug use than countries with more liberal policies (e.g., the Netherlands) (Degenhardt et al. 1988).

It's important to look at these numbers. Forty-three percent of Americans have tried pot, as opposed to 20 percent of the Dutch, despite their more lenient policies (MacCoun and Reuter 2001). (In Holland, possession and production for personal use are considered misdemeanors, punishable by a fine only.) Also, interestingly, after California opened up its medical marijuana program, teen cannabis use fell (MPP 2008), proving that making a drug more available in a specific framework does not necessarily yield rampant abuse of that drug.

Cannabis is the most popular illicit drug in the world. An estimated 162 million adults worldwide, 52 million in Asia, and somewhere between 11 and 20 million Americans are regular users (United Nations 2006). According to the most recent available data, 3.5 million U.S. citizens report smoking marijuana daily or near-daily, 14.5 million report smoking the drug at least once a month, and more than 100 million have tried it at least once in their lives (Substance Abuse and Mental Health Services Administration 2008). That's nearly 43 percent of the American population aged twelve years and older admitting to the federal government about their illegal drug use. The numbers are most likely much higher.

Because millions of people around the world are using cannabis, the sensible course of action is to find ways to minimize its harmful impact. Most useful medications have recommended doses and toxic doses, as well as methods of ingestion that minimize harm and maximize therapeutic results. Harm-reduction strategies should include not only utilizing vaporizers to diminish pulmonary disease, but also a careful reexamination of our drug laws. It is illogical that the most harmful consequence of cannabis use is a blow delivered by our legal system. There's a great Jimmy Carter quote I love: "Penalties against possession of a drug should not be more damaging to an individual than the use of the drug itself."

Yet somehow we persist in punishing the pot smokers, adding them to the heap of imprisoned Americans. Our nation now leads every other country on the planet in one thing: more prisoners. One percent of American adults are in jail. Both per capita and in absolute terms, we put more of our own nation in prisons than any other. In 2009, half of all federal prisoners in the United States were serving sentences for drug offenses (Mendoza 2010). U.S. spending on the drug war tops $100 billion annually. Each prisoner costs $45,000 per year. That is very expensive public housing.

As long as cannabis is illegal, there will be a black market for its sale and distribution. And underground means unregulated. Despite intensive eradication efforts, domestic marijuana production has increased tenfold over the past twenty-five years, from 2.2 million pounds in 1981 to 22 million pounds in 2006. American gang members are the primary retail distributors of most illegal drugs, and they have increased their ranks to nearly 1 million, growing 20 percent from 2005 to 2008, according to the Justice Department (2009), which reports that gangs are responsible for up to 80 percent of the crime in many communities. Mexican drug cartels make 70 percent of their profits from marijuana sales. There is no question in anyone's mind that the Mexican gangs and the warfare that is waged on both sides of our borders is primarily marijuana-driven. Legalize cannabis, and this mess most likely goes away.

The other important issue here is children's access to pot. All surveys of teenagers show that it is getting easier for them to acquire marijuana as time goes on; teens have an easier time buying it than purchasing cigarettes or alcohol. Dealers don't card. Liquor stores do. Also, dealers may interest kids in purchasing other drugs besides marijuana. What the Netherlands figured out a long time ago is that if you separate cannabis from the harder drugs, you can have an impact on which drugs teenagers end up using. In Holland, they have one quarter as many cocaine users as we have in America. Less than 2 percent of the adult population has ever used cocaine. Lifetime cannabis use in the Dutch population aged twelve years and over is less than half of what it is in America (Degenhardt et al. 2008). (For more on the Dutch, please see chapter 39.) It is quite possible that a harm-reduction-based drug policy could keep our country healthier.

What I hope to outline in the pages that follow is a comprehensive assessment of cannabis, its risks and benefits, including the ramifications of our current drug policy. I have gathered experts from around the world to come together and teach what I could not, to share their knowledge with you all. I hope you learn as much as I learned in the process of editing this book.

PART ONE

An Overview of Cannabis

Hemp is of first necessity to the wealth and protection of the country. The greatest service which can be rendered any country is to add a useful plant to its culture.

THOMAS JEFFERSON

Make the most you can of the Indian hemp seed and sow it everywhere.

GEORGE WASHINGTON

We shall, by and by, want a world of hemp more for our own consumption.

JOHN ADAMS

Introduction to Part One

Cannabis is one of humankind's oldest cultivated crops. It is a 38-million-year-old plant, older than humanity, and it is our job to learn how to share the earth with it. We have coevolved on this planet with cannabis and other intoxicating plants for thousands of years, and we have naturally occurring substances in our brains and bloodstream that mimic the cannabinoids. Comprised of specific receptors in our brains for our own internal cannabis, the endocannabinoid system is capable of altering mood, anxiety level, and, more intriguing, the inflammation and immune responses. There is no doubt in my mind that this area of study will continue to blossom and grow, resulting in crucial benefits to our medical knowledge and armamentarium of disease-fighting therapies.

The very basic idea of plant-as-medicine dates back to before recorded history. In the past few decades, we have seen a return to herbal remedies and treatments. Despite the pharmaceutical industry's attempts at taking over, synthesizing, and standardizing a plant's chemical components, plant-based medications are the cornerstone of the practice of medicine, and shamanism is still practiced in many cultures throughout the world.

Cannabis has been a medicine since at least 2800 BCE, and until the 1940s, it was listed in America's pharmacopeia. Remains of a ritual object that contained charred hemp seeds, dating back at least 5,000 years, have been excavated in Romania. As discussed in chapter 2, the Yanghai Tombs near Turpan, China, were excavated to reveal the 2,700-year-old grave of a Caucasoid shaman whose accoutrements included a large cache of cannabis, superbly preserved by climatic and burial conditions. The cannabis, female plants only, was presumably employed by this culture as a medicinal or psychoactive agent, or an aid to divination (Russo et al. 2008).

The earliest known hemp-based textiles, woven fabrics dating back to 7000 BCE, were discovered in northern China. In India, evidence for cannabis use dates to between 1400 and 2000 BCE; and in Egypt, remnants of a cannabis plant were found on the mummified Ramses II, circa 1200 BCE. In the millennium before Christ, hemp was our planet's largest agricultural crop—a major industry providing fabric for clothing and sails, rope, paper, canvases, medicine, lamp oil, and food.

In America, cannabis was a patent medicine, an ingredient in numerous tinctures and extracts throughout the 1800s and early 1900s. In the 1930s, Harry Anslinger (the man who almost single-handedly smeared cannabis and is largely responsible for its illegality) opted for a new name for the plant, one that would be unfamiliar to Americans: *marijuana*. Mexican migrant workers who smoked it were demonized by his tirades against the "loco weed," which he insisted would make them insane and dangerous, raping our white women and wreaking violent havoc on us all. Add to that the Southern black jazz musicians who were known to smoke their mezz, and you have a recipe for xenophobia and racism dictating drug policy. (And not much has changed in that regard. Blacks and Latinos have always been arrested and jailed disproportionately for all drug policy offenses.) In 1937, with the passage of the Marihuana Tax Stamp Act, this medicine—cannabis—was turned into an illegal drug—marijuana.

I prefer to use the word cannabis, when speaking medically at least, for a few reasons. Back when it was a patent medicine found in tinctures and salves, this was its name. The word *marijuana* was coined by a politician looking to scare the public with a new, foreign-sounding word, to align the drug with immigrants and away from the doctors who'd been prescribing cannabis for centuries. Also, because we have receptors in our brains for this drug, and these cannabinoid receptors can be stimulated to diminish pain, nausea, and muscle spasms, the drug deserves to be given a medically based name. To me, reverting to the original word *cannabis* helps signify a restoration of this medicinal plant to the people who can benefit from its use.

There is a healing potential in nonordinary states of consciousness. Cannabis, MDMA, and psilocybin are all psychoactive medicines—powerful tools that physicians and patients may benefit from, but they are also considered recreational drugs with a significant potential for abuse. Whether harmful or helpful, they deserve careful study, if for no other reason than because millions of people worldwide are using them.

But the National Institute on Drug Addiction (NIDA), the scientific body meant to study these substances, has put up roadblocks every step of the way, making it nearly impossible for scientists and physicians to examine the therapeutic worth of smoked cannabis.

Simply put, NIDA will fund only studies looking at risks, not benefits. Puritanical influences die hard, and there are tremendous fear-based policies and politics at work here, perhaps a natural reaction left over from our earlier incarnations as hunters and gatherers, to tread softly where "poisonous" plants are concerned. (The Greek word *pharmacon* means both medicine and poison, and, as Michael Pollan reminded us in *The Botany of Desire,* the word *toxic* is embedded within *intoxication*.) But fear should not trump knowledge. Data from international studies as well as the few goverment-sponsored American studies show that cannabis is remarkably safe and has many potential therapeutic applications.

This plant has thousands of uses. Even if you discount the flowering tops that can be ingested as medicine or relaxant, there is still the stalk of the plant, better known as hemp, the potential answer to many of our ecological problems. Hemp is a renewable energy source that grows easily and naturally all over America, without pesticides or soil erosion. It has the potential to replace fossil fuels. It is the raw material for paper that could help end deforestation. Instead of plastic bags made from petroleum products that end up in our treetops and in the "plastic vortex" at sea, we could be using hemp-based cellophane that is biodegradable. Instead of styrofoam that sits in our landfills for generations, we could be using compostable hemp-based cellulose.

Cannabis seeds (delicious toasted) are a complete-protein vegetarian food. They also make good feed for livestock and poultry. Hempseed oil, unlike flaxseed oil, has the exact ratio (3:1) of the essential fatty acids omega 6 to omega 3, required by our bodies. It tastes better than flaxseed oil (I make a mean shallot hempseed oil vinaigrette!) and won't create essential fatty acid deficiencies over time if used as continuously as flaxseed oil can (Schwab 2006). Besides being a nutritious food, hempseed oil, once used to light Lincoln's oil lap, is a biodeisel fuel that could help to end our dependence on foreign oil. Any one of these indications (medicine, food, fuel) would be enough to earn cannabis the respect and attention it deserves, yet our society continues to demonize and vilify it, outlawing it primarily because it makes people giddy. It makes them laugh. As a psychiatrist, I must tell you: This is insanity.

1

The Subjective Effects of Cannabis

Matthew G. Kirkpatrick and Carl L. Hart, Ph.D.

In April 2006, a Michigan police officer and his wife baked brownies containing confiscated marijuana. Following consumption, the officer made a panicked 911 emergency call, which subsequently became a popular national news story and an Internet sensation. The following is an excerpt from the call:

Caller: I think I'm having an overdose, and so is my wife.
Dispatch: Overdose of what?
Caller: Marijuana. I don't know if there was something in it. Can you please send rescue?
Dispatch: Do you guys have a fever or anything?
Caller: No, I'm just—I think we're dying.
Dispatch: How much did you guys have?
Caller: I don't know. We made brownies. And I think we're dead. Time is going by really, really, really, really slow.

The above provides an illustration of some of the potential *subjective effects* produced by marijuana. Subjective effects simply refers to subjectively experienced changes in one's physiological and/or psychological state following drug administration. In the above example, one subjective effect clearly experienced by the caller was increased anxiety.

9

Interestingly, although the caller was unquestionably distressed about his medical well-being, listeners to the call often found it hilarious. Indeed, it became a national joke, as evidenced by local newscasters making fun of the caller and YouTube clips with titles such as, "Cop eats pot brownies. Thinks he's dying. Idiot." and "Dumb Cop Brownies." One question is, why were so many people amused by the caller's predicament rather than being gravely concerned for his and his wife's health? Is it because most people are insensitive to others' apparent suffering? We think not. Rather, we believe that many individuals have obtained a fair amount of education about the effects produced by marijuana. Based on this education, rational people recognize that the caller's reaction may have been a lack of experience with marijuana-related subjective effects, and that the likelihood of death following ingestion of marijuana is low.

SOURCE OF MARIJUANA EDUCATION

It is not surprising that many members of our society are informed about some of the effects produced by marijuana. It was mentioned in the Introduction to Part One, but bears repeating here, that an estimated 3.5 million U.S. citizens report smoking marijuana daily or almost daily, 14.5 million report smoking the drug at least once a month, and more than 100 million have tried it at least once in their lives (SAMHSA 2008). This means that approximately one half of the U.S. adult population has personally experienced marijuana-related effects at some point in their lives. Others, who have not personally indulged, have seen humorous depictions of the effects produced by marijuana smoking in the popular media for more than sixty years. Of course, there are caveats to this type of information. For example, in the 1930s the majority of the popular portrayal of marijuana-associated effects was exaggerated and inaccurate. Moreover, anecdotal evidence from personal marijuana use experience fails to offer a comprehensive understanding of the drug's effects.

This is so, in part, because numerous extraneous and/or uncontrolled factors accompanying marijuana use may influence the observed drug effects. For instance, in the case of the Michigan police officer and his wife, we do not know how much of the drug they ingested, how much prior experience they had with the drug, what their expectations were of marijuana-related effects before they consumed the drug, and whether they had ingested any other drugs in combination with the marijuana-laced brownies. All these factors are known to influence the subjective effects of not only marijuana, but other psychoactive drugs as well.

One way to increase the confidence in our knowledge about the subjective effects of marijuana is to study the effects of the drug in a laboratory setting, where extraneous variables can be limited. Although these investigations are often conducted in tandem with other research questions, such as investigating a drug's abuse potential (e.g., how likely is it that the drug will be abused?), physiological effects (does the drug alter cardiovascular measures?), and cognitive effects (does the drug alter memory?), the study of drug-related subjective effects is, by itself, quite useful. For instance, systematically investigating the subjective experiences produced by a drug provides a powerful tool for profiling these effects and directly comparing drug effects both within a single drug class (e.g., morphine versus heroin) and between drug classes (e.g., marijuana versus cocaine). This profiling has been important in classifying novel drug compounds as well as providing a greater degree of specificity in our understanding of the drugs themselves. Importantly, direct comparisons of oral delta-9-tetrahydrocannabinol (delta-9-THCl; one of over sixty known cannabinoids in the marijuana plant) and smoked marijuana have provided further evidence that this single cannabinoid is primarily responsible for the typical user's "high" (Hart et al. 2002a; Wachtel et al. 2002).

As mentioned above, there are many factors that influence the subjective effects of any drug, including marijuana. In this chapter we will focus on two important factors:

- The route of administration. The way an individual takes marijuana (e.g., smoked or orally) strongly influences the time course and intensity of the drug's effects. For marijuana, the smoked route of administration is by far the most common.
- The individual's marijuana use history. The amount and frequency of marijuana use influences the subjective effects of the drug. For instance, long-term frequent marijuana users may become *tolerant* to some of marijuana's effects.

SUBJECTIVE EFFECTS IN THE LABORATORY

Since childhood we have learned to apply verbal labels to subjectively experienced mood states (e.g., happy, sad, angry). Researchers can use self-report questionnaires to exploit this ability by requiring study participants to match their drug-induced changes in sensations and mood to a set of standardized statements and adjectives (for an in-depth discussion, see Fischman and Foltin

1991). Although there are several standardized questionnaires, this chapter focuses on data from studies employing the Visual Analog Scale (VAS), because the majority of controlled laboratory studies have included this measure. The VAS is a multi-item self-report questionnaire, often administered on a computer, that consists of a series of individually presented lines labeled "Not at all" at one end and "Extremely" at the other end. Centered above each line is a sentence or adjective describing a mood (e.g., "I feel Anxious," "I feel Friendly"), a drug effect (e.g., "I feel High," "I feel a Good Drug Effect"), or a physiological indicator (e.g., "I feel Hungry," "My heart is beating faster than usual").

Many of the subjective effects of marijuana are reliably produced in the laboratory and correspond with anecdotal reports. For instance, one of the most robust findings across studies in experienced marijuana users is that euphoria is consistently increased shortly after consuming the drug. Because *euphoria* can be a vague, imprecise term, researchers use multiple VAS items to approximate this subjective effect. In various studies individuals reported increased ratings of "High," "Good Drug Effect," and "Stoned" following administration of smoked marijuana (Ilan et al. 2005) or oral delta-9-THC (Haney et al. 2007). Other positive subjective effect ratings, such as "Stimulated" and "Mellow" are also consistently increased (Hart et al. 2002a). In addition, subjective-effect ratings probing physiological states (e.g., "Hungry" and "Dry-mouthed") are acutely increased by smoked marijuana or oral delta-9-THC administration (Ilan et al. 2005; Haney et al. 2007). Importantly, many of the above subjective effects are delta-9-THC-concentration-dependent. That is, the larger the concentration of delta-9-THC in the marijuana, the greater the ratings on these subjective-effect items.

Even though the effects of smoked marijuana and oral delta-9-THC can be quite similar, the intensity of these effects (as well as the speed of onset and overall time course) can differ based on the route by which the drug is administered. Most users of marijuana smoke the drug. By this route, marijuana smoke is inhaled and absorbed through the lungs. Because the lungs have a large surface area and many blood vessels leading directly to the brain, the onset of psychoactive effects produced are rapid, occurring within seconds. Due to this rapid onset, experienced smokers can easily titrate their dose to achieve the desired subjective effects. In other words, this gives smokers a great deal of control over their acute marijuana experience, potentially maximizing positive drug effects and minimizing negative effects. Typically, the effects following smoked administration are relatively short-lived, lasting no longer than one to two hours.

By contrast, marijuana (or delta-9-THC) taken by mouth produces a slower onset of effects. After oral ingestion, the drug must move from the stomach to the small intestine, where it is absorbed into the bloodstream. Before reaching the bloodstream, however, some of the drug is metabolized (or broken down) by the liver. Once in the bloodstream, the drug moves to the heart and then to the brain. Because the drug does not travel directly to the brain following oral ingestion, the onset of psychoactive effects is delayed. Peak psychoactive effects (or subjective effects) following oral administration usually occur approximately one-and-a-half hours after ingestion.

In practical terms, this means that the user is less able to titrate the dose taken. In some cases, as illustrated in our example at the start of the chapter, because psychoactive effects are delayed, some inexperienced users may continue to ingest large amounts of drug in an effort to facilitate a more rapid onset of effects. Of course, a major concern with this strategy is that by the time psychoactive effects are initially experienced, there may still be a large amount of drug in the stomach, which will be continuously released over an extended period. Indeed, some delta-9-THC-related effects have been reported to persist for as long as up to eight hours after a single oral administration of the drug to infrequent users (Curran et al. 2002). This might help explain why the Michigan police officer and his wife had such an extremely negative drug experience.

Now that you have a basic understanding of some common routes by which marijuana is administered, it should be clear that the onset of effects are most rapid following smoked administration, while effects are most delayed after oral administration. Accordingly, the subjective effects produced by oral ingestion of marijuana last longer than those produced by smoking the drug. It is important to note that although the onset and offset of drug effects vary depending on the route of administration, the effects produced by marijuana are qualitatively similar despite the route of administration. As such, the user may experience marijuana-associated positive (e.g., euphoria) as well as deleterious (e.g., anxiety) effects regardless of the route by which the drug is used.

THE IMPORTANCE OF THE INDIVIDUAL'S HISTORY OF MARIJUANA USE

In his landmark study of case reports, Becker (1953) suggested that before individuals are able to experience marijuana-associated positive subjective effects, they must go through a process in which they learn to recognize and interpret psychoactive effects produced by the drug. As one acquires more experience with using marijuana, one becomes more competent in identifying marijuana-related subjective effects, suggesting that the "marijuana experience" will be viewed differently depending on one's marijuana use history. For instance, while an experienced marijuana user might report an enjoyable "high" after smoking the drug, the novice might report an unpleasant feeling. Although there is little experimental evidence to support Becker's arguments, it is clear that an individual's marijuana use history influences their response to the drug. For example, it is likely that frequent marijuana smokers (for the purpose of this chapter, those who smoke four to seven days per week) compared with infrequent smokers (those who smoke less than once per week) may exhibit *tolerance* to many marijuana-related effects.

Tolerance is usually characterized by the need for an increased amount of drug to obtain the desired effects and simply means that the user has become physiologically and/or psychologically accustomed to the potential effects of the drug. Most importantly, frequent users may be able to tolerate an amount of marijuana large enough to produce negative subjective effects in infrequent users. Thus, before making any broad claims about the subjective effects of marijuana, any investigation should take into account the individual's marijuana use history.

Much of the experimental evidence on tolerance in marijuana users is centered on the potential negative effects produced by moderate to large concentrations of delta-9-THC. In the laboratory, these negative subjective effects are most commonly associated with infrequent marijuana smokers. For example, researchers have reported elevated ratings of "Impaired," "Confused," "Sluggish," and decreased ratings of "Clear-headed" in infrequent users after they had smoked marijuana (Azorlosa et al. 1992). Consistent with these data, Kirk and de Wit (1999) observed that infrequent marijuana users reported a decreased "Drug Liking" following a large dose of oral delta-9-THC compared with placebo, indicating that they may have found the effects of the larger dose somewhat aversive.

By comparison, these negative subjective effects are rarely reported in studies examining marijuana-related effects in frequent smokers. For example, in the study by Kirk and de Wit, frequent smokers did not report a decreased "Drug Liking" after taking the large dose. Furthermore, in their study of daily marijuana smokers, Hart and colleagues (2001) observed dramatic increases on ratings probing *positive* subjective effects (e.g., euphoria) after participants had smoked a marijuana cigarette, whereas *negative* subjective-effect ratings were not significantly altered. The above suggests that THC-related tolerance develops in different ways to positive vs. negative effects.

SUBJECTIVE EFFECTS AND ABUSE POTENTIAL

The likelihood that a drug will be abused,* or used chronically above and beyond therapeutic use, is often called the drug's *abuse potential*. The abuse potential of smoked marijuana is well documented. According to the 2007 Treatment Episode Data Set, marijuana accounted for about 16 percent of all drug treatment admissions in the United States. Many researchers have suggested that the acute positive subjective effects produced by a given drug contribute to that drug's abuse potential (Fischman and Foltin 1991). Although it seems intuitive that the more euphoria a drug produces, the more likely the drug will be abused, empirical evidence examining the potential role of subjective effects in determining marijuana abuse potential has been mixed.

In a typical laboratory investigation of marijuana-associated abuse potential, participants are offered a choice between the opportunity to consume the drug and an alternative, such as money. Selection of the drug under these conditions is referred to as *self-administration*. Using similar procedures, Hart and colleagues (2005) examined the abuse potential and subjective effects of oral delta-9-THC in frequent marijuana users. They reported dose-related increases in both positive subjective effects and choice to administer delta-9-THC capsules. Furthermore, the investigators found significant correlations between capsule choice and four subjective effects: "Good Drug Effect," "Friendly," "High," and "Mellow," suggesting that these positive subjective effects may play a role in maintaining oral delta-9-THC self-administration.

Studies of smoked marijuana administration, however, have produced conflicting results. For instance, Ward and colleagues (1997) observed delta-9-THC-concentration-related increases in positive subjective effects, such as "High" and "Good Drug Effect," but this concentration-related effect did not extend to marijuana self-administration. That is, although participants chose more active marijuana compared to placebo marijuana, their choice

---

*The term *abuse*, as it is used throughout this chapter, encompasses the *Diagnostic and Statistical Manual of Mental Disorders*, fourth edition (DSM-IV-TR), and International Statistical Classification of Diseases and Related Health Problems (ICD-10) definitions of substance abuse and dependence. DSM-IV-TR and ICD-10 terms are used to avoid the use of pejorative terms and terms that have multiple meanings.

was neither concentration-dependent nor predicted by their subjective-effect ratings. This is consistent with observations from other marijuana self-administration studies (Kelly et al. 1994; Haney et al. 1997).

There is also evidence indicating that marijuana self-administration continues despite a reduction in self-reported subjective effects. For example, Hart and colleagues (2002b) maintained frequent marijuana smokers on oral delta-9-THC in an effort to reduce the positive subjective effects of smoked marijuana and thus reduce choice to self-administer marijuana. They found that oral delta-9-THC maintenance markedly reduced positive subjective effects (e.g., "Good Drug Effect") but did not alter choice to self-administer marijuana. In other words, the abuse potential of marijuana was unaffected by the decrease in positive subjective effects, indicating that the marijuana-related subjective effects and self-administration are dissociable. The dissociation of drug-related self-administration and subjective effects has been well documented by several investigators using different classes of drugs (Johanson and Uhlenhuth 1980; Fischman et al. 1990; Comer, Collins, and Fischman 1997) and underscores the importance of assessing multiple measures of drug effects when evaluating a drug to determine its abuse potential.

CONCLUSION

From the systematic study of marijuana in the laboratory, we have gained a more realistic and nuanced understanding of the subjective effects of marijuana and its primary psychoactive component, delta-9-THC. In any evaluation of marijuana-related effects on subjective mood (whether marijuana is used in the laboratory or at home), it is important to account for the route by which the drug is taken, amount of drug ingested, and experience of the individual user. According to epidemiological data, marijuana has a low to moderate potential for abuse. Results from some laboratory studies have indicated that marijuana-related subjective effects and self-administration are dissociable, making it more difficult to predict the drug's abuse potential by assessing only subjective responses after drug administration. Nevertheless, a considerable increase in negative subjective effects might limit further intake of the drug, although fewer empirical data addressing this issue are available.

2
Early/Ancient History

Chris Bennett

The role of cannabis in the ancient world was manifold. It was a food, a fiber, a medicine, and a magically empowered religious sacrament. In this article the focus is on archaic references to cannabis use as both a medicine and a sacrament, rather than as a source of food or fiber, and its role in a variety of ancient cultures in this context is examined.

Oxford archaeologist Andrew Sherrat points to the earliest evidence of cannabis as a sacrament via the use of cannabis incenses at a gravesite of a group known as the Proto-Indo-Europeans, the Kurgans, who occupied what is now Romania five thousand years ago. The discovery at the site of a smoking cup that contained remnants of charred hemp seeds documents that three thousand years before Christ, humanity had already been using cannabis for religious purposes for millennia. From remnants of the charred hemp seeds, we can see that the combustible (and psychoactive) parts of the plant—namely flowers and leaves—had been consumed, and the hard, shell-like residue of the seeds left behind. Sherrat also points to even older ceramic tripod bowls—believed to have been ancient incense burners for cannabis, due to the use of hemp cords to place impressions upon them—as further indications of humanity's primordial relationship with cannabis.

It was likely that the primordial cannabis cult arose from an even earlier group and spread out, reaching all the way from the Orient to throughout the Middle East and into Europe, India, and Africa. Considering this, it is not surprising to find that *canna,* the root word for *cannabis,* occurs in the

Indo-European language, the primordial dialect that accounts for similarities in the English, German, Latin, Greek, Persian, and Sanskrit languages. *Canna* came to refer to the long canelike stocks of the multipurpose cannabis crop grown in the ancient world for both its fibrous and its pharmacological properties, and the term *cane* itself is derived from *canna* and can originally be identified with the multipurpose hemp stalk.

Possibly still earlier than the Indo-European use of cannabis is the role that hemp played in the even more ancient traditions of the indigenous people of the Orient.

CANNABIS IN CHINA

The earliest reference to the use of marijuana as a medicine is believed to have been made sometime around 2800 BCE,* as it is mentioned in the medical compendium *Pen Ts'ao* of the legendary Chinese emperor Shen-Nung. Shen-Nung determined that the female plant, being a very high source of yin, contained the most potent medicine, and prescribed *chu-ma* (female hemp, as opposed to *ma,* hemp) for the treatment of absentmindedness, constipation, malaria, beriberi, rheumatism, and menstrual problems. Shen-Nung, known as the Father of Chinese Medicine, was so thoroughly impressed with the beneficial effects of *chuma,* he deemed it one of the Superior Elixirs of Immortality.

Throughout the centuries, Chinese physicians continued to prescribe marijuana, and as they became more familiar with the effects of the plant, new discoveries were made about its properties. One such discovery was made in 200 CE by the early and well-known Chinese surgeon Hua T'o. Almost two thousand years ago, Hua T'o is reputed to have performed such complicated operations as "organ grafts, resectioning of intestines, laparotomies (incisions into the loin), and thoracotomies (incisions into the chest)" (Abel 1980). Moreover, these dangerous and complicated surgeries were rendered painless by an anesthetic prepared from cannabis resin and wine known as *ma-yo.*

Ancient Chinese shamans showed their awareness of the medical powers of cannabis symbolically, by carving serpents into a stalk of hemp and using it as a magic wand for healing ceremonies.

China's ancient use of cannabis flowers and leaves was not limited to medicine, as ancient Taoist references record that the herb was used for mys-

---

*Although the *Pen Ts'ao* is widely believed to have been compiled around this time, no original copies of the text have survived. The oldest copy of the *Pen Ts'ao* dates to about 100 CE and was compiled by an anonymous author who claimed to have incorporated the more ancient material into his own medical compendium.

tical purposes as well. A Taoist priest wrote in the fifth century BCE that cannabis was employed by "necromancers, in combination with Ginseng, to set forward time and reveal future events" (Schultes and Hofmann 1979).

As mentioned in the Introduction to Part One, in the 2006 *Journal of Ethnopharmacology* article "A New Insight into Cannabis sativa (Cannabaceae) Utilization from 2,500-year-old Yanghai Tombs, Xinjiang, China," the authors discuss rare, well-preserved archaeological specimens of cannabis and conclude, "Based on the shamanistic background of the deceased man and ancient customs, it is assumed that the Cannabis was utilized for ritual/medicinal purposes" (Jiang et al. 2006).

ANCIENT MIDEAST HISTORY

It is widely believed that cannabis was brought to the Mideast by Caucasian tribes that lived on the borders between what is now Russia and China. Likely these tribes, now known under the collective title of the Scythians, took to their use of cannabis from the same Asian tribes that pushed them out of their homeland.

The Scythians played a very important part in the ancient world from the seventh to first centuries BCE. They were expert horsemen and were one of the earliest peoples to master the art of riding and to use horse-drawn covered wagons. This early high mobility is probably why most scholars credit them with the spread of cannabis knowledge throughout the ancient world.

Marijuana was an integral part of the Scythian cult of the dead, wherein homage was paid to the memory of their departed leaders. In a famous passage written in about 450 BCE, Herodotus describes the funeral rites that took place when a king died among the Scythians. After burial, he recorded, the Scythians would purify themselves by setting up small tepeelike structures covered by rugs, which they would enter to inhale the fumes of hemp seeds (and the resinous flower calyxes surrounding the seeds) thrown onto red-hot stones: "On a framework of three sticks, meeting at the top, they stretch pieces of woolen cloth, taking care to get the joints as perfect as they can, and inside this little tent they put a dish with red-hot stones in it. Then they take some of the hemp seed, creep into the tent, and throw the seeds on to the hot stones. At once it begins to smoke, giving off a vapor unsurpassed by any vapor bath one could find in Greece. The Scythian enjoy it so much they howl with pleasure." (It is most likely that the seeds described by Herodotus were seeded buds, and the charred seeds found by archaeologists were what was left over from the burned buds.)

Herodotus's ancient records of the Scythian hemp rites were thought to be mythical but were later verified in 1929 with the discovery of a Scythian tomb in Pazyryk, western Altai, by S. I. Rudenko. It contained censers used for vaporizing cannabis plant matter over heated stones, and a tentlike structure for holding the fumes of the smoldering plants (Rudenko 1970).

In ancient Mesopotamia, cannabis was used medicinally, and oils and incenses were prepared from the plant because its "aroma was pleasing to the Gods" (Meissner 1925). In the second quarter of the first millennium BCE, the word *qunabu* (*qunapy, qunnubu, qunbu*) begins to turn up referring to a source of oil, fiber, and medicine (Barber 1989). In our own time, numerous scholars have come to acknowledge *qunubu* as an early reference to cannabis* (Meissner 1932–33; Benetowa 1936; Benet 1975; Schultes and Hofmann 1979; Abel 1982).

Apparently cannabis was used in topical lotions as well. An Assyrian medical tablet from the Louvre collection has been transliterated: "So that god of man and man should be in good rapport:—with hellebore, cannabis and lupine you will rub him" (Russo 2007).

Recipes for cannabis incense, regarded as copies of much older versions, were found in the cuneiform library of the legendary Assyrian king Assurbanipal, and records from the time of his father, Esarhaddon, refer to cannabis, "*qunubu,*" as one of the main ingredients of the "sacred rites."

Mesopotamian use went far beyond the spiritual. The medicinal properties of the plant were well known, as noted in the groundbreaking 2007 paper by cannibinoid expert Ethan Russo, "Clinical Cannabis in Ancient Mesopotamia: A Historical Survey with Supporting Scientific Evidence."

Dr. Russo records that numerous topical applications of cannabis for medical purposes can be found throughout ancient Mesopotamian documents: "Cannabis was used with the plant El in petroleum to anoint swelling . . . [and] was also employed as a simple poultice." More interestingly, records of topical ointments used in the treatment of an ancient malady called Hand of Ghost, now thought to be epilepsy, included cannabis as a key ingredient. Ancient Mesopotamian preparations that included cannabis were also used in the treatment of certain diseases of the chest and lungs, stomach problems, skin lesions, lice, swollen joints, and a variety of other maladies (Russo 2007).

---

*L. Lewin in 1882 suggested that *qunubu* was derived from the East Iranian word for cannabis, *konaba*, and through the Scythians spreading the use of the plant throughout much of the ancient world, the word eventually became our modern *cannabis*.

Similar topical preparations of cannabis were used for both healing and spiritual purposes throughout the ancient world. In Egypt, where cannabis was known by the name *sm-sm-t,* the healing herb was believed to have been a creation of the sun god, Ra, and was used in ceremonies honoring the dead (Graindorge 1992).

According to Lise Mannich (1989), the literal translation of *sm-sm-t* is "the Medical Marihuana Plant." Egyptian medical texts that include references to cannabis include the Ramesseum III Papyrus (1700 BCE), Eber's Papyrus (1600 BCE), the Berlin Papyrus (1300 BCE), and the Chester Beatty VI Papyrus (1300 BCE). Possibly due to the sticky and adhesive quality of honey, a number of Egyptian topical medical preparations required it as an admixture to cannabis-based medicines. According to the ancient papyri, such topical cannabis preparations were used to treat ingrown toe- and fingernails and inflammations of the vagina (Ghalioungui 1963).

For more than a century, various researchers have been trying to bring attention to potential cannabis references in the Hebrew Scriptures ("Old Testament"). Like the ancient Greeks, the biblical Israelites were surrounded by marijuana-using peoples. A British physician, C. Creighton, concluded in 1903 that several references to marijuana can be found in the Hebrew Scriptures. Examples are the "honeycomb" referred to in the Song of Solomon 5:1, and the "honeywood" in I Samuel 14:25–45 (*Consumer Reports* 1972). Of the historical material indicating the Hebraic use of cannabis, the strongest and most profound piece of evidence was established in 1936 by Sula Benet (a.k.a. Sara Benetowa), a Polish etymologist from the Institute of Anthropological Sciences in Warsaw. In 1975 Benet stated, "In the original Hebrew text of the Old Testament there are references to hemp, both as incense, which was an integral part of religious celebration, and as an intoxicant."

Through comparative etymological study, Benet documented that in the Hebrew Scriptures and their Aramaic translation, the Targum Onculos, hemp is referred to as *q'neh bosm* (variously translated as *kaneh bosem, keneh bosem, kaniebosm*) and is also rendered in traditional Hebrew as *kannabos* or *kannabus.* The root *kan* in this construction means "reed" or "hemp," while *bosm* means "aromatic." This word appears in Exodus 30:23, Song of Songs 4:14, Isaiah 43:24, Jeremiah 6:20, and Ezekiel 27:19.

Benet's etymological research regarding the Hebrew terms *q'neh bosem* and *q'neh* was based on tracing the modern word *cannabis* back through history to show the similarities between the cognitive pronunciation of *cannabis* and *q'eneh bosem*,* as well as comparing the term to the names used for cannabis by contemporary kingdoms, such as the Assyrian and Babylonian term for the plant, *qunubu*. In fact, the term *q'neh bosem* is the Hebrew transliteration of an earlier Indo-European term for the plant, *canna*. This term left traces through the vernacular *an*, seen in various modern terms for *c'an'nabis*, such as the Indian *bh'a'ng*, the French *ch'an'vre*, the Dutch *c'an'vas*, and the German *h'an'f*.

This use of an Indo-European word in the Semetic language shows that the ritual use of cannabis came to the Hebrews from foreign sources and as an item of trade; it retained the core aspects of its original name. Indeed, in both the Jeremiah and Ezekiel references referred to by Benet, cannabis is identified as coming from a foreign land. As the additional references noted by Benet indicate, when put into the context of the biblical storyline, this foreign association with the plant may in fact have been the cause of its disfavor among the ancient Hebrews. Initially it was deemed to be favorable; it was part of a list of ingredients in a holy anointing oil, which when bestowed upon a chosen individual made him "the anointed one" (in Hebrew this is rendered as *Messiah* and later, in Greek, as *Christ*). But this love affair was not to last. As linguist and mythologist Carl Ruck, along with his equally educated coauthors, have also noted:

> Chrismation was a mode of administering healing balms. In the Old Testament, chrismation involves pouring the anointing oil over the head, which functions to purify (obviously in a spiritual sense, not to cleanse physically) and to confer power, strength, or majesty. Its most common occurrence is the coronation of kings, which sometimes is accomplished by Yahweh, himself; but priests and prophet-shamans are also anointed, as also are objects to set them aside from profane use. In *Exodus* 30,23 *sq.*, Yahweh specifies the ingredients for the chrism, making clear that such unguents contained herbal additives to the oil: *Cannabis sativa* (*kaneh bosm,* usually translated "aromatic cane") is combined with perfuming spices (cinnamon, cassia, and myrrh) in oil. The psychoactivity of the "spices" in the anointing oil, in addition to the *Cannabis,* deserves attention. Cinnamon and cassia are mild to moderate stimulants. Myrrh is reputed to have medical properties. To elaborate on Old Testament references to cannabis, the root phrase that

---

*Another example of analogous pronunciation of this kind is found with the Semetic term *kinamon,* the source of our modern *cinnamon.*

represents cannabis, *kaneh bosm,* is often translated as "calamus." This mis-
translation starts as early as the Septuagint. *Kaneh bosm* occurs also in *Song
of Songs* 4.14, where it grows in an orchard of exotic fruits, herbs, and spices
and in the *Song of Songs* as an ethnobotanical encomium of the entheogen.
It occurs also in Isaiah 43.24 where Yahweh lists it amongst the slights not
received in sacrifice, and *Jeremiah* 6.20, where Yahweh, displeased with his
people, rejects such an offering; and *Ezekiel* 27.19, where it occurs in a cata-
logue of the luxurious items in the import trade of Tyre. Benet concludes
that these references confirm that hemp was used by the Hebrews as incense
and intoxicant. This conclusion has since been affirmed by other scholars.
(Ruck 2001)

These passages are particularly telling of how the disappearance of cannabis from the Hebrew Scriptures came about. In Isaiah 43:24—"Thou
hast bought me no sweet* cane [*q'neh*] with money, neither hast thou filled
me with the fat of thy sacrifices: but thou hast made me to serve with thy
sins, thou hast wearied me with thine iniquities"—Yahweh condemns the
Hebrews for not bringing him cannabis or enough of the lavish animal sacrifices common in the Hebrew Scriptures.

A further reading of the texts shows that these items are being sacri-
ficed in honor of competing deities. This situation is compounded through
the words of the monotheistic reformer Jeremiah: "To what purpose
cometh there to me incense from Sheba, and the sweet cane [*q'neh*] from a
far country? Your burnt offerings [are] not acceptable, nor your sacrifices
sweet unto me" (Jer. 6:20). Here, just prior to the final fall of Hebrew
kingdoms, the pagan and foreign associations with the plant finally drive
it underground. But it must be understood that from the time of Moses
and throughout the kingdom period, the use of cannabis in a ritual context had continued.

This theme is more fully explored and expanded upon in my own
book *Sex, Drugs, Violence and the Bible,* coauthored with Neil McQueen
(Forbidden Fruit Publishing, 2001). Following in the footsteps of Benet's
research, we were able to follow the history of the sacred anointing oil into
the early Christian period, particularly among heretical Gnostic Christian
sects, who, along with pagan cults, were brutally banned at the inception of
the Dark Ages and the rise of Catholicism.

---

*In the original Hebrew, "sweet" in this context can also refer to scent.

As noted, the term *Christ* itself is a Greek rendering of the Hebrew *Messiah,* and this means the "anointed one," making reference back to the original anointing oil as described in Exodus 30:23. Indeed, even in the Christian Scriptures, Jesus does not baptize any of his own disciples, but rather, in the oldest of the synoptic Gospels, Jesus sends out his followers to heal with the anointing oil: "They cast out many devils, and anointed with oil many that were sick, and healed them" (Mark 6:13). Likewise, after Jesus's passing, James says, "Is any one of you sick? He should call the elders of the church to pray over him and anoint him with oil in the name of the Lord" (James 5:14).

It should also be understood that in the ancient world, diseases such as epilepsy were attributed to demonic possession, and to cure somebody of such an illness, even with the aid of certain herbs, was the same as exorcism, or miraculously healing them. Interestingly, cannabis has been shown to be effective in the treatment of not only epilepsy, but many of the other ailments that Jesus and the disciples healed people of, such as skin diseases (Matt. 8:1–4, 10:8, 11:5; Mark 1:40–45; Luke 5:12–14, 7:22, 17:11–19), eye problems (John 9:6–15), and menstrual problems (Luke 8:43–48).

According to ancient Christian documents, even the healing of cripples could be attributed to the use of the holy oil. "Thou holy oil given unto us for sanctification . . . thou art the straightener of the crooked limbs" (Acts of Thomas). One ancient Christian text, the Acts of Peter and the Twelve Apostles, which is older than the New Testament and estimated to have been recorded in the second century CE, has Jesus giving the disciples an "unguent box" and a "pouch full of medicine" with instructions for them to go into the city and heal the sick.

As Jesus and his followers began to spread the healing knowledge of cannabis around the ancient world, the singular *Christ* became the plural term *Christians,* that is, those who had been smeared or anointed with the holy oil. As the New Testament explains: "The anointing you received from him remains in you, and you do not need anyone to teach you. But as his anointing teaches you about all things and as that anointing is real, not counterfeit—just as it has taught you, remain in him" (I John 2:27). The Christians, the "smeared" or "anointed ones," received "knowledge of all things" by this "anointing from the Holy One" (I John 2:20). Thereafter, they needed no other teacher and were endowed with their own spiritual knowledge. According to Ruck (2003), "Residues of cannabis, moreover, have been detected in vessels from Judea and Egypt in a context indicating its medicinal, as well as visionary, use."*

In the first few centuries CE, Christian Gnostic groups such as the Archontics, Valentians, and Sethians rejected water baptism as superfluous, referring to it as an "incomplete baptism" (The Paraphrase of Shem). In the tractate Testimony of Truth, baptism by water is rejected with a reference to the fact that Jesus baptized none of his disciples (Rudolph 1987). Being "anointed with unutterable anointing," the so-called sealings recorded in the Gnostic texts, can be seen as a very literal event: "There is water in water, there is fire in chrism" (Gospel of Philip); "The anointing with oil was the introduction of the candidate into unfading bliss, thus becoming a Christ" (Mead 1900).

Chadwick (1967) observes, "The oil as a sign of the gift of the Spirit was quite natural within a semetic framework, and therefore the ceremony is probably very early. In time the biblical meaning became obscured." In the Gospel of Philip it is written that the initiates of the empty rite of Baptism "go down into the water and come up without having received anything. . . . The anointing [chrisma] is superior to baptism. For from the anointing we were called 'anointed ones' [Christians], not because of the baptism. And Christ also was [so] named because of the anointing, for the Father anointed the son, and the son anointed the apostles, and the apostles anointed us. [Therefore] he who has been anointed has the All. He has the resurrection, the light . . . the Holy Spirit. . . . [If] one receives this unction, this person is no longer a Christian but a Christ."

The apocryphal book The Acts of Thomas refers to the ointment's

---

*An archaeological dig in Bet Shemesh near Jerusalem has confirmed that cannabis medicine was in use in the area up until the fourth century. Thus it would stand to reason that it was used for these purposes throughout the intervening Christian period. In the case of the Bet Shemesh dig, the cannabis had been used as an aid in childbearing, both as a healing balm and an inhalant. Scientists commenting on the find noted that cannabis was used as a medicine as early as the sixteenth century BCE, in Egypt (Abel 1980). This find garnered some attention, as can be seen from a 1992 article titled "Hashish Evidence Is 1,600 Years Old" from the Associated Press: "Archaeologists have found hard evidence that hashish was used as a medicine 1,600 years ago, the Israel Antiquities Authority said yesterday. Archaeologists uncovered organic remains of a substance containing hashish, grasses and fruit on the abdominal area of a teenage female's skeleton that dates back to the fourth century, the antiquities authority said in a statement. Anthropologist Joel Zias said that although researchers knew hashish had been used as a medicine, this is the first archaeological evidence."

entheogenic effects as being specifically derived from a certain plant: "Holy oil, given us for sanctification, hidden mystery in which the cross was shown us, you are the unfolder of the hidden parts. You are the humiliator of stubborn deeds. You are the one who shows the hidden treasures. You are the plant of kindness. Let your power come by this [unction]."

Although the idea that Jesus and his disciples used a healing cannabis ointment may seem far-fetched at first, when weighed against the popular alternative (one that is held by millions of believers) that Jesus performed his healing miracles magically, through the power invested in him by the omnipotent Lord of the Universe, the case for ancient accounts of medicinal cannabis seems a far more likely explanation. When one considers that Jesus himself may have healed and initiated disciples with such topical cannabis preparations, the modern reintroduction of cannabis-based medicines becomes, if not a miracle, at least a profound revelation.

In light of this profound history, some have come to see the use of cannabis as a freedom-of-religion issue. But after fifteen years of researching the cross-cultural history of cannabis, and following its use from the Stone Age to present, I have come to see that the right to use cannabis is even more fundamental than religious freedoms, for humanity created religion, but no matter what god you believe in, you had better believe that god created cannabis. Even from an atheistic standpoint, from the cross-cultural perspective, as possibly our oldest cultivated crop, cannabis has had a evolutionary partnership with humanity that stretches back more than ten thousand years. Indeed, humanity has a natural indigenous right to all the plants of the Earth, all people and all plants, and any law that stands in the way of that natural relationship is an abomination to both God and nature.*

---

*Preservation is an issue that must be addressed, as extinction of a species threatens our collective inheritance. Endangered species must be protected for the benefit of all.

3
Recent History

David Malmo-Levine

"But if it's so harmless and helpful, why is it illegal?"—an often-asked question these days. Those familiar with the history of the origins of cannabis prohibition must overcome the common and comfortable (but evidence-free) fantasy regarding "health concerns," and instead reply "Racism and monopoly."

The prohibition of cannabis is a game of hierarchy, megalomania, and monopoly over medicine and sacrament, of classic divide-and-conquer of the masses. It's difficult to say where exactly this game begins, but more than one cannabis historian claims it begins with Moses.

In Exodus 30:23, *kanna-bosm* is identified as an ingredient in the holy anointing oil—the oil that gives the terms *christ* and *messiah* ("the anointed one") their meaning. In Exodus 30:33 it is explained that any nonpriest who uses the holy cannabis oil is condemned to die in the desert (Bennett and McQueen 2001). Later variations include penalties for using cannabis while "worshiping the wrong gods" and later still, using cannabis while "worshiping the devil," along with harsh penalties for those convicted.

Modern-day *kanna-bosm* prohibition is no different, in either its false pretexts, its ferocity, or its co-opting by those in power.

Drug prohibition in North America began with opium prohibition in Canada, stemming from a racist riot against Asians in Vancouver in 1907. It continued with the corporate-engineered closing of herbal medicine schools beginning in 1910 (see page 30). It then shifted to the racist and corporate efforts to criminalize cannabis on a national level, first in Canada in 1923, and then in the United States in 1937. If the details of these events became common knowledge, they would result in a revolution in North American drug policy.

KING AND THE ANTI-ASIAN RIOT

To fully understand the origins of cannabis prohibition, one must first study the origins of opium prohibition. From early on in the campaign to prohibit cannabis, it was mislabeled a narcotic, solidifying its guilt by association (opium is a narcotic). The mass media promoted racist stereotypes and played on parental anxiety, thereby shaping public opinion and transforming a botanical-medicine-trusting population into a drug-phobic one. In this sense, opium prohibition created a path for cannabis prohibition to follow.

On September 7, 1907, an economic depression hit Vancouver, Canada, and the local community of white supremacists—the Asiatic Exclusion League, along with some of the area's newspapers—decided to hold a mass meeting. The protesters marched down Hastings Street, and by the time they reached City Hall at Hastings and Main, the crowd had grown to eight thousand. Rather than blame fast-and-loose bankers, irresponsible government, or tight-fisted employers for their economic misfortune, they blamed competition from the Chinese and Japanese, who worked harder for less pay.

They also blamed politicians who would let more immigrants into the country. After a few fiery speeches and the burning of Lieutenant-Governor Dunsmuir in effigy, fifteen thousand marched down to Chinatown, where they smashed windows with rocks, wrecked many stores, and beat up the Chinese. The Japanese people fought back and saved their community from similar destruction (Morley 1961).

The Chinese community asked for compensation from the Canadian government. Ottawa sent future prime minister (then deputy minister of labor) William Lyon Mackenzie King to Vancouver. King visited Vancouver and spoke to some Chinese Christian clergymen and merchants interested in anti-opium legislation. In his report on the riot, King noted that two of the stores requesting compensation were opium dens, and that Canada should not compensate "an industry so inimical to our national welfare." King suggested that the government should "render impossible, save in so far as may be necessary for medicinal purposes, the continuance of such an industry" as opium distribution (MacFarlane 1986). These "oriental clubs," by the way, had been servicing the hardest-working Canadians—the gold-mining, railroad-building, poorly paid Chinese Canadians—for twenty years. The dens paid their taxes and helped the locals get a good night's sleep (MacFarlane 1986).

Not content to leave the recommendation in his riot report, King wrote a July 3, 1908, report titled "The Need for the Suppression of the Opium Traffic in Canada," wherein he wrote, "The habit of smoking opium was making headway, not only among white men and boys, but also among women and girls" (King 1908). This pushed buttons by heightening fears over racial mixing, creating parental hysteria.

King then wrote the Anti-Opium Act of 1908—North America's first national drug prohibition law—and, taking his own advice, helped pass this law, which banned opium sales by Chinese people across Canada.

The race-based monopoly worked like this: (1) Chinese people weren't allowed to become pharmacists until 1947 (Yee 2006), and (2) labels on the white pharmacists' opium bottles indicated that they were dealing in "medicinal opium," not recreational opium (Boyd 1991). The fact that both labeled opium and unlabeled opium had the same effect didn't seem to matter. It is even possible that the Chinese merchants could get better-quality opium than the white botanical druggists. Irrationally questioning the credentials of nonelite herb distributors or the quality of their merchandise is a recurring theme in drug prohibition and drug monopoly history. The theft of brown-skinned people's herbal medicines by white-skinned people in the form of "labeled" medications and patented formulas is another.

CANNABIS: THE MOST POPULAR PATENT MEDICINE?

The use of cannabis as an antispasmodic, analgesic, and a sedative, was widespread between 1850 and 1940 (Grinspoon 1996). Researchers have documented over six hundred pre-1937 cannabis medicines, including one popular brand, Piso's. The Hazeltine Corporation was founded in 1869 and soon became famous for its cough medicine, Piso's Cure for Consumption (tuberculosis). In fact, the product became so popular that, in time, the company actually changed its name to The Piso Company (antiquecannabisbook .com).

According to author Christian Rätsch, "Scientific medicine utilized cannabis as a universal remedy. In the nineteenth century, a variety of hashish preparations could be obtained without a prescription" (Rätsch 2001).

FLEXNER AND THE CLOSING OF THE
PRO-HERB MEDICAL SCHOOLS

The United States of the eighteen hundreds was a time of great experimentation in all branches of medicine. During this time, pioneers such as Samuel Thomson, Alva Curtis, and Dr. Benedict Lust opened up colleges and schools focusing on herbs and other aspects of medicine. The Flexner report brought all that experimentation to an end. This was a book-length study of medical education in the United States and Canada, written by the professional educator Abraham Flexner and published in 1910 under the aegis of the Carnegie Foundation. In fact, the report was partially conceived by Charles Eliot (of the Rockefeller Foundation, General Education Board, and the Institute) and Simon Flexner (also of the Rockefeller Institute)—who suggested his brother as author (Brown 1979). One of the recommendations of the report was that those who gave money to medical schools stop sponsoring the herbal schools, because they didn't have the proper "laboratories and texts" (Flexner 1910; gaiagarden .com).

Three years after publishing his report, Abraham Flexner went to work for the Rockefeller Institute, implementing the recommendations in his report for over two decades (Jonas 1989). This influential report contributed greatly to the decline of alternative medicine, including herbology (drpelletier.com). By 1932, Arthur Dean Bevan, the head of the American Medical Association's committees on medical education, stated he was "grateful" to Flexner for enabling them "to put out of business" the eclectic medical schools in existence in 1910 (Brown 1979).

Like Flexner, Mackenzie King also went to work for Rockefeller (Chernow 1998), just six years after completing his monopolization of the opium industry. Even more interesting, it was in 1900 (seven years before the race riot in Vancouver) that Rockefeller began putting money into eugenics—a "science" based on genetics created to justify racism (Marrs 2000).

HEARST, ANSLINGER, AND MURPHY

The first laws against cannabis in the United States were passed in border towns with Mexico, such as the ordinance passed in El Paso in 1914 (Sloman 1979). Designed allegedly to control cannabis, the law succeeded only in providing a weapon the local government could beat Mexicans with (Mann

2001). William Randolph Hearst was an up-and-coming newspaper tycoon, owning twenty-eight newspapers by the mid-1920s. In 1915, Pancho Villa's men took over Babicora, a million-acre ranch in Mexico owned by Hearst (Swanberg 1961). Hearst then dropped the words *cannabis* and *hemp* from his newspapers and began a propaganda campaign against "marijuana," (following in Anslinger's footsteps); it was the favored relaxant of Villa's men (Conrad 1994; Marez 2004).

Harry Anslinger was chosen to be the head of the Federal Bureau of Narcotics in 1930 by his wife's uncle, Andrew Mellon (Sloman 1979). Anslinger would receive tremendous positive newspaper coverage for his new war on cannabis, cocaine, and opiates—much of this from Hearst's newspapers (Silver 1979). In 1937, Anslinger would select lurid newspaper stories from his famous "gore file" and read them out loud while testifying to the House Ways and Means Committee: "Negro raped a girl eight years of age. Two Negroes took a girl fourteen years of age and kept her for two days in a hut under the influence of marihuana. Upon recovery she was found to be suffering from syphilis. . . . Colored students at the University of Minnesota partying with female students (white) smoking and getting sympathy with their stories of racial persecution. Result—pregnancy" (Sloman 1979; Grey 1998).

Emily Murphy, Canada's first female judge, wrote a series of racist articles for *Macleans* magazine entitled "The Grave Drug Menace," which she later expanded into a book called *The Black Candle* (Anthony and Solomon 1973; Oscapella 2004). The magazine—and book—along with a series of anti-Asian and anti-opium propaganda published in Canadian newspapers between 1920 and 1922—led to more anti-opium laws and the first anti-marijuana legislation in Canada in 1922 and 1923.

FDR, MELLON, AND ROCKEFELLER

By 1937, when the Marijuana Tax Act (which would effectively outlaw cannabis if passed) was being debated, there were no herbalism schools—no "alternative medicine" schools of any kind—left to provide a champion to speak on behalf of cannabis. And the supposedly left-wing President Roosevelt was no help, according to one researcher, because FDR (who signed the 1937 Marijuana Tax Act into law) had been on J. D. Rockefeller Jr.'s payroll since his first days in politics (Bealle 1949). Rockefeller—America's first billionaire and owner of Standard Oil, the largest oil company in the United States—had successfully eliminated or bought out any potential opponent to the oil industry's attempts at outlawing their natural competitor, hemp. Rockefeller's attack on herbalism with the Flexner report of 1910 made Andrew Mellon's attack on cannabis in the '20s and '30s possible.

Andrew Mellon owned Alcoa, Gulf Oil, and the Mellon Bank (Lundberg 1968). In the 1920s, Mellon financed DuPont's takeover of General Motors, and DuPont owned chemicals used by Hearst's paper-making factories. Hearst, along with Congressman Robert Doughton and Senator Prentiss Brown (both DuPont allies), combined their strength and passed the Marijuana Tax Act with little opposition. The DuPont 1937 Annual Report stated, "The revenue raising power of government may be converted into an instrument for forcing acceptance of sudden new ideas of industrial and social reorganization" (Conrad 1994). The "revenue raising" they were talking about was a tax act that was designed to avoid handing out any tax stamps—a prohibition pretending to be a tax. With hemp rope gone, DuPont's new invention, nylon, would be one of the synthetic "sudden new ideas" accepted by North American citizens. The hemp-free paper made from trees using Dupont's chemicals would be another.

The same "outlaw the natural to monopolize the synthetic" business strategy would work with fuel. According to one researcher, with today's enzyme technology, hemp ethanol could be produced for $1.37 per gallon plus the cost of the raw material, with technological improvements and tax credits reducing the price by another dollar or so per gallon (Castleman 2001). The cost of the raw material would decrease as hemp was grown for more products, providing more free (or nearly free) hemp stalks as a "waste product." Could you imagine paying under 50 cents per gallon (United States) or 15 cents per liter (Canadian) for your hemp ethanol? Rockefeller and Mellon could envision it, but they preferred their vision of dirty-fuel monopolies for Standard Oil and Gulf Oil rather than clean-fuel farms for prosperous farmers. It was crucial to their business model that hemp became illegal and stayed illegal.

IT GOES ON AND ON . . .

Race continues to play a role, in that police choose whom to arrest and scapegoat (drugwarfacts.org). Ads against cannabis use are sponsored by The Partnership for a Drug-Free America, with donors in the pharmaceutical industry, as well as all the old antihemp team: Chevron and ExxonMobil (both previously Standard Oil), Hearst, and DuPont, who donate $30,000 to $100,000 yearly. Rockefeller's Chase Manhattan and Citibank sometimes provide up to $15,000 per year to The Partnership for a Drug-Free America, while General Motors and even Ford (once a proponent of hemp) give double that (sourcewatch.org).

Election campaign contributions also ensure that hemp remains prohibited or overregulated. The oil and gas industry donated $4,529,926 to the Bush presidential campaigns (opensecrets.org). From 1992 to 2002, energy giant Enron contributed a total of $3,021,108 to the Republican National Committee, the National Republican Congressional Committee, the National Republican Senatorial Committee, Bush-Quayle '92, and George W. Bush 2000 (freerepublic.com). Not that the Bush administration wasn't already comfortable with the oil industry; as most people know, George Sr. was once a Texas oilman, and Dick Cheney ran Halliburton—the massive oil well construction and services corporation. Former Secretary of State Condoleezza Rice worked at (Rockefeller's) Chevron—they even named a tanker after her!

And much like the racist monopoly with opium, various cannabis products, such as the famous hashish of Afghanistan and the ganja of Jamaica, remain illegal while the British firm GW Pharmaceuticals and the German Bayer Corporation (once Standard Oil's largest business partner) enjoy a monopoly of legal cannabis products with their Sativex cannabis tincture spray. For those familiar with cannabis, economics, and racism, it would appear that white people have rationalized themselves into another medicinal monopoly, using false concerns over smoke and euphoria and a lack of labeling as justification.

THE TREE OF LIFE AND HEAVEN OR HELL

I'm no Christian fundamentalist, but the choices we face are so stark that only a biblical metaphor will capture their true essence. The reality of the situation is that we could all live in a world where harmless people would no longer fear persecution and imprisonment, where climate change could be reversed through hemp-fuel carbon sinks, where oil wars would be nonexistent, and where pollution would be a crime worth punishment. This is a world where simple pleasures, happiness, and euphoria—from whatever source—would be deemed worthy of protection, where culturally rich and politically active cannabis cafes flourished everywhere. The alternative is to continue to prohibit the tree of life—the sacred *kanna-bosm*—and continue down our current road to a hellish situation.

The medicine and fuel economies are worth hundreds of billions of dollars in North America alone. If we cannabis activists ever wonder why our letter-writing campaigns are unsuccessful and misunderstood, it could be because those in power fully understand us, but are ignoring us. The reason cannabis is still illegal is that some rich white men continue to make a killing off this game. The actual origins are not men, but the twin devils of greed and ignorance sitting on their shoulders, two devils with flaming swords, guarding God's tree, whispering into the ears of the powerful.

If cannabis is ever to be re-legalized, activists and those in the mass media must learn and teach its true history and expose this satanic game for what it is.

RECOMMENDED READING

antiquecannabisbook.com

 http://antiquecannabisbook.com/chap1/Pre1937.htm. Accessed April 27, 2010.

 http://antiquecannabisbook.com/chap15/QPiso.htm. Accessed April 27, 2010.

www.drpelletier.com

gaiagarden.com

 www.gaiagarden.com/art/history_herbal_medicine4.html. Accessed April 27, 2010.

 www.drugwarfacts.org/racepris.htm. Accessed April 27, 2010.

sourcewatch.org

 www.sourcewatch.org/index.php?title=Partnership_for_a_Drug_Free_America. Accessed April 27, 2010.

opensecrets.org

 www.opensecrets.org

freerepublic.com

 www.freerepublic.com/focus/f-news/1638383/posts. Accessed April 27, 2010.

For more on hemp as a fuel, please see the following article by David Malmo-Levine: http://hemp-ethanol.blogspot.com/2008/01/original-hemp-field.html. Accessed April 27, 2010.

4
The Botany of *Cannabis*

Lyle E. Craker, Ph.D., and Zoë Gardner

In many locations, the plant genus *Cannabis* has become synonymous with the recreational drug marijuana. While *Cannabis* plants are grown and used for food, fiber, fuel, medicine, and shelter (Brown 1998a, Guy 2004) in different areas of the world, primary cultivation, especially in the United States, is for the psychoactive chemical constituents known as cannabinoids. These cannabinoids have been demonstrated to be effective in the treatment of an assortment of human disease conditions (Russo 2004), but they have also been deemed addictive and dangerous substances with no therapeutic value (NIDA 2007). Thus, species of *Cannabis* are considered to be both a botanical blessing and a scourge to society.

As a plant with a long history of cultivation and use (Russo 2004; Schultes 1970; Wills 1998), *Cannabis* has been dispersed from origins in Central Asia, the northwest Himalayas, and, quite possibly, China (Nelson 1996; Schultes 1970) to a number of habitats throughout the tropical and temperate regions of the world (Russo 2004; Wills 1998) by populations enthralled by the intoxicating resin and the functional applications of the fibers and the extractable oil from the fruit (achenes, commonly known as seeds) (Clarke 1993; Schultes 1970). This dichotomy of uses for *Cannabis* as a medicinal and recreational drug and as a fiber and oil source has continuously stimulated public and scientific interest and curiosity in the value of the plant, leading to earlier reviews on the botany and other aspects of the plant (Brown 1998b; Boyce 1912; Clarke 1993; Guy 2004; Joyce and Curry 1970;

Walton 1938). *Cannabis* is a member of the Cannabaceae family along with the genus *Humulus* (hops) and the genus *Celtis* (hackberry and sugarberry).

NOMENCLATURE

Complete taxonomic classification within the genus *Cannabis* remains under considerable dispute. Some authorities (Small and Cronquist 1976; Quimby 1974) claim that all *Cannabis* plants grown for fiber or resin or other purposes belong to the species *C. sativa,* with subspecies, such as *C. sativa* subspecies *indica,* to differentiate among types. Other authorities (Schultes and Hofmann 1991) insist that morphological differentiation (narrower leaflets, thinner cortex, and more branches) and lack of cannabinoids within plants of European origin, as compared with plants in India, indicate two species, *C. sativa* (historically identified as the source of hemp fibers) and *C. indica* (historically identified as the source of canabinoid-containing resin). Additional species have been distinguished: *C. ruderalis* (wild/naturalized accessions) and *C. chinensis* (currently thought to be a subset of *C. indica*) have been proposed due to differentiation in phenotypic traits of the plants (Schultes and Hofmann 1991). A recent investigation on allozyme (an enzyme that differs by one amino acid from other forms of the same enzyme) variation within 157 populations of *Cannabis* (Hillig 2005) strongly suggests that the genus *Cannabis* consists of only two species, *C. sativa* and *C. indica.*

The relationships within *Cannabis* species and the production of fiber and cannabinoids, however, are not completely understood, making absolute assignment of *C. sativa* as the source of fiber and *C. indica* as the source of the resin unwarranted until more complete chemotaxonomic data is available. The movement and selection of plants by growers and others has certainly led to a number of environmental and cultivated variants of *Cannabis,* as the plants became adapted to growth in various locations and growers chose and seeded plants (accessions) with desirable characteristics. Strains of *Cannabis* approved for industrial hemp production in Europe and elsewhere have been selected to produce only minute amounts of psychoactive constituents, while strains of *Cannabis* used for medicinal and recreational use have been selected for production of cannabinoids (Small and Marcus 2002). A study of ninety-seven *Cannabis* accessions (de Meijer et al. 2003) indicated that plants produced for delta-9-tetrahydrocannabidiol (THC) and cannabidiol (CBD) demonstrated a continuous variation in content of these constituents among the accessions with no phenotypic characteristic (physical appearance) that could accurately separate those with high THC from those with low THC content. All species of *Cannabis* can seemingly be bred to produce fiber or cannabinoids.

BOTANICAL HISTORY

Historically, botanical interest in *Cannabis* undoubtedly began as the plant became recognized as a source of food, fiber, and medicine. Archaeological evidence indicates use of the plant in China as a fiber some twelve thousand years ago (Nelson 1996; Schultes 1970). Early use as medicine is documented by inclusion of the plant in the first known Chinese materia medica (treatise on medical remedies), *Pen Ts'ao* (accredited to Emperor Shen Nung, 2737 and 2697 BCE), in which people were advised to cultivate the female plant for its greater medicinal properties (Schultes 1970). As the plant moved from country to country in trade, first to Asian counties such as India, Korea, and Japan, cultivation was initiated by farmers as demand for the product increased. Over subsequent years, several rituals were developed for cultivation of the plant, most likely to ensure the growth of the female plant to be used for the resin produced.

After contact with the Indian subcontinent by the Indo-Europeans, cultivation of *Cannabis* was spread throughout the Middle East and Europe for both fiber and resin. *Cannabis* was a fiber crop in America in prehistoric times (Schultes 1970), and the plant was prevalent in America before the arrival of European explorers. Early cultivators of *Cannabis,* including George Washington and Thomas Jefferson, provided extended notes on planting, harvesting, and expected yields, indicating a familiarity with the botany of the plant (Nelson 1996). After America outlawed the cultivation and use of marijuana, it became "hidden" among other crops, forested areas, and enclosed structures to prevent discovery. Yet, despite the efforts at restriction on the growth of *Cannabis* by local, state, and federal governments, American growers are estimated to have produced 22.3 million pounds of marijuana with a value of $35.8 billion in 2006 (Gettman 2006).

Growing in the wild, *Cannabis* plants usually have limited growth, generate small seeds, and produce small amounts of oil, fiber, or resin, as compared with cultivated species, due to lack of soil nutrients. To maximize development and productivity, the *Cannabis* plant, which is known as a "heavy feeder," needs lots of mineral nutrients, levels that can be supplied under cultivated conditions. Other environmental variables, such as temperature, light, water availability, and plant spacing, also affect the growth and development of the *Cannabis* plant, causing variations in plant appearance and productivity

(Bósca and Karus 1998; Clarke 1993; Potter 2004). To maximize quality production for use of the plant for medicinal purposes and to ensure quality and "hidden" production of the plant for recreational use, *Cannabis* is often produced hydroponically in a greenhouse or enclosed room where the environmental conditions can be controlled (Clarke 1993; Potter 2004). Of the current *Cannabis* crop grown in America, 17 percent is thought to be cultivated inside buildings under controlled conditions (Gettman 2006). To meet the need for specialized equipment for controlled growth, various equipment suppliers offer hydroponic equipment and instructions designed to produce vigorously growing plants.

MORPHOLOGY

Cannabis is a rapidly growing dioecious (male and female reproductive organs on different plants), wind pollinated, annual herb that in some plant selections can reach heights of twenty feet (six meters) (figures 4.1 and 4.2). Seeds, which readily germinate within a week, develop two seed leaves (cotyledons) that are approximately one-half inch (1.7 cm) long, slightly unequal in size, and broader at the tip than the base (Clarke 1993; Stearn 1970). The first true leaves, which form as a pair on opposite sides of the stem at right angles to and approximately an inch above the cotyledons, consist of two narrow, serrated leaflets (blades) two to four inches (5 to 10 cm) long connected to the plant stalk by a distinct petiole (Clarke 1993). The next pair of leaves, formed at right angles to the first pair, can be unifoliate (one leaflet per leaf) or palmate (multiple leaflets arising at a single point on the end of the petiole) (figure 4.3). The number of leaflets per leaf generally increases as new leaves form on the stem until a maximum of ten or eleven leaflets per leaf is reached.

The stem, which is sometimes hollow, is angular and pubescent (covered in small hair-like structures) (Stearn 1970). If the plant has adequate growing space, the axillary buds (growing points located where the leaf joins the stem) will form branches. If vegetative growth conditions are favorable, the stem will increase in height by two inches per day when exposed to the long daylight periods of summer. While some selections of *Cannabis* are day-neutral (flower under any day length), most are classified as short-day plants (they need a long dark period, usually fourteen hours or more) and shift from vegetative to generative (reproductive) growth upon exposure to short daylight periods. With the change to reproductive growth, the leaf pairs change from leaves opposite each other on the stem to an alternate, spiral

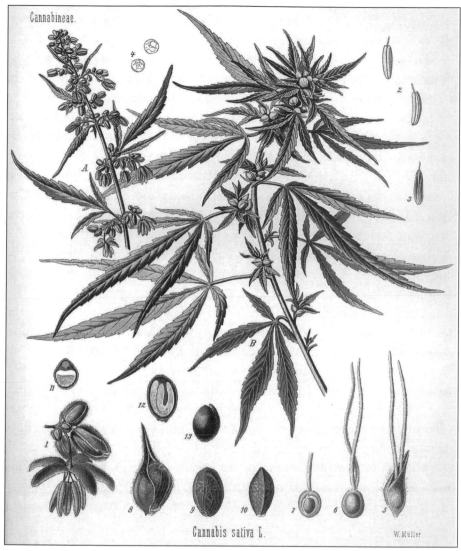

Figure 4.1. Cannabis sativa *plants and selected reproductive parts. Source: Köhler, FE. 1914. Köhler's Medizinal-Pflanzen In Naturgetreuen Abbildungen Mit Kurz Erläuterndem Texte. Gera-Untermhaus*

A. Male *Cannabis sativa* plant in flower
B. Female *Cannabis sativa* plant in flower
1. Male flower
2, 3. Anthers from male flowers
4. Pollen grains
5. Female flower (calyx with two pistils)
6. Female flower with calyx removed
7. Cross-section of ovary after pollination
8. Ripe seed (achene) with calyx
9, 10. Ripe seed (achene)
11, 12. Cross-sectional views of seeds (achenes)
13. Seed (achene) with seedcoat removed

arrangement (a single leaf on one side of the stem and the next leaf higher on the stem is not directly above the lower leaf) (Potter 2004).

During vegetative growth, male and female plants of *Cannabis* cannot be distinguished from each other with any certainty, although the female plant tends to be more stocky and flower later than the male plant (Raman 1998). As the plants enter the reproductive phase, however, the density of leaves on the upper part of the plants begins to differ, with the male plant having fewer leaves than the female plant. The male plant forms flowers in long, loose clusters (six to twelve inches long) from buds within claw-shaped bracts on branches at the top of the plant, while the female plant forms flowers in tight, crowded clusters from buds within tubular-shaped bracts. In male flowers, the bracts are formed from five relatively short pubescent sepals (small leaflike structures), a half-inch long or less, that are a yellowish, greenish, or whitish in color (Clarke 1993). The female flowers are borne in pairs, and each individual flower is enclosed in green colored bracts (calyx formed by sepals).

The upper leaves, unfertilized flower heads, and flower bracts of the female plant are the primary source of cannabinoids in *Cannabis* (Russo 2004). The cannabinoids are enclosed in tiny (just visible to the eye) glandular trichomes (globe-shaped structures, supported on short stalks) found on bracts and floral leaves and unstalked, glandular trichomes (peltate trichomes) found on vegetative leaves and pistillate (flower) bracts (Hammond and Mahlberg 1977; Raman 1998; Starks 1990) and produce the sticky resin containing cannabinoids and terpenes (figure 4.4).

Maximum cannabinoid-producing trichomes occur on the flowering part of the *Cannabis* plant during the late flowering period. The flowering head and other vegetative tissues (lower leaves and stems) of the plant

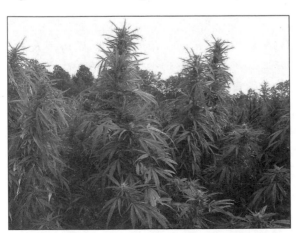

Figure 4.2. Cannabis *plants growing outdoors*

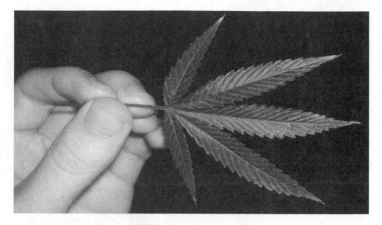

Figure 4.3. A typical Cannabis *leaf*

can also develop three other types of trichomes (unicellular curved, squat unicellular, and bulbous) that do not produce cannabinoids. The number of resin-producing trichomes is higher in female plants than on male plants, especially on the bracts.

APPLICATIONS

Pollination occurs when pollen grains move from the male to the female flower by floating in the wind or by the purposeful transfer of pollen to create specific crosses (mating the same or two different strains to develop desirable features) (Green 2005). Following fertilization (the fusion of the male and female gametophytes, sperm and egg, respectively), the female flower develops seeds (achenes) over fourteen to thirty-five days. The male plant usually dies after shedding pollen, but the female plant, fertilized or unfertilized, continues to mature for another two to five months. Monoecious plants (having both male and female flowers on the same plant) occasionally occur, but this is not a normal occurrence except in specially selected varieties.

In new plantings from seed, an essentially equal number of male and female plants can be expected, although extreme stress, such as that produced by nutrient excesses or deficiencies, temperature extremes, altered light cycles, or mutilation may increase the number of female plants in the population (Clarke 1993). *Cannabis* plants can also be grown from vegetative cuttings (asexual reproduction, also known as cloning, in which a small part of a plant is used to develop a complete plant) (Clarke 1993; Potter 2004). The use of vegetative cuttings is used to preserve unique

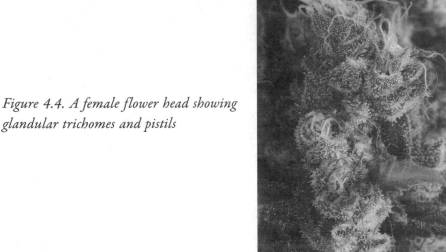

Figure 4.4. A female flower head showing glandular trichomes and pistils

characteristics, as the new plant will have the same genotype (genetic composition) and thus the potential for the same phenotypic characteristics as the plant it was taken from, though a different environment may change the plant appearance and chemistry. Offspring of sexually propagated plants (those grown from seed) will have genotypes different from the parent plants, as inheritable characteristics (genes) that determine the plant phenotype come from both the male and the female plant. Planned plant crosses (mating of male and female plants by transfer of pollen from a specific male to a specific female) are used to develop new varieties.

Cannabis plants used for fiber production are strains that produce only very small quantities of cannabinoids (Rannali 1999; Schultes 1970). To produce the best fibers, these plants are best grown in cold or temperate regions and harvested in the juvenile (vegetative) stage of growth. As the plant ages, the bast fibers (fibers that run the length of the stem, produced in the inner bark) undergo lignification (a hardening that makes the fibers brittle) (Potter 2004). Monoecious plants are preferred for fiber production because the plants all mature at the same time, enabling mechanical harvest. Seeds to be used as a fixed (fatty) oil source (nonnarcotic), food, or propagation material are harvested only after the seeds have matured. Many seeds usually fall to the ground before harvest, as the achenes held in the flower pods are loose, and the pods have a tendency to dehisce (discharge seeds) upon ripening.

Cannabis plants grown for medicinal or recreational products are harvested for the resin produced by the leaves and bracts of the flowering tops (Nelson 1999). To maximize the number of glands and resin production, male plants are frequently removed from the production location to prevent flowers on the female plants from producing seeds. The lack of seed formation induces the female plants to produce more flowers, leading to increased resin production, frequently with higher cannabinoid content than resin from plants with seeds (ElSohly et al. 1984). The plant material used for recreational purposes produced from nonseed flowering tops of female plants is known as sinsemilla and is valued for high THC content, enhanced appearance, and a more intense aroma, as compared with other similar products obtained from plants allowed to form seeds (Hanrahan 2001; Rosenthal 1984). Dried, crushed flowers and small upper leaves used as the recreational drug are commonly known as marijuana, while the resin collected by brushing the glandular trichomes from the plant tissues and used as a recreational drug is commonly known as hashish.

CONCLUSION

As plants closely associated with humans for several thousand years, *Cannabis* species have undergone morphological and chemical changes through plant selection and breeding to adapt the botany of the plant to meet the needs of the populace. The closeness and overlapping of traits among the species has made differentiation difficult and created confusion among taxonomists (Schultes 1970; Schultes and Hofmann 1991). Differences among *Cannabis* types suggest that some were selected and improved to produce fibers, while other types were selected and improved for production of cannabinoids. Such selection of desirable types continues and has led to plants that can grow in different environments and produce more resin or fiber than wild types of *Cannabis* (de Meijer, van der Kamp, and van Eeuwijk 1992, 1993; Hillig 2005; Russo 2004; Schultes 1970).

Considerable efforts in breeding and selection have produced *Cannabis* varieties and cultivars that are uniquely suited for production of medicinal or psychoactive compounds, fibers, and fixed oils. Examination of medicinal applications of *Cannabis* has been renewed in the past twenty years, with botanical selections now being made to meet that need (Guy 2004). Having been in close association with humans for thousands of years, the *Cannabis* plant continues to be botanically adaptable to meet the requirements of the societies in which the plant is grown.

5
Cannabis Grow Revolution

Danny Danko, Senior Cultivation Editor, *High Times* Magazine

Gardening is civil and social, but it wants the vigor and freedom of the forest and the outlaw.

HENRY DAVID THOREAU

From my observations based on traveling to cannabis fairs and pot gardens worldwide for a number of years, growing cannabis for personal use is on the rise as more people discover the virtues of creating their own "homegrown." Police crackdowns push consumers away from the black market while economic downturns convince more of them to become self-sufficient smokers. The same pressures have driven pot seed breeders and advanced cultivators to create new hybrids, growing techniques, and stealth products to stay one step ahead of the authorities.

The real secret is that growing cannabis for your own use is quite simple; provide the proper environment, including lighting, nutrients, humidity, air movement, and pest control, and the plants will produce many ounces for a small fraction of current prices.

Stick to the easiest ways to grow at first, using a loose potting soil or a soilless mix in two- to four-gallon buckets with holes in the bottom for drainage. A lower wattage (250–400-Watt) HID (High Intensity Discharge) grow light or a few compact fluorescents are perfectly adequate for a closet or small grow area. Larger rooms will require HIDs with higher wattages, such as 600-Watt or 1,000-Watt HPS (High-Pressure Sodium) or MH (Metal Halide) bulbs and ballasts. Higher wattages produce stronger lighting but also more heat. New advancements in light-emitting diode (LED) technology look somewhat promising, and initial test results show that their future is bright. LEDs drastically reduce power consumption and heat, creating usable lumens without the typical drawbacks of other light systems.

INDICA VS. SATIVA

The cannabis we smoke can be generally classified as either indica, sativa, or more often, a hybrid or combination of the two. (*Cannabis ruderalis* is a low-THC variety native to Eastern Europe and Russia that grows wild but does not lend itself to being smoked.)

Indicas, which originated in the Hindu Kush region of Central Asia, are characterized by their short stature and fatter leaf structure. Traditionally, these plants were grown and bred for making hashish. The buds are covered with the glandular trichomes that we sometimes refer to as crystals or kif. The trichomes are sifted away from the leaf and buds and then pressed together to make hashish. Indicas tend to give their users a lethargic feeling, sometimes referred to as "couch-lock" or "stoned."

Sativas are the taller, longer-flowering variety native to equatorial regions with a longer growing season. The leaves are typically thinner and longer and the buds tend to be thinner and more elongated as well. Sativa plants were traditionally bred for hemp purposes, as well as for medicinal applications from smoking and brewing tea. Less trichome production is augmented by the characteristic sativa high, known as racy and "electric." This "up" high was described by veterans returning from Vietnam who smoked the Vietnamese, Thai, and Laotian sativas of Southeast Asia. Some pure sativas have been known to induce paranoia and heart-racing in unsuspecting smokers.

Pot aficionados know that different hybrids exhibit unique characteristics of flavor, scent, and intoxication. The qualities expressed by strains of cannabis vary greatly from catatonic to giddy, and from stoned to high. Personal preference plays an enormous role, and humans have bred the cannabis they most enjoy repeatedly. Many connoisseurs consider sativas to be a daytime smoke and indicas primarily as a nightcap. Most of what is smoked is a hybrid of the two, typically not more than 60 percent of one over the other.

MALES VS. FEMALES

The buds we smoke are the dried flowers of the female cannabis plant. Males are basically useless to anyone but breeders, who collect the pollen from male flowers to pollinate female flowers to produce seeds. For pot-production purposes, male plants should be discarded as soon as they're discovered to prevent seeding your entire crop of females.

During the early stages of flowering, males will begin to show their sex at the plant node—the area where the leaf meets the main stem. Male flowers will protrude like the tip of a spear and then droop down, resembling a tiny bunch of bananas. If they are allowed to continue growth after this point, the "bananas" will open, spilling their pollen to the wind and ruining your dreams of growing seed-free pot (sinsemilla). Show no mercy.

Females will also start showing their sex in early flowering. Pear-shaped bracts form at the nodes, and white hairs emerge from them. These hairs are a sure sign of a female plant, but you must beware of hermaphrodites. Some plants show their sex as females but actually have male flowers as well that can ruin a crop. Always check developing flowers for signs of hermaphrodite behavior and be sure to nip it in the bud by getting rid of those meddlesome plants whenever you encounter them.

SOIL VS. HYDROPONICS

Traditionally, plants are grown in soil or soilless potting mixes that mimic natural earthy loam. Advances in hydroponics, or the growing of plants with their roots immersed in a nutrient solution, allow cultivators to increase the rate of growth as well as final yields. Roots growing in a hydroponic system typically grow bigger plants faster than the same roots in a soil-type medium.

Hydroponic growing should be considered an advanced technique because much more data must be taken into account; water temperatures, nutrient levels, and pH (the acidity or alkalinity of the nutrient solution) must all be monitored several times daily for optimal growth. Soil growing is much more forgiving; problems can be spotted and fixed over a matter of days, as opposed to hydroponic problems, which must be dealt with more quickly. Beginners should almost always start with plants in a soil-type potting mix to ensure success.

Recent advanced techniques in hydroponics prove interesting to growers. Aeroponics, in which roots are constantly misted with nutrient solution, was pioneered by NASA for long-term space exploration and exhibits astonishingly fast growth rates in optimal lab-like conditions. Also, new 360-degree grow units take advantage of the full light footprint of their air-cooled grow bulbs by rotating the plants fully around the light source.

Hydroponic growers are also perfecting ways to use organic nutrients, with the most interesting subset being aquaponics, in which fish farms stacked below hydro trays feed plant roots in a symbiotic relationship, creating both plant and animal produce for local markets.

I always recommend a soilless mix or coco coir (a renewable product made from hulled shells of coconuts). These mediums hold roots, yet allow plenty of oxygen to reach them without the typical hassles of hydroponic growing, such as water temperature fluctuations or clogged tubes. Coco coir requires a slightly different nutrient and pH profile, and watering must take place more often than with soil, but I find it to be the best of both worlds and one of the most ecological ways to grow indoors.

VEGETATIVE VS. FLOWERING GROWTH

Cannabis plants grow in two distinct stages: vegetative and flowering (reproductive). Seedlings under proper light will grow taller, spreading their branches and creating more growing shoots until the light cycle is shortened to twelve hours per day or less. Outdoors, this occurs naturally as summer turns to fall, but indoor flowering must be induced by the grower.

This means that if you don't reduce the amount of light, the plant will continue to grow vegetatively and never flower, leaving you with a lot of lumber, leaves, and sticks, but no buds. The only time when this practice is useful is when growing mother plants from which to take cuttings, or clones, of vegetative plants in perpetuity. I've seen twenty-year-old mother plants in gardens, but they're quite rare.

Indoor plants begin their lives under eighteen to twenty-four hours of light per day. When they have attained the desired height, a timer reduces the amount of light to half the twenty-four-hour period. If the twelve-hour dark period remains uninterrupted, the plant will gradually shift from upward and outward growth and begin to form flowers, which eventually turn into the buds we prize.

This transition, however, is gradual, and the plant will continue to stretch for the first several weeks of flowering. The hybrids typically grown by most cultivators flower for forty-five to sixty-five days, but some pure sativas have been known to have flowering times of three months or more.

Vegetative and flowering plants have completely different food requirements, so you must tailor the nutrients used during each stage to the proper formula. During the vegetative stage, a nitrogen-heavy nutrient, such as liquid fish and seaweed, is necessary, while flowering requires more potassium and phosphorous-based foods such as bat guano. It's crucial to know your N/P/Ks (ratios of nitrogen, phosphorous, and potassium)!

INDOOR VS. OUTDOOR

In general, pot grown outdoors is less highly regarded than its indoor-cultivated counterpart. This is because outdoor pot tends to be leafier and less fully developed, due primarily to its being grown on a much larger scale. It's infinitely easier to properly manicure a few ounces than hundreds of pounds. Nonetheless, great pot can be grown outside, as long as several factors are met.

Wind and rain can destroy cannabis plants quickly. Wind degrades THC and terpenes, bruising trichomes and breaking branches. Always create a windbreak or use a greenhouse to protect outdoor plants. Rain, especially late in the flowering stage, can create molds that will quickly consume your cannabis tops, or colas. At the first sign of any spreading mold, harvest the plants and discard affected branches; healthy buds will soon rot if left exposed to molds and moisture. Water plants at their roots, and cover them during rainy or humid weather.

Indoor plants require a whole different system of growing. The best indoor bud is grown in rooms that use a combination of intake and outtake fans in conjunction with charcoal filters to clean the odor. Negative pressure creates a constant supply of new cool, fresh air. Spent hot air is vented elsewhere, sometimes even heating the house or a pool.

Pot plants indoors need constant supervision for pest control. Without natural predators, vegetarian bugs such as spider mites, thrips, and white flies can have a field day on uninspected leaves. Organic insect sprays and predatory bugs help keep pest populations from devastating crops. Branches may also need to be staked to strengthen them. Lighting must never be too close or too far from the plant tops; between one and two feet is about right for most indoor grow lighting applications.

ORGANIC VS. CHEMICAL: FERTILIZATION

Like all plants, cannabis needs nutrients to grow. Besides the basic N/P/K profile, several other micronutrients must be present, some in quite minuscule amounts, for proper growth.

The difference between chemically based nutrients and organic ones is determined by how the plant foods are derived. Concentrated salts formulas such as Miracle-Gro, developed in a laboratory, are typically not considered organic. Nutrients derived from a recently living organism, such as bat guano or liquid fish or seaweed, are.

Growing organic pot requires that your medium and plant foods come from natural sources, not synthetic salt compounds dreamed up in a lab. Don't get me wrong, great pot can be grown with General Hydroponics' three-part formula, but it'll never be organic or medical grade, burning cleanly with all flavors and odors intact and at their peak.

Some growers claim that the plants can't possibly tell the difference between the elemental molecules they take up and thus believe that "organic" is a sham and a waste of money. Organic growers will swear their buds are safer and better tasting. The truth is somewhere in between.

Organic nutrients typically smell a bit more than their chemical counterparts, but the final product is worth the trouble. Plus, there are issues such as the environmental impact of draining all those chemical salts into our water supply and sewers. All in all, organic growing using freshly brewed compost teas and natural nutrients is cheaper, easier, and healthier for people and the planet. Sounds like a no-brainer to me.

All plants, organic or otherwise, must be flushed for the final two weeks of their growth to leach out salts and minerals they've collected throughout their life cycle. Plain water, with no added nutrients, is used to water the plants, which sometimes even develop yellowing leaves toward the end. But don't fret; this is an essential step, and the loss of green in the leaves translates into less "green" taste in the buds. If more growers would flush their plants, it would improve the quality of marijuana around the world.

ORGANIC VS. CHEMICAL: PEST CONTROL

Another bone of contention among growers is the use of potentially harmful pesticides. Some swear by pyrethrum "bombs" and chemical sprays, while others lean toward natural neem oil or predatory insects and nematodes that fight and destroy the pests we hate such as spider mites, white flies, and thrips. Most would agree that the latter are safer for the finished product than the former, but growers sometimes find themselves quite overwhelmed by pest issues. Many more resort to nuclear tactics than are willing to admit it.

A combination of good grow-room hygiene practices, such as checking the undersides of plant leaves daily and rinsing them occasionally with a mild pest treatment, will surely keep most insect attacks at bay. Also, eternal vigilance against pests can lead to many other discoveries, such as a pH problem or an overfertilized plant. My recommendation is to use the least-harmful ways possible at all times, whether nutrients, pest control, or sanitation in general. Well-cared-for plants produce better-tasting pot, and no amount of rinsing can wash off the residue of some of the available products out there. Keep it simple, and keep it green!

THE MEDICAL MARIJUANA REVOLUTION

Lately, a whole new realm of growing has emerged, especially in California, where Proposition 215 has allowed medical use of marijuana for over ten years. These growers are creating medicine for themselves and fellow patients, and their attention to detail is astounding. Strains are selected for specific medical needs, such as alleviation of nausea from chemotherapy or eye pressure for sufferers of glaucoma. Indeed, these growers are laying the groundwork for the future of medicinal marijuana research.

Along with the medical marijuana growers' quest for better genetics and more information comes a new domestic production of hashish. Patients searching for relief of extreme pain and debilitating symptoms need stronger medicines. Growers utilize the trimmings from their harvests, previously thrown out or used to make cannabis foods, to create "bubblehash" or ice-water-extracted trichomes. Bubblehash gets its name from the way it bubbles and melts when heated; the potency of this U.S.-produced hashish rivals the strongest imports from Morocco or India.

The hashish is a concentrated concoction of trichome heads and stalks. This is where the THC and other essential oils, known as terpenes, are primarily located. The glandular trichomes are broken from the leaves using ice water and agitation and collected on a screen. After drying, the paste crumbles and turns to a more sand-like consistency. When smoked, it can overpower the user and cause serious coughing fits. This type of product should only be used by a seasoned cannabis consumer. With bubblehash, remember to sip and not chug.

THE FUTURE OF CANNABIS

More states in the United States are passing laws allowing the medical use of marijuana, and majorities of voters clearly advocate the decriminalization of recreational cannabis use by adults. The will of the people continues to defeat the propaganda of the drug warriors. Doctors', nurses', and patients' voices are finally being heard, and the groundswell of support for marijuana law reform has reached a fever pitch. Truly, we are nearing the tipping point.

Growing pot as a hobby and practice has spread throughout the planet. Our recent Global Harvest Report (*High Times,* December 2009) highlighted such far-ranging places as Spain and Australia, South Africa and Malawi. Personal experience and anecdotal evidence suggests that cannabis cultivation is on the rise throughout Eastern Europe, Asia, and beyond.

Smart cultivators will develop a stable of mother plants and share the material with their like-minded compatriots. The time of hoarding strains is over. Medicinally, the best cannabis for each individual ailment will be isolated and developed to further soothe the selected symptoms.

From my perspective, the growers of the future are armed with more technology, information, and genetic material than ever before. Techniques continue to develop and become perfected, with cannabis cultivators sharing their experiences safely and anonymously. The Internet has created a forum for growers to work together, solving each others' problems with solutions derived from collective experiences. As these alliances develop and thrive, strains and techniques make their way around the globe, spreading this powerful plant and her cultivation "secrets" far and wide.

6

The Endocannabinoid System

Gregory L. Gerdeman, Ph.D., and
Jason B. Schechter, Ph.D.

Recent years have been witness to a huge surge in scientific research with a focus on both the workings of marijuana and its biological targets of action. Much has been learned about pot's effects on our nervous system; and, in the process, the extensive study of cannabis has elucidated many marvelous insights into how our brains function. Worldwide scientific inquiry has revealed a remarkable physiological endocannabinoid system, active not just in the brain but throughout our bodies, which seemingly works in many ways to maintain both our overall health and our sense of well-being.

The use of cannabis is demonstrably ancient (Russo et al. 2008), but the study of endocannabinoids and their actions is both young and constantly expanding. New and even surprising discoveries seem to occur with regularity, and findings about the function and evolution of endocannabinoid signaling reveal new complexity as to how cannabis is likely to influence human health and disease. Medical potential for the cannabinoids is now evidenced on many biological levels—ranging from genes to behavior—and for numerous indications that were entirely unexpected merely twenty years ago.

Not wanting to get carried away with broad claims of panacea, we will touch only casually on some of these biological effects and therapeutic applications, many of which are covered more formally elsewhere in this book. We also confess to a sprinkling of speculative commentary, which was born from our general study of cannabinoid pharmacology and which we feel is on solid scientific ground. Our aim is to introduce the cellular and molecular physiology of endocannabinoids and their receptors—players that form the molecular context of how and why cannabis elicits its myriad effects in the body.

THE CANNABINOID RECEPTORS

Marijuana affects the body because its constituent bioactive compounds—especially, but not exclusively, delta-9-THC—bind to and activate tiny molecular *receptors* encoded by our genes. These cannabinoid-capturing receptors are proteins that are "expressed" on the membranous surfaces of cells. It is precisely because they selectively bind cannabinoid-shaped molecules that these little receivers are collectively called *cannabinoid receptors*, and the many different cells and tissue types in our bodies that express these cannabinoid receptors are responsible for the diversity of physiological effects generated by marijuana intake (Iverson and Snyder 2000; Kofalvi 2008; Reggio 2009; figure 6.1).

In the brain, various neurological effects depend on what particular brain areas and networks the cannabinoid-sensitive cells participate in. For example, some networks of neurons are responsible for mediating our short-term memory. Other networks regulate anxiety. Still others regulate compulsive behavior, or our sleep cycles, or how hungry we are and when. *Where* the receptors are located is a major determinant of what the particular effect of cannabinoid exposure will be (Piomelli 2003).

The brain and other nervous system tissues express cannabinoid receptors called, simply, CB1. A second receptor—called CB2—has been identified primarily in certain cells of our immune system. Thus, most of the mental and perceptual influences of cannabis can be attributed to CB1 receptor activation rather than CB2. CB2 receptors, in contrast, appear to be responsible for the ability of cannabinoids such as THC, cannabidiol (CBD), and the terpenoid β-carophyllene (Gertsch et al. 2008) to reduce inflammation and various types of pain (Pacher, Batkai, and Kunos 2006).

How *do* we know such things? Ever since Drs. Mechoulam and Gaoni isolated delta-9-THC from hash oil (Gaoni and Mechoulam 1964), it has been clear that THC is of paramount importance in many—but not all—of the effects of cannabis on the body and mind. Other cannabinoids present in cannabis are similar in molecular structure to THC, as are most synthetic drugs that mimic marijuana's effects. These were clues that a specific receptor system

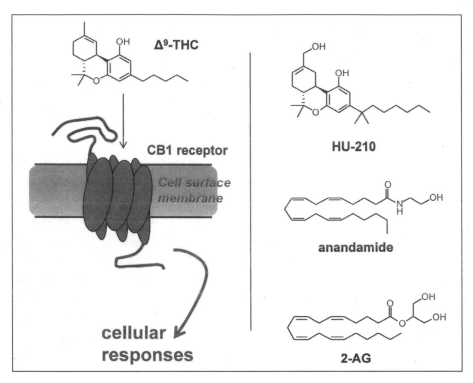

Figure 6.1. Chemical structures of cannabinoids, including Δ⁹-THC and its much more potent synthetic analog HU-210, which has been used experimentally. The chemical structures of the eCBs, anandamide and 2-AG, are quite different, but anandamide has been shown to fold over on itself to resemble THC in three dimensions.

is involved. That is, the *shape* of the molecule was realized to be important because it acts as a molecular key to a specific biological lock—the cannabinoid receptors (Howlett et al. 2002; Iverson and Snyder 2000).

When THC enters the brain from the bloodstream, it binds to the CB1 receptors in multiple brain areas, altering the intrinsic function of these areas and the circuits they participate in. To test this hypothesis experimentally, some of the THC-like drugs produced in the 1980s were designed to be weakly radioactive. These so-called hot drugs light up (on film) and thus are able to reveal the cannabinoid receptors that the drugs are binding to (Devane et al. 1988).

Using this method, scientists are able to see which neurons throughout the brain are most sensitive to THC. These and other clever techniques are helping us understand precisely *where* in the brain marijuana acts to elicit its effects. It turns out, the brain is simply teeming with CB1 receptors, consistent with marijuana having wide-ranging influences on mental function (Herkenham et al. 1990; Glass, Dragunow, and Faull 1997). Observing where the receptors are located is one step toward understanding cannabinoid activity. Another equally important approach is to study those receptors at the molecular level, in order to ask the question: what do they do? This was the quest that identified the endocannabinoids (see Mechoulam chapter 7) and is providing tremendous new insight into neural function and homeostatic regulation.

THE ENDOCANNABINOIDS

The internal physiological signals that drive the function of our CB1 and CB2 receptors are a family of molecules present in the brain and other tissues—not just in humans, but all over the animal kingdom (McPartland et al. 2006). Quite independent from the cannabis plant, these native molecules borrow from its name nonetheless. They are called, collectively, the endogenous cannabinoids—or *endocannabinoids*—just as *endorphin* is an abbreviation of "endogenous morphine" (Snyder and Childers 1979).

In a loose sense, the endocannabinoids (often abbreviated as eCBs) have been called the "marijuana of the brain," although this is a deceptive metaphor since, unlike marijuana, the eCBs are an integral part of our regular physiological processes (Nicoll and Alger 2004). It is far more accurate to say that within the cannabis plant's ancestral lineage, compounds evolved that are remarkable biochemical mimics of our own *endo*cannabinoids. In actuality, the eCBs appeared much earlier in evolutionary history than did the cannabis plant, as indicated by their presence in so many diverse and early life forms, including even rudimentary marine organisms (McPartland et al. 2006; Elphick and Egertová 2009).

There are currently two well-studied and readily detectable eCBs in our bodies: anandamide and 2-arachidonylglycerol (2-AG). Each of these eCB compounds is generated in our cells by specific enzymes in response to the appropriate activation signals. In other words, cells generate and release anandamide or 2-AG when they receive particular electrochemical signals telling them to do so. In the brain, for example, if one neuron (an electrical cell of the brain) unleashes a barrage of excitatory electrical activity toward another neuron, the target neuron may respond by generating and releasing eCBs from its own cellular membrane (figure 6.2).

The eCBs travel "backward" across the synaptic cleft—the gap separating the two neurons—where they find CB1 receptors waiting. Through the molecular signaling of these strategically located CB1 receptors (on presynaptic axon terminals), the release of other, more principal neurotransmitters is momentarily paused. In this manner, the eCBs act as negative feedback, to say, "Whoa! That's enough input, slow down now!" Because of the unexpectedly reversed directionality of eCBs—traveling opposite the conventional neurotransmitter

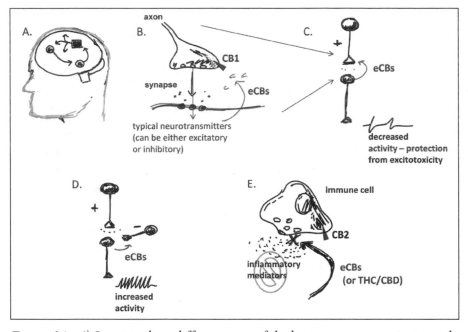

Figure 6.2. A) Imagine three different areas of the brain: one communicates to the next through many neurons, which send long processes (axons) to form connections (synapses) with the surface of target cells in the next brain area. B) At synapses, conventional neurotransmitters are released from the ends of axons and bind to receptors on target cells. The eCBs work in reverse, and bind to CB1 receptors on axon terminals, turning down the level of neurotransmitter release. C) When cannabinoids inhibit release from excitatory neurons (+), the net result is a decreased activity and protection from possible excitotoxicity. D) When eCBs target inhibitory neurons (-), the net result is an increased activity that alters synchrony with other neurons in the network. E) When cannabinoids activate CB2 receptors on immune cells, there is a decrease in the release of inflammatory mediators, and cell migration is also inhibited in certain cells. (This is a simplified description: a full consideration of cannabinoid actions on either the immune or nervous systems is beyond the scope of this article.)

pathway across synapses—the eCBs have been dubbed "retrograde messengers" (Gerdeman et al. 2003b; Piomelli 2003; Wilson and Nicoll 2002).

This groundbreaking scientific discovery has revealed a fascinating method by which a large number of brain cells appear to work: namely, a given neuron releases eCBs in order to continuously regulate and tune its own synaptic inputs (Katona and Freund 2008; Hashimotodani, Ohno-Shosaku, and Kano 2007; Gerdeman 2008a; Heifets and Castillo 2009). Such a process, whereby the synaptic connections between neurons are malleably weakened or strengthened, is referred to as *synaptic plasticity*— a mechanism by which learning and memory occurs at the cellular level (Kandel 2006; LeDoux 2002). Accordingly, pathologies of mental function, ranging from autism to OCD, may be due to genetic or environmental disruption of the cellular machinery of different forms of synaptic plasticity throughout the brain. It seems reasonable to consider that the psychotherapeutic potential of targeting the widespread, plasticity-regulating CB1 receptors may likewise be far-reaching.

The feedback mechanism of eCB-mediated synaptic plasticity is important not just for computational processes (how we think and feel and learn), but as a matter of cellular survival. Too much excitement can be deadly to the cells of the brain. An apparent and major function of eCBs—and therefore a significant effect of the cannabinoids found in cannabis—is *neuroprotection*, protecting the brain cells from too much excitation (Melis et al. 2006; Marsicano et al. 2003; Monory 2006). Known as "excitotoxicity," this overstimulation has been proven to be a serious contributor to the brain-damaging consequences of stroke, epilepsy, and a great many diverse neurological disorders. A key action of eCB release in the brain, therefore, is a cellular protectionism, countering the ravages of neuronal excitotoxicity (figure 6.2; Katona and Freund 2008; Mechoulam and Lichtman 2003).

NEURONAL FREQUENCY AND SYNCHRONY: SETTING TEMPO WITH ECBS

What we have just described is how eCBs are used by the brain to *dampen* patterns of electrical communication. Thus, one of the therapeutic effects of cannabis is to mimic this property. Yet this is far from the whole story of how CB1 receptors help choreograph brain activity. In some neural circuits, the eCBs are used in an opposite way, to *release* the neuron from *inhibitory* input, allowing it to fire its electrical signal at a less-restrained frequency.

This phenomenon is known as *disinhibition,* and is another way that eCB-mediated synaptic plasticity appears to be adaptive for healthy brain function (figure 6.2). In a brain area called the *amygdala,* for example, the release of eCBs appears to be a key mechanism by which memories of aversive experiences are encoded and extinguished (Marsicano et al. 2002; Phan et al. 2008). eCB activity in the amygdala may facilitate one's ability to move past prior emotional traumas. For this reason, there is a lot of talk about the potential utility of cannabinoids (including herbal cannabis) as a legitimate treatment for some cases of post-traumatic stress disorder (PTSD). In another brain area called the *hippocampus,* tightly controlled eCB signaling allows cells to fire in a coordinated synchrony, setting up the brain rhythms that are important for orienting oneself in physical space (Robbe et al. 2006; Gerdeman 2008a).

This supports one cellular model of how marijuana acts to interrupt spatial memory: that is, by simultaneously flooding *all* the cells in this hippocampal rhythmic engine with THC. The so-called *somatic* symptoms of the marijuana high—such as feelings of floating, sinking into one's seat, or altered balance—are likely due to similar effects in the THC-sensitive circuitry in the motoric center of our brain—the *cerebellum* (Heifets and Castillo 2009; Safo, Cravatt, and Regehr 2006).

Depending, therefore, on the precise cellular distribution of CB1 receptors in a given brain region, eCBs might either *inhibit* neuronal activity, by slowing down *excitatory* synapses onto that neuron, or *disinhibit* (excite) neuronal activity by slowing down *inhibitory* synapses. Both of these are physiologically relevant actions that contribute greatly to normal brain function. The fact that CB1 receptors can orchestrate the tempo of many brain cells in either direction—faster or slower—surely helps explain how cannabis can have such wide-ranging, and even opposing, perceptual effects in different individuals under varying circumstances.

The story of eCBs is not just about the brain, however, and there is an emerging concept of eCBs as "master regulators" of homeostasis, via actions throughout the body (see table opposite). For example, while eCBs enhance feeding behaviors via actions in the hypothalamus ("the munchies"), they also regulate metabolism and lipogenesis (Di Marzo and Matias 2005; Pacher, Batkai, and Kunos 2006). This presents distinct implications for the clinical treatment of human metabolic disorders. Endocannabinoids also regulate blood pressure (Mach and Steffens 2008), body temperature (Wenger and Moldrich 2002), and fertility (Maccarrone 2009), enhance bone density (Bab and Zimmer 2008), and regulate digestion by modulating the nervous system of the gut (Wright, Duncan, and Sharkey 2008).

TABLE 6.I. THE INFLUENCE OF CANNABIS ON VARIOUS PARTS AND SYSTEMS OF THE BODY

Cannabis influences cellular function throughout the body, because of the widespread roles of endocannabinoids in modulating physiology. This table presents a partial survey of eCB actions in various brain areas and other systems, highlighting pathological states for which cannabinoid receptors may represent promising therapeutic targets.

Brain area or other tissue system	Proposed physiological role of endocannabinoid system (with *diseases of relevance*)
Brain: excitatory synapses	In multiple brain areas, activation of CB1 receptors dampens excitation, thereby protecting neurons from excitotoxicity (*epilepsy, stroke, acute head trauma, etc.*) (Panikashvili et al. 2001; Marsicano et al. 2003; Monory et al. 2006)
Brain: microglia	ECBs prevent *neuroinflammation* by inhibiting both the release of inflammatory mediators and microglia migration. Neuroinflammation is key to both autoimmune disorders (*multiple sclerosis*, etc.) and neurodegenerative diseases (*Alzheimer's, Parkinson's, Huntington's diseases, etc.*) (Centonze et al. 2007; Wolf, Tauber, and Ullrich 2008; Pryce, Jackson, and Baker 2008)
Brain: hippocampus	ECS regulates synchrony of neuronal ensembles, enabling us to process context of self within our psychophysical environment. It is possible that similar coordination of network rhythmicity occurs in frontal areas of the cerebral cortex, helping govern the construction of various sensory and cognitive patterns (Robbe et al. 2006; Katona and Freund 2008; Gerdeman 2008a).
Brain reward network: VTA, nucleus accumbens, others	ECBs act in these areas as a hedonic signal, by which we feel pleasure and learn to repeat behaviors that are rewarding to us (*addiction involves maladaptive overlearning of rewarded behaviors*) (De Vries and Schoffelmeer 2005; Mahler, Smith, and Berridge 2007; Gerdeman et al. 2003b).
Brain: amygdala	Release of eCBS helps relieve memories of past traumatic events, and may minimize the perception of fearing personal harm more generally (*PTSD*) (Marsicano et al. 2002; Phan et al. 2008; Heifets and Castillo 2009).
Brain: basal ganglia	Subcortical brain network important for the selection and execution of motor routines. The learning of habitual memories may involve CB1 receptors in this network; think of such things as riding a bike or learning an instrument, for example, or an unwanted behavioral tic (*Parkinson's disease, Tourette syndrome, obsessive-compulsive disorder, various dyskinesias*) (Yin and Knowlton 2006; Gerdeman et al. 2003b; Gerdeman, Schechter, and French 2006; Gerdeman and Fernandez-Ruiz 2008b; Hilario et al. 2007; Kreitzer and Malenka 2007).

TABLE 6.1 (continued)

Brain area or other tissue system	Proposed physiological role of endocannabinoid system (with *diseases of relevance*)
Brain: hypothalamus	Neurons that synthesize and release some neurohormones (via the pituitary gland) use eCBs to regulate their own activity. Some of these cells may mediate *stress-relieving* effects of cannabis. Appetite-promoting effects of cannabinoids—"munchies"—are also mediated by neurons of the hypothalamus, relevant for *wasting* and *cachexia* (Hill and Gorzalka 2009; Malcher-Lopes et al. 2006; Wenger and Moldrich 2002).
Brainstem/ midbrain	Scarcity of receptors in areas controlling respiration contributes to marijuana's remarkable safety profile. Special pain center (the PAG) initiates analgesia by releasing eCBs (a sort of "top-down" control over pain perception). Cannabis also likely mediates its potent anti-*nausea* effects through parts of the brainstem (Hohmann and Suplita 2006; Darmani and Crim 2005).
Immune system	Reduced inflammatory mediators and inhibition of autoimmune responses contribute to beneficial properties for *multiple sclerosis (MS)*. Potent *antioxidant* properties of cannabinoids are also likely to support healthy immune function (Hampson et al. 1998; Pryce, Jackson, and Baker 2008; Wolf, Tauber, and Ullrich 2008).
Gut	CB1 and CB2 receptors are both active in controlling gastric motility through the enteric nervous system (aka the "brain of the gut"). Possible relevance to *irritable bowel syndrome, Crohn's disease*) (Russo 2004; Wright, Duncan, and Sharkey 2008).
Cardiovascular system	Many complicated roles of ECS, including regulation of blood pressure through multiple mechanisms. THC has been found to prevent *atherosclerosis* in animals. An "endocannabinoid deficiency" has been proposed to explain recurrent *migraine* in some people (Russo 2004; Sarchielli et al. 2007; Mach and Steffens 2008).
Bone	CB2 receptors in bone have been found to increase bone density and growth (*osteoporosis* is a disease caused by loss of bone density) (Bab and Zimmer 2008).
Fat, adipose tissue	ECS plays important roles in metabolic regulation of fat stores (*metabolic syndrome, diabetes mellitus*) (Pacher, Batkai, and Kunos 2006; Di Marzo and Matias 2005).
Peripheral nervous system (sensory fibers)	CB1 receptors on nociceptor sensory nerves inhibit primary *pain* signals (relevant to *spasticity* pain in MS and others et al.) (Kelly and Donaldson 2008; Agarwal et al. 2007)

The notion has emerged that multiple pathological conditions might be envisioned as syndromes of "endocannabinoid deficiency" (Russo 2004; Sarchielli et al. 2007). A growing body of evidence even indicates that the eCB system provides innate protection against tumor growth and/or metastasis, via multiple mechanisms, suggesting potentially valuable anticancer uses for cannabinoids in clinical medicine (Alexander, Smith, and Rosen 2009; Wang et al. 2008; Velasco et al. 2007).

In addition, some important homeostatic, and thus arguably therapeutic, properties of the eCBs are mediated by CB2 receptors residing on our immune cells (Munro, Thomas, and Abu-Shaar 1993). Among other functions, these cells are called upon to promote inflammation after an injury or in the course of fighting an infection—an important and adaptive mechanism of sustaining health. However, immune action can also be a detriment to our well-being, as untoward inflammation may quickly become a source of pain and tissue damage, presenting obstacles to efficient healing. Activation of CB2 receptors—either by eCBs released from surrounding tissues or from multiple active molecules found in marijuana—tells the immune cells to slow down the release of these chemical mediators of inflammation (figure 6.2).

This process is directly analogous to what we described above for the brain, whereby eCBs exert a dampening influence on the release of neurotransmitters. Throughout the body (including the brain, where immune cells are called *microglia*), the presence of cannabinoids tells immune cells to put the brakes on releasing compounds responsible for causing inflammation (Stella 2009; Wolf, Tauber, and Ullrich 2008). Research suggests that cannabinoids (which are also potent antioxidants) might be especially useful in minimizing inflammatory responses in the brain itself, symptoms of which are believed to be key to many serious neurodegenerative diseases ranging from Alzheimer's dementia, to Parkinson's disease, to other related motor disorders (Ashton and Glass 2007; Centonze et al. 2007).

REFRAMING THE DISCUSSION:
THE "ENDOCANNABINOID SYSTEM"

All the endogenous cannabinoids, the CB1 and CB2 receptors that are activated by them, and the complement of enzymes that synthesize and degrade these compounds, are collectively known as the *endocannabinoid system,* or ECS. With the elaboration of all these molecular players in the ECS, recent years have seen an explosion of discovery. Whereas for decades the scientific study of marijuana advanced only in a modest number of laboratories, there are now thousands of researchers worldwide striving to elucidate the molecular physiology of cannabinoid receptors.

What are the therapeutic possibilities for the cannabinoids, and how might they be developed into useful medicines? Such questions are hotly pursued by a field that now largely focuses less on cannabis per se and more on the nature of the ECS and how it could be manipulated to prolong or block eCB signaling. The diverse and growing body of eCB research suggests that if we did not have a functioning ECS, we would tend to live shorter, less healthy lives. Essentially every physiological system identified in our bodies is in some way modulated by eCBs, no doubt again a reflection of the ancient evolutionary origins of these homeostatic signaling molecules and their receptors.

From the rich folkloric history of this distinctive herb, the twenty-first century field of cannabinoid research now branches into quite new directions (Russo 2007). It is no longer controversial to say that the future, not just the past, holds many intriguing possibilities for cannabinoid-based medicines. With time, research will prove some of them more promising than others. At any rate, in today's world of critical ecological balance, the future of cannabinoid botanicals as an environmentally sustainable source of medicine surely must be discussed not only with intelligence and compassion, but also with a mature appreciation and natural reverence for the endocannabinoid system that seems to contribute a great deal to the physiological balance of our body and mind.

7
Anandamide and More

Raphael Mechoulam, Ph.D., and Lumír Hanuš

About forty-five years ago I (R. Mechoulam) applied for my first grant from the National Institutes of Health (NIH). I had joined the Weizmann Institute of Science in Rehovot in Israel and had started research on various topics in the field of natural products. One of the topics I proposed to work on was the isolation and identification of the active component of *Cannabis sativa,* the marijuana plant. I was turned down. I was told that NIH did not support research on marijuana as it was not an American problem—it was used mostly in Mexico and South America. About a year later, Dr. Dan Efron, then head of pharmacology at the National Institute of Mental Health, changed his mind.

A U.S. senator whose son had been seen smoking pot had called NIH and wanted to know whether the drug would affect his son's brain. But NIH knew nothing about marijuana. Efron recalled then that somebody from Israel had asked for a grant and was actually working in this area. Efron flew over, promised to support our research—which NIH then generously did for decades—and took with him the "world" supply of tetrahydrocannabinol (THC), the active component of marijuana, which we had just isolated and identified. Much of the early work in the United States in the cannabis field was done with the material that Efron presumably smuggled out of Israel into the United States.

Why was research on cannabis so neglected? For decades, the three major psychoactive plant drugs—illicit in most of the Western world—were opium, cocaine, and cannabis. Morphine had been isolated from opium early in the nineteenth century (Sertürner 1817), and its very complicated structure was elucidated in the 1920s by Sir Robert Robinson (Gulland and Robinson 1925). Cocaine was isolated from coca leaves in the middle of the nineteenth century (Gaedcke 1855), and the famous chemist Richard Willstätter had been able to describe its unusual structure in the last decade of the nineteenth century (Willstätter 1898).

The availability of pure materials made possible biochemical, pharmacological, and clinical work with these important alkaloids. Modern scientists refrain from work on mixtures—and crude plant extracts are complicated mixtures—as the results of such research are difficult to reproduce and interpret. As the active constituent(s) of cannabis was not available in pure form, there was very little modern biological and clinical work on it.

A further difficulty was a legal one. As cannabis was an illicit substance, it was not readily available to most scientists. Even if obtained legally, research with it was a laboratory nightmare. In many countries special security precautions had to be undertaken. In most universities, researchers could not follow the security regulations effectively, and pharmaceutical companies did not want the presumed notoriety of "trying to make money out of marijuana." From a scientific point of view, cannabis research had effectively been suppressed.

I was not aware of these legal problems. I obtained hashish from the police—surprisingly, they were also unaware that they were not supposed to give it to me for research—and went happily ahead isolating the cannabis constituents. My friend Dr. Yehiel Gaoni joined me, and we collaborated for

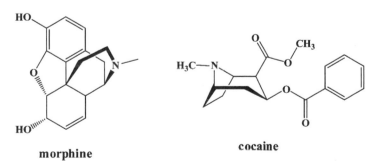

Figure 7.1. The complicated chemical structures of morphine and cocaine

six or seven years. We isolated most of the major typical constituents of the plant, which we named cannabinoids (there were over a hundred of them) (Hanuš 2009). (For a review of the early work, see Mechoulam 1970.)

These were tested in rhesus monkeys by Habib Edery and Yona Grunfeld (Edery et al. 1971) from the nearby Biological Research Institute. They found that only one constituent caused effects that paralleled the marijuana effects in cannabis smokers. The active constituent was delta-9-tetrahydro-cannabinol (delta-9-THC) (Gaoni and Mechoulam 1964). Another constituent, cannabidiol (CBD) (Mechoulam and Shuo 1963), which causes no marijuana-type effects, is now known to produce a variety of other effects. It is a potent anti-inflammatory drug, it arrests the onset of autoimmune diabetes, ameliorates cognitive, and motor impairments due to bile duct ligation. These effects have been shown in mice. In humans, it has been shown to reduce the number of epileptic attacks and to lower anxiety. It is also being investigated as an anti-schizophrenic drug.

THE PLANT CONSTITUENTS

The group of secondary plant products, known as cannabinoids, are specific to the *Cannabis sativa* plant. Of the one hundred-plus cannabinoids known, all are variations on the same chemical theme: a resorcinol ring (substituted with an alkyl side chain on the C-5 position) attached to a terpene with ten carbons (a monoterpene).

Why does the cannabis plant produce these compounds? This is actually a general question in botany. Most plants produce specific compounds typical for a family or a genus or even a single species. They are known as secondary metabolites. These are in addition to the primary metabolites, such as proteins, sugars, and lipids, which are found in all living organisms. Why has nature evolved this difference? Animals protect themselves from foreign protein attacks—be they microbes, viruses, or parasites—with their well-developed immune systems. Plants do not have immune systems; they protect themselves with specific secondary metabolites, which may be toxic to some predatory insects or parasites. These metabolites have additional tasks; they may attract insects necessary for pollination, for example. But we do not know the reason the cannabis plant produces its one-hundred-odd cannabinoids. It certainly does not do this to please *Homo sapiens*!

Although the plant cannabinoids have closely related chemical structures, only very few cause the well-known "high." Delta-9-THC is the major psychoactive constituent (Mechoulam 1970). Cannabinol (CBN), which actually may be an oxidation product of delta-9-THC, also has some activity. The psychoactive isomer of delta-9-THC, named delta-8-THC (due to the position of the double bond), is usually present in minute amounts only. Cannabidiol (CBD), a major component in most plant varieties, does not cause the typical marijuana high, but it causes a plethora of other effects. It is a potent anti-inflammatory substance, blocks the development of diabetes type 1, and modulates sleep in rats, just to name a few of its effects (for a review, see Mechoulam 2007). Tetrahydrocannabivarin, which differs from THC only in the length of the side chain, actually antagonizes the effects of THC. Most of the other plant constituents have not been thoroughly

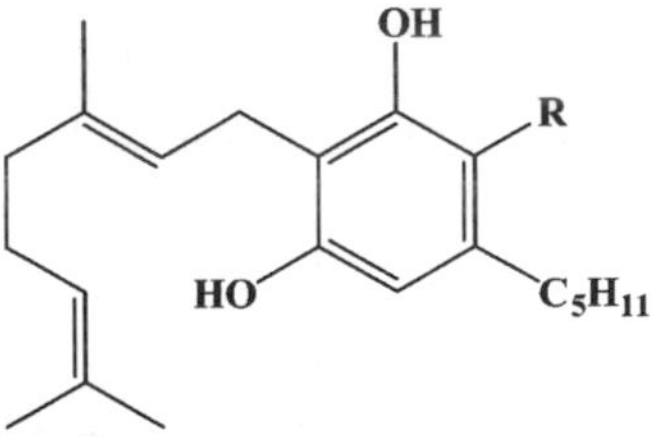

R = H, cannabigerol (CBG)
R = COOH, cannabigerolic acid (CBGA)

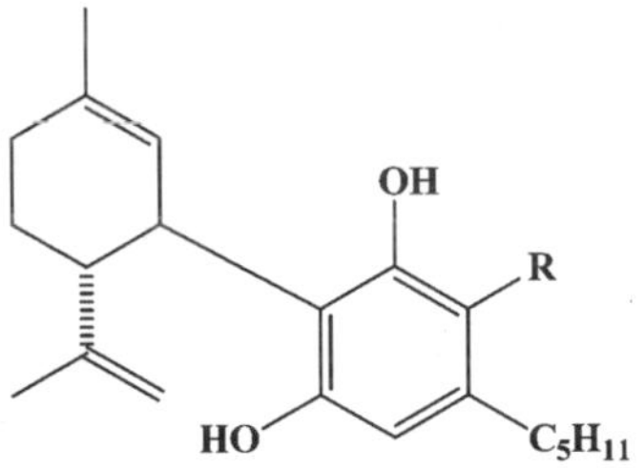

R = H, cannabidiol (CBD)
R = COOH, cannabidiolic acid (CBDA)

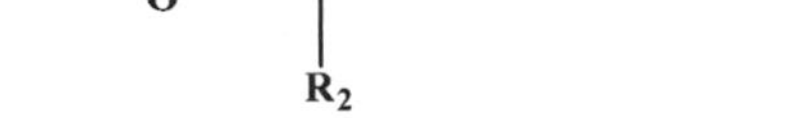

$R_1 = R_2 = H, \Delta^9$-THC
$R_1 = COOH, R_2 = H, \Delta^9$-THCA

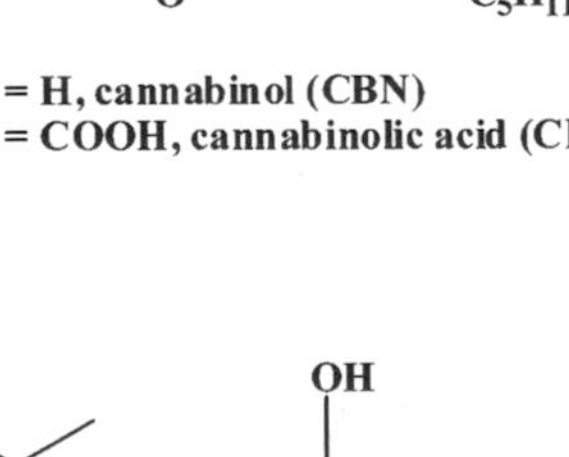

R = H, cannabinol (CBN)
R = COOH, cannabinolic acid (CBNA)

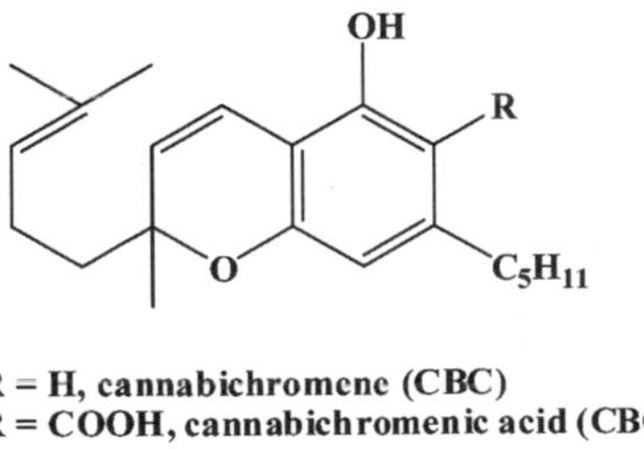

R = H, cannabichromene (CBC)
R = COOH, cannabichromenic acid (CBCA)

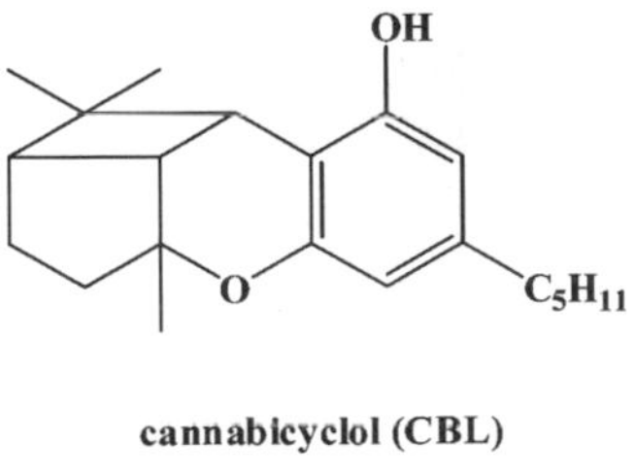

cannabicyclol (CBL)

Figure 7.2

examined for their biological activities. Are we missing a potential chemical treasure trove?

Many, possibly all, the plant cannabinoids are originally formed as their acids (see figure 7.2). On the plant's surface, they start losing their acidic function—this chemical reaction is called decarboxylation (figure 7.3)—which continues to take place when the plant is harvested and dried. If the plant is smoked, the rest of these acids, if still present, fully decarboxylate. The cannabinoid acids are not psychoactive, but some of them are anti-inflammatory.

Industrial hemp, which is a variety of *Cannabis sativa,* contains very low amounts of THC (up to 0.3 percent) (Small and Marcus 2003). It is used for the very strong cords that can be made from it. The ancient Greeks and Romans certainly knew and used industrial hemp. Dioscorides, whose book on plant drugs was the standard text for almost two millennia, recommended covering inflamed body parts with soaked cannabis roots (Dioscorides 2000). One can assume that the fun-loving Greeks and Romans were unaware of the variety that forms THC. We assume that they would have used hashish and marijuana had they known about their psychoactivity. (For a historical review on the medical use of cannabis, see Mechoulam 1986.)

The cannabinoids in the plant are formed following a standard pathway. Apparently, first the plant synthesizes cannabigerolic acid (Mechoulam and Gaoni 1965), which then, by oxidation and cyclization, forms cannabichromenic acid (Shoyama et al. 1968), cannabidiolic acid (Krejčí 1995), and THC acid (Korte, Haag, and Claussen 1965). Surprisingly, THC acid is not formed from cannabidiolic acid by a simple cyclization, but follows a special enzymatic pathway (Taura et al. 1995).

The next step in the cannabis saga was the development of laboratory syntheses of the cannabinoids. Chemists see an intellectual challenge in competing with nature in building new molecules. But in many cases this

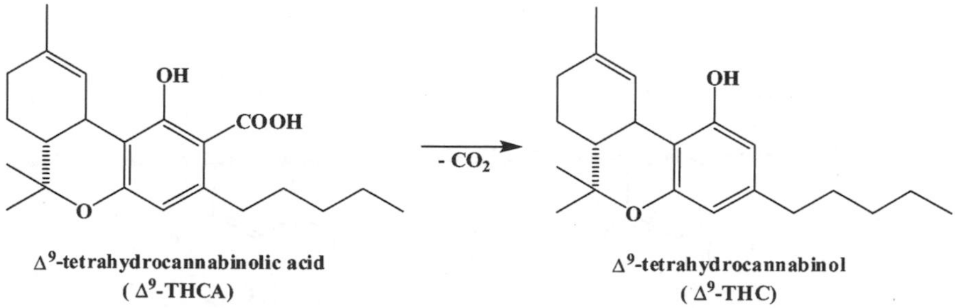

Δ⁹-tetrahydrocannabinolic acid
(Δ⁹-THCA)

$- CO_2$

Δ⁹-tetrahydrocannabinol
(Δ⁹-THC)

Figure 7.3

challenge is accompanied by the desire to design routes for the production of better analogs of active products. Several syntheses of THC and cannabidiol have been reported, and some of them are still in use after more than forty years (for reviews, see Mechoulam 1973; Mechoulam, Parker, and Gallily 2002). Our synthetic procedure is illustrated in figure 7.4 (Mechoulam, Braun, and Gaoni 1967).

The next step in the study of cannabinoids was the evaluation of their metabolism. The mammalian body gets rid of many small foreign molecules by converting them into water-soluble molecules that can be excreted in the urine. This is indeed the route followed in the metabolism of cannabinoids. In the early 1970s, almost simultaneously, four groups discovered the initial metabolic steps: THC is first converted into 11-hydroxy-delta-9-THC, which then is further oxidized into an acid, which finally binds to a sugar, becoming slightly soluble in water (see figure 7.5, and for a review, see Agurell et al. 1986). The intermediate acid formed may, however, dissolve in body fats and remain there for many weeks, being slowly released. Indeed, urine analyses for this acid may be positive for weeks after a person has smoked a single cannabis joint.

By the mid 1970s, the major goals of cannabis research in chemistry had been reached. The constituents of the plant were known, their structure and

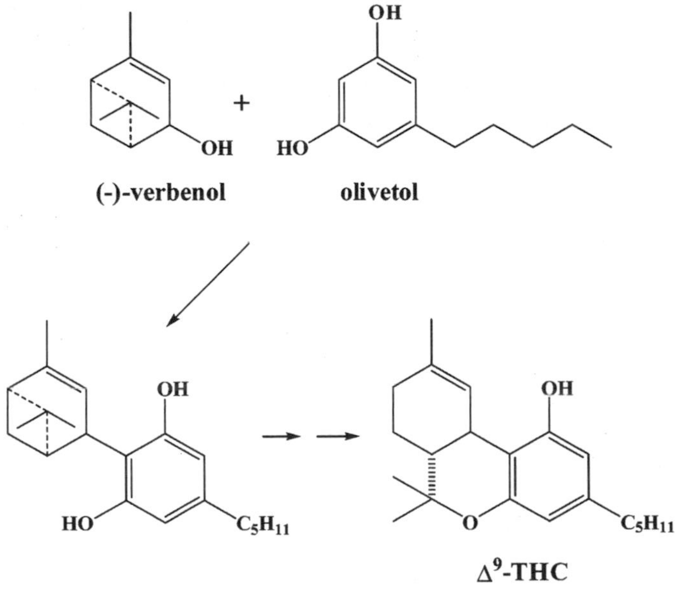

$$\Delta^9\text{-THC}$$

Figure 7.4

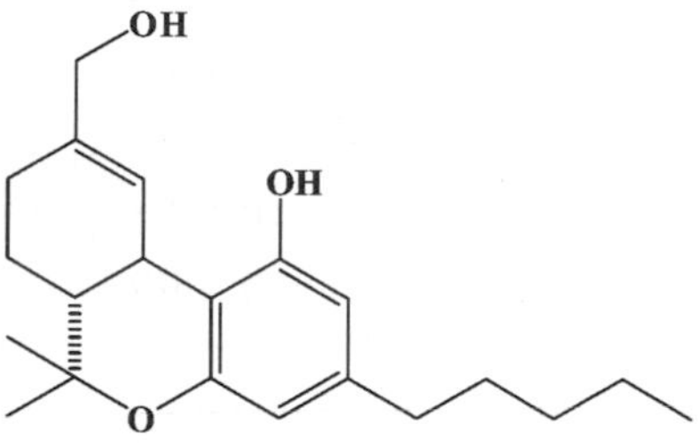

Hydroxy-Δ^9-THC

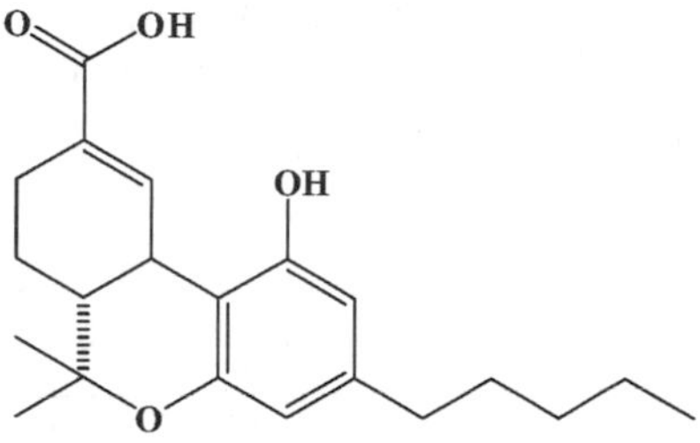

acid metaboliote of Δ^9-THC

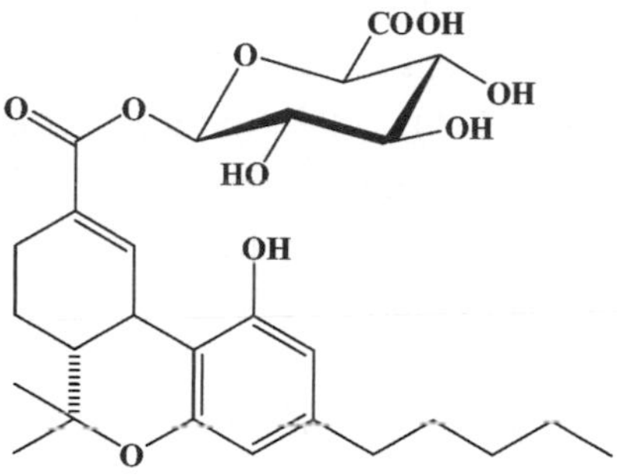

sugar metabolite of Δ^9-THC

Figure 7.5

stereochemistry had been elucidated, syntheses had been developed, and their metabolism was well established. Biologists were investigating their activity in a variety of tissues, organs, and animals. Surprisingly, however, very little was known about the mechanism of action of THC.

The reasons for this baffling situation were both conceptual and technical. The conceptual problem related to THC activity had been raised by an Oxford group, which had pointed out that the cannabinoids belong to the group of biologically active lipid-soluble molecules, and that their effects could be nonspecific, comparable with the chronic effects of anesthetics and solvents (Paton 1975). Hence, following this line of thought, it was possible to explain the action of THC without postulating the existence of a receptor.

The technical problem was due to the fact that THC can exist in two steric forms, named enantiomers. Natural (–) THC has a specific steric form—that is, it is a single enantiomer. The second form, (+) THC, can be synthesized in the laboratory. It was noted that THC is active in both enantiomeric forms (although with a different level of potency), and this was incompatible with action on a receptor, which also has one specific steric form and will usually bind one enantiomer only. However, all the work on the stereospecificity of cannabinoid action had been performed with THC synthesized according to a procedure published by our group based on commercial starting material, α-pinene (Mechoulam, Braun, and Gaoni 1967). We knew that commercial pinene was not stereochemically pure and therefore led to stereochemically impure products. Hence, the lack of streospecificity could be due to the presence of minor amounts of the active (–) stereoisomer in the presumed pure synthetic (+) isomer.

So we repeated the synthesis with stereochemically pure starting material and tested the unnatural (+) THC produced. As expected, it had no (–) THC-like activity. This observation meant that natural (–) THC could possibly have a receptor. However, the bottom line of this scientific mixup was that the search for a cannabinoid receptor was delayed by nearly two decades.

THE ENDOCANNABINOIDS

In 1988 Allyn Howlett, with her then-graduate student William Devane, brought out the first evidence that a cannabinoid receptor existed in the brain (Devane et al. 1988). We assumed that a cannabinoid receptor is not formed in the brain for the sake of a plant constituent. Presumably, an endogenous brain ligand existed, which would stimulate the cannabinoid receptor and lead to physiological effects. As THC is a lipophilic compound, we also assumed that any putative endogenous agonist would be a lipid, and we therefore employed isolation methods developed for lipids. We extracted pig brains, as it is known that many porcine lipids are also present in humans.

Identification of a physiologically active constituent in a plant extract is based on separation of the components of the plant extract, followed by their biological evaluation in an appropriate assay. Such feedback data should be obtained by relatively rapid in vitro assays. As Bill Devane had now joined our lab as a postdoctoral fellow, we chose to study the binding to the cannabinoid receptor for which we had already developed a labeled ligand (Devane et al. 1992a).

The isolation problems were at first almost insurmountable. Chromatography fractions of porcine brain that bound to the cannabinoid receptor started to lose their activity rapidly. We know now that this was due to the lack of stability of the endogenous cannabinoid ligand. Ultimately we had a minuscule amount of material, which, however, was enough for an NMR spectrum. The spectrum we obtained was typical for polyunsaturated long-chain fatty acids. We believe that this was the turning point of the project—we had an active polyunsaturated fatty acid derivative. Indeed, further mass spectral work led to the structure as known today, namely N-arachidonoyl ethanolamide (Devane et al. 1992b). The endogenous material paralleled THC in inhibition of a typical electrically evoked twitch response, an assay developed by Roger Pertwee, a collaborator on the project. We decided to name the new brain-derived ligand anandamide, based on the word *ananda* (supreme joy in Sanskrit).

In 1993, Munro in Cambridge isolated a second receptor in the spleen that was absent in the brain (Munro, Thomas, and Abu-Shaar 1993). The two receptors are now known as the CB1 and CB2 receptors. We assumed that the new receptor was activated by a second agonist, and we went ahead trying to isolate a "peripheral" endocannabinoid ligand. Indeed, in 1995 we reported a new endocannabinoid, 2-arachidonoyl glycerol (2-AG), closely related to anandamide both chemically and pharmacologically (Mechoulam et al. 1995). A Japanese group later reported that they had also identified 2-AG (Sugiura et al. 1995). We know now that anandamide and 2-AG activate both receptors.

Anandamide and 2-AG (figure 7.6) remain the major endocannabinoids identified and have been the object of thousands of investigations. They are involved in a large number of biochemical reactions and physiological processes, which are discussed in detail in other chapters. I will present one example only. Traumatic brain injury leads to a local and transient accumulation of 2-AG at the site of injury. Neuroprotection exerted by the administration of synthetic 2-AG suggests that the formation of 2-AG may serve as a molecular regulator of this pathological event, attenuating the brain damage (Panikashvili et al. 2001). 2-AG exerts its neuroprotective effect after traumatic brain injury, at least in part, by inhibition of NF-κB activation. NF-κB, a protein, is known to lead to inflammation (Panikashvili et al. 2005). 2-AG also inhibits the expression of proinflammatory cytokines and lowers endothelin (ET-1)–induced vasoconstriction after brain injury (Chen et al.

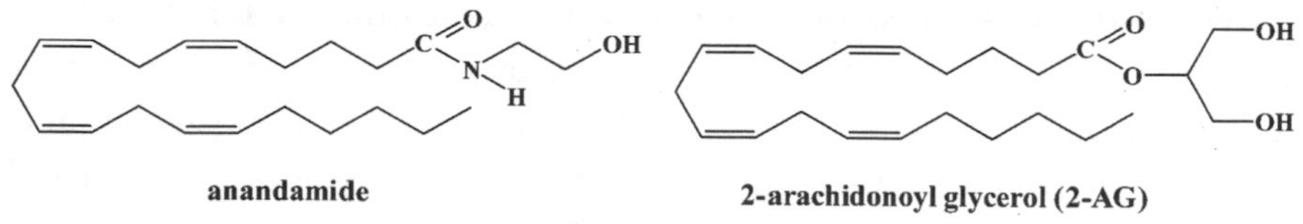

anandamide   2-arachidonoyl glycerol (2-AG)

Figure 7.6

2000). The cytokines and ET-1 are endogenous proteins that lead to a variety of physiological reactions. Thus, we showed that 2-AG plays a neuroprotective role following several different pathways.

Chemists have synthesized numerous novel compounds that bind specifically, as agonists or antagonists, to either the CB1 or CB2 receptor. CB1 agonists are of little therapeutic value due to their potent THC-like psychoactivity. However, CB1 antagonists lower appetite, and one such compound, named rimonabant, was actually on the market as an anti-obesity drug. Unfortunately, as the CB1 receptor also lowers anxiety, the antagonist rimonabant caused enhanced anxiety and was taken off the market. It is possible, however, that CB2 agonists may someday be introduced as therapeutic agents in neurological diseases and as anti-osteoporosis drugs, as the CB2 receptor apparently blocks some neurological changes due to disease and also enhances bone formation.

Anandamide and 2-AG are derivatives of the fatty acid arachidonic acid, bound to ethanolamine or glycerol. Their identification led to investigations into the possible existence of related fatty acid derivatives. Indeed, in our laboratory we found that arachidonoyl serine (arachidonic acid bound to the amino acid serine), present in the brain, which does not bind to the cannabinoid receptors, is a vasoconstrictor (Milman et al. 2006), and oleoyl serine (oleic acid bound to serine) enhances the activity of osteoblasts (bone-forming cells) and lowers the activity of osteoclasts (bone-absorbing cells) (Mechoulam and Bab 2008). Many other groups have found numerous related compounds with a variety of activities. Thus, the Piomelli group in California has found that oleoyl ethanolamide lowers appetite (Gaetani, Oveisi, and Piomelli 2003), and there are many reports on the anti-inflammatory activity of palmitoyl ethanolamide (Hoareau et al. 2009). Recently Walker's group in Indiana reported the presence of a long list of related fatty acid amides with amino acids present in brain (Tan 2009). It is safe to assume that the mammalian body does not produce compounds without a physiological reason. Many of these compounds presumably possess biological properties that remain to be discovered.

We will end with a speculation. The endocannabinoids have been reported to affect a large number of pathological conditions and, in our view, can be seen as a part of a general protective network that works in conjunction with the immune system and with various other physiological systems to protect against various kinds of damage, such as head trauma. Research over the next few years may hopefully give support to this assumption.

8

Cannabis Laws in the United States

Allen St. Pierre, Director of NORML

This chapter was updated May 14, 2010. Please reference www.norml.org for ongoing updates to cannabis laws in the United States.

Despite the general cultural acceptance and economic popularity of cannabis in modern America—government data indicates that nearly 30 million citizens consume cannabis annually, and cannabis traditionally ranks as a top-five domestic cash crop—there exists today a disparate patchwork of city, state, and federal penalties that target citizens who consume cannabis.

Since 1965, nearly 20 million citizens have been arrested in the United States on cannabis-related charges—nine out of ten for simple cannabis possession. Every thirty-eight seconds in the United States a citizen is arrested for cannabis; there were 848,000 cannabis arrests in 2008 alone.

Cannabis laws in the United States vary widely. Whether an individual caught by law enforcement with a small amount of cannabis will be treated lightly with a small civil fine or arrested and pulled into the criminal justice system, depends largely upon one factor: geography.

If a cannabis consumer possessing a single ounce of cannabis begins a cross-country automobile journey in Portland, Maine (where cannabis has been decriminalized since 1978), that ounce of cannabis will have changed its legal status dozens of times while crossing the United States on the way to the other Portland in Oregon (where cannabis was first decriminalized in the United States, in 1973). However, if these erstwhile travelers from Portland to Portland were to interface with law enforcement, and their cannabis were to be lawfully discovered in states such as Indiana, Iowa, Kansas, Utah, South Dakota, or Idaho, then the cannabis-possessing "criminals" would be readily arrested, prosecuted, and face potential incarceration of up to two years.

In Ohio a citizen can possess up to one hundred grams (three and half ounces) of cannabis and face only a $100 fine, which is treated as inconsequentially as a minor traffic violation. If a cannabis consumer were to be caught in neighboring Indiana with the same amount of cannabis, they'd be promptly arrested and prosecuted as a cannabis dealer based simply on the weight.

Also, there are a number of large American cities that have decriminalized the minor possession of cannabis for adults, including Ann Arbor, Columbia, Madison, Milwaukee, Missoula, Seattle, and Topeka. In January 2008, the city of Seattle issued a report regarding the city's adoption of a policing program (Initiative 75 or I-75)* that makes cannabis arrests low law enforcement priorities.

> There is no evidence of any adverse effect of the implementation of I-75 including specifically:
>
> 1. No evident increase in marijuana use among youth and young adults;
> 2. No evident increase in crime;
> 3. No adverse impact on public health.
>
> There is some evidence of arguably positive effects from I-75 in the following substantive areas examined:
>
> 1. Fewer adults experiencing the consequences of involvement in the criminal justice system due to their personal use of marijuana; and,
> 2. A small reduction in the amount of public safety resources dedicated to marijuana possession cases and a corresponding slight increase in availability of these resources for other public safety priorities.

Thirteen states (whose populations amount to one-third of the entire U.S. population, 120 million citizens—Alaska, California, Colorado, Maine, Massachusetts, Minnesota, Mississippi, Nebraska, Nevada, New York, North

---

*Initiative 75 was the successful 2003 voter initiative in Seattle that made cannabis arrests the lowest of police priorities.

Carolina, Ohio, and Oregon) have decriminalized small amounts of cannabis. Additionally, fourteen states (and Washington, D.C.) since 1996, representing one fifth of America's total population (approximately 90 million citizens), recognize the medical benefits of cannabis and have, despite opposition from the federal government, adopted "medical marijuana" patient-protection laws (Alaska, California, Colorado, Maine, Maryland, Michigan, Montana, Nevada, New Mexico, Oregon, Washington, and the District of Columbia by binding voter initiative; Hawaii, Rhode Island, and Vermont by legislation).

Historically, the top five states for all cannabis arrests are California, New York, Texas, Illinois, and Georgia. The top five states for cannabis arrests per capita in 2002 (national average equals 239 cannabis arrests per 100,000 citizens): Nebraska (460 cannabis arrests per 100,000), Louisiana (400), Wyoming (385), Kentucky (365), and Illinois (360).

According to The Sentencing Project in Washington, DC, approximately 48,000 persons are currently incarcerated in America's jails and prisons having been prosecuted on cannabis-only related offenses. A 2005 economics paper by Harvard professor Jeffrey Miron indicates that the federal and state governments annually spend $8 billion trying to enforce cannabis prohibition laws in the United States.

Clearly, the physical location in America where a person is caught possessing cannabis is crucial in determining the individual's potential criminal and civil penalties.

How much marijuana are we talking about?

- One regular-sized "joint" weighs about .5 grams (slightly less than a commercially purchased tobacco cigarette).
- One "blunt" weighs about 3 grams (which is approximately the size of a tobacco cigar).
- One ounce of dried marijuana can be held in palmed hands (and equals about fifty to sixty rolled "joints," or about the same as two packs of cigarettes).
- One pound of marijuana (16 ounces), uncompressed, is approximately the size of a small pillow.
- One kilo (equaling 2.2 pounds) is a popular size to smuggle marijuana, which after being compressed is equal in size and shape to a building brick.

A complete and updated listing of state and federal laws, as well as annual arrest and crop reports regarding cannabis in the United States, are published by the National Organization for the Reform of Marijuana Laws (NORML), based in Washington, D.C. (888-67-NORML, www.norml.org).

LISTING OF STATE-BY-STATE
(AND FEDERAL) CANNABIS LAWS AND PENALTIES

Key: D = Decriminalized

M = Medical Marijuana

Alabama

Possession of marijuana is a criminal, arrestable offense. For possession of an amount of one kilogram (2.2 pounds) or less, the crime is a misdemeanor, punishable by up to one year in jail and a fine of up to $2,000. For possession of any amount over one kilogram, the crime is a felony, punishable by one to ten years in prison and a fine of up to $5,000.

The sale, cultivation, or manufacture of marijuana is a felony offense. If the amount is one kilogram or less, the mandatory minimum sentence is three years in prison and a fine of up to $25,000. For an amount greater than one kilogram but less than one hundred pounds, the sentence is a minimum of five years in prison and a fine of up to $50,000. For an amount up to five hundred pounds, the sentence is a minimum of fifteen years in prison and a fine of up to $200,000. Any amount of one thousand pounds or greater is punishable by life without the possibility of parole.

The penalties for sale of marijuana are enhanced if the sale takes place within a three-mile radius of a school or public housing project, adding five years to the sentence for the sale. Sale to minors (under eighteen years old) can increase the penalty by ten years to life in prison, and no suspension or probation can be granted to this sentence.

The possession or sale of drug paraphernalia is a misdemeanor punishable by up to one year in jail and a fine of up to $2,000. If the paraphernalia is sold to a minor at least three years younger than the seller, the penalty becomes a felony and is punishable by two to twenty years in prison and a fine of up to $10,000. Any conviction for possession, sale, manufacture, or cultivation also results in the suspension of the offender's driver's license for a period of six months.

Alaska (D, M)

Possession of one ounce or less of marijuana in the privacy of the home is legal. The status of possessing an amount between one ounce and four ounces is unclear, pending clarification by the courts. Possession of four ounces or more of marijuana is a felony punishable by up to five years in prison and a fine of up to $50,000.

Possession of fewer than twenty-five plants is protected under the Alaska Constitution's right to privacy (see *Ravin v. Alaska*). Possession of twenty-five or more marijuana plants is "misconduct involving a controlled substance in the fourth degree" and is punishable by a fine of up to $50,000 or five years in prison.

Any possession within five hundred feet of school grounds or a recreation center or possession on any school bus is a felony punishable by up to five years in prison and a fine of up to $50,000.

Sale, delivery, or manufacture of marijuana of less than one ounce is a misdemeanor and is punishable by up to one year in jail and a fine of up to $5,000. For amounts of one ounce or greater, the crime is a felony that can be punished with a sentence of up to five years in prison and a fine of up to $50,000.

It is an affirmative defense to possession, manufacture, or delivery that the offender is a patient or caregiver who is registered with the state for medical use of marijuana.

Maintaining any structure or dwelling, including vehicles, to use for keeping and distributing marijuana is a felony offense and punishable by up to five years in prison and a fine of up to $50,000.

Alaska has legal protections for medical cannabis patients.

Summary: Fifty-eight percent of voters approved Ballot Measure #8 on November 3, 1998. The law took effect on March 4, 1999. It removes state-level criminal penalties on the use, possession, and cultivation of marijuana by patients who possess written documentation from their physician advising that they "might benefit from the medical use of marijuana." Patients diagnosed with the following illnesses are afforded legal protection under this act: cachexia; cancer; chronic pain; epilepsy and other disorders characterized by seizures; glaucoma; HIV or AIDS; multiple sclerosis and other disorders characterized by muscle spasticity; and nausea. Other conditions are subject to approval by the Alaska Department of Health and Social Services. Patients (or their primary caregivers) may legally possess no more than one ounce of usable marijuana, and may cultivate no more than six marijuana plants, of which no more than three may be mature. The law establishes a confidential state-run patient registry that issues identification cards to qualifying patients.

Amendments: Yes. Senate Bill 94, which took effect on June 2, 1999, mandates all patients seeking legal protection under this act to enroll in the state patient registry and possess a valid identification card. Patients not enrolled in the registry will no longer be able to argue the "affirmative defense of medical necessity" if they are arrested on marijuana charges.

Medical Marijuana Statutes: Alaska Stat. §§ 17.37.10 - 17.37.80 (2007).

Arizona

The possession of marijuana is a criminal offense. For possession of an amount less than two pounds, the sentence can range from six to eighteen months and a fine of $750 to $150,000. Possession of two or more pounds but less than four pounds is punishable by nine months to two years in jail and a fine of $750 to $150,000. Possession of four pounds or more is punishable by eighteen months to three years in prison and a fine of $750 to $150,000.

Any person convicted of personal possession or use of marijuana is eligible for probation. The court is required to suspend the imposition or execution of the sentence. The person on probation is required to participate in an appropriate drug treatment or education program and may be required to attend a more stringent treatment program for a second offense. Persons convicted of a third or subsequent offense are not eligible for probation. Persons on probation must also submit to urine drug tests as a condition of their probation, with the only exception being made for those who use marijuana under a prescription.

The penalties for possession for sale of less than two pounds of marijuana are eighteen months to three years in prison and a $750 to $150,000 fine. For amounts of less than four pounds, the penalties increase to thirty months to seven years in prison and a $750 to $150,000 fine. Possession for sale of four pounds or more is punishable by four to ten years in prison and a $750 to $150,000 fine.

Production or cultivation of less than two pounds of marijuana is punishable by nine months to two years in jail and a $750 to $150,000 fine. For less than four pounds, the penalties increase to eighteen months to three years in prison and a $750 to $150,000 fine. Production of cultivation of four pounds or more is punishable by thirty months to seven years in prison and a $750 to $150,000 fine.

Sale or delivery for sale of less than two pounds of marijuana is punishable by thirty months to seven years in prison and a fine of $750 to $150,000. Sale or delivery of two pounds or more is punishable by four to ten years in prison and a fine of $750 to $150,000.

Possession or sale within three hundred feet of a school, on any public property within one thousand feet of any school, at any school bus stop, or on any bus transporting pupils to or from school adds an additional one year to the sentence and requires a minimum fine of $2,000.

Possession and sale of paraphernalia is punishable by six to eighteen months in jail and a fine of up to $150,000.

Arkansas

The penalty for possession of one ounce or less of marijuana is a misdemeanor and is punishable by up to one year in prison and a fine of up to $1,000. The court may defer the proceedings and grant probation for no less than one year. Upon granting probation, the court may require drug treatment. If the terms of the probation are fulfilled, the court can discharge and dismiss the proceedings. There is a rebuttable presumption that any possession greater than one ounce is possession for sale.

Possession for sale or cultivation of marijuana is a felony. For amounts greater than one ounce, the punishment is four to ten years in prison and a fine of up to $25,000. For amounts of ten pounds or more the sentence can range from five to twenty years in prison and a fine of $15,000 to $50,000. For any amounts of one hundred pounds or more, the punishment is six to ten years in prison and a fine of $15,000 to $100,000. Second convictions of possession, sale, delivery, or cultivation can result in sentences up to twice that allowed for first offenses.

Any sale to a minor at least three years younger than the seller can double the above penalties. Any sale within one thousand feet of a school, public park, community or recreation center, public housing, daycare center, church, skating rink, or video arcade increases the penalty for the offense by ten years. Minors convicted of any drug offense are subject to a driver's license suspension of six months. Possession or use of drug paraphernalia in furtherance of a felony violation is punishable by three to ten years in prison and a fine of up to $10,000.

California (D, M)

Possession of 28.5 grams (one ounce) or less of marijuana is not an arrestable offense. As long as the offender can provide sufficient identification and promises to appear in court, the officer will not arrest the offender. Upon conviction of the misdemeanor charge, the offender is subject to a fine of $100. Possession of greater than 28.5 grams is punishable by up to six months in jail and a fine of up to $500.

Possession of 28.5 grams or less of marijuana on school grounds when the school is open is punishable by up to ten days in jail and a $500 fine. Possession of greater than 28.5 grams or more of marijuana in a school zone is punishable by up to six months in jail and a fine of up to $500.

The cultivation or processing of any amount of marijuana is punishable by up to sixteen months in state prison. There is an exception to the cultivation prohibition for patients or patients' caregivers who possess or cultivate for personal use by the patient upon approval of a physician.

The laws regarding possession and cultivation of marijuana do not apply to patients or patients' primary caregivers who possess or cultivate marijuana for the personal medical use of the patient, upon the recommendation or approval of a physician. Selling marijuana in any amount is punishable by two to four years in the state prison. Giving away less than 28.5 grams is a misdemeanor and is punishable by a fine of up to $100.

Sale of marijuana to a minor is punishable by three to five years in prison. For anyone under the age of twenty-one convicted of any of the above offenses, the state may suspend the offender's driver's license for up to one year. Possession of paraphernalia is a civil fine of $200 to $300 for the first offense and goes up to $5,000 to $6,000 for a fifth or subsequent violation within a five-year period.

Summary: Fifty-six percent of voters approved Proposition 215 on November 5, 1996. The law took effect the following day. It removes state-level criminal penalties on the use, possession, and cultivation of marijuana by patients who possess a "written or oral recommendation" from their physician that he or she "would benefit from medical marijuana." Patients diagnosed with any debilitating illness where the medical use of marijuana has been "deemed appropriate and has been recommended by a physician" are afforded legal protection under this act. Conditions typically covered by the law include but are not limited to: arthritis; cachexia; cancer; chronic pain; HIV or AIDS; epilepsy; migraine; and multiple sclerosis. No set limits regarding the amount of marijuana patients may possess and/or cultivate were provided by this act, though the California Legislature adopted guidelines in 2003.

Amendments: Yes. Senate Bill 420, which was signed into law in October 2003 and took effect on January 1, 2004, imposes statewide guidelines outlining how much medicinal marijuana patients may grow and possess. Under the guidelines, qualified patients and/or their primary caregivers may possess no more than eight ounces of dried marijuana and/or six mature (or twelve immature) marijuana plants. However, S.B. 420 allows patients to possess larger amounts of marijuana when such quantities are recommended by a physician. The legislation also allows counties and municipalities to approve and/or maintain local ordinances permitting patients to possess larger quantities of medicinal pot than allowed under the new state guidelines.

Senate Bill 420 also mandates the California Department of State Health Services to establish a voluntary medicinal marijuana patient registry and issue identification cards to qualified patients. To date, however, no such registry has been established.

Senate Bill 420 also grants implied legal protection to the state's medicinal marijuana dispensaries, stating, "Qualified patients, persons with valid identification cards, and the designated primary caregivers of qualified patients . . . who associate within the state of California in order collectively or cooperatively to cultivate marijuana for medical purposes, shall not solely on the basis of that fact be subject to state criminal sanctions."

Medical Marijuana Statutes: California Compassionate Use Act 1996, Cal. Health & Saf. Code, § 11362.5 (1996) (codifying voter initiative Prop. 215).

Cal. Health & Saf. Code, §§ 11362.7 - 11362.83 (2003) (codifying SB 420).

Contact Information: For more information on California's medical marijuana law, please contact:

California NORML
2215-R Market Street #278
San Francisco, CA 94144
(415) 563-5858
www.canorml.org.

For detailed information on California county or municipal medical marijuana guidelines, please visit: www.canorml.org/prop/local215policies.html.

Colorado (D, M)

Possession of one ounce or less of marijuana is a petty offense. The offender receives a summons to appear in court, and upon a promise to appear in court, the offender is to be released from detention. The maximum penalty for a violation is $100. Failure to appear at the specified time and location results in the increase of the charges to a misdemeanor. Displaying or using the marijuana in public results in the added penalty of up to fifteen days in jail.

Possession of greater than one ounce is a misdemeanor, punishable by six to eighteen months in jail and a fine of $500 to $5,000, plus a $600 surcharge. Possession of greater than eight ounces of marijuana is a felony, punishable by one to three years in prison and a fine of $1,000 to $100,000 and a surcharge of $1,125. Generally, subsequent convictions of possession of over one ounce double the possible penalties.

Transfer of less than one ounce of marijuana for no consideration is considered possession and is punished as such. Any other transfer, sale, manufacture, or cultivation is a felony, punishable by two to four years in prison and a fine of $2,000 to $500,000 and a $1,500 surcharge. Any transport of greater than one hundred pounds is punishable by eight to twenty-four years in prison and a fine of $5,000 to $1,000,000. Any transfer to a minor is also a felony punishable by two to four years in prison and a fine of $2,000 to $500,000. Any sale within one thousand feet of a school or public housing area increases the penalties to eight to twenty-four years in prison and a fine of $10,000 to $1,000,000.

Patients who possess written documentation from their physician recommending the use of marijuana and are registered with the state and issued an identification card may legally possess no more than two ounces of marijuana or no more than six marijuana plants.

Any convictions for drug offenses that involve diversion from the prison system require a mandatory sixteen to forty-eight hours of community service. Any felony convictions involving possession or sale of marijuana also result in the suspension of the offender's driver's license for a period of up to one year. Possession or sale of paraphernalia is a petty offense punishable by a fine of up to $100.

Summary: Fifty-four percent of voters approved Amendment 20 on November 7, 2000, which amends the state's constitution to recognize the medical use of marijuana. The law took effect on June 1, 2001. It removes state-level criminal penalties on the use, possession, and cultivation of marijuana by patients who possess written documentation from their physician affirming that he or she suffers from a debilitating condition and advising that they "might benefit from the medical use of marijuana." (Patients must possess this documentation prior to an arrest.) Patients diagnosed with the following illnesses are afforded legal protection under this act: cachexia; cancer; chronic pain; chronic nervous system disorders; epilepsy and other disorders characterized by seizures; glaucoma; HIV or AIDS; multiple sclerosis and other disorders characterized by muscle spasticity; and nausea. Other conditions are subject to approval by the Colorado Board of Health. Patients (or their primary caregivers) may legally possess no more than two ounces of usable marijuana, and may cultivate no more than six marijuana plants. The law establishes a confidential state-run patient registry that issues identification cards to qualifying patients. Patients who do not join the registry or possess greater amounts of marijuana than allowed by law may argue the "affirmative defense of medical necessity" if they are arrested on marijuana charges.

Medical Marijuana Statutes: C.O. Const. art. XVIII, §14 (2001) (codified as §0-4-287 art. XVIII).

Colo. Rev. Stat. § 18-18-406.3 (2001) (interpreting the provisions of the ballot initiative and constitutional amendment).

Colo. Rev. Stat. § 25-1.5-106 (2003) (originally enacted as § 25-1-107(1) (jj) (2001)) (describing the powers and duties of the Colorado Department of Public Health).

Contact Information: Application information for the Colorado medical marijuana registry is available online or by writing:

Colorado Department of Public Health and Environment
HSVR-ADM2-A1
4300 Cherry Creek Drive South
Denver, CO 80246-1530
Phone: 303-692-2184
www.cdphe.state.co.us/hs/medicalmarijuana/fullpacket.pdf

On June 10, 2010, after Governor Bill Ritter signed House Bill 1284 into law, Colorado became the fourth state to allow state-sanctioned medical cannabis dispensaries, joining Maine, New Jersey, New Mexico, Rhode Island, and Washington, D.C.

Connecticut

Possession of up to four ounces of marijuana is punishable by up to one year in jail and a fine of up to $1,000 for the first offense. A subsequent offense is punishable by up to five years in prison and a fine of up to $3,000. Possession of four ounces or more of marijuana is punishable by up to five years in prison and a fine of up to $2,000 for a first offense. Subsequent offenses are punishable by up to ten years in prison and a fine of up to $5,000. Possession of any amount within 1,500 feet of a school adds a two-year minimum mandatory sentence to run consecutively with any other sentence imposed.

Cultivation, delivery, or sale of marijuana is punishable by up to seven years in prison and a fine of up to $25,000. Sale to a minor adds a two-year mandatory minimum sentence to run consecutively with any other sentence. Sale within 1,500 feet of a school, public housing project, or daycare center adds a three-year mandatory minimum sentence to run consecutively with any other sentence.

Possession of paraphernalia is punishable by up to three months in jail and a fine of up to $500. If the possession of paraphernalia occurs within 1,500 feet of a school, an additional one-year mandatory minimum sentence is imposed to run consecutively with any other sentence.

Delaware

Conviction of any violation involving marijuana allows the court to recommend to the licensing boards within the state that the offender's license to practice or carry on his profession be suspended or revoked. Possession of any amount of marijuana is a misdemeanor, punishable by up to six months in jail and a fine of $1,150. If the possession or sale of marijuana occurs within one thousand feet of a school, the penalty can be up to fifteen years in prison and a fine of up to $250,000, and if it occurs within three hundred feet of a church, park, or recreation area, the penalty can be up to fifteen years in prison and a fine of up to $250,000.

Manufacture or delivery of marijuana in any amount is a felony, punishable by up to five years in prison and a fine of $10,000. If the sale of marijuana is made to a person under the age of twenty-one, the punishment can be up to five years in prison. If the person is under sixteen years of age, there is a mandatory minimum sentence of six months imposed. If the person is under fourteen years of age, there is a mandatory one-year minimum sentence imposed.

If marijuana is purchased from a minor under twenty-one years old, the sentence can be up to five years in prison. If purchased from a minor under sixteen years old, there is a six-month mandatory minimum sentence imposed, with a maximum sentence of five years. If marijuana is purchased from a minor under fourteen years old, a mandatory minimum sentence of one year and no more than five years will be imposed.

It is a felony to traffic in marijuana, and all violations have mandatory minimum sentences. For greater than five pounds, the minimum sentence is two years and a fine of $25,000. For one hundred pounds or more, the minimum sentence is four years and a fine of $50,000. For five hundred pounds or more, the minimum sentence is eight years and a fine of $100,000.

The use or possession of paraphernalia is a misdemeanor punishable by up to one year in jail and a fine of up to $2,300. The sale of paraphernalia is a felony punishable by up to two years in prison. Sale or delivery of paraphernalia to a minor is punishable by up to five years in prison.

District of Columbia

Possession of any amount of marijuana is a misdemeanor and is punishable by up to six months in jail and a fine of up to $1,000. First-time offenders are eligible for probation and dismissal of the charges upon successful completion of the probation contract.

The cultivation, sale, or delivery of any amount of marijuana is punishable by up to one year in jail and a fine of up to $10,000. If the distribution occurs within one thousand feet of a school, pool, playground, arcade, library, youth center, or public housing, or if the distribution is made to a minor, the penalties can be doubled.

Upon conviction of a drug offense, the offender's driver's license can be suspended from six months to two years. The possession of paraphernalia is punishable by up to thirty days in jail and a $100 fine. The sale of paraphernalia is punishable by up to six months in jail and a fine of up to $1,000 unless the sale is made to a minor, in which case the penalty increases to a possible eight years in prison and a fine of up to $15,000.

Summary: Ballot initiative 59, first passed by the voters in 1998 with 69 percent of the vote, will permit seriously ill individuals to legally use marijuana for medical treatment when recommended by a licensed physician.

The Congress has thirty legislative days either to override the measure, or to allow it to become law. Current expectations are the measure will become law, with regulations issued by the District of Columbia City Council to define the dispensary system authorized by the initiative, by the end of 2010.

Federal Government

Possession of marijuana is punishable by up to one year in jail and a minimum fine of $1,000 for a first conviction. For a second conviction, the penalties increase to a fifteen-day mandatory minimum sentence with a maximum of two years in prison and a fine of up to $2,500. Subsequent convictions carry a ninety-day mandatory minimum sentence and a maximum of up to three years in prison and a fine of up to $5,000.

Distribution of a small amount of marijuana, for no remuneration, is treated as possession. Manufacture or distribution of less than fifty kilograms of marijuana is punishable by up to five years in prison and a fine of up to $250,000. For fifty kilograms or more, the penalty increases to a possible twenty years in prison and a fine of up to $1,000,000. Manufacture or distribution of one hundred kilograms or more carries a penalty of five to forty years in prison and a fine of up to $2,000,000. For one thousand kilograms or more, the penalty increases to ten years to life in prison and a fine of up to $4,000,000.

Distribution of greater than five grams of marijuana to a minor under the age of twenty-one doubles the possible penalties. Distribution within one thousand feet of a school, playground, or public housing, or within one hundred feet of a youth center, public pool, or video arcade also doubles the possible penalties.

The sale of paraphernalia is punishable by up to three years in prison. The sentence of death can be carried out on a defendant who has been found guilty of manufacturing, importing, or distributing a controlled substance if the act was committed as part of a continuing criminal enterprise—but only if the defendant is:

1. The principal administrator, organizer, or leader of the enterprise or is one of several such principal administrators, organizers, or leaders, and

2. The quantity of the controlled substance is sixty thousand kilograms or more of a mixture or substance containing a detectable amount of marijuana, or sixty thousand or more marijuana plants, or if the enterprise received more than $20 million in gross receipts during any twelve-month period of its existence.

Florida

Possession of twenty grams or less of marijuana is a misdemeanor, punishable by up to one year in jail and a fine of up to $1,000. Possession of greater than twenty grams of marijuana is a felony, punishable by up to five years in prison and a fine of up to $5,000.

The delivery of twenty grams or less of marijuana for no consideration is a misdemeanor and is punishable by up to one year in jail and a fine of up to $1,000. Sale, delivery, or cultivation of any other amount up to twenty-five pounds is a felony and punishable by up to five years in prison and a fine of up to $5,000.

Sale, delivery, or cultivation of greater than twenty-five pounds is considered trafficking, and all trafficking offenses have mandatory minimum sentences. For less than two thousand pounds or fewer than two thousand plants, there is a mandatory minimum sentence of three years and a fine of $25,000. For less than ten thousand pounds or fewer than ten thousand plants, there is a mandatory minimum sentence of seven years and a fine of $50,000. For ten thousand pounds or ten thousand plants or greater, the mandatory minimum sentence is fifteen years in prison and a fine of $200,000.

Any sale or delivery occurring within one thousand feet of a school, college, public park, public housing, daycare center, or church is punishable by up to fifteen years in prison and a fine of $10,000. The possession of paraphernalia is a misdemeanor, punishable by up to one year in jail and a fine of up to $1,000. Conviction of a drug-related offense also requires suspension of the offender's driver's license for at least six months but not longer than two years.

Georgia

Possession of less than one ounce of marijuana is a misdemeanor and can be punished by up to one year in jail and a fine of up to $1,000. However, upon a first drug conviction, the offender may be placed on probation, and upon successful completion the proceedings against him may be discharged.

Possession of one ounce or more is a felony and is punishable by one to ten years in prison.

Any cultivation, manufacture, or distribution is a felony, punishable by one to ten years in prison. Any possession, manufacture or distribution of greater than fifty pounds is considered trafficking, and all trafficking offenses carry mandatory minimum sentences. For amounts greater than fifty pounds but less than two thousand pounds, the sentence is a minimum of five years in prison and a $100,000 fine. For two thousand pounds to less than ten thousand pounds, the minimum sentence is seven years in prison and a fine of $250,000. For ten thousand pounds or more, the minimum sentence is fifteen years and a $1,000,000 fine.

The use of any communication facility, such as a telephone or radio, during any drug felony may add one to four years to the sentence and a fine of $30,000. Distribution or possession within one thousand feet of any school, park, playground, recreational center, or drug-free commercial zone is punishable by up to twenty years in prison and a fine of up to $20,000, for the first conviction. A second conviction is punishable by five to forty years in prison and a fine of up to $40,000.

Upon a first conviction of a drug offense, the offender's driver's license is suspended for at least six months and will be reinstated only upon completion of a drug-use program. For a second conviction, the suspension will be at least one year; and for a third conviction, the suspension will be at least two years. Professional licenses can also be suspended upon a drug conviction.

Hawaii (M)

Possession of less than one ounce of marijuana is a misdemeanor offense, punishable by up to thirty days in jail and a fine of up to $1,000. Possession of one ounce or more is a misdemeanor punishable by up to one year in prison and a fine of up to $2,000. Any possession of amounts of one pound or more are felonies. The possible sentence for possession of one pound or more is up to five years in prison and a fine of up to $10,000. Possession of two pounds or more is punishable by up to ten years in prison and a fine of up to $25,000. Possession of twenty-five pounds or more is punishable by up to twenty-five years in prison and a fine of up to $50,000.

For first-time offenders, the court can defer proceedings, place the accused on probation, and, upon completion of the probationary period, the court can dismiss the charges.

For cultivation of twenty-five plants or more, the possible sentence can be up to five years in prison and a fine of up to $10,000. For fifty plants or more, the sentence can be up to ten years in prison and a fine of up to $25,000. For one hundred plants or more, the sentence can be up to twenty years in prison and a fine of up to $50,000.

Sale or distribution of less than one ounce of marijuana is a misdemeanor, punishable by up to one year in prison and a fine of up to $2,000. Sale or distribution of any amount greater than one ounce is a felony. For one ounce or more, the sentence can be up to five years in jail and a fine of up to $10,000. For one pound or more, the sentence can be up to ten years in prison and a fine of up to $25,000. For five pounds or more, the penalty rises to a possible twenty years in prison and a fine of up to $50,000.

It is an affirmative defense to any marijuana-related offense that the person distributing or possessing the marijuana was authorized to do so for medical purposes.

Any marijuana found in a vehicle results in all the occupants of the vehicle being charged with its possession, unless the marijuana was found on the person of one of the occupants.

Summary: Governor Ben Cayetano signed Senate Bill 862 into law on June 14, 2000. The law took effect on December 28, 2000. The law removes state-level criminal penalties on the use, possession, and cultivation of marijuana by patients who possess a signed statement from their physician affirming that he or she suffers from a debilitating condition and that the "potential benefits of medical use of marijuana would likely outweigh the health risks." Patients diagnosed with the following illnesses are afforded legal protection under this act: cachexia; cancer; chronic pain; Crohn's disease; epilepsy and other disorders characterized by seizures; glaucoma; HIV or AIDS; multiple sclerosis, and other disorders characterized by muscle spasticity; and nausea. Other conditions are subject to approval by the Hawaii Department of Health. Patients (or their primary caregivers) may legally possess up to 3 ounces of usable marijuana, and may cultivate no more than seven marijuana plants, of which no more than three may be mature. The law establishes a mandatory, confidential state-run patient registry that issues identification cards to qualifying patients.

Amendments: No, although Hawaii has a separate statute allowing patients arrested on marijuana charges to present a "choice of evils" defense arguing that their use of marijuana is medically necessary.

Medical Marijuana Statutes: Haw. Rev. Stat. §§ 329-121 to 329-128 (2008).

Contact Information: Administrative rules for Hawaii's medical marijuana program are available online from the Drug Policy Forum of Hawaii website at: www.dpfhi.org.

Application information for the Hawaii medical marijuana registry is available by writing or calling:
Hawaii Department of Public Safety
919 Ala Moana Boulevard
Honolulu, HI 96814
(808) 594-0150

Idaho

It is a crime to be under the influence of marijuana in a public place or to use marijuana in a public place, punishable by up to six months in jail and a fine of up to $1,000.

The penalty for possession of three ounces or less of marijuana is up to one year in jail and a fine of up to $1,000. Possession of greater than three ounces is a felony and punishable by up to five years in prison and a fine of up to $10,000.

The penalty for cultivation, sale, or distribution of less than one pound (or fewer than twenty-five plants) is a prison term of up to five years and a fine of up to $15,000. Cultivation, sale, or distribution of amounts greater than one pound are all subject to mandatory minimum sentences. The maximum possible punishment for any cultivation, sale, or delivery is fifteen years in prison and a fine of up to $50,000. For amounts of one pound or more (or more than twenty-four plants), the punishment is a mandatory minimum sentence of one year in prison and a fine of not less than $5,000. Cultivation, sale, or distribution of five pounds or more (or more than forty-nine plants) is punishable by a mandatory minimum prison term of three years and a fine of not less than $10,000. For amounts of twenty-five pounds or more (or more than ninety-nine plants), the punishment is a mandatory minimum sentence of five years in prison and a fine of not less than $15,000.

Any sale to a minor, at least three years younger than the seller, doubles the possible prison sentence. Any sale on premises where minors are present is punishable by up to five years in prison and a fine of up to $5,000.

It is also a crime to be present in a place where the person knows that there is illegal drug activity taking place and is punishable by up to ninety days in jail and a fine of up to $300.

Possession of paraphernalia is punishable by up to one year in jail and a fine of up to $1,000. Sale or manufacture of paraphernalia is punishable by up to nine years in prison and a fine of up to $30,000.

Any second conviction for a drug offense can double the possible penalties.

Illinois

Possession of 2.5 grams or less of marijuana is a misdemeanor, punishable by up to thirty days in jail and a fine of up to $1,500. Possession of greater than 2.5 grams is punishable by up to six months in jail and a fine of up to $1,500. Possession of greater than ten grams is punishable by up to one year in jail and a fine of up to $2,500.

All possession of greater than thirty grams is considered a felony. Possession of greater than thirty grams is punishable by one to three years in prison and a fine of up to $25,000. For a subsequent conviction, the penalty increases to two to five years in prison and a fine of up to $25,000. For possession of greater than five hundred grams, the penalty is two to five years in prison and a fine of up to $25,000. For possession of greater than two thousand grams, the penalty is three to seven years in prison and a fine of up to $25,000. For any possession of an amount greater than five thousand grams, the penalty is four to fifteen years in prison and a fine of up to $25,000.

The cultivation of no more than five marijuana plants is a misdemeanor, punishable by up to one year in jail and a fine of up to $2,500. Cultivation of more than five plants is a felony, punishable by one to three years in prison and a fine of up to $25,000. Cultivation of more than twenty plants is punishable by two to five years in prison and a fine of up to $25,000. The penalty for cultivation of more than fifty plants is three to seven years in prison and a fine of up to $100,000.

Casual delivery of marijuana is treated as possession. Manufacture or delivery of 2.5 grams or less is considered a misdemeanor and is punishable by up to six months in jail and a fine of up to $1,500, unless activity occurred in school zone, then up to one year in jail and a fine of up to $2,500. Manufacture or delivery of greater than 2.5 grams is punishable by up to one year in jail and a fine of up to $2,500 (in a school zone: one to three years in prison and a fine of up to $25,000). For manufacture or delivery of greater than ten grams, the penalty is one to three years in prison and a fine of up to $25,000 (in a school zone: two to five years in prison and a fine of up to $50,000). For manufacture or delivery of more than thirty grams, the penalty is two to five years in prison and a fine of up to $50,000 (in a school zone: three to seven years in prison and a fine of up to $100,000). The penalty for manufacture or delivery of greater than five hundred grams is three to seven years in prison and a fine of up to $100,000 (in a school zone: four to fifteen years in prison and a fine of up to $200,000). The penalty for manufacture or delivery of greater than two thousand grams is four to fifteen years in prison and a fine of up to $150,000. Any manufacture or delivery of amounts greater than five thousand grams is punishable by six to thirty years in prison and a fine of up to $200,000.

Bringing more than 2,500 grams into the state for manufacture or delivery is considered trafficking and the penalties are doubled. Any sale to a minor at least three years younger than the seller also doubles the penalty and fine. When convicted of a drug-related offense, the court may impose an additional fine of at least the full street value of the marijuana seized.

For any first conviction for possession of less than thirty grams, cultivation of any amount or manufacture or delivery of less than fifty plants, the court can defer judgment, place the offender on probation for twenty-four months, and, upon successful completion of the probation, the court can discharge the proceedings.

Indiana

The possession of thirty grams or less of marijuana is a misdemeanor punishable by up to one year in jail and a fine of up to $5,000. For first offenders, the court may consider a conditional discharge. For possession of more than thirty grams, the penalties range from six months to three years in prison and a fine of up to $10,000.

The cultivation, delivery, or sale of thirty grams or less is a misdemeanor, punishable by up to one year in jail and a fine of up to $5,000. Cultivation or delivery of more than thirty grams is a felony, punishable by six months to three years in prison and a fine of up to $10,000. For cultivation or delivery of any amount of ten pounds or more the penalties range from two to eight years in prison and a fine of up to $10,000.

Any sale within one thousand feet of a school, public park, or a family housing complex, or any sale on a school bus, is punishable by two to eight years in prison and a fine of up to $10,000. Sale to a minor is punishable by six months to three years in prison and a fine of up to $10,000.

Possession of paraphernalia can be a misdemeanor if it is committed "recklessly" and is punishable by imprisonment for a fixed term of not more than one year and a fine of not more than $5,000. There is no mention in the statute of what "recklessly" means.

Possession of paraphernalia can be a felony if the person has a previous judgment or conviction under the statute, and it is punishable by imprisonment for a fixed term of one and one-half years and a fine of not more than $10,000.

Knowingly visiting a place where drugs are used is a misdemeanor, punishable by up to six months in jail and a fine of up to $1,000. A person convicted of dealing or possessing marijuana will have his operator's license suspended, his existing motor vehicle registration suspended, and his ability to register motor vehicles suspended.

Iowa

The possession of any amount of marijuana is a misdemeanor, punishable by up to six months in jail and a fine of up to $1,000. For a second offense the penalties increase to up to one year in jail and a fine of up to $1,500. Subsequent offenses are punishable by up to two years and a fine of $500 to $5,000. There is the possibility for conditional discharge for possession charges. Possession within one thousand feet of a school, public park, swimming pool, or recreation center adds an additional one hundred hours of community service to the sentence.

Manufacture or delivery of fifty kilograms or less of marijuana is punishable by up to five years in prison and a fine of $750 to $7,500. The penalty for manufacture or delivery of greater than fifty kilograms is up to ten years in prison and a fine of $1,000 to $50,000. Manufacture or delivery of greater than one hundred kilograms is punishable by up to twenty-five years in prison and a fine of $5,000 to $100,000. For any manufacture or delivery of any amount greater than one thousand kilograms, the sentence can be up to fifty years in prison and a fine of up to $1,000,000.

Sale to a minor carries a five-year mandatory minimum sentence with a twenty-five-year maximum sentence. Sale within one thousand feet of a school or public park carries a ten-year mandatory minimum sentence with a twenty-five-year maximum sentence. Possession or sale of paraphernalia is a simple misdemeanor punishable by up to thirty days in jail and a fine of

$50 to $500. Second or subsequent offenses are punishable by up to three times the sentence for first offenses. For juveniles convicted of drug charges, driver's licenses are suspended for up to one year.

Kansas

Possession of any amount of marijuana for personal use is punishable by up to one year in jail and a fine of up to $2,500. For a second conviction the penalty increases to ten to forty-two months in jail and a fine of up to $100,000.

Possession with intent to sell or actual sale is punishable by fourteen to fifty-one months in jail and a fine of up to $300,000. Probation is possible for sentences of less than thirty-two months. Sale or possession with intent within one thousand feet of a school is punishable by forty-six to eighty-three months in prison and a fine of up to $300,000.

Manufacture of a controlled substance is punishable by 138 to 204 months in prison.

Possession of paraphernalia for personal use is punishable by up to one year in jail and a fine of up to $2,500. Possession of paraphernalia that would be used for planting or growing more than five marijuana plants is punishable by ten to forty-two months in jail and a fine of up to $100,000.

Kentucky

Possession of less than eight ounces of marijuana is a misdemeanor, punishable by up to one year in jail and a fine of up to $500. For subsequent offenses, the penalties increase to one to five years in jail and a fine of $1,000 to $10,000. Possession of eight ounces or more is considered possession with intent to sell and is charged as trafficking.

Sale or delivery (trafficking) of less than eight ounces is punishable by up to one year in jail and a fine of up to $500. The penalties for sale or delivery of eight ounces or greater are one to five years in prison and a fine of $1,000 to $10,000. Sale or delivery of five pounds or more is punishable by five to ten years in prison and a fine of $1,000 to $10,000.

Any sale to a minor is punishable by five to ten years in prison and a fine of $1,000 to $10,000 for a first offense, and ten to twenty years in prison and a fine of $1,000 to $10,000 for a second or subsequent offense.

Any sale within one thousand yards of a school is punishable by one to five years in prison and a fine of $1,000 to $10,000.

Cultivation of less than five plants is punishable by up to one year in jail and a fine of up to $500. For subsequent offenses, the penalties increase to one to five years in prison and a fine of $1,000 to $10,000. For cultivation of five plants or more, the penalties are one to five years in prison and a fine of $1,000 to $10,000. For subsequent offenses the penalties increase to five to ten years in prison and fines of $1,000 to $10,000.

Possession of paraphernalia is a misdemeanor for the first offense, punishable by up to one year in jail and a fine of up to $500. Subsequent offenses are punishable by one to five years in prison and a fine of $1,000 to $10,000. Minors convicted of drug offenses are also subject to suspension of their driver's licenses for one year for the first offense and two years for the second offense.

Louisiana

Possession of any amount of marijuana is punishable by up to six months in jail and a fine of up to $500 for a first offense. For a second offense the penalties increase to up to five years in prison and a fine of up to $2,000. A third or subsequent offense increases the penalty to up to twenty years in prison.

Cultivation or sale, or possession with intent to distribute less than sixty pounds of marijuana is punishable by five to thirty years in prison and a fine of up to $50,000. For greater than sixty pounds of marijuana, the penalty increases to ten to sixty years in prison and a fine of up to $50,000 to $100,000. For greater than two thousand pounds, the punishment ranges from twenty to eighty years in prison and a fine of $100,000 to $400,000. For greater than ten thousand pounds, the penalty increases to fifty to eighty years in prison and a fine of $400,000 to $1,000,000.

Any sale to a minor at least three years younger than the seller doubles the possible penalties. For felony possession or sale within one thousand feet of a school, religious building, or public housing the penalty includes a mandatory minimum sentence of at least one half of the maximum penalty for the offense. Possession or sale of paraphernalia is punished by up to six months in jail and a fine of up to $500 for the first offense. For a second offense, the penalty increases to up to one year in jail and a fine of up to $1,000. For a third offense, the penalty is up to five years in prison and a fine of up to $5,000.

Maine (D, M)

Possession of less than 1.25 ounces is a civil violation, punishable by a fine of $200 to $400. Possession of 1.25 ounces or more is considered evidence of intent to distribute and is punished as such (see below). Possession of a usable amount of marijuana is lawful if at the time of the possession the person has an authenticated copy of a medical record demonstrating that the person has a physician's recommendation.

Cultivation of five plants or less of marijuana is punishable by up to six months in jail and a fine of up to $1,000. For more than five plants, the penalties increase to up to one year in jail and a fine of up to $2,000. For more than one hundred plants, the possible punishment is up to five years in prison and a fine of up to $5,000. For any amount of plants greater than five hundred, the penalties increase to up to ten years in prison and a fine of up to $20,000.

The penalty for sale of marijuana is up to one year in jail and a fine up to $2,000. The penalties increase to up to five years in prison and a fine of up to $5,000 if the sale was made to a minor or if it occurred within one thousand feet of a school or on a school bus.

Possession of greater than one pound of marijuana is considered trafficking and is punishable by up to one year in jail and a fine of up to $2,000.

Possession and personal use of paraphernalia is a civil violation punishable by a fine of $200. The sale of paraphernalia is punishable by up to six months in prison and a fine of up to $1,000, unless the sale was to a minor, in which case the penalty increases to up to one year in jail and a fine of up to $2,000. Upon conviction, the court may suspend or revoke the professional license of the offender.

Summary: Sixty-one percent of voters approved Question 2 on November 2, 1999. The law took effect on December 22, 1999. It removes state-level criminal penalties on the use, possession, and cultivation of marijuana by patients who possess an oral or written "professional opinion" from their physician that he or she "might benefit from the medical use of marijuana." Patients diagnosed with the following illnesses are afforded legal protection under this act: epilepsy and other disorders characterized by seizures; glaucoma; multiple sclerosis and other disorders characterized by muscle spasticity; and nausea or vomiting as a result of AIDS or cancer chemotherapy. Patients (or their primary caregivers) may legally possess no more than one and one-quarter ounces of usable marijuana, and may cultivate no more than six marijuana plants, of which no more than three may be mature. Those patients who possess greater amounts of marijuana than allowed by law are afforded a "simple defense" to a charge of marijuana possession. The law does not establish a state-run patient registry.

Amendments: Yes. Senate Bill 611, which was signed into law on April 2, 2002, increases the amount of useable marijuana a person may possess from one and one-quarter ounces to two and one-half ounces. Question 5, approved by 59 percent of voters on November 3, 2009, mandates the Department of Health to enact rules within 120 days establishing a confidential patient registry and identification card system, and allowing for the dispensing of medicinal cannabis via state-licensed nonprofit dispensaries. The act also expands the list of qualifying illnesses for which a physician may recommend medical cannabis to include: "A. cancer, glaucoma, positive status for human immunodeficiency virus, acquired immune deficiency syndrome, hepatitis C, amyotrophic lateral sclerosis, Crohn's disease, agitation of Alzheimer's disease, nail-patella syndrome or the treatment of these conditions; B. a chronic or debilitating disease or medical condition or its treatment that produces intractable pain, which is pain that has not responded to ordinary medical or surgical measures for more than six months; C. a chronic or debilitating disease or medical condition or its treatment that produces one or more of the following: cachexia or wasting syndrome; severe nausea; seizures, including but not limited to those characteristic of epilepsy; or severe and persistent muscle spasms, including but not limited to those characteristic of multiple sclerosis; or D. any other medical condition or its treatment approved by the department as provided."

Medical Marijuana Statutes: Me. Rev. Stat. tit. 22, § 2383-B(5), (6) (1999) (amended 2001).

Me. Rev. Stat. tit. 22, § 2383-B(3)(c) (amended 2001) (increasing amount of marijuana a patient may posses to two and one-half ounces).

Contact Information: Brochures outlining Maine's medical marijuana law are available from:

www.mainecommonsense.org

Maine Citizens for Patients Rights
P.O. Box 1074
Lewiston, ME 04243

Maryland

Possession or use of any amount of marijuana is punishable by up to one year in jail and a fine of up to $1,000.

Cultivation, delivery, or sale of less than fifty pounds of marijuana is punishable by up to five years in prison and a fine of up to $15,000. For fifty pounds or more, the penalties increase to a five-year mandatory minimum sentence and a fine of up to $100,000. If the sale occurs within one thousand feet of a school, while the school is in session, or on a school bus, the penalty is up to twenty years in prison and a fine of up to $20,000.

Bringing five to forty-five kilograms of marijuana into the state is punishable by up to ten years in prison and a fine of up to $10,000. Transporting forty-five kilograms or more into the state is punishable by up to twenty-five years in prison and a fine of up to $50,000.

Possession, use, or sale of paraphernalia is a criminal fine of $500 for the first offense. For a second or subsequent offense, the penalties increase to a term of up to two years in prison and a fine of up to $2,000. For any second or subsequent conviction, the sentence may double from that for a first offense.

Massachusetts (D)

Possession of one ounce or less of marijuana is a civil offense, subject to a $100 fine like a traffic ticket. Offenders under eighteen will be required to attend a drug-awareness program or pay a $1,000 fine. Possession of more than one ounce of marijuana is punishable by up to six months in jail and a fine of up to $500. For first-time offenders, the court will sentence the offender to probation, and upon successful completion of the probation period, the offender's record will be sealed. For subsequent offenses, probation may still be possible.

Cultivation, delivery, or sale of less than fifty pounds of marijuana is punishable by up to two years in prison and a fine of up to $5,000. For fifty pounds or more, the penalty increases to a mandatory minimum of one year in prison and a possible range of thirty-six months to fifteen years in prison and a fine of $500 to $10,000. For cultivation or sale of one hundred pounds or more, the mandatory minimum sentence is three years and up to fifteen years in prison, along with a fine of $2,500 to $25,000. For two thousand pounds or more, the penalties increase to a mandatory minimum five-year sentence up to fifteen years in prison and a fine of $5,000 to $50,000. For any amount of ten thousand pounds or more, the mandatory minimum sentence is ten years with up to fifteen years in prison possible and a fine of $20,000 to $200,000.

Sale of marijuana within one thousand feet of a school adds another two-year mandatory minimum sentence for sale and can go as high as an additional fifteen years in prison and a fine of $1,000 to $10,000. The manufacture or sale of paraphernalia is punishable by one to two years in prison and a fine of $500 to $5,000, unless the sale was to a minor, in which case the penalty is three to five years in prison and a fine of $1,000 to $5,000.

Michigan (M)

The penalty for the use of marijuana is up to ninety days in jail and a fine of up to $100. Possession of marijuana in any amount is punishable by up to one year in jail and a fine of up to $2,000, unless the possession occurred in a public or private park, which increases the penalty to a possible two years in prison. Conditional discharge is available in all use and possession cases. Distribution of marijuana without remuneration is a misdemeanor, punishable by up to one year in jail and a fine of up to $1,000. For cultivation of less than twenty plants or sale of less than five kilograms, the punishment is up to four years in jail and a fine of up to $20,000. For cultivation of twenty or more plants or sale of five kilograms or more, the punishment is up to seven years in prison and a fine up to $500,000. Cultivation of two hundred or more plants or sale of forty-five kilograms or more is punishable by up to fifteen years in prison and a fine up to $10,000,000.

The sale of paraphernalia is punishable by up to ninety days in jail and a fine of up to $5,000. The arrest for sale of paraphernalia is preceded by a cease and desist order, and if the order is complied with, it is a complete defense to the charges.

Ann Arbor: The penalty for being caught with marijuana is $25 for the first offense, $50 for the second, and $100 for the third or subsequent offense (and no incarceration or probation). However, laws do not apply on university property, for instance, in the dorms; the university has a much more strict policy on possession and/or use.

Summary: Sixty-three percent of voters approved Proposal 1 on November 4, 2008. The law took effect on December 4, 2008. It removes state-level criminal penalties on the use, possession, and cultivation of marijuana by patients who possess written documentation from their physicians authorizing the medical use of marijuana. Patients diagnosed with the following illnesses are afforded legal protection under this act: Cancer, glaucoma, positive status for human immunodeficiency virus, acquired immune deficiency syndrome, hepatitis C, amyotrophic lateral sclerosis, Crohn's disease, agitation of Alzheimer's disease, nail patella, or the treatment of these conditions. Patients are also offered legal protection if they have a chronic or debilitating disease or medical condition or treatment of said condition that produces one or more of the following: cachexia or wasting syndrome; severe and chronic pain; severe nausea; seizures, including but not limited to those characteristic of epilepsy; or severe and persistent muscle spasms, including but not limited to those characteristic of multiple sclerosis. Patients (or their primary caregivers) may possess no more than twelve marijuana plants kept in an enclosed, locked facility or 2.5 ounces of usable marijuana. The law establishes a confidential state-run patient registry that issues identification cards to qualifying patients. The state officially began accepting applications for the program on April 6, 2009.

Valid medical marijuana registry cards from other medical marijuana states are recognized in this state, as long as the cardholder is in compliance with the possession limits imposed on cardholders in this state.

Amendments: Yes. Administrative rules for the program took effect on April 4, 2009. A copy of the regulations is available here.

Medical Marijuana Statutes: Michigan Medical Marihuana Act, Mich. Comp. Law §§ 333.26421 - 333.26430 (2008).

Contact Information:
> Michigan Medical Marihuana Program (MMMP)
> Michigan.gov/mmp

> Michigan Medical Marijuana Association
> http://michiganmedicalmarijuana.org

Minnesota

The penalty for possession of a small amount (less than 42.5 grams) of marijuana is a fine of up to $200 and possible requirement of drug education. Possession of 42.5 grams or more of marijuana is punishable by up to five years in prison and a fine up to $10,000. Possession of ten kilograms or more of marijuana increases the penalty to a fine up to $250,000 and up to twenty years in prison. Possession of fifty kilograms or more is punishable by up to twenty-five years in prison and a fine up to $500,000. For any possession of one hundred kilograms or more, the penalty is up to thirty years in prison and a fine up to $1,000,000.

Possession of greater than 1.4 grams in a motor vehicle (except in the trunk) is punishable by up to one year in prison. Conditional discharge is a possibility for first-time offenders.

For distribution of a small amount of marijuana (42.5 grams or less) for no remuneration, the penalty is a fine of up to $200 and possible requirement of drug education. For sale of any amount less than five kilograms, the punishment is up to five years in prison and a fine of up to $10,000. Sale of five kilograms or more is punishable by up to twenty years in prison and a fine up to $250,000. For sale of twenty-five kilograms or more, the penalties increase to a possible twenty-five years in prison and a fine up to $500,000. Sale of fifty kilograms or more is punishable by up to thirty years in prison and a fine up to $1,000,000.

The penalty for sale to a minor is up to twenty years in prison and a fine up to $250,000. Sale within a school zone, park zone, or public housing area, or near a drug treatment facility, increases the penalty to up to fifteen years in prison and a fine up to $100,000. The importing of fifty kilograms or more into the state is punishable by up to thirty-five years in prison and a fine up to $1,250,000. Driver's licenses can be suspended for thirty days if the offense was committed while driving a motor vehicle.

Mississippi (D)

Possession of thirty grams or less of marijuana is punishable by a fine of $100 to $250 for the first offense. For possession of greater than thirty grams, the penalty increases to a fine of up to $3,000 and up to three years in prison. The penalty for possession of 250 grams or more is two to eight years in prison and a fine up to $50,000. For possession of five hundred grams or more, the penalty is six to twenty-four years in prison and a fine up to $500,000. For possession of five kilograms or greater, the penalty is ten to thirty years in prison and a fine up to $1,000,000. There are additional penalties for possession in any part of a motor vehicle except the trunk.

Sale or delivery of less than one ounce is punishable by up to three years in prison and a fine up to $3,000. Sale of one ounce or more is punishable by up to twenty years in prison and a fine up to $30,000. For sale of one kilogram or more, the penalty is up to thirty years in prison and a fine of $5,000 to $1,000,000. For sale of more than ten pounds, the penalty is life in prison without the possibility of parole.

Sale to a minor doubles the penalty. Sale within 1,500 feet of the buildings of a school, church, public park, ballpark, gymnasium, youth center, or movie theater also doubles the penalties available. Possession of thirty grams or less of marijuana in the passenger compartment of a car is a misdemeanor with a fine of no more than $1,000 and no more than ninety days in county jail. For second or subsequent offenses of over thirty grams of marijuana, the penalty increases to twice the amount available to first offenders. A second conviction within two years for possession of thirty grams or less carries a fine of $250 and not less than five or more than sixty days in county jail. For drug convictions, the offender's driver's license is suspended for six months.

Missouri

Possession of thirty-five grams or less of marijuana is a misdemeanor, punishable by up to one year in jail and a fine up to $1,000. Possession of greater than thirty-five grams is a felony and is punishable by up to seven years in prison and a fine of up to $5,000. Possession of greater than thirty kilograms is considered trafficking and the penalty is five to fifteen years in prison. Possession of one hundred kilograms or more carries a penalty of ten years to life in prison.

Sale or manufacture of five grams or less of marijuana is a felony, punishable by up to seven years in prison and a fine of up to $5,000. Sale of greater than five grams carries a penalty of five to fifteen years in prison. Sale of greater than thirty kilograms is punishable by ten years to life in prison, and sale of one hundred kilograms or more is punishable by ten years to life in prison with no probation or parole.

Any sale to a minor increases the penalties by five to fifteen years in prison. Any sale within two thousand feet of a school or within one thousand feet of a public housing project increases the penalties to ten years to life in prison. The possession of paraphernalia is a misdemeanor, punishable by up to one year in jail and a fine of up to $1,000. The sale of paraphernalia is punishable by up to five years in prison and a fine of up to $5,000. Senate Bills 5 and 21 altered the state's forfeiture laws. Most notably, they require that law enforcement report all seizures to the prosecuting attorney or the attorney general, who must then make an annual report of the activity to the Department of Public Safety and the state auditor. In addition, no property may be transferred to a federal agency without judicial approval, and any agency making a seizure must file an annual audit with the state auditor's office. Failure to comply is punishable by a fine of up to $1,000.

Montana (M)

Possession of sixty grams or less of marijuana is a misdemeanor, punishable by up to six months in jail and a fine of $100 to $500 for the first conviction. For subsequent convictions, the penalties increase to up to three years in prison and a fine up to $1,000. Possession of greater than sixty grams carries a sentence of up to twenty years in prison and a fine up to $50,000.

Production or manufacture of one pound or less of marijuana is punishable by up to ten years in jail and a fine up to $50,000. For amounts greater than one pound or more than thirty plants, the penalty includes a two-year mandatory minimum sentence to life in prison and a fine up to $50,000. Subsequent convictions can double the possible sentence.

Sale or distribution of marijuana carries a penalty of one year to life in prison and a fine up to $50,000. Sale to a minor carries an additional penalty of two years to life in prison and a fine up to $50,000. Any sale within one thousand feet of a school also adds an additional three years to life in prison and a fine up to $50,000.

All dangerous-drug convictions require the offender to attend a dangerous-drug information course. There is also the possibility of alternative sentencing such as fines, drug treatment, community service, or probation if the court feels that incarceration is not warranted. The penalty for possession or sale of paraphernalia is up to six months in jail and a fine up to $500.

Summary: Sixty-two percent of voters approved Initiative 148 on November 2, 2004. The law took effect that same day. It removes state-level criminal penalties on the use, possession, and cultivation of marijuana by patients who possess written documentation from their physicians authorizing the medical use of marijuana. Patients diagnosed with the following illnesses are afforded legal protection under this act: cachexia or wasting syndrome; severe or chronic pain; severe nausea; seizures, including but not limited to seizures caused by epilepsy; or severe or persistent muscle spasms, including but not limited to spasms caused by multiple sclerosis or Crohn's disease. Patients (or their primary caregivers) may possess no more than six marijuana plants. The law establishes a confidential state-run patient registry that issues identification cards to qualifying patients.

Valid medical marijuana registry cards from other medical marijuana states are recognized in this state, so long as the cardholder is in compliance with the possession limits imposed on cardholders in this state.

Amendments: No.

Medical Marijuana Statutes: Montana Medical Marijuana Act, Mont. Code Ann. §§ 50-46-1 to 50-46-2 (2007).

Contact Information: www.dphhs.mt.gov/medicalmarijuana

Nebraska (D)

Possession of one ounce or less of marijuana is an infraction, and the offender receives a citation and is subject to a $100 fine and possible referral to a drug education course for the first offense. For a second offense, the penalty increases to a possible five days in jail and a fine of $200. For subsequent offenses, the fine increases to $300 and a possible seven days' jail time. For possession of greater than one ounce, the penalty is up to seven days in jail and a fine up to $500. Possession of greater than one pound is punishable by up to five years in prison and a fine up to $10,000.

The penalty for distribution of marijuana is up to twenty years in prison and a fine up to $25,000. The penalty increases for sale to minors and sale within one thousand feet of a school, college, or playground, or within one hundred feet of a youth center, public swimming pool, or video arcade to the next-higher classification of offense.

Possession of paraphernalia is punishable by a fine of $100 for the first offense. For the second offense, the fine increases to $200 to $300, and for subsequent offenses, the fine increases to $200 to $500. Sale of paraphernalia is punishable by up to six months in jail and a fine up to $1,000.

Nevada (D, M)

Possession of marijuana by persons twenty-one years of age or older is a misdemeanor and is punishable by a fine of $600 or possible drug treatment. For a second offense, the fine increases to $1,000. For a third offense, the punishment is up to one year in jail and a fine of up to $2,000. A fourth offense changes the classification to a felony and is punishable by one to four years in prison and a fine of up to $5,000.

Possession of marijuana by persons under twenty-one years of age of less than one ounce of marijuana is a felony, punishable by one to four years in prison and a fine of up to $5,000. Probation is usually granted in lieu of imprisonment for first and second offenses; for third offenses, there is a presumption of imprisonment.

Cultivation, delivery, or sale of less than one hundred pounds of marijuana is punishable by one to six years in prison and a fine of up to

$20,000 for the first offense. For a second offense, the penalty increases to two to ten years in prison and a fine up to $20,000. For a third or subsequent offense, the penalty increases to three to fifteen years in prison and a fine up to $20,000. Cultivation, delivery, or sale of one hundred pounds or more is punishable by up to five years in prison and a fine up to $25,000. For amounts of two thousand pounds or greater, the penalty increases to two to twenty years in prison and a fine up to $50,000. For amounts greater than ten thousand pounds, the penalty can be up to life in prison, with the possibility for parole after a minimum of five years and a fine up to $200,000.

It is an affirmative defense to any charge of possession, delivery, or production of marijuana that the person is engaged in the medical use of marijuana if the amount is no more than one ounce of usable marijuana, three mature plants, or four immature plants.

Any sale to a minor is punishable by one to twenty years in prison for the first offense, and up to life for a second offense. Sale within one thousand feet of a school, video arcade, public pool, or youth center doubles the possible penalty.

Possession of paraphernalia is punishable by up to six months in jail and a fine up to $1,000. Sale of paraphernalia is punishable by one to four years in prison and a fine up to $5,000.

Summary: Sixty-five percent of voters approved Question 9 on November 7, 2000, which amends the states' constitution to recognize the medical use of marijuana. The law took effect on October 1, 2001. The law removes state-level criminal penalties on the use, possession, and cultivation of marijuana by patients who have "written documentation" from their physician that marijuana may alleviate his or her condition. Patients diagnosed with the following illnesses are afforded legal protection under this act: AIDS; cancer; glaucoma; and any medical condition or treatment to a medical condition that produces cachexia, persistent muscle spasms or seizures, severe nausea or pain. Other conditions are subject to approval by the health division of the state Department of Human Resources. Patients (or their primary caregivers) may legally possess no more than one ounce of usable marijuana, and may cultivate no more than seven marijuana plants, of which no more than three may be mature. The law establishes a confidential state-run patient registry that issues identification cards to qualifying patients. Patients who do not join the registry or possess greater amounts of marijuana than allowed by law may argue the "affirmative defense of medical necessity" if they are arrested on marijuana charges.

Amendments: No.

Medical Marijuana Statutes: Nev. Rev. Stat. §§ 453A.010 - 453A.240 (2008).

Contact Information: Application information for the Nevada medical marijuana registry is available by writing or calling:

> Nevada Department of Health and Human Services,
> Nevada State Health Division
> 1000 East Williams St., Ste. 209
> Carson City, NV 89701
> 775-687-7590

New Hampshire

Possession of any amount of marijuana is a misdemeanor and is punishable by up to one year in jail and a fine up to $2,000.

Manufacture or distribution of less than one ounce of marijuana is punishable by up to three years in prison and a fine up to $25,000. For one ounce or more, the penalty increases to a possible seven years in prison and fine up to $100,000. Manufacture or distribution of five pounds or more is punishable by up to twenty years in prison and a fine up to $300,000.

Penalties for sale or distribution within one thousand feet of a school are up to two times the possible prison term and fine. Upon conviction of a person aged fifteen to eighteen years for possession with intent to sell, an additional penalty of one- to five-year driver's license suspension may be imposed. For persons aged fifteen to eighteen years convicted of possession or use, the offender's driver's license is suspended for ninety days to one year. For persons over the age of eighteen convicted of possession with intent to sell, the driver's license suspension may be for as long as life. Sale or manufacture of paraphernalia is a misdemeanor, punishable by up to one year in jail and a fine up to $2,000.

New Jersey

Possession of fifty grams or less of marijuana or being under the influence of marijuana is a disorderly persons offense, punishable by up to six months in jail and a fine of up to $1,000. Possession of greater than fifty grams is punishable by up to eighteen months in jail and a fine of up to $25,000. Any possession within one thousand feet of a school adds an additional one hundred hours or more of community service to the sentence.

Manufacture or distribution of less than one ounce of marijuana is punishable by up to eighteen months in jail and a fine up to $10,000. For amounts of one ounce or more, the penalty increases to three to five years in prison and a fine up to $25,000. Manufacture or sale of five pounds or more or cultivation of ten to fifty plants is punishable by five to ten years in prison and a fine up to $150,000. For amounts of twenty-five pounds or greater, or cultivation of greater than fifty plants, the penalties increase to ten to twenty years in prison and a fine up to $300,000.

If you are growing marijuana and caught with over ten plants, the presumption of operating a narcotics manufacturing facility occurs, which is a first-degree felony carrying ten to twenty years.

Sale or distribution of marijuana within one thousand feet of school property or on a school bus adds the imposition of a minimum sentence. For less than one ounce of marijuana, the minimum sentence imposed is between one-third and one-half of the total sentence or one year, whichever is greater. For one ounce or more, the minimum sentence imposed is between one-third and one-half of the total sentence or three years, whichever is greater. An additional fine of up to $150,000 may also be imposed for these violations.

Sale or distribution of marijuana within five hundred feet of public housing, a public park, or a public building increases the possible penalties. For sale of less than one ounce, the penalty increases by three to five years in prison and a fine up to $15,000. Sale or distribution in these zones of one ounce or more is punishable by five to ten years in prison and a fine up to $150,000.

Distribution to minors or pregnant females increases the penalty to twice the possible sentence. Use or possession of paraphernalia is punishable by up to six months in jail and a fine up to $1,000. Distribution of paraphernalia is punishable by up to eighteen months in jail and a fine up to $10,000. Any distribution of paraphernalia to a person less than eighteen years of age is punishable by three to five years in prison and a fine up to $15,000.

Summary: Governor Jon Corzine signed the New Jersey Compassionate Use Medical Marijuana Act into law on January 18, 2010. The law takes effect six months after this date. The law mandates the state to promulgate rules governing the distribution of medical cannabis to state-authorized patients. These rules shall address the creation of up to six state-licensed "alternative treatment centers." Patients diagnosed with the following illnesses are afforded legal protection under this act: cancer, glaucoma, seizure and/or spasticity disorders (including epilepsy), Lou Gehrig's disease, multiple sclerosis, muscular dystrophy, HIV/AIDS, inflammatory bowel disease (including Crohn's disease), any terminal illness if a doctor has determined the patient will die within a year. Other conditions are subject to approval by the state Department of Health. Patients authorized to use marijuana under this act will not be permitted to cultivate their own cannabis, and are limited to the possession of two ounces of marijuana per month.

For More Information:
New Jersey NORML
www.normlnj.org

Coalition for Medical Marijuana—New Jersey
www.cmmnj.org

New Mexico (M)

Possession of one ounce or less of marijuana is a petty misdemeanor, punishable by up to fifteen days in jail and a fine of $50 to $100 for the first offense. For subsequent offenses, the penalty increases to a possible one year in jail and a fine of $100 to $1,000. Possession of greater than one ounce is punishable by up to one year in jail and a fine of $100 to $1,000. For possession of eight ounces or greater, the penalty increases to up to eighteen months in jail and a fine up to $5,000.

For a first offense, manufacture or distribution of one hundred pounds or less of marijuana is punishable by up to eighteen months in prison and a fine up to $5,000. For subsequent offenses, the penalty increases to a possible three years in prison and a fine up to $5,000. For amounts greater than one hundred pounds, the penalty can be up to three years in prison and a fine up to $5,000. For subsequent offenses, the penalty increases to a possible nine years in prison and a fine up to $10,000.

Distribution to a minor is punishable by up to three years in prison and a fine up to $5,000 for the first offense and up to nine years in prison and a fine up to $10,000 for subsequent offenses. Distribution of one hundred pounds or less within a drug-free school zone is punishable by up to three years in prison and a fine up to $5,000 for the first offense and up to nine years in prison and a fine up to $10,000 for subsequent offenses. For distribution of greater than one hundred pounds within a drug-free school zone, the penalty increases to up to nine years in prison and a fine up to $10,000 for the first offense and up to eighteen years in prison and a fine up to $15,000 for subsequent offenses.

Possession of paraphernalia is punishable by up to one year in jail and a fine of $50 to $100. Delivery of paraphernalia is punishable by up to one year in jail and a fine up to $1,000, unless the delivery was to a minor at least three years younger than the offender, in which case the penalty increases to a possible eighteen months in jail and a fine up to $5,000.

Summary: Governor Bill Richardson signed Senate Bill 523, "Lynn and Erin Compassionate Use Act," into law on April 2, 2007. The new law took effect on July 1, 2007. The law mandates the state Department of Health by October 1, 2007, to promulgate rules governing the use and distribution of medical cannabis to state-authorized patients. These rules shall address the creation of state-licensed "cannabis production facilities," the development of a confidential patient registry and a state-authorized marijuana distribution system, and "define the amount of cannabis that is necessary to constitute an adequate supply" for qualified patients.

Amendments: Yes. In January 2009, the New Mexico Department of Health finalized rules governing the production, distribution, and use of medicinal cannabis under state law. Patients registered with the state Department of Health and who are diagnosed with the following illnesses are afforded legal protection under these rules: Arthritis, severe chronic pain, painful peripheral neuropathy, intractable nausea/vomiting, severe anorexia/cachexia, hepatitis C infection currently receiving antiviral treatment, Crohn's disease, Post-traumatic Stress Disorder, Amyotrophic Lateral Sclerosis (Lou Gehrig's disease), Cancer, Glaucoma, Multiple sclerosis, damage to the nervous tissue of the spinal cord with intractable spasticity, epilepsy, HIV/AIDS, and hospice patients.

Other conditions are subject to approval by the Department of Health. Patients may legally possess six ounces of medical cannabis (or more if authorized by their physician) and/or 16 plants (four mature, twelve immature) under this act.

State regulations also authorize nonprofit facilities to apply with the state to produce and dispense medical cannabis. State licensed producers may grow up to 95 mature plants at one time.

Medical Marijuana Statutes: Lynn and Erin Compassionate Use Act, N.M. Stat. Ann. § 30-31C-1 (2007).

Contact Information: Please contact the Medical Cannabis Program Coordinator at (505) 827-2321 or medical.cannabis@state.nm.us or visit www .nmhealth.org/marijuanahtml for more information.

New York (D)

Possession of twenty-five grams or less of marijuana is punishable by a fine of $100 for the first offense. For the second offense, the penalty increases to a $200 fine, and for subsequent offenses the fine increases to $250 and a maximum of fifteen days in jail time may be imposed. Possession of greater than twenty-five grams or possession of any amount in public where the marijuana is burning or open to public view is a class B misdemeanor and is punishable by up to three months in jail and a fine up to $500.

For possession of greater than two ounces, the penalty increases to a possible one year in jail and a fine up to $1,000. Possession of greater than eight ounces increases the penalties to a possible one to one-and-a-half years in prison and a fine up to $5,000. The penalties for possession of greater than sixteen ounces are one to two-and-a-half years in prison and a fine up to $5,000. For possession of any amount greater than ten pounds, the penalty is one to five-and-a-half years in prison and a fine up to $5,000.

Delivery or manufacture of two grams or less of marijuana for no remuneration is punishable by up to three months in jail and a fine up to $500. For delivery or manufacture of twenty-five grams or less, the penalty is up to one year in jail and a fine up to $1,000. For amounts greater than twenty-five grams, the penalty increases to one to one-and-a-half years in jail and a fine up to $5,000. Delivery or manufacture of greater than four ounces is punishable by one to two-and-a-half years in prison and a fine up to $5,000. For any amount greater than sixteen ounces, the penalty increases to one to five-and-a-half years in prison and a fine up to $5,000.

Any sale or delivery to a minor is punishable by one to two-and-a-half years in prison and a fine up to $5,000. Possession or sale of paraphernalia is punishable by up to one year in jail or a fine up to $1,000.

North Carolina (D)

Possession of one-half ounce or less is punishable by up to thirty days in jail, most likely suspended. Possession of greater than one-half ounce is punishable by one to 120 days in jail, with a possibility of community service or probation in lieu of jail. Possession greater than 1.5 ounces increases the penalties to up to twelve months in jail.

Manufacture, cultivation, sale, or delivery of less than five grams for no remuneration (payment, barter, or exchange of any kind) is considered possession and not sale. For amounts of ten pounds or less, the penalty is up to twelve months in jail.

Penalties for sale, delivery, or manufacture are increased if the sale occurs within three hundred feet of a school zone if the offender is over twenty-one and if the sale was made to a minor or to a pregnant woman. Possession of paraphernalia is punishable by up to six months in jail.

North Dakota

Possession of less than one-half ounce of marijuana is a misdemeanor, punishable by up to thirty days in jail and a fine of up to $1,000. Possession of one-half ounce or more is punishable by up to one year in jail and a fine of up to $2,000. First convictions for possession of one ounce or less of marijuana can be expunged from the record after two years if no further criminal violations occur. Possession of greater than one ounce of marijuana is punishable by up to five years in prison and a fine up to $5,000.

Possession of less than one-half ounce while operating a motor vehicle is punishable by up to one year in jail and a fine of up to $1,000. Sale, distribution, or manufacture of less than one hundred pounds of marijuana is punishable by up to ten years in prison and a fine up to $10,000. For amounts of one hundred pounds or more, the penalty increases to a possible twenty years in prison and a fine up to $10,000.

Penalties for sale or distribution increase if the sale occurs within one thousand feet of a school.

All convictions also require the offender to undergo a drug addiction evaluation.

Ohio (D)

Possession of less than one hundred grams of marijuana is a citable offense only, with a fine of $100. Possession of one hundred grams or more is punishable by a fine of up to $250. For possession of two hundred grams or more, the penalty increases to a possible sentence of six months to one year in jail. Possession of one thousand grams or more is punishable by one to five years in prison. Any possession of less than five thousand grams does not carry the presumption of prison, which leaves available the possibility of probation. Possession of five thousand grams of marijuana or more is punishable by one to five years in prison. For any amount of twenty thousand grams or more, the penalty increases to a mandatory minimum sentence of eight years in prison.

Delivery of twenty grams or less, for no remuneration, is considered possession and is punished with a fine of $100. Sale or distribution of less than two hundred grams carries a penalty of six to eighteen months in jail. Sale or distribution of two hundred grams or more is punishable by one to five years in prison. Sale or distribution of six hundred grams or greater carries a mandatory minimum sentence of six months and a possible two- to eight-year sentence.

Sale to minors, sale within one thousand feet of a school, sale within one hundred feet of a juvenile, and previous felony drug convictions all increase the penalty for the sale or distribution of marijuana. Possession of paraphernalia is punishable by up to thirty days in jail and sale of paraphernalia is punishable by up to ninety days in jail.

For all drug convictions, including minor misdemeanors, the offender's driver's license is also suspended for a period of six months to five years. Professional licenses are also suspended.

Oklahoma

Possession of any amount of marijuana is punishable by up to one year in jail for the first offense and two to ten years in prison for subsequent offenses. Conditional discharge is available to first-time offenders. Cultivation of one thousand plants or less is punishable by two years to life in prison and a fine up to $20,000. Cultivation of greater than one thousand plants is punishable by twenty years to life in prison and a fine up to $50,000.

Sale or delivery of less than twenty-five pounds is punishable by two years to life in prison and a fine of $20,000. For sale or delivery of twenty-five pounds or more, the penalties increase to four years to life in prison and a fine of $25,000 to $100,000. Sale or delivery of one thousand pounds or more is also punishable by four years to life in prison, but the fine increases to $100,000 to $500,000. Any sale to a minor doubles the penalties. Sale within two thousand feet of schools, public parks, or public housing doubles the available penalties and carries a mandatory minimum sentence of 50 percent of the imposed sentence.

A person eighteen years of age or over who delivers/sells drug paraphernalia to a person under eighteen years of age shall, upon conviction, be guilty of a felony, which causes a driver's license suspension for six months to three years. Any person convicted of any offense described in this section shall, in addition to any fine imposed, pay a special assessment trauma-care fee of one hundred dollars to be deposited into the Trauma Care Assistance Revolving Fund.

If a person who has never been previously convicted of offenses under any statute of the United States or of any state relating to narcotic drugs, marijuana, or stimulant, depressant, or hallucinogenic drugs pleads guilty to or is found guilty of possession of a controlled dangerous substance, the court may, without entering a judgment of guilt and with the consent of such person, defer further proceedings and place him on probation upon such reasonable terms and conditions as it may require, including the requirement that such person cooperate in a treatment and rehabilitation program of a state-supported or state-approved facility, if available.

Any student loan, grant, fellowship, teaching fellowship, or other means of financial assistance authorized by and/or under the control of the Oklahoma State Regents for Higher Education, any operating board of regents of Oklahoma universities or colleges, or any employee or employees of any university, college, or other institution of higher learning, whether such loan, grant, fellowship, teaching fellowship, or other means of financial assistance be financed by state or federal funds, or both, may be revoked or terminated by the person or persons authorizing and/or controlling same for any of the following reasons: unlawful manufacture, preparation, delivery, sale, offering for sale, barter, furnishing, giving away, possession, control, use, or administering of narcotic drugs, marijuana, barbiturates, or stimulants.

Oregon (D, M)

Possession of less than one ounce of marijuana is punishable by a fine of $500 to $1,000. Possession of one ounce or more is punishable by up to ten years in prison. Conditional discharge is possible for possession offenses.

Possession of greater than 110 grams is considered a commercial drug offense and penalties are substantially greater, depending on the prior record of the offender.

Delivery of less than five grams, for no remuneration, is punishable by a fine of $500 to $1,000. Delivery for no remuneration of less than one ounce is punishable by up to one year in jail and a fine of up to $5,000. Any sale of marijuana is punishable by up to ten years in prison and a fine of up to $100,000.

Possession of one ounce or less or cultivation of three plants or fewer is lawful for any person who possesses a registry identification card indicating that the person is a patient who uses marijuana for medicinal purposes. This is an affirmative defense to any charges of possession or cultivation within the amount limits.

If you are over seventeen years old and deliver any amount of marijuana to a minor who is at least three years younger than you (whether or not you receive something for it), you have committed a class A felony punishable by a maximum sentence of twenty years and a $100,000 fine.

Any sale to a minor, at least three years younger than the offender, or any sale within one thousand feet of a school is punishable by up to twenty years in prison and a fine of up to $300,000.

Manufacturing any amount of marijuana is a very serious offense. "Manufacturing" means growing even one plant and packaging, repackaging, labeling, or relabeling marijuana. Manufacturing marijuana is a class A felony punishable by a maximum sentence of twenty years in prison and a $100,000 fine.

Knowingly maintaining, visiting, or even staying at a place where people are using, storing, or selling marijuana is a class A misdemeanor punishable by up to a year in jail and a $5,000 fine. However, if the amount of marijuana is one ounce or less, and it is just kept or used on the premises, the fine is $100 and not a criminal conviction.

Any manufacture of marijuana is punishable by up to twenty years in prison and a fine of up to $300,000. Sale of paraphernalia is punishable by up to one year in jail and a fine of up to $5,000. A conviction for manufacturing, possessing, or delivering marijuana, or for driving under the influence of marijuana, will result in a six-month driver's license suspension, unless the court finds compelling circumstances not to order the suspension of driving privileges.

Summary: Fifty-five percent of voters approved Measure 67 on November 3, 1998. The law took effect on December 3, 1998. It removes state-level criminal penalties on the use, possession, and cultivation of marijuana by patients who possess a signed recommendation from their physician stating that marijuana "may mitigate" his or her debilitating symptoms. Patients diagnosed with the following illnesses are afforded legal protection under this act: cachexia; cancer; chronic pain; epilepsy and other disorders characterized by seizures; glaucoma; HIV or AIDS; multiple sclerosis and other disorders characterized by muscle spasticity; and nausea. Other conditions are subject to approval by the Health Division of the Oregon Department of Human Resources. Patients (or their primary caregivers) may legally possess no more than three ounces of usable marijuana, and may cultivate no more than seven marijuana plants, of which no more than three may be mature. The law establishes a confidential state-run patient registry that issues identification cards to qualifying patients. Patients who do not join the registry or possess greater amounts of marijuana than allowed by law may argue the "affirmative defense of medical necessity" if they are arrested on marijuana charges.

Amendments: Yes. House Bill 3052, which took effect on July 21, 1999, mandates that patients (or their caregivers) may only cultivate marijuana in one location, and requires that patients must be diagnosed by their physicians at least 12 months prior to an arrest in order to present an "affirmative defense." This bill also states that law enforcement officials who seize marijuana from a patient pending trial do not have to keep those plants alive. Last year the Oregon Board of Health approved agitation due to Alzheimer's disease to the list of debilitating conditions qualifying for legal protection.

In August 2001, program administrators filed established temporary procedures further defining the relationship between physicians and patients. The new rule defines attending physician as "a physician who has established a physician/patient relationship with the patient; . . . is primarily responsible for the care and treatment of the patients; . . . has reviewed a patient's medical records at the patient's request, has conducted a thorough physical examination of the patient, has provided a treatment plan and/or follow-up care, and has documented these activities in a patient file."

Also, Senate Bill 1085, which took effect on January 1, 2006, raises the quantity of cannabis that authorized patients may possess from seven plants (with no more than three mature) and three ounces of cannabis to six mature cannabis plants, 18 immature seedlings, and 24 ounces of usable cannabis. However, those state-qualified patients who possess cannabis in amounts exceeding the new state guidelines will no longer retain the ability to argue an "affirmative defense" of medical necessity at trial. Patients who fail to register with the state, but who possess medical cannabis in amounts compliant with state law, still retain the ability to raise an "affirmative defense" at trial.

Other amendments to Oregon's medical marijuana law redefine "mature plants" to include only those cannabis plants that are more than twelve inches in height and diameter, and establish a state-registry for those authorized to produce medical cannabis to qualified patients.

Medical Marijuana Statutes: Oregon Medical Marijuana Act, Or. Rev. Stat. § 475.300 (2007).

Contact Information: Application information for the Oregon medical marijuana registry is available online or by writing:

Oregon Department of Human Services
800 NE Oregon St.
Portland, OR 97232
(503) 731-4000
http://egov.oregon.gov/DHS/ph/ommp/index.shtml

Oregon Cannabis Patients registry: 1 (877) 600-6767

Pennsylvania

Possession of thirty grams or less of marijuana is a misdemeanor, punishable by up to thirty days in jail and a fine of up to $500. The penalties for possession of greater than thirty grams increase to a possible one-year prison term and a fine up to $5,000.

Delivery for no remuneration of thirty grams or less of marijuana is treated as possession with a possible penalty of thirty days in jail and a fine up to $500. Cultivation, delivery, or sale of one thousand pounds or less is punishable by up to five years in prison and a fine of up to $15,000. For amounts greater than one thousand pounds, the penalty increases to a possible ten years in prison and a fine up to $100,000. The court is authorized to increase the fines beyond the maximum to exhaust the proceeds of the crime. Sale or distribution to a minor by a person over the age of twenty-one doubles the possible penalties.

Delivery of marijuana within one thousand feet of a school or within 250 feet of a recreational playground is punishable by two to four years in prison. Possession or sale of paraphernalia is punishable by up to one year in jail and a fine up to $2,500, unless the sale was to a minor, in which case the possible penalties double. For first offenders, the court may grant probation without verdict.

Any second or subsequent drug conviction increases the possible penalties to twice those for first-time offenders.

Rhode Island (M)

Possession of less than one kilogram of marijuana is punishable by up to one year in jail and a fine of $200 to $500.

Driving while in possession of marijuana is penalized by suspension of the offender's driver's license for six months for the first offense and for one year for subsequent offenses.

Manufacture or delivery of less than one kilogram of marijuana is punishable by up to thirty years in prison and a fine of $3,000 to $100,000. Delivery to a minor at least three years younger than the offender adds an additional two to five years in prison and a fine up to $10,000. Sale or possession within three hundred yards of a school, public park, or playground doubles the possible penalties.

Convictions for possession, manufacture, or sale of one kilogram or more carry mandatory minimum sentences. For five kilograms or less, the penalty is a mandatory minimum sentence of ten years in prison with a maximum of fifty years and a fine of $10,000 to $500,000. For more than five kilograms, the penalty is a mandatory minimum sentence of twenty years in prison with a maximum of life in prison and a fine of $25,000 to $100,000.

For sentences of probation with no imprisonment, the offender is required to undergo a drug abuse evaluation, attend a drug education course, and perform one hundred hours of community service.

Summary: The Edward O. Hawkins and Thomas C. Slater Medical Marijuana Act took effect immediately upon passage on January 3, 2006. The law removes state-level criminal penalties on the use, possession, and cultivation of marijuana by patients who possess "written certification" from their physician stating, "In the practitioner's professional opinion, the potential benefits of the medical use of marijuana would likely outweigh the health risks for the qualifying patient." Patients diagnosed with the following illnesses are afforded legal protection under this act: cachexia; cancer; glaucoma; Hepatitis C; severe, debilitating, chronic pain; severe nausea; seizures, including but not limited to, those characteristic of epilepsy; or severe and persistent muscle spasms, including but not limited to, those characteristic of multiple sclerosis or Crohn's disease; or agitation of Alzheimer's disease. Other conditions are subject to approval by the Rhode Island Department of Health. Patients (and/or their primary caregivers) may legally possess 2.5 ounces of cannabis and/or twelve plants, and their cannabis must be stored in an indoor facility. The law establishes a mandatory, confidential state-run patient registry that issues identification cards to qualifying patients. Patients who do not register with the Department of Health, but have received certification from their physician to use medicinal cannabis, may raise an affirmative defense at trial.

Valid medical marijuana registry cards from other medical marijuana states are recognized in this state, so long as the cardholder is in compliance with the possession limits imposed on cardholders in this state.

Amendments: Yes. In June 2007, the Rhode Island House and Senate enacted legislation eliminating the sunset clause of the The Edward O. Hawkins and Thomas C. Slater Medical Marijuana Act, making the provisional program permanent

Medical Marijuana Statutes: The Edward O. Hawkins and Thomas C. Slater Medical Marijuana Act, R.I. Gen. Laws § 21-28.6 (2006).

Contact Information: www.health.state.ri.us
Application Forms are available at www.health.ri.gov/hsr/mmp/index.php or by visiting room 104 at the Health Department, 3 Capitol Hill, Providence.

More helpful information can be found here: http://ripatients.org.

South Carolina
Possession of one ounce or less is punishable by up to thirty days in jail and a fine of $100 to $200 for a first offense. For subsequent offenses the penalties increase to up to a year in jail and a fine of $200 to $1,000.

Convictions for a first offense are eligible for conditional discharges. Possession of greater than one ounce is considered evidence of intent to sell and is punished as such.

Sale or delivery of less than ten pounds of marijuana is punishable by up to five years in prison and a fine up to $5,000. Sale or delivery of ten pounds or more is considered trafficking, and all trafficking offenses are subject to mandatory minimum sentences. For trafficking of less than one hundred pounds, the mandatory minimum sentence is one year with a maximum of ten years and a fine of $10,000. For sale or delivery of less than two thousand pounds the mandatory minimum sentence is twenty-five years in prison and a fine of $25,000. For less than ten thousand pounds the penalty is also a minimum of twenty-five years in prison, and the fine increases to $50,000. For amounts of ten thousand pounds or more, the mandatory minimum is twenty-five years with a maximum of thirty and a fine of $200,000.

Sale to a minor or within a one-half-mile radius of a school, public park, or playground is a separate offense and carries a penalty of up to ten years in prison and a fine up to $10,000.

Cultivation of fewer than one hundred marijuana plants is punishable by up to five years in prison and a fine of up to $5,000. Cultivation of one hundred marijuana plants or more is punishable by a mandatory minimum sentence of twenty-five years in prison and a fine of $25,000. For more than one thousand plants, the mandatory minimum stays at twenty-five years, but the fine increases to $50,000. For greater than ten thousand plants, the mandatory minimum sentence is twenty-five years, with a maximum of thirty years and a fine of $200,000.

Possession of paraphernalia is punishable by a civil fine of $500.

South Dakota

Possession of two ounces or less of marijuana is a misdemeanor and is punishable by up to one year in jail and a fine up to $1,000. Possession of less than eight ounces is punishable by up to two years in prison and a fine up to $2,000. For less than one pound, the penalty increases to a possible five years in prison and a fine up to $5,000. Possession of ten pounds or less carries up to ten years in prison and a fine up to $10,000. For amounts over ten pounds, the penalty is up to fifteen years in prison and a fine up to $15,000.

A positive urine test or other evidence of recent marijuana use is considered possession and is punished as such.

Inhabiting a room where marijuana is being stored or used is punishable by up to one year in jail and a fine of up to $1,000.

Transferring less than one-half ounce of marijuana for no remuneration is punishable by not less than fifteen days and not more than one year in jail and a fine up to $1,000. Cultivation, delivery, or sale of one ounce or less is punishable by up to two years in prison and a fine up to $2,000. For amounts less than eight ounces, the penalties increase to a possible five years in prison and a fine up to $5,000. Cultivation, delivery, or sale of less than one pound carries a penalty of up to ten years in prison and a fine up to $10,000. For any amounts of one pound or more, the penalty increases to a possible fifteen years in prison and a fine up to $15,000.

All convictions for sale, cultivation, or distribution carry a mandatory minimum sentence of thirty days for the first offense and one year for the second or subsequent offense.

Any sale to a minor is punishable by up to ten years in prison and a fine of up to $10,000. Any sale within one thousand feet of a school or within five hundred feet of a youth center, public pool, or video arcade carries a penalty of a five-year mandatory minimum prison sentence.

The use or possession of paraphernalia is punishable by up to thirty days in jail and a fine up to $200.

Tennessee

Possession, delivery, or sale of one-half ounce or less is punishable by up to one year in jail and a fine up to $2,500.

For delivery or sale of amounts over one-half ounce the penalty increases to one to six years in prison and a fine up to $5,000. Delivery or sale of ten pounds or more is punishable by two to twelve years in prison and a fine up to $5,000. For amounts of seventy pounds or more, the penalty increases to eight to thirty years in prison and a fine up to $200,000. Delivery or sale of three hundred pounds or more carries a penalty of fifteen to sixty years in prison and a fine up to $500,000.

Any sale to a minor or any sale within one thousand feet of a school increases the penalty classification one level.

Cultivation of ten to nineteen plants is punishable by two to twelve years in prison and a fine up to $50,000. For cultivation of twenty to ninety-nine plants, the penalty increases to three to fifteen years in prison and a fine up to $100,000. For 100 to 499 plants, the penalty increases to eight to thirty years in prison and a fine up to $200,000. Cultivation of five hundred or more plants is punishable by fifteen to sixty years in prison and a fine up to $500,000.

For all first convictions for misdemeanor drug offenses, there is a mandatory minimum fine of $250. For second convictions, the mandatory minimum increases to $500 and for subsequent convictions, it increases to $1,000. For all first convictions of felony drug offenses, there is a mandatory minimum fine of $2,000, increasing to $3,000 for second convictions and to $5,000 for any subsequent convictions.

The use or possession of paraphernalia is punishable by up to one year in jail and a fine up to $2,500. Sale of paraphernalia carries a penalty of one to six years in prison and a fine up to $3,000.

Texas

Possession of two ounces or less of marijuana is punishable by up to 180 days in jail and a fine up to $2,000.*

Possession of greater than two ounces is punishable by up to one year in jail and a fine up to $4,000. For greater than four ounces, the penalty increases to 180 days to two years in jail and a fine up to $10,000. Possession of greater than five pounds carries a penalty of two to ten years in prison and a fine up to $10,000. For greater than fifty pounds, the penalties increase to two to twenty years in prison and a fine up to $10,000. For any amount greater than two thousand pounds, the penalty is five to ninety-nine years and a fine up to $50,000.

The penalty for delivery, without remuneration, of one-quarter of an ounce or less is up to 180 days in jail and a fine up to $2,000. For delivery or sale of one-quarter of an ounce or less, the penalty is up to one year in jail and a fine of up to $ 3,000. For delivery or sale of amounts greater than one-quarter ounce of marijuana the penalty increases to 180 days to two years in jail and a fine up to $10,000. Sale or delivery of greater than five pounds is punishable by two to twenty years in prison and a fine up to $10,000. The penalty for delivery or sale of greater than fifty pounds is five to ninety-nine years in prison and a fine up to $10,000. For any amount of two thousand pounds or greater, the penalty is a mandatory minimum ten to ninety-nine years in prison and a fine up to $100,000.

---

*With no prior felony convictions, if a person is convicted of possession of less than one pound of marijuana, a judge must impose a sentence of probation with mandatory drug treatment. If no treatment center exists within the jurisdiction, the judge may waive the treatment requirement. The judge can also waive all fines.

Any sale to a minor is punishable by two to twenty years in prison and a fine up to $10,000. Sale within one thousand feet of a school or within three hundred feet of a youth center, public pool, or video arcade increases the penalty classification to the next highest level.

Repeat Misdemeanor Offenses:
- If charged with a Class A misdemeanor and defendant has been before convicted of a Class A misdemeanor or any degree of felony = ninety days to one year; $4,000
- If charged with a Class B misdemeanor and defendant has been before convicted of a Class A or Class B misdemeanor or any degree of felony = thirty days to 180 days; $2,000
- If charged with a Class C misdemeanor and defendant has been before convicted under one or a combination of the two above three times and the prior offense was committed within twenty-four months of incident = more than 180 days; $2,000

Repeat Felony Offenses:
- If charged with a state jail felony punishable and defendant has previously been finally convicted of two state jail felonies, on conviction the defendant shall be punished for a third-degree felony.
- If charged with a state jail felony punishable and defendant has previously been finally convicted of two felonies, and the second previous felony conviction is for an offense that occurred subsequent to the first previous conviction having become final, on conviction the defendant shall be punished for a second-degree felony.
- If charged with a state jail felony or of a third-degree felony and defendant has been once before convicted of a felony, on conviction he shall be punished for a second-degree felony.
- If charged with a second-degree felony and the defendant has been once before convicted of a felony, on conviction he shall be punished for a first-degree felony.
- If it is a first-degree felony and defendant has been once before convicted of a felony, on conviction he shall be punished by imprisonment in the institutional division of the Texas Department of Criminal Justice for life, or for any term of not more than ninety-nine years or less than fifteen years. In addition to imprisonment, an individual maybe punished by a fine not to exceed $10,000.

Utah

Any conviction results in a six-month driver's license suspension.

Possession of less than one ounce of marijuana is punishable by up to six months in jail and a fine up to $1,000. For possession of one ounce or more, the penalty increases to up to one year in jail and a fine up to $2,500. Amounts of one pound or more carry a penalty of up to five years in prison and a fine up to $5,000. Possession of greater than one hundred pounds is punishable by one to fifteen years in prison and a fine up to $10,000.

The penalty for sale or delivery of marijuana is up to five years in prison and a fine up to $5,000. Sale in the presence of a minor or sale within one thousand feet of a school, public park, amusement park, recreation center, church, synagogue, shopping mall, sports facility, theater, or public parking lot increases the level of the offense to the next highest degree.

Possession of paraphernalia is punishable by up to six months in jail and a fine up to $1,000. The penalty for sale of paraphernalia is up to one year in jail and a fine up to $2,500, unless the sale was to a minor, in which case the penalty increases to up to five years in prison and a fine up to $5,000.

Vermont (M)

Possession of less than two ounces of marijuana is punishable by up to six months in jail and a fine up to $500 for the first offense. For a second offense the penalty increases to a possible two years in prison and a fine up to $2,000. There is a possibility of deferred sentencing for first offenders. For possession of two ounces or more, the penalty is up to three years in prison and a fine up to $10,000. Possession of one pound or more is punishable by up to five years in prison and a fine up to $100,000. Possession of ten pounds or more carries a penalty of up to fifteen years in prison and a fine up to $500,000.

Cultivation of more than three plants is punishable by up to three years in prison and a fine up to $10,000. For more than ten plants, the penalties increase to a possible five years in prison and a fine up to $100,000. Cultivation of more than twenty-five plants carries a penalty up to fifteen years in prison and a fine up to $500,000.

Sale or delivery of less than one-half ounce of marijuana is punishable by up to two years in prison and a fine up to $10,000. For amounts of one-half ounce or more, the penalties increase to a possible five years in prison and a fine up to $100,000. Sale or delivery of one pound or more carries a penalty of up to fifteen years in jail and a fine up to $500,000.

Anyone over eighteen who delivers marijuana to a minor who is at least three years his junior faces an additional penalty of up to five years in prison and a fine up to $25,000. Any sale of marijuana to a minor or any sale on school grounds or on a school bus carries an additional sentence of up to ten years in prison.

Sale of paraphernalia is punishable by up to one year in jail and a fine of up to $1,000

Summary: Senate Bill 76 became law without Gov. James Douglas' signature on May 26, 2004. The law took effect on July 1, 2004. The law removes state-level criminal penalties on the use, possession, and cultivation of marijuana by patients diagnosed with a "debilitating medical condition." Patients diagnosed with the following illnesses are afforded legal protection under this act: HIV or AIDS, cancer, and multiple sclerosis. Patients (or their primary caregiver) may legally possess no more than two ounces of usable marijuana, and may cultivate no more than three marijuana plants, of which no more than one may be mature. The law establishes a mandatory, confidential state-run registry that issues identification cards to qualifying patients.

Amendments: Yes. Senate Bill 7, which took effect on July 1, 2007, expands the definition of "debilitating medical condition" to include: "(A) cancer, multiple sclerosis, positive status for human immunodeficiency virus, acquired immune deficiency syndrome, or the treatment of these conditions, if the disease or the treatment results in severe, persistent, and intractable symptoms; or (B) a disease, medical condition, or its treatment that is chronic, debilitating, and produces severe, persistent, and one or more of the following intractable symptoms: cachexia or wasting syndrome; severe pain; severe nausea; or seizures."

The measure also raises the quantity of medical cannabis patients may legally possess under state law from one mature and/or two immature plants to two mature and/or seven immature plants. Senate Bill 7 also amends state law so that licensed physicians in neighboring states can legally recommend cannabis to Vermont patients.

Medical Marijuana Statutes: Therapeutic Use of Cannabis, Vt. Stat. Ann. tit. 18, §§ 4471- 4474d (2003).

Contact Information:
Marijuana Registry
Department of Public Safety
103 South Main Street
Waterbury, Vermont 05671
802-241-5115
www.safeaccessnow.org/article.php?id=2012

Virginia

Possession of marijuana is punishable by up to thirty days in jail and a fine up to $500 for the first offense and up to one year in jail and a fine up to $2,500 for subsequent offenses.

Cultivation of marijuana is punishable by five to thirty years in prison and a fine up to $10,000. A conviction for manufacturing marijuana must include proof that the marijuana was being grown for a purpose other than the grower's personal use.

The delivery or sale of one-half ounce of marijuana or less is punishable by up to one year in jail and a fine up to $2,500. For greater than one-half ounce, the penalties increase to a possible one to ten years in prison and a fine up to $2,500. Sale or delivery of greater than five pounds carries a penalty of five to thirty years in prison. Any amount of one hundred kilograms or greater is punishable by a mandatory minimum sentence of twenty years in prison with a possible maximum of life in prison and a fine of up to $1,000,000.

Any sale to a minor carries a penalty of ten to fifty years in prison and a fine of up to $100,000. Any sale within one thousand feet of a school, school bus, school bus stop, recreation center, public library, or state hospital is punishable by one to five years in prison and a fine up to $100,000.

Transporting five pounds or more into the state with the intent to sell carries a sentence of five to forty years in prison, with a three-year mandatory minimum sentence, and a fine of up to $1,000,000.

Probation with deferred proceedings is possible for first offenders in some instances.

The sale of paraphernalia is punishable by up to one year in jail and a fine up to $2,500, unless the sale was to a minor, in which case the penalty increases to one to five years in prison and a fine up to $2,500.

Washington (M)

Possession of less than forty grams is punishable by up to ninety days in jail and a fine up to $1,000. For amounts of forty grams or more the penalties increase to up to five years in prison and a fine up to $10,000.

Cultivation, delivery, or sale of marijuana is punishable by up to five years in prison and a fine up to $10,000. Any sale to a minor at least three years younger than the offender doubles the possible penalties.

It is an affirmative defense to violations of marijuana-related laws that the person, possessing no more than is necessary for personal medical use for up to sixty days, has valid documentation and meets all criteria as a qualifying patient or as a primary caregiver.

Possession, manufacture, or delivery of paraphernalia is punishable by up to ninety days in jail and a fine up to $1,000. Any convictions of a misdemeanor carry a twenty-four-hour mandatory minimum jail sentence and a mandatory minimum fine of $250. For any subsequent convictions the possible prison sentence doubles. For drug offense convictions of juveniles, the offender's driver's license is suspended for one year.

Summary: Fifty-nine percent of voters approved Measure 692 on November 3, 1998. The law took effect on that day. It removes state-level criminal penalties on the use, possession, and cultivation of marijuana by patients who possess "valid documentation" from their physician affirming that he or she suffers from a debilitating condition and that the "potential benefits of the medical use of marijuana would likely outweigh the health risks." Patients diagnosed with the following illnesses are afforded legal protection under this act: cachexia; cancer; HIV or AIDS; epilepsy; glaucoma; intractable pain (defined as pain unrelieved by standard treatment or medications); and multiple sclerosis. Other conditions are subject to approval by the Washington Board of Health. Patients (or their primary caregivers) may legally possess or cultivate no more than a 60-day supply of marijuana. The law does not establish a state-run patient registry.

Amendments: Yes. Senate Bill 6032, mandated the Department of Health to "adopt rules defining the quantity of marijuana that could reasonably be presumed to be a sixty-day supply for qualifying patients." In October 2008, the department finalized guidelines allowing patients to cultivate up to 15 cannabis plants and/or possess up to 24 ounces of usable marijuana. The new limits took effect on November 2, 2008.

Patients who possess larger quantities of cannabis than those approved by the Department will continue to receive legal protection under the law if they present evidence indicating that they require such amounts to adequately treat their qualifying medical condition.

Senate Bill 6032 also affirmed changes previously recommended by the state's Medical Quality Assurance Commission to expand the state's list of qualifying conditions to include Crohn's disease, hepatitis C, and any "diseases, including anorexia, which result in nausea, vomiting, wasting, appetite loss, cramping, seizures, muscle spasms, and/or spasticity, when these symptoms are unrelieved by standard treatments or medications."

It also limits the ability of police to seize medicinal cannabis that is "determined . . . [to be] possessed lawfully [by an authorized patient] under the . . . law."

Additional Amendments: Yes. Senate Bill 5798 allows additional health care professionals, including naturopaths, physician's assistants, osteopathic physicians, osteopathic physicians assistants, and advanced registered nurse practitioners to legally recommend marijuana therapy to their patients. The new law will take effect on June 10, 2010.

Medical Marijuana Statutes: Wash. Rev. Code §§ 69.51A - 69.51A.901 (2007).

Contact Information: Fact sheets outlining Washington's medical marijuana law are available from:

Washington State Department of Health
1112 SE Quince St.
P.O. Box 47890
Olympia, WA 98504-7890
(800) 525-0127 or (360) 236-4052
Attention: Glenda Moore
www.doh.wa.gov

ACLU of Washington, Drug Reform Project
(206) 624-2184
www.aclu-wa.org/detail.cfm?id=182

West Virginia

Possession of marijuana is punishable by ninety days to six months in jail and a fine up to $1,000. Possession with intent to manufacture or deliver a controlled substance is a felony and can result in imprisonment of not less than one year and not more than five years, or a fine of $15,000 dollars, or both.

Conviction of possession of less than fifteen grams triggers an automatic conditional discharge. Conditional discharge does not apply to a defendant who has previously been convicted of any offense relating to narcotic drugs or marijuana.

Cultivation, delivery, or sale is punishable by one to five years in prison and a fine up to $15,000. Sale to a minor or sale within one thousand feet of a school requires a two-year mandatory minimum sentence for the sale.

Transportation of marijuana into the state with the intent to deliver is punishable by one to five years in prison and a fine up to $15,000. Subsequent offenses double the possible penalties. Operating an illegal drug paraphernalia business is punishable by six months to one year in jail and a fine up to $5,000.

Wisconsin

Possession of marijuana is punishable by six months in jail and/or a fine of $1,000 for the first offense, and for second or subsequent offenses (includes *any* prior controlled substance conviction), three-and-a-half years in jail and a fine of $10,000. Conditional discharge is available for first offenders. Possession within one thousand feet of a school, school bus, public park, public pool, youth center or community center adds an additional one hundred hours of community service to the sentence for possession.

Manufacture/distribution/delivery/possession with intent of two hundred grams or less of marijuana is punishable by three-and-a-half years in prison and a fine of $10,000. For amounts greater than two hundred grams, the penalty increases to six to fifteen years in prison and a fine of $10,000 to $25,000.

If a person seventeen years of age or over delivers a controlled substance to a person seventeen years of age or under who is at least three years his or her junior, the applicable maximum term of imprisonment may be increased by five years. Sale within one thousand feet of a school, school bus, public park, public pool, youth center, community center, treatment facility, jail, or public housing project adds five years to the maximum possible prison term.

Distribution or sale on a public transit vehicle also increases the maximum possible prison sentence by five years.

Possession of paraphernalia is punishable by up to thirty days in jail and a fine up to $500. Delivery or possession with intent to distribute is punishable by up to ninety days in jail and a fine up to $1,000, unless the sale or delivery was to a minor, in which case the penalties increase to a possible nine months in jail and a fine up to $10,000.

Upon conviction of a drug offense, the offender's driver's license is suspended for six months to five years.

Wyoming

Using or being under the influence of marijuana is punishable by up to ninety days in jail and a fine up to $100. Possession of three ounces or less of marijuana is punishable by up to one year in jail and a fine up to $1,000. Possession of greater than three ounces carries a penalty of up to five years in prison and a fine up to $10,000. Any possession within five hundred feet of a school increases the fine by $500. First offenders may be placed on conditional probation and may have the proceedings discharged.

Cultivation of marijuana is punishable by up to six months in jail and a fine of up to $1,000. Sale or delivery of marijuana is punishable by up to ten years in prison and a fine up to $10,000. Sale to a minor at least three years younger than the offender doubles the possible prison sentence. Sale within five hundred feet of a school requires a mandatory minimum sentence of two years in prison and a fine up to $1,000.

Second and subsequent offenses are subject to double the possible penalties.

9

On Ending Prohibition

Ethan Nadelmann, J.D., Ph.D.

This is a slightly edited transcript of a speech given by Ethan Nadelmann at the NAACP Centennial Conference held at the Manhattan Hilton Hotel in New York on July 13, 2009.*

Good afternoon to all of you.

Let me begin by saying that the views I hold are held by people who are white, black, brown, yellow, red, and everything in between. They are held by Republicans, Democrats, and Independents. They are held by people who have been addicted to drugs, people who love drugs, people who've lost loved ones to drugs, people who have no problem with drugs, people who have been behind bars, and people in law enforcement, and they are opposed by people from all those categories as well. I just want to be clear that this is only a point of view—one to which I hope you will all open your minds and hearts.

When I talk about the harms of the drug war, I am not coming at it, first and foremost, as someone concerned with racial justice. Rather, I am primarily concerned with human rights. As a human rights activist, however, you cannot escape the fact that the war on drugs is not just a human rights issue but a direct assault on racial justice as well.

---

*The original speech can be viewed by going to www.youtube.com and entering "End the Drug War Now" into the search bar.

Just look at the numbers. In the United States today we have less than 5 percent of the world's population, but almost 25 percent of the world's incarcerated population. We rank first in the world in the per capita incarceration of our fellow citizens. The Russians and the Belarusians keep huffing and puffing trying to keep up, but they can't do it. We are number one in the world when it comes to locking up our fellow citizens. When it comes to locking up people for drug charges, we went from fifty thousand people in 1980 to over five hundred thousand people today, never mind the hundreds of thousands more locked up on parole or probation violations related to drug offenses. In America, we lock up more people for violating a drug law than all of Western Europe locks up for all charges combined—and they have 100 million more people than we do. Do any of you think that would be possible if the vast majority of the people behind bars in this country were white?

If the vast majority of those people were white, we would not be leading the world in incarceration rates. Something happens in your mind when you see a television program or a photograph of the prison population and see that it is made up of overwhelmingly black and brown men. There's this little thing that clicks and goes, "That's okay, that's right." The movement for reform would be moving a lot faster than it is right now if the vast majority of people being corralled into prisons were white.

When you look at the history of America, you can look from slavery, to Jim Crow, to the war on drugs. No better system has ever been created to imprison millions of people, disproportionately black and brown, to dehumanize them, give them a number, take them away from their homes, put them in remote communities, dissolve their identity, and treat them as second- and third- and fourth-class citizens for the rest of their lives. That is what the war on drugs is doing today.

This has got to change. To change it means struggling with ourselves as well. It is important to remember that the war on drugs is not just a matter of white people putting black people behind bars. The war on drugs that emerged in the 1970s, 1980s, and 1990s was a bipartisan struggle and a biracial struggle; the people who supported the original crack powder laws were not just white but black as well; the people who opposed needle exchange programs to stem the spread of AIDS were white *and* black; the people who bought into drug war hysteria were white *and* black. That means, quite frankly, that we have to look deep within ourselves and our fears, deep down, and allow ourselves to feel uncomfortable. Only through critical self-examination can we uproot this from American society.

I want each one of you to please think back twenty years, when crack was devastating inner-city communities. Were you the one saying, "Lock 'em up! Put 'em behind bars"? When people were saying that we needed needle exchange programs to stop the spread of AIDS, were you the one saying, "I don't want to give a needle to a junkie, why would I enable their addiction?" Were you the one saying these things, and only now, a few tens of millions of arrests later, do you understand that wasn't the appropriate response?

There is a price to a slow learning curve. When other nations understood what was right twenty years ago, we were slow. The price of our slowness is an incarcerated population that leads the world and hundreds of thousands of people who have died or are now living with HIV/AIDS. Now more than ever, we cannot afford a slow learning curve. We have to understand that no matter how much we hate drugs, the punitive war on drugs is not the answer. Criminalization and the criminal justice system are not answers for what is primarily a health issue. It is always a mistake to call in our oppressors to save ourselves from ourselves.

Twice as many people get busted for marijuana today as was true twenty-five years ago. The 1.8 million people getting arrested on drug charges each year are disproportionately black. If they had been arresting as many people for marijuana twenty-five years ago as they are today, the man who currently occupies the White House might well have been arrested. Would that man have made it to the White House had he been arrested as a youth? How many people are being derailed, and how much promise wasted, because of our slow learning curve?

When we were ran a ballot initiative in California in 2008 to shift resources from prison and parole to treatment and rehabilitation, Alice Huffman (the director of the NAACP in California) signed onto it. When my organization led the effort to repeal the Rockefeller drug laws in New York, [the new NAACP director] Ben Jealous sent out an alert not just to New York members, but to NAACP's national membership, because he knew those laws were part of a systemic problem. Will you be part of the collective movement to end this war on people?

We can't just tinker around the edges of our ideological roadblock. I repeat, no matter how much you hate drugs, no matter how much you have seen the worst that drugs can do, the war on drugs, the criminal justice system, and the criminalization approach cannot and will not be the right way. It does not make sense to put our limited resources in the hands of the prison-industrial complex, allowing it to absorb a hundred billion dollars a year that should be directed toward treatment, education, health care, and housing.

I hope and I pray that as more reforms arise and as people start talking about drug policy more sensibly, not just giving lip service, that we all recognize a moral obligation to reduce the role of criminalization and the criminal justice system in drug policy as much as possible. We are never going to be a drug-free society. There has never been a drug-free society, and there never will be a drug-free society. Our challenge as human beings and communities is to accept that reality and to learn how to live with drugs so that they cause the least possible harm, and in some cases the greatest possible good. Our obligation is to uproot our fears and actively fight for drug policies grounded in science, compassion, health, and human rights.

Thank you very much.

PART TWO

Risks of Use and Harm Reduction

Penalties against possession of a drug should not be more damaging to an individual than the use of the drug itself, and where they are they should be changed.

JIMMY CARTER

I now have absolute proof that smoking even one marijuana cigarette is equal in brain damage to being on Bikini Island during an H-bomb blast. . . . If adults want to take such chances (with marijuana) that is their business.

RONALD REAGAN

I wouldn't call myself a pothead. I mean, I enjoy it once in a while. There's nothing wrong with that. Everything in moderation.

JENNIFER ANISTON

Introduction to Part Two

It is human nature to search for ways to alter our consciousness. Most animals, and every society, every culture, and nearly every indigenous tribe have devised methods to induce altered states. (The only exception seems to be the Inuit/Eskimos, at least until alcohol arrived on their scene.) Pursuing altered states, though natural, is inherently a risky venture. The top three drugs used in America are alcohol, tobacco, and cannabis. Cigarettes kill 1,200 Americans every day, and 5.4 million a year worldwide. Thirty-five thousand Americans die yearly as a direct result of alcohol use. Alcohol is more addictive, more toxic to the brain and liver, and more closely associated with violence (domestic abuse, sexual assault, homicide, suicide), and impairs driving significantly more than cannabis. Acetaldehyde, the major byproduct of alcohol metabolism, is toxic and carcinogenic.

In medicine, the most basic evaluation all physicians are taught to perform is the risk/benefit analysis. All medicines have indications and caveats for their judicious use. Some medications are potent but toxic. They exert their desired effects but exact a heavy toll. Other medications have a wider therapeutic index, so that higher doses are not necessarily as dangerous as those of other drugs. Given that most human beings do attempt to alter themselves, it makes sense, from a medical perspective, to choose the least dangerous method.

Cigarettes, poor nutrition, and alcohol are the first three leading causes of death in America. Cananabis is nowhere on this list. Say what you will about marijuana, one thing you can't say is that pot kills. No practical lethal dose has ever been established; no fatal overdose has ever been recorded. Almost all drugs, both legal and illegal, pose greater health risks than cannabis. By any comparison, cannabis is significantly safer than the two most commonly used drugs—alcohol and tobacco—but it is not entirely without risk. Lung irritation and psychiatric symptoms are two of the biggest concerns of use. It is wise to recommend that people with personal or family histories of psychosis and people with lung disease not smoke cannabis.

The following chapters delineate not only the acute and chronic harms inherent in cannabis use, but provide options for diminishing these harms. Harm reduction is a philosophy that accepts the inevitability of drug use and does not insist on abstinence. It is a practical, pragmatic framework upon which to build a therapeutic structure. Seatbelts, motorcycle helmets, and condoms are all good examples of harm-reduction products. They make risky behavior a bit safer and reduce the potential for harmful outcomes.

In the case of cannabis, one of the most important harm-reduction tools available is the vaporizer. This is a device that heats cannabis to the temperature required to release the psychoactive components of the plant into a vapor without burning it. Because the cannabis is vaporized, there is no combustion. This markedly reduces the amount of irritating particulate materials that get inhaled, resulting in much less inflammation and damage to the lining of the lungs.

In America, the most likely harm one might experience as a result of using cannabis is getting arrested. Harry Levine's chapter 16 on the inherent racism of America's drug policy and Richard Glen Boire's chapter 18 on the collateral harms stemming from a conviction are a sobering, eye-opening look at the myriad potential negative consequences once this chain of events is set into motion. As I mention elsewhere (see the introduction to part 4), the fact that smoking pot is illegal, and therefore must be hidden, ends up creating a layer of psychopathology that wasn't necessarily there to start. The obsessive rituals involved with hiding and covering up, the shame that stems from the secrecy, the anxiety created from the clandestine requirements, all make the drug-taking experience more adrenaline-charged, and thereby potentially more reinforcing and addicting. The guilt causes dissonance that needs to be quelled, and the pleasure causes a desire, or even a compulsion, to repeat the act.

With regard to cannabis and addiction, I have certainly come across patients—in my private practice and also at Bellevue Hospital in New York City, where I used to work—who felt that they wanted to stop smoking pot, or perhaps just to smoke more moderately, and yet were having a hard time making the changes necessary to do so. For some pot smokers, daily use becomes a compulsion, an ingrained habit with diminishing rewards. Learning this lesson takes time, and modifying cannabis consumption can be quite challenging for some. But there are also those who can walk away from this drug and never look back, and still more who have figured out a way to reduce harm and maximize gain, and so have made peace with whatever their use pattern may be.

In the same way that not everyone who drinks alcohol becomes an alcoholic, not every pot smoker turns into a habitual "stoner." The probability of becoming dependent on various abuse-able substances, according to an Institute of Medicine report in 1999, is as follows: cannabis 9 percent, alcohol 15 percent, cocaine 17 percent, opiates 23 percent, nicotine 32 percent. In a 2002 review by Anthony, cannabis ranked eleventh in dependence potential after heroin, cocaine, tobacco, methadone, barbiturates, alcohol, benzodiazepines, amphetamines, buprenorphine, and ketamine. You'll notice that two of these substances are unscheduled, and many more are prescription medications.

There are cannabis addicts in treatment, yes, but not in the numbers our government would have you believe. Many Americans are forced to choose drug treatment as their sentence or as part of a plea bargain, and yet they are not necessarily addicted to cannabis. Roughly 70 percent of Americans in drug treatment for cannabis are there courtesy of our criminal justice system (Copeland and Maxwell 2007). In this book I have chosen to present a fairly conservative chapter on addiction, painting a grimmer picture than may be necessary, because I don't want to put a rosy face on the issue. But in terms of the physical phenomenon of tolerance, dependence, and withdrawal, cannabis is not even in the same ballpark as most other drugs of abuse. There is minimal discomfort or risk following abrupt cessation, unlike alcohol withdrawl—the DTs carry a 30 percent chance of death. When examining the psychological components of addiction, it gets more complicated.

The idea that people want what they want, right up until they get it, is eternal. Addiction is manifest by a compulsive desire to do something even though wc know wc shouldn't. We discount the negative consequences and carry on with the behavior. For many drug users the promise of an altered state, and expectations of a better frame of mind are projected onto the experience, which may or may not occur. People get pleasure from it, or it relieves their pain—psychic and physical. But there is usually a downside. They get self-conscious, or tongue-tied, or have trouble remembering something, or can't get off the couch. Opportunities for optimism abound, but not always getting the pleasure or relief expected makes the experience a partial intermittent reinforcer. And any behavioral researcher will tell you that is the strongest reinforcer there is. So the fact that pot is a "mixed bag" in this regard may enhance its addictive quality.

Then there are the rituals of use: many of my patients smoke every night before bed, or before every yoga class, for example. I have some patients who jokingly refer to cannabis as their "maintenance medication" and believe strongly that it does "maintain" them, for better or for worse. It is hard to tease apart the many pros and cons that result from their use.

Another layer of ritualized use comes in the accoutrements of smoking: the bongs, papers, scales, screens, pipes, and the hiding places where all these things belong. These accessories become fetishes, adding to the reinforcing properties of the ritual. The rituals that surround drug use help reinforce the learned behavior. Rituals are in and of themselves soothing and satisfying. The progression to a predictable outcome lessens anxiety for many.

Performing the rituals provides much of the pleasure—sometimes more than the actual taking of the drug. But the drug use itself helps reinforce the rituals, infusing them with meaning and enhancing the pleasure of completion. The mutually reinforcing stimulus augments the process of learning, the strength of the pair bonding. (In this way, cannabis addiction resembles obsessive compulsive disorder, in which rituals are performed to lessen anxiety.)

For many, pot smoking is a way to demarcate time, or to mark a transition, for instance between work and home, productivity and relaxation. In the way many Americans come home from work and have a beer, some will have a joint. Drug use becomes a transition marker: this is "me time," celebrating independence, solitude, and freedom.

I spend time in my private practice encouraging my patients to find other means of delineating their time and space: a warm bath, a steaming cup of tea, meditation, exercise, journaling, stretching, music. The trick is to find soothing substitutes that create that sense of irresponsibility, of being unreachable, of resting and recharging the batteries without becoming incapacitated.

An important hallmark of addiction is lying about and hiding the behavior. There's a great joke about not believing the data from studies on rats with alcoholism until those rats start hiding their bottles. Addictions are all about secrets, hiding, duping delight (enjoying being altered around others without their knowing it), and shame. The problem here is that since cannabis is illegal, most smokers need to hide their use already. In this case, drug use can give a ready rationale for self-hatred, guilt, and a sense of failure. It is here that the compulsive behavior becomes a foundation for masochism. Mental health comes through self-love and acceptance. If you accept and honor the relaxing behavior, whatever it may be, and treat it as a sacrament, sanctifying and sanctioning it, it is more likely to normalize in frequency. It is important to analyze the pattern of use and its effect on your functioning. Harm-reduction psychotherapy can help to balance the benefits and harms, and adjust the use for the best functional output and outcome.

One more important thing about addiction: In European countries especially, many young people who experiment with cannabis do it by combining it with tobacco in a spliff. They end up addicted to cigarettes in the bargain. Tobacco is inherently much more addictive than cannabis—actually it is the most addictive drug around—and its negative health consequences are well known and accepted. I believe (as does Mario Lap, whose chapter on Dutch drug policy is included in this book) that it is important for European countries to disentangle these two drugs.

Despite the risks inherent in using cannabis, I do believe, in general, that it is possible to healthfully integrate altered states into one's lifestyle. I believe that as healthy adults we can moderate our drug and alcohol use in a way that is judicious, sanctified, and beneficial to our health and well-being. There are countless patients who can benefit from medical marijuana, and many more who may be better off with cannabis than with alcohol, cigarettes, or prescription drugs. It is a worthy goal, this healthy integration of altered states, one that requires careful thinking, analyzing, planning, and most of all, discussing. Ideally, risk reduction occurs in a medical model, a framework that includes a physician's consultation. One way to maximize benefit and minimize harm is to use cannabis under medical supervision, or perhaps a better way to state it, with medical evaluation and collaboration.

10
Medical Risks and Toxicology

William Holubek, M.D.

Marijuana is the most commonly used illicit drug in the United States. According to the 2003 National Survey of Drug Use and Health, 94 million Americans (40 percent of the population) aged twelve years and older have tried marijuana (NIDA 2005). Most people using marijuana feel it is safe (McGuigan 2006).

Toxicology is the study of how a substance produces its chemical and clinical effects on an organism, both harmful and beneficial. In this chapter, we will discuss some of the scientific and research data focusing on specific toxicities and medical risks of marijuana use.

TERMINOLOGY

Cannabis sativa is a female hemp plant that contains a large number of chemicals called cannabinoids. Some of the major cannabinoids include cannabinol, cannabidiol, and tetrahydrocannabinol. The primary psychoactive agent is delta-9-tetrahydrocannabinol (THC). THC is found in all parts of the plant, but its concentration is highest in the flowers, followed by the leaves, stems, and seeds. More specifically, THC concentrates in the trichomes of the plant, which are small outgrowths or appendages of a plant that contain a resin.

The term *marijuana* refers to the mixture of dried leaves and flowers.

Hashish, or hash, is produced by collecting the resin-containing trichomes and pressing or cooking them into a solid mass. Hashish oil, also known as honey oil, refers to the actual resin that is isolated through extraction procedures, usually involving solvents. It is important to make these distinctions because the THC content differs between these sources. A typical marijuana cigarette contains about 0.5 to 5 percent THC, whereas hashish contains about 2 to 20 percent THC, and hashish oil about 15 to 50 percent THC (Hall and Solowij 1998). Therefore, two equal doses (amounts) of a marijuana product may in fact have very different concentrations of THC. Some authors state that the marijuana available today may contain more THC than marijuana used in past several decades; however, the data to support this statement is lacking, so this remains a debated issue today (NIDA 2005; Hall and Solowij 1998; Taylor 1988).

PHARMACOKINETICS AND PHARMACODYNAMICS

Pharmacokinetics is a term used to describe what happens to a chemical or substance once it is in the body. It pertains to how a substance is absorbed, where in the body it gets distributed, how it gets metabolized, and how it is excreted. *Pharmacodynamics,* on the other hand, deals with the relationship between the amount of substance in one's body and the apparent clinical effects one experiences.

Absorption

THC can be absorbed in many ways, but inhalation is the most common route. The absorption rate of THC via inhalation is rapid, with levels detectable within seconds. The amount of THC in a single marijuana cigarette that can be extracted by smoking varies substantially from about 20 to 70 percent, depending on how much is lost in sidestream smoke and combustion (Hall and Solowij 1998; McGuigan 2006). Devices such as a pipe or a bong can increase the total amount of THC one can extract from marijuana, but it is the bioavailability of THC that determines the actual amount that gets absorbed into the bloodstream. The bioavailability of inhaled THC varies from 5 to 24 percent. This appears to be affected by the amount inhaled, the depth of inhalation, and the length of time that the breath is held (Grotenhermen 2003).

Oral ingestion of THC results in more variable absorption rates. Many factors can influence these times, including stomach contents, amount of THC ingested, and co-ingestion of other drugs that may influence gastric function, such as diphenhydramine (Benadryl) and opioids (Grotenhermen 2003; McGuigan 2006).

Other routes of THC administration, including ophthalmologic, rectal, sublingual, and dermal, have been studied. The resulting bioavailability is highly variable.

Distribution

Once THC is absorbed, it is rapidly distributed to tissues and organs that have a high blood supply, such as the liver, kidneys, heart, fat, and muscle. THC is a lipophilic molecule, meaning it likes fatty tissues, so over time it redistributes from the blood and accumulates in the liver and other fatty tissues. Brain concentrations of THC appear to be relatively low during peak psychoactive effects, as shown in a rat model (Gill and Jones 1972). However, one of the THC metabolites, 11-hydroxy-THC, appears to enter the brain's circulation much better and faster than THC itself, which may account for this finding (Grotenhermen 2003).

THC crosses the placenta and is detected easily in the blood of the fetus. Fetal concentrations of THC reach about 10 to 30 percent of that of maternal concentrations. THC is also found in breast milk and can concentrate up to eight times more than the maternal concentration in chronic marijuana users (Grotenhermen 2003).

Metabolism

THC is metabolized in the liver to nearly 100 compounds. The primary metabolite is 11-hydroxy-THC, which also produces psychoactive effects. This compound is further metabolized to THC-carboxylate, which is inactive. 11-hydroxy-THC has a short half-life, meaning it does not exist in the bloodstream for a long period. After smoking one marijuana cigarette, the peak plasma 11-hydroxy-THC concentration occurs in approximately thirteen minutes. THC-carboxylate has a much longer half-life, and its peak plasma concentration occurs in approximately two hours.

The ratio of THC to its metabolites changes over time. For example, one hour after smoking a marijuana cigarette, the THC-to-11-hydroxy-THC ratio is 3:1, while the THC-to-THC-carboxylate ratio is 1:2. Approximately three hours later, the ratios are 2:1 and 1:16, respectively. This illustrates the comparatively longer half-life of THC-carboxylate. Current research is trying to use these ratios to estimate time of marijuana use and whether a person is a chronic user (Grotenhermen 2003).

When THC is orally ingested, the times to peak plasma concentrations are more variable; however, the ratios are similar after about three hours.

Excretion

When speaking about excretion, we need to define the term "elimination half-life." This describes the time necessary to remove half of the measurable amount of a substance in the blood. After five elimination half-lives, elimination is virtually complete.

THC and its metabolites are excreted mainly in the feces but also in the urine. Studies have shown that within seventy-two hours following a single oral ingestion of THC, approximately 50 percent is excreted in the feces and 15 percent in the urine. Following intravenous THC administration, approximately 25 to 35 percent is excreted in the feces and 15 percent in the urine. Based on pharmacokinetic principles, inhalation of THC is thought to produce results similar to intravenous administration. Within five days, about 80 to 90 percent of THC is excreted from the body (McGuigan 2006).

Time and Clinical Effect

A typical marijuana cigarette contains about 500 to 1,000 mg of cannabis plant material, of which 1 to 15 percent is THC (5 to 150 mg). Typically, an occasional user may only require 2 to 3 mg to experience a pleasurable feeling or "high" (Hall, Solowij, and Lemon 1994). The onset of clinical psychoactive effects occurs within minutes, and a peak blood concentration occurs in an average of eight minutes (McGuigan 2006). The time to peak "high" after smoking 19 mg of THC in a cigarette is between twenty and thirty minutes and returns to baseline after about four hours. Similar results are obtained from intravenous administration of 5mg of THC (Grotenhermen 2003).

Oral ingestion of THC results in a significantly slower time to clinical psychoactive effects (about one to three hours) and peak plasma concentration (about two to four hours). The time to peak "high" after oral ingestion of 20 mg of THC in a cookie is between two and four hours and returns to baseline after about six hours (Grotenhermen 2003; McGuigan 2006).

DRUG TESTING

The elimination half-life and urinary detection of THC and its metabolites show extreme individual variation. THC-carboxylate is the primary urinary metabolite, and it has a urinary excretion half-life of two to three days, ranging from 0.9 to 9.8 days (McGuigan 2006). Oral or intravenous administration of THC results in an elimination half-life of THC, 11-hydroxy-THC, and THC-carboxylate ranging from twenty-five to thirty-six hours, twelve to thirty-six hours, and twenty-five to fifty-five hours, respectively. The elimination half-lives of THC metabolites are much longer than that of THC itself (Grotenhermen 2003).

There are many methods that can be used to detect the presence of THC and its metabolites, but the EMIT (enzyme immunoassay technique) assay is commonly used as a screening test for marijuana use. There are different types of EMIT assays with different cutoff levels for a positive result, ranging from 20 ng/mL to 200 ng/mL (Schwartz and Hawks 1985). The lower the cutoff value, the more sensitive the test, and the longer urine will test positive. After a single dose of THC, positive urinary detection of THC metabolites occurs usually for three to five days, but for as long as twelve days (Grotenhermen 2003).

Urinary excretions of THC metabolites in chronic users of marijuana steadily decrease, but then appear to fluctuate around some EMIT detection values for a variable period. This fluctuation in excretion patterns results in alternating positive and negative urine screens. Light marijuana users (defined as weekly use or less) will have a negative urine test usually within 8.5 days (range 3 to 18 days), but can still test positive up to an average of 12.9 days (range 3 to 29 days). Heavy marijuana users, defined as daily use, will have their first negative urine test after 19.2 days on average (range 3 to 46 days), but can still test positive up to an average 31.5 days later (range 4 to 77 days) (Ellis et al. 1985). This illustrates the extreme variation in excretion patterns between individuals. Chronic users of marijuana can take up to one month (on average) to have consistently negative urine screens.

There is a tremendous amount of information available on techniques and products that claim to help beat or fool urine drug screens (Gombos 1998). Some of these masking techniques include diluting urine to decrease the drug concentration, changing the urine color to decrease its colorimetric detection, or binding the drug or its metabolites, rendering it undetectable (Heard and Mendoza 2007). These products include diuretics, vitamins, zinc, and niacin, to name a few. Some of these products and techniques can have life-threatening consequences and should not be attempted (Heard and Mendoza 2007; Mittal et al. 2007).

GENERAL TOXICITY

To date, there have been no substantiated deaths related solely to marijuana use (Grotenhermen 2003). The lethal dose of THC has been studied in different animal models. The LD-50 is the dose at which 50 percent of subjects die.

In rats, the LD-50 of oral THC is 800 to 1,900 mg/kg; however, there have been no reported deaths in dogs given oral doses up to 3,000 mg/kg or monkeys given oral doses up to 9,000 mg/kg (Grotenhermen 2003). Intravenous administration of THC, however, results in a much lower LD-50 of 130 mg/ kg in the dog and monkey (Hall, Solowij, and Lemon 1994).

A typical marijuana cigarette (also referred to as a "joint" or "cone") can contain anywhere from 0.5 to 1 gram of marijuana plant matter, of which THC content varies from 1 to 15 percent (5 to 150 mg), depending on multiple variables including the strain of plant, growing conditions, and preparation (Caldicott et al. 2005; Hall, Solowij, and Lemon 1994). A light marijuana user may need only 2 to 3 mg of THC to obtain a "high," while some very heavy users in Jamaica have been reported to smoke up to 420 mg per day (Hall, Solowij, and Lemon 1994).

Although marijuana is most commonly inhaled, reports of intravenous use of marijuana have been described. These cases have resulted in a wide spectrum of clinical effects including life-threatening low blood pressure, kidney failure, gastroenteritis, abdominal pain, liver injury, and blood cell abnormalities (Payne and Brand 1975).

Cardiovascular Toxicity

The cardiovascular system comprises both the heart (cardiac system) and the blood vessels (vascular system). THC has effects on both these systems. In human subjects, THC causes an elevation in blood pressure (hypertension) while one is lying flat, but upon standing, blood pressure decreases (orthostatic hypotension). The hypertension results in part from a constriction of blood vessels (called vasoconstriction) that can have effects on many organs in the body including the heart, brain, and kidney (Moussouttas 2004).

A relaxation or dilation of the blood vessels (vasodilation) plays a major role in the development of orthostatic hypotension, which most likely causes the head "rush" sensation experienced upon standing, similar to the effect one obtains from using amyl nitrite. Thus, marijuana users should use caution when standing up quickly, as this can result in a brief loss of consciousness (passing out). THC also increases heart rate (tachycardia) within minutes of use; it returns to baseline after about three hours. Some studies also suggest an association with the development of abnormal cardiac rhythms (arrhythmias) (Fisher et al. 2005; Kosior et al. 2001; Singh 2000).

The heart receives oxygen mainly through blood delivered by the coronary arteries. High blood pressure or increased heart rate in individuals with coronary artery disease causes an increased demand for oxygen by the heart muscle (myocardium). If the heart does not receive enough oxygen, an individual may experience symptoms including chest discomfort and shortness of breath. This is called angina. Stable angina is defined as angina that occurs predictably during periods of exercise and is relieved by rest. Lack of oxygen delivery to the heart (such as blockage or vasoconstriction of a coronary artery) results in death of heart muscle, known as a heart attack or myocardial infarction.

It seems intuitive that the effects of THC on the cardiovascular system (hypertension and tachycardia) may precipitate adverse cardiac effects by increasing the myocardial oxygen demand, as explained above. People with stable angina developed chest discomfort during a stress test 48 percent sooner after smoking a marijuana cigarette (containing 19.8 mg THC) compared to 8 percent sooner when smoking a placebo marijuana cigarette (containing only 0.05 mg THC) (Aronow and Cassidy 1974). However, it is probably true that smoking anything would decrease the exercise time to developing angina because the act of burning a cigarette produces carbon monoxide, which transforms normal hemoglobin into carboxyhemoglobin. Carboxyhemoglobin does not deliver oxygen very well to the myocardium, and so angina develops sooner. This theory proved correct when people who smoked a non-nicotine lettuce leaf cigarette showed a shorter exercise time to developing angina compared to not smoking (Aronow and Rokaw 1971).

So how does smoking a high-nicotine cigarette compare to smoking a marijuana cigarette with respect to developing angina? One study compared subjects smoking one marijuana cigarette (containing 18.9 mg THC) and those smoking one high-nicotine cigarette (containing 1.8 mg nicotine) with nonsmoking controls. Both groups experienced angina in shorter amounts of time when compared to not smoking; however, this effect was greater in the marijuana smokers (50 percent decrease in exercise time) than the high-nicotine smokers (23 percent decrease) (Aronow and Cassidy 1975).

Although it remains unclear if the magnitude of these cardiovascular effects by THC can clinically increase one's risk for a heart attack, one study suggests an increased relative risk of developing a heart attack in the first hour after smoking marijuana (Caldicott et al. 2005; Mittleman et al. 2001).

Neurological Toxicity
The neurological effects of THC vary from person to person. Some common neurological effects include feelings of euphoria, relaxation, disinhibition, alterations in perception, time distortion, and intensified sensory experiences.

These effects appear to be dose-dependent, meaning the more one uses, the more intense effects one experiences. However, large doses of THC can produce some unwanted neurological effects including paranoia, confusion, amnesia, delusions, hallucinations, anxiety, and agitation. Drowsiness and lethargy were reported in a patient who swallowed twenty-six balloons of hashish oil, one of which ruptured (Lopez et al. 1974).

Some marijuana users develop a psychiatric condition known as schizophrenic psychosis; however, population studies have concluded that this likely occurs in people who were already predisposed to developing this condition, and that marijuana use may bring it out earlier (Grotenhermen 2003). A more thorough discussion on mental health risks and cognitive impairments caused by cannabis is covered separately in chapters 12 and 13 of this book.

The cardiovascular effects of THC described earlier (tachycardia and hypertension) can have deleterious effects on the brain. Constriction of blood vessels in the brain (cerebral vasoconstriction) can cause ministrokes (called transient ischemic attacks or TIAs) and strokes (called cerebral vascular accidents or CVAs). There are case reports of healthy people under the age of thirty-five years who have developed TIAs and CVAs either while or shortly after using marijuana (Caldicott et al. 2005; Moussouttas 2004; Zachariah 1991). The association between marijuana use and stroke needs further study and remains controversial.

Pulmonary Toxicity

Since marijuana is most commonly smoked, the pulmonary system is directly affected. Marijuana smoke contains many of the same substances found in a tobacco cigarette, including tar, carcinogens, hydrogen cyanide, carbon monoxide, polycyclic aromatic hydrocarbons, and particulate matter (Taylor 1988). Inhalation of these substances can have deleterious effects on pulmonary function, ultimately leading to the development of bronchitis (inflammation of the mucous membranes lining the major airway leading to the lungs).

In addition, the actual mechanics of smoking marijuana may place an individual at risk for other specific pulmonary injuries, including pneumothorax (collection of air or gas within the chest that causes the lung to collapse) and pneumomediastinum (collection of air or gas within the middle portion of the chest). Both these clinical entities result from increased pressure within the chest wall (barotrauma). Forceful breath-holding (trying to exhale against a closed mouth or glottis), otherwise known as a Valsalva maneuver, is performed not only by marijuana smokers but also by freebase and crack cocaine users. This smoking technique increases the risk of developing these life-threatening injuries (Goodyear, Laws, and Turner 2004; Panacek et al. 1992). (Please see Mitch Earleywine's chapter 11 for a more in-depth analysis of these issues.)

Marijuana and Pregnancy

Marijuana is the most common illicit drug used by women of childbearing age in most Western societies (Hurd et al. 2005). THC does cross the placenta and enters the circulation of the developing fetus, reaching concentrations of about 10 to 30 percent of maternal concentration (Grotenhermen 2003). Studying the effects of marijuana use in pregnancy, however, is very difficult for many reasons. Marijuana use is usually self-reported and cannot be substantiated. There are numerous confounding factors that can also affect the fetus, such as socioeconomic status, concomitant tobacco and alcohol use, genetic factors, and marijuana impurities and adulterants.

One of the most common ways to determine whether maternal drug use has an effect on fetal development is to assess for changes in fetal growth. The studies published thus far suggest an association between prenatal marijuana use and a decrease in head circumference and fetal weight and length; however, one study actually reported an increase in fetal weight (Fried and Smith 2001; Hurd et al. 2005). Some studies suggest an increased incidence of preterm labor with marijuana use, while other studies fail to show this possible association (Fried and Smith 2001). There also appears to be evidence for cognitive and behavioral abnormalities in the offspring of those mothers who abuse marijuana (Hurd et al. 2005). One study looked at marijuana use and the incidence of sudden infant death syndrome (SIDS) and could not find a statistically significant risk but concluded that it may be a "weak risk factor" (Scragg et al. 2001). The consequences of maternal marijuana use on fetal growth are continually being studied, and many remain controversial.

Cyclical Hyperemesis

Cyclical hyperemesis is a condition characterized by bouts of severe nausea and vomiting (hyperemesis) and colicky abdominal pain lasting several days; it recurs in a cyclical fashion every few weeks to months. This syndrome has recently been described in chronic marijuana users across a spectrum of ages with no psychiatric illness or major medical problems (Allen et al. 2004). The symptoms can be severe enough to require medical attention and, in some cases, hospital admission. These patients also describe a temporary relief of their symptoms with hot baths or showers. The validity of these complaints being associated with marijuana use is made stronger by the fact that when these patients stopped using marijuana, the symptoms stopped; when they started using marijuana again, the symptoms returned. This syndrome has been reported by others (Roche and Foster 2005), but its existence as a legitimate diagnosis is still controversial (Byme, Hallinan, and Wodak 2006).

Infants and Children

Pediatric exposures to marijuana have been reported in infants and toddlers ranging from age 8 months to 3.5 years old. These cases have resulted in varying degrees of decreased consciousness, hypotonia (decreased muscle tone), hyporeflexia (decreased muscle reflexes), apnea (temporary cessation of breathing), and opisthotonic-like movements (severe muscle contractions of the back and neck) (Appelboam and Oades 2006; Johnson, Conradi, and McGuigan 1991). Few patients in these studies received mechanical ventilation (artificial respiration or intubation), and all patients recovered without sequelae. Although no deaths have been reported, infants and children exposed to marijuana appear to require careful attention to their respiratory and neurological status.

Adulterants

Adulterants are added substances that make a product impure. Marijuana cigarettes are commonly adulterated with other drugs to enhance particular effects. For example, marijuana can be adulterated with phencyclidine (PCP) to enhance hallucinogenic effects. These PCP-adulterated marijuana cigarettes are known by slang terms including *wet, illy, embalming fluid, water,* and *amp.* There are many perceptions among marijuana users that lead to confusion and dangerous practices. The term *embalming fluid* was once a common slang term for PCP; however, uninformed users may actually take this term literally and dip cigarettes in formalin (the liquid form of formaldehyde) (Holland et al. 1998; erowid.org). Some common adulterants and their associated U.S. slang terms are listed in the table on page 151. Slang terms may overlap depending on the part of the country in which they are used.

MANAGEMENT OF MARIJUANA INTOXICATION

Marijuana intoxication alone is rarely life-threatening. Patients may develop mild anxiety or paranoia that can be managed with reassurance and by surrounding the patient with a quiet, nonthreatening environment (McGuigan 2006).

The clinical presentation of marijuana intoxication can vary greatly

TABLE 10.1. MARIJUANA ADULTERANTS
AND THEIR ASSOCIATED SLANG TERMS
(TEXAS POLICE CENTRAL, 2007)

Adulterant	Slang term
alcohol	B-40, Herb and Al
cocaine or crack	banano, buda, caviar, champagne, chronic, cocktail, dirty joint, fry daddy, geek, gimmie, juice joint, jumbos, oolies, p-dogs, primo, thirty-eight, torpedo, turbo, woolies, yeola
cocaine and PCP	Jim Jones
hashish oil	Thai sticks
heroin or opium	A-bomb, atom bomb, Buddha, canade, love boat
insecticides	fuel, whack
PCP	amp, chippy, clicker, clickums, dank, donk, dust blunt, embalming fluid, fry, illy, killer weed, leak, love boat, squirrel, super grass, water, wet, zoom
sedatives	rompums

depending on the presence of an adulterant (see table above) or co-ingestant. Heroin and other opiates can cause life-threatening respiratory depression, while cocaine and PCP can cause life-threatening behaviors, hyperthermia, and cardiac manifestations. These conditions must be identified and treated accordingly.

MARIJUANA AND CANCER

The association between cancer risk and marijuana use is controversial. Many marijuana smokers also tend to be tobacco smokers, and some marijuana smokers mix tobacco with marijuana prior to smoking. These are just two important confounding factors that make the results of these studies difficult to interpret.

Cancer development (carcinogenesis) is a complex process ultimately leading to malignant tumor formation. Mutagens are compounds that have the potential to cause cancer by inducing mutations (or changes) in genetic material, while carcinogens are compounds that are known to cause cancer. Tobacco smoke contains many known human carcinogens including phenols, polycyclic aromatic hydrocarbons, and nitrosamines, and smoking tobacco is the leading cause of cancer-related death worldwide (Das 2003; Pfeifer et al. 2002; Sasco,

Secretan, and Straif 2004). Marijuana smoke contains both mutagens and several known human carcinogens, similar to those found in tobacco smoke (Hall and Solowij 1998; Hashibe, Ford, and Zhang 2002; Taylor 1988).

In fact, some studies found the concentration of these carcinogens to be higher in marijuana smoke than tobacco smoke (Taylor 1988). The technique of smoking a marijuana cigarette increases the exposure to these carcinogens per cigarette, as marijuana smokers tend to inhale a greater volume of smoke, inhale more deeply, and hold their breath longer. On the other hand, marijuana smokers tend to smoke far fewer marijuana cigarettes per day compared to the number of tobacco cigarettes smoked by tobacco smokers.

When comparing the cells lining the airway of the lungs (bronchial epithelium) of marijuana smokers with nonsmokers, molecular changes consistent with increased risk of developing cancer are seen in the marijuana smokers (Hall and Solowij 1998; Hashibe, Ford, and Zhang 2002). Another study reported not only an increased prevalence of abnormal lung tissue in those that smoked tobacco alone and marijuana alone, but those that smoked both marijuana and tobacco had an even greater increase in abnormal lung tissue, suggesting an additive effect (Fligiel et al. 1997).

Case series and a hospital-based case-control study report an association between marijuana use and the development of premalignant oral lesions and upper and lower respiratory tract squamous cell carcinoma (Hashibe, Ford, and Zhang 2002). However, another study following younger patients did not find any increase in overall cancer incidence, but did find an elevated risk of prostate and cervical cancers (Sydney et al. 1997). And yet another study found no association between marijuana use and oral squamous cell carcinoma (Rosenblatt et al. 2004).

Although tobacco smoking is a known cause of cancer, and marijuana smoke contains carcinogens similar to those in tobacco smoke, the literature relating cancer risk with marijuana use is unclear, and to date remains controversial. (Please also see Mitch Earleywine's chapter 11 for more on this.)

CONCLUSION

Marijuana is the most widely used illicit drug in the United States, and its perceived risk is low and no deaths have been reported due to marijuana use alone. The effects of chronic marijuana use on the developing fetus remain uncertain. Current evidence suggests an association with myocardial infarction, but the relationship between cancer and marijuana use is still unsettled. Large, well-controlled studies are necessary to resolve the many controversial issues of the health effects of marijuana use.

11
Pulmonary Harm and Vaporizers

Mitch Earleywine, Ph.D.

Debates about recreational and medical use of marijuana often turn to discussions about the health of the lungs. Marijuana smoke contains many of the same gases and particles found in tobacco smoke. The noxious gases include carbon monoxide, carbon dioxide, ammonia, acetaldehyde, acetone, and benzene. Potentially toxic particles include naphthalene, dimethylphenol, and benzopyrene. The heat associated with smoke can also create inflammation, adding to the potential negative effects of these substances. Although serious lung problems are rare in marijuana smokers who do not use cigarettes, the potential for marijuana-induced pulmonary troubles seems high.

Research on cannabis and the respiratory system focuses on lung cancer, lung function, and respiratory symptoms like coughing, wheezing, and sputum production. A review of this literature reveals that rates of lung cancer in marijuana smokers who do not use cigarettes is comparable to the rates in nonsmokers, but lung function impairments and respiratory symptoms are possible. Harm-reduction techniques, including a switch from smoked to vaporized or edible cannabis, appear to be worth the effort for regular users.

LUNG CANCER

As public service announcements consistently remind Americans, the smoke from the tobacco and marijuana plants are comparable. Some irritants,

153

including naphthalene, acetaldehyde, and ammonia, are even more concentrated in marijuana smoke than in tobacco smoke. In addition, many marijuana users inhale the smoke more deeply and hold their hits longer, giving toxins a greater chance to deposit on lung tissue (Earleywine 2005; Iversen and Snyder 2000). These points would suggest that smoking marijuana should increase the risk for lung cancer.

Despite all these concerns, Dr. John Morgan has consistently asked "Where are the bodies?" That is, if marijuana is supposed to cause all these horrible problems, where are the cases of marijuana-induced lung damage? Currently, multiple studies show no definitive increases in rates of lung cancer among people who smoke marijuana but not tobacco. For example, a retrospective study of over 64,000 patients showed no increases in risk for many types of cancer once researchers controlled for alcohol and cigarette use (Sidney et al. 1997).

A case-control study compared over 1,000 people with lung or upper aerodigestive tract cancers to over 1,000 controls and showed no link between marijuana use and oral, laryngeal, or lung cancers (Hashibe et al. 2006). A large review of epidemiological studies also showed no link between marijuana use and lung cancer (Hashibe et al. 2005). In short, marijuana smokers who do not smoke cigarettes get lung cancer no more often than people who don't smoke marijuana.

These unaltered rates of lung cancer in marijuana smokers seem odd given the parallels between marijuana smoke and tobacco smoke. Recent theorizing suggests that key differences between the two plants might account for the absence of marijuana-induced lung cancer (Melamede 2005). Cannabis smoke contains cannabinoids but no nicotine; tobacco smoke contains nicotine but no cannabinoids. Nicotine's activity in lung cells actually increases the chances of cancer, while the cannabinoids might decrease these chances.

The processes involved are complicated, but they essentially arise because respiratory tissue has many nicotine receptors but no cannabinoid receptors. Damaged cells in the respiratory system often die off. New cells replace the damaged ones, keeping the respiratory system functioning. In the presence of nicotine, however, cells become less likely to die. Although keeping cells alive certainly sounds like a good thing, nicotine can even prevent damaged cells from dying. This increased presence of damaged cells makes cancer more likely.

In contrast, cannabinoids do not preserve damaged lung cells, permitting the natural replacement of these cells with new, functional ones. In addition, cannabinoids can decrease inflammation and tumor growth in ways that nicotine cannot. Thus, despite many similarities between cannabis and tobacco smoke, key differences in their components make tobacco smoke potentially more carcinogenic.

LUNG FUNCTION

Cannabis could still harm the respiratory system without creating lung cancer. Researchers have also examined lung function in cannabis users. One study shows no deficits, but others reveal evidence of obstructed airflow even in those who do not smoke cigarettes. A large study performed in Los Angeles (Tashkin et al. 1997) examined chronic obstructive pulmonary disease (COPD), a disorder of the lung airways. This work relied on a measure of the volume of air that people can force from their lungs in one second (forced expiratory volume in one second; FEV1). People who can force more air from their lungs have fewer obstructions in their respiratory tracts.

Consumers of tobacco cigarettes invariably show increasing obstruction each year that they smoke, suggesting blocked airways. In contrast, Tashkin's 1997 data showed that people who had smoked up to three marijuana joints per day (but no cigarettes) for an average of fifteen years did not differ significantly from those who did not smoke at all. Tobacco smokers in this study showed significant impairment on the FEV1 measure. These results suggest that cannabis use may not lead to COPD.

Other work performed in Tuscon revealed blocked airways in people who smoke "nontobacco" cigarettes. An initial study (Bloom et al. 1987) looked at FEV1 as well as other measures of lung function, including FEVC (forced expired vital capacity—a measure of the total amount of air forced out in one breath). Smokers of "nontobacco" cigarettes showed no deficits in FEV1, but their ratio of FEV1 to FEVC was significantly smaller than the same ratio in nonsmokers, but only in men. Decreases in this ratio often precede COPD. A longitudinal follow-up of this sample (Sherrill et al. 1991) confirmed deficits in this same ratio.

A study of New Zealanders who smoked cannabis daily or almost daily showed deficits in this same measure (Taylor et al. 2000). A follow-up of this New Zealand sample found that the results were no longer statistically significant once confounding variables were included (Taylor et al. 2002). Only further work can help resolve these conflicting results, though it is my sincere hope that users will turn to safer methods of administration that will make COPD and lung airway problems less likely.

BRONCHOSCOPE EXAMINATIONS
AND BIOPSIES

Another approach to examining pulmonary consequences in marijuana users involves examination with a bronchoscope. This assessment technique can reveal damage that occurs prior to obvious deficits in lung function. Visual inspection of the lungs revealed that people who smoked five joints a week for two years had more redness, swelling, and mucus. People who smoked both cannabis and tobacco had particularly bad symptoms (Roth et al. 1998). Thus, even without creating COPD or cancer, marijuana can create alterations in the airways that nonsmokers do not experience.

Biopsies taken from some of these same people revealed that marijuana smokers had more abnormal lung cells. Many lung cells normally have cilia, small hairs that help clear the lungs of particles. In cannabis smokers, many of these ciliated cells had transformed into cells more similar to skin. The changes were particularly common among people who smoked both cannabis and tobacco. These sorts of cellular transformations are particularly alarming because they may herald the development of lung cancer. In fact, this work sounded the alarm for the search for marijuana-induced lung cancer, but as mentioned above, the anticarcinogenic effects of the cannabinoids might have saved regular users from developing lung cancer.

RESPIRATORY ILLNESSES

Aside from these other problems, smoking cannabis could still have the potential to create other respiratory illnesses. Researchers report mixed evidence for marijuana-induced increases in colds, flu, or bronchitis. A review of a large sample of hospital records revealed that 36 percent of daily marijuana smokers saw a physician for respiratory symptoms over six years. Slightly fewer (33 percent) of the nonsmokers sought treatment for the same problems (Polen 1993). This difference was statistically significant given the large sample size. Nevertheless, the idea that smoking marijuana increases one's risk of respiratory problems from 33 percent to 36 percent is unlikely to lead people to make dramatic changes in behavior.

Other research (Tashkin et al. 1987; Sherrill 1991) reveals more symptoms of bronchitis, including chronic cough and phlegm production, in heavy marijuana smokers. The sample from New Zealand discussed above revealed higher rates of symptoms like tightness in the chest, wheezing, shortness of breath, and increased sputum production in daily cannabis users (Taylor et al. 2000). A large Internet survey suggested that comparable measures of respiratory symptoms increased with marijuana use and rose even more with concurrent cigarette smoking (Earleywine and Smucker Barnwell 2007). Thus, although marijuana smoking does not appear to create lung cancer, it can alter measures of respiratory symptoms.

HEALTHIER LUNGS FOR CANNABIS SMOKERS

Drug lore suggests that certain strategies may minimize marijuana's potential to harm the lungs. Oral administration, using vaporizers, refraining from holding hits, never smoking leftover resin, and using stronger marijuana can potentially decrease respiratory symptoms and airflow problems. Abstaining from cigarettes is another obvious step toward improving lung health.

ORAL ADMINISTRATION

Obviously, eating products made with marijuana or hashish will have no smoke-induced impact on the respiratory system. Any drug taken orally has a slower onset of effects than the same drug inhaled, and cannabis is no exception. Medical users seeking rapid relief from symptoms may find this approach too slow. Monitoring dosage can also require experimentation. Small doses taken on an empty stomach can still require hours of digestion before peak effects. Eating a subsequent dose before the initial dose has reached its peak impact can lead to effects with a greater intensity and duration than desired.

Edible marijuana products have become widely available at medical dispensaries in California. Relevant cookbooks and instructional DVDs are also available. Most remedies recommend making a tincture by placing marijuana in a glass jar, covering it with an alcoholic spirit like vodka, and waiting six to eight weeks for the cannabinoids to dissolve. A quicker alternative requires cooking finely ground marijuana with oil or butter to extract the fat-soluble cannabinoids. Recommendations range from ⅛ to ½ ounce of marijuana per ¼ cup of oil or butter. Cooking times range from twenty to forty-five minutes. Shorter cooking times should release fewer flavonoids and minimize the grassy taste. Chefs can then use these oils or butters in any recipe. Fans of marijuana tea are numerous and outspoken, but THC is not water soluble, making this technique for oral ingestion inefficient.

VAPORIZERS

Vaporizers heat cannabis to temperatures that release cannabinoids in a fine mist without creating the toxins associated with combustion (Gieringer, St. Laurent, and Goodrich 2004; Hazekamp et al. 2006). Although vaporizers are not common knowledge in popular culture, a recent photograph of one appeared in the *New England Journal of Medicine* (Okie 2005), and information about the machine is becoming more available. A clinical study that administered cannabis to participants in the laboratory shows that using the vaporizer leads to blood levels of THC comparable to smoking a joint but without raising expired carbon monoxide (Abrams 2007). A large survey of marijuana smokers also revealed that those who vaporize are less likely to report respiratory symptoms like coughing, wheezing, and increased phlegm (Earleywine and Smucker Barnwell 2007).

These studies inspired an intervention trial in this laboratory funded by the Marijuana Policy Project for which we are recruiting non-cigarette-smoking cannabis users who report at least two respiratory symptoms like coughing, wheezing, or increased sputum production. Participants complete measures of lung function, respiratory symptoms, and cannabis use, and then receive a free vaporizer to use. They return one month later to complete the same assessments. These data should help establish if the vaporizer can decrease respiratory problems.

Water pipes (bongs) are so ubiquitous that they deserve comment here. Because water pipes cool the smoke, they have the potential to decrease the negative effects of heat, including inflammation. Nevertheless, despite popular belief, water pipes do not appear to decrease the amount of tar and particles in smoke (Doblin 1994). A detailed analysis of the smoke extracted from water pipes, an early version of the vaporizer, and standard joints examined the ratio of THC to tars. Although THC is not water soluble, the water appeared to trap some of the THC, leading to less total THC and an unfavorable ratio of THC to tars. The ratio of THC to tars was actually superior in the standard joint. Unfortunately and again despite popular belief, the decrease in THC may lead some users to smoke more cannabis through a water pipe than they might with a standard joint. Smoking more may create increased deposits of tar and particles in the lungs. Thus, the water pipe is not a panacea for all cannabis-induced respiratory problems.

HOLDING HITS

An additional strategy for reducing respiratory problems associated with smoking marijuana concerns the length of time users keep smoke inside their bodies. The common habit of holding smoke in the lungs for long periods likely increases tar deposits, which undoubtedly add to respiratory problems. Although many experienced users swear by this habit, two studies reveal that holding "hits" longer does not create greater changes in mood (Zacny and Chait 1989; Zachny 1991).

Announcing this result in large crowds has gotten me pelted with objects, so let please let me provide some details. Researchers had marijuana smokers take a hit and either blow it out immediately or hold it for up to twenty seconds. Holding hits did not create a larger impact on mood. Unfortunately, it did increase the amount of carbon monoxide in their lungs. Holding hits after smoking a placebo weed did create a lightheaded, dizzy experience of consciousness easily confused with marijuana's effects (Block, Farinpour, and Braverman 1992). In short, any extra "high" associated with holding hits probably stems from simply holding one's breath. Users who are committed to holding their breath should probably exhale the marijuana smoke first. Otherwise, exhaling soon after inhaling should produce identical subjective experiences with markedly less potential for respiratory injury.

RESIN

The resinous glands of the marijuana plant can be rich in cannabinoids. The black residue that remains in smoking instruments after continued use is also known as resin. Because heat destroys cannibinoids, it is unlikely that this resin is psychoactive. Nevertheless, many users swear that smoking this substance creates a psychoactive effect. Anecdotal evidence suggests that users turn to this substance when marijuana is not available.

Although no published data address the issue, this habit could be extremely detrimental given the exposure to heat and burned material. The amount of tars in the black residue lining smoking apparatus is likely much higher than in cannabis, and it appears to require higher temperatures to release smoke. Its THC content is also likely to be small. Increased availability of cannabis as well as education on the potential drawbacks of this behavior may help decrease the prevalence of this problematic habit.

STRONGER MARIJUANA

Given the limited fear of lethal overdose, marijuana with larger percentages of THC may offer some respiratory benefits. Although warnings that stronger marijuana is more dangerous abound, no research that actually assesses potency can support this assertion. Stronger cannabis may lead to smoking smaller amounts to achieve desired effects. Smoking smaller quantities could provide some protection against the health problems normally associated with inhaling smoke. Smokers tend to take smaller, shorter puffs when using more potent marijuana (Heishman, Stitzer, and Yingling 1989). Smoking less would decrease the amount of tars and noxious gases inhaled, limiting the risk for mouth, throat, and lung damage (Matthias et al. 1997).

ABSTAINING FROM CIGARETTES

Public service announcements have inundated cigarette smokers with information on the dangers of the habit of smoking. The impact of marijuana on measures of respiratory problems appears more severe in those who smoke cigarettes. Measures of lung function, including FEV1 and FVC, are invariably impaired in cigarette smokers. Their reports of respiratory symptoms, including coughs, wheezing, and increased sputum production, are also invariably higher. Many studies show additive effects where smoking marijuana and tobacco is markedly worse than using either alone. When combined with behavioral interventions, nicotine replacement and pharmacotherapy can help cigarette smokers quit (Reid et al. 2007).

CONCLUSION

Data and theory suggest that simple changes in the use of marijuana can minimize respiratory complications. Adults who vaporize high-potency marijuana and do not hold their hits, smoke the burned resin that appears on pipes, or smoke cigarettes are less likely to experience coughs, wheezing, shortness of breath, or other symptoms.

Although these strategies can increase the safety of cannabis as far as respiratory symptoms are concerned, pulmonary problems are not the only potential negative consequences of the plant. Approximately 10 percent of marijuana users develop symptoms of dependence (see Earleywine 2005 for a review). Cannabis can lead to impaired driving skills (Liguori 2007), and heavy use in adolescence might create deviant brain structure (Wilson et al. 2000), as well as decreases in intelligence (Fried, James, and Gray 2002). The techniques for respiratory safety offer no protection against these negative consequences. Nevertheless, these strategies do help counter one of the most common arguments against medical and recreational marijuana use.

12
Cannabis and Cognition

Caroline B. Marvin and
Carl L. Hart, Ph.D.

Cannabis, which comprises delta-9-tetrahydrocannabinol-containing products including marijuana and hashish, is the most widely used illicit drug in the world (Anthony and Helzer 1995), with nearly 150 million people reporting annual use (UNODCCP 2002). While most users of cannabis consume the drug infrequently and without apparent negative consequences, the popular view of cannabis users has varied over the years. For example, the 1936 film *Reefer Madness* depicted the alleged dangers of cannabis use, with the drug severely compromising users' cognitive functioning and turning mild-mannered teenagers into violent, sex-crazed criminals.

Today this cautionary tale has turned into a cult classic, mocked and spoofed for its exaggerated claims. But while our understanding of the effects of cannabis use has evolved considerably, arguably some of the "madness" remains. For example, recent scientific and media attention has focused on the connection between cannabis use and psychosis (Moore et al. 2007; McLaren et al. 2009), a link for which causal evidence is scarce. More generally, our understanding of the neuropsychological (i.e., cognitive) consequences of marijuana intoxication remains controversial; despite intense research attention, there is limited consensus regarding cannabis-related cognitive effects. In this chapter, we explore the scientific research in this area, identifying areas of congruence and discrepancy and discussing the ways in which we can be more precise in our understanding of the effects of cannabis on cognition.

RELEVANT CANNABINOID NEUROPHARMACOLOGY

Over the past two-and-a-half decades, basic research data has provided a better understanding of neurobiological mechanisms mediating and/or modulating the effects of cannabinoids, such as delta-9-tetrahydrocannabinol (THC) and related compounds. A comprehensive review of cannabinoid neuropharmacology is beyond the scope of this chapter, but a brief overview might provide clues to how cannabis-related effects on cognition are accomplished.

Cannabinoids bind to two types of receptors: cannabinoid receptor 1 and cannabinoid receptor 2 (CB1 and CB2). These receptors are much more abundant than opioid receptors (Sim 1996), indicating that the potential actions of cannabinoids are widespread. CB2 receptors are found mainly outside of the brain in immune cells, suggesting that cannabinoids may play a role in the modulation of the immune response. CB1 receptors are found throughout the body but primarily in the central nervous system. The highest density of CB1 receptors has been found in cells of the basal ganglia, the primary components of which include the caudate nucleus, putamen, and globus pallidus (for review, see Pertwee 1997 and Herkenham 1995). Cells of the basal ganglia are involved in learning and memory.

Other regions that also contain a larger number of CB1 receptors include the cerebellum, which coordinates fine body movements; the hippocampus, which is involved in aspects of memory storage; and the cerebral cortex, which regulates the integration of higher cognitive functions. This suggests that endogenous cannabinoid activity modulates a broad range of behaviors relevant for cognition.

DIRECT EFFECTS OF CANNABIS ON COGNITION

Cannabis has been shown to negatively affect cognitive performance in a variety of domains, including psychomotor control (Casswell and Marks 1973), attention (Meyer et al. 1971), and executive function (Ramaekers 2006; see Table 12.1 on pages 170–73). One of the most consistent findings, however, is that memory performance is compromised following consumption (Abel 1971). Cannabis-related deleterious effects on memory have been reported in the scientific literature for at least four decades (Melges et al. 1970; Tinklenberg et al. 1970), and recent data confirm previous findings

(D'Souza et al. 2004; Ilan, Smith, and Gevins 2004). For example, Hunault and colleagues (2009) investigated the effects of smoked marijuana on cognitive performance of infrequent users. Following baseline assessments, participants smoked one marijuana cigarette and then completed various cognitive tasks. Marijuana disrupted performance on immediate memory tasks and caused participants to perform more slowly. Curran and colleagues (2002) conducted a similarly designed study but used oral THC rather than smoked marijuana and found that the drug impaired immediate memory performance of the infrequent smokers studied.

Beyond these fairly consistent effects on memory, researchers have also investigated cannabis-related effects on complex cognitive functioning, including risk taking, decision making, and planning (Ramaekers 2006; Lane et al. 2005). Tasks assessing these domains require participants to make choices based on predicted outcomes. Lane and colleagues (2005) evaluated risk taking in infrequent marijuana users and found that marijuana increased risky monetary choice selection. Ramaekers and colleagues (2006) studied the performance of a similar sample of marijuana users on a task that measures executive function and planning and reported that participants made fewer correct decisions during marijuana intoxication. Together, the data indicate that cannabis produces temporary deficits in multiple cognitive domains when infrequent users are tested. One question is whether similar decrements are observed when frequent users are evaluated.

Using methods like those employed in the studies described above, Hart and colleagues (2001) studied near-daily marijuana users and found that cannabis produced only limited effects on a wide range of cognitive tasks. Participants required more time to complete some tasks, and they tended to make more premature responses following drug administration. However, accuracy performance on attention, memory, visuospatial processing, reasoning, flexibility, and mental calculation tasks was not altered. Vadhan and colleagues (2007) reported similar findings when they assessed decision-making using a contingency-based gambling task in a sample of frequent users. During acute marijuana intoxication, participants' speed of performance was slowed, but accuracy was unaffected. These findings suggest that the effects of cannabis on cognition are muted in frequent users.

As is illustrated by the examples above, the impact of cannabis intoxication on cognitive performance may vary as a function of cannabis use history. Unfortunately, this issue has received relatively limited attention in the literature. In a discussion of why findings from the Ramaekers (2006) and Hart et al. (2001) studies diverged, Nordstrom and Hart (2006) posited that tolerance played a role in the apparent conflicting results. Participants in the study by Ramaekers and colleagues reported using cannabis approximately three times per month, whereas participants in the Hart study reported almost daily (i.e., six days per week) cannabis use. These use differences might have accounted for the disparity in cognitive performance during cannabis intoxication.

In an effort to better understand this issue, Ramaekers and colleagues (2009) conducted a follow-up study, during which they investigated cannabis-related effects on cognitive performance of frequent and infrequent users. The authors reported that cannabis significantly impaired performance on tasks assessing perceptual motor control, motor inhibition, and divided attention among occasional cannabis users. In contrast, among frequent users, cognitive performance was largely unaffected. These findings are thus consistent with the hypothesis of Nordstrom and Hart (2006) that frequent users are tolerant to many cannabis-related performance-impairing effects.

The reader should be aware that although tolerance seems to develop to cannabis-related cognitive effects, it might not necessarily occur in other domains, including positive subjective effects and cardiovascular measures. The reason for this nonuniform tolerance is unclear, but some have offered persuasive speculations. Schuster and colleagues (1966) hypothesized that tolerance develops to drug effects that may have a negative impact on an organism's ability to perform reinforced behaviors, for example, the ability to think clearly or walk steadily, but does not develop to drug effects that have no bearing on reinforcement delivery, for example, experiencing subjective effects such as "drug liking" or "feeling high."

As an illustration of this point, recently Hart and colleagues (in press) examined the cognitive and neurophysiological functioning of daily marijuana smokers following administration of smoked marijuana (to date this study has not been published). They found that while the drug produced limited effects on cognitive performance, it produced dramatic transient electroencephalographic (EEG) and evoked potential (EP) alterations. These findings were partially inconsistent with those obtained by Ilan and colleagues (2005), who used identical procedures but a different study sample (i.e., infrequent marijuana smokers), and reported that both cognitive performance and neurophysiological measures were disrupted. Thus, the data show that while frequent users did not develop tolerance to cannabis-related brain alterations, they did develop tolerance to cannabis-related cognitive effects, that is, effects that would negatively impact their ability to perform.

LONG-TERM EFFECTS OF CANNABIS
ON COGNITION

The above discussion focuses on the acute cognitive effects of cannabis in frequent and infrequent users, in other words, how cognition is affected—or unaffected— in the minutes and hours following administration. Researchers have also assessed the chronic effects of cannabis, investigating how regular use of the drug over a period of months or years might affect cognition. Importantly, these effects are measured absent acute intoxication.

A better understanding of the long-term effects of cannabis use on cognition is important with regard not only to recreational use but also to medical use. Thus, in addition to our desire to gain a greater understanding of the cognitive effects of cannabis more generally, it has become important to better ascertain what the chronic consequences of medical marijuana use might be if the drug is to be prescribed by doctors as a long-term treatment. The studies discussed in this section look at frequent users and investigate whether regular use of cannabis might have enduring effects on cognition, unrelated to a state of acute intoxication.

As was the case in our discussion of acute effects, the findings of studies evaluating the chronic effects of cannabis on cognition are nuanced and often inconsistent. Some researchers have found cannabis-related impairments in complex cognitive functions such as mental flexibility, decision making, and executive function (Whitlow et al. 2004; Pope and Yurgelun-Todd 1996), while others have not (Solowij et al. 2002; Fletcher et al. 1996; see Table 12.2 on pages 174–77). However, as we found in our review of acute effects, the most consistent chronic effects of cannabis on cognition relate to learning and memory. Grant and colleagues (2003) conducted a meta-analysis of eleven studies investigating the long-term effects of cannabis on cognition and found effect sizes suggesting decrements in participants' ability to learn and remember information.

However, the meta-analysis revealed no consistent effects in all other neuropsychological domains examined, including verbal/language, perceptual/motor, abstraction/executive, and attention. It should be noted that the inclusion criteria used in this meta-analysis were relatively strict, requiring that studies included a group of "cannabis only" users as well as appropriate controls. Additional requirements were that the cannabis users were drug-free on the days of testing, that the periods of abstinence from cannabis prior to testing were noted, that the studies provided sufficient information for calculating effect size, that valid neuropsychological tests were used as outcome measures, and that the studies addressed participants' potential use of other substances as well as their neurological and psychiatric histories. Few studies met these criteria, suggesting that there are important methodological issues that should be considered when interpreting research in this area.

One issue to consider is the testing itself. Performance on neuropsychological tests is mediated by general intellectual ability and education, with higher IQ and greater educational experience often correlating with better performance (Diaz-Asper, Schretlen, and Pearlson 2003; Van der Elst et al. 2004). This effect can be readily observed with tasks measuring learning and memory ability, in which participants are often asked to learn and then recall or recognize a set of words, which may be biased toward certain educational experiences and backgrounds. For example, versions of the Rey Auditory Verbal Learning Test (RAVLT) and Buschke's Selective Reminding Test (BSRT) include words such as *axe, kettle, stool, discrete, county,* and *grant.*

While these words may be familiar to many participants, they are indicative of a particular acculturation and educational experience and may not be commonly used by some participants. There is a question, therefore, as to whether standard tests such as these measure recall ability equally well in all participants. It has been posited that including words in recall lists that were more familiar to a particular drug-using population—for instance, words associated with the drug or with related paraphernalia—might result in greater recall, and, more generally, in more accurate assessment of memory function (Harrison Pope, personal communication). To our knowledge, such alternate word lists have not been studied among drug-using samples, but this may be an interesting avenue of research.

Regardless of the particular word lists and tasks used, it is clear that participants' intellectual abilities affect their performances on neuropsychological tests. In many of the studies of acute effects we reviewed previously, individual differences in IQ were not confounding factors. Most of these studies used within-subject designs, meaning that a participant was tested under a placebo condition and during marijuana intoxication, and the two test results were compared. It is virtually impossible to employ within-subject designs when evaluating the cognitive effects of chronic cannabis use. Instead, researchers use between-subject designs, during which neuropsychological tests are administered to control participants (nonusers or infrequent users) and frequent users, and the results are compared. In such cases, individual differences in IQ become extremely relevant.

The findings of Bolla and colleagues (2002) illustrate this point. These researchers compared the neuropsychological performances of light (mean eleven marijuana cigarettes per week), moderate (forty-two marijuana cigarettes per week), and heavy (ninety-four marijuana cigarettes per week) marijuana users after twenty-eight days of abstinence and found that as the average number of marijuana cigarettes smoked per week increased, participants' performance was altered in a variety of domains, including verbal memory, visual learning and memory, executive functioning, manual dexterity, and psychomotor speed.

Interestingly, this effect was somewhat dependent on IQ. That is, among those with lower IQ scores, users who smoked more often performed considerably more poorly on multiple tasks than those who smoked less often. In contrast, among participants with higher IQ scores, increased marijuana use was associated with fewer decrements and even with better performance on multiple tasks. These results demonstrate that the mediating influence of IQ is important to consider when evaluating long-term effects of cannabis on cognition. Of course, as is the case with most studies of the chronic effects of cannabis on cognition, participants' premorbid IQs (their IQs prior to initiation of cannabis use) were not ascertained.

Without information about the intellectual capabilities of participants before their initiation of drug use, we cannot fully determine whether their regular cannabis use affected their cognitive performance. Fried and colleagues (2004) aimed to address this limitation by examining a group of participants who had been evaluated since birth as part of a prospective study. The authors compared the results of neuropsychological tests administered to these participants when they were preteens (ages nine to twelve; presumably, marijuana use among participants at this age was rare) to the results of similar tests administered to these same participants when they were young adults (ages seventeen to twenty-one) and found that the young adults who were currently frequent marijuana users exhibited reduced performance in multiple domains, including vocabulary, concept formation/abstract reasoning, and attention.

However, when the authors controlled for premorbid intellectual functioning, these deficits did not persist, indicating that cognitive performance was compromised prior the initiation of marijuana use. One limitation of the study design, however, is that participants were not instructed to abstain from marijuana for a prolonged period and had typically smoked marijuana during the twenty-four hours prior to cognitive testing.

This lack of an appropriate abstinence period introduces a potential confound, as it does not allow for a sufficient washout period, which is important when we consider the extent to which marijuana remains in the body following use. Unlike with most recreational drugs, the active component of marijuana (THC) and its metabolites have an extended terminal half-life; it can take as long as twenty-five to thirty-six hours for 50 percent of the drug to be removed from the body. One accepted minimum pharmacological guideline is that investigators should allow at least five half-lives to elapse following a participant's last use of cannabis before initiating any testing (i.e., an approximately 180-hour or one-week interval). Of course, if study participants are heavy cannabis users, intertest intervals should be increased.

One reason that regular users should be viewed differently relative to infrequent users is because more drug metabolites will have accumulated in their bodies over time, and abrupt discontinuation of drug use most likely will lead to symptoms of withdrawal. Cannabis withdrawal syndrome may include a variety of symptoms such as increased deficits in cognitive performance, anxiety, restlessness, depression, irritability, disrupted sleep, and decreased food intake (Kouri, Pope, and Lukas 1999; Haney et al. 2003, 2004). These symptoms have been reported to begin one day after cessation of drug use, to peak between days two and six, and to persist for four to fourteen days, depending on an individual's level of cannabis use (Budney et al. 2003).

To ensure that the effects observed are not related to residual drug effects or withdrawal symptoms, some researchers have required participants to remain abstinent from marijuana for an extended period, sometimes as long as twenty-eight days, and have verified abstinence either by requiring regular urine toxicology screens or admitting participants into an inpatient unit. For example, Pope and colleagues (2001) examined the cognitive performance of current frequent users, those who had used marijuana at least five thousand times in their lives, and who were smoking on a daily basis prior to the study. They compared the performance of current frequent users to that of former frequent users (individuals with the same past use history as current users but who had used infrequently in the past three months), and to controls (individuals who had used marijuana fewer than fifty times).

Pope and colleagues required participants to be abstinent from marijuana for twenty-eight days and asked that participants perform a battery of neuropsychological tasks after zero, one, seven, and twenty-eight days of abstinence.

Current frequent users performed worse than controls on word recall on days zero, one, and seven, and this decreased performance was associated with the concentration of 11-nor-9-carboxy-delta-9-tetrahydrocannabinol, a metabolite of marijuana, in participants' blood upon entry into study. There were no significant differences between controls and former frequent users, suggesting that the decreased performance seen in current users may have been related to residual drug or withdrawal effects. Furthermore, by day twenty-eight, there were no significant differences among all three groups on word recall as well as a variety of other cognitive tasks, including those assessing attention, mental flexibility, and memory, indicating that whatever cognitive differences may have existed among current users did not endure following prolonged abstinence.

Finally, no review of the cognitive effects of marijuana would be complete without a discussion of brain-imaging data. A growing number of studies have combined neuropsychological testing and brain-imaging techniques to examine differences in cognitive performance and brain activation between cannabis users and nonusers. For example, Eldreth and colleagues (2004) used positron emission tomography (PET) and a task measuring executive function to investigate brain activation and cognition in a group of frequent users who had been abstinent for twenty-five days.

The researchers found hyperactivity in the hippocampus and hypoactivity in the left perigenual anterior cingulate cortex and the left lateral prefrontal cortex among users as compared to controls. Despite these differential brain activations, there were no differences between users and nonusers on cognitive performance. Other researchers have found similar changes in brain activation but no cognitive performance differences between cannabis users and controls (Jager et al. 2006; Kanayama et al. 2004). While we recognize the promise of using neuroimaging techniques to better inform our understanding of cannabis-associated effects on cognitive functioning, the above observations emphasize the importance of carefully examining the major behavior of interest—cognitive performance. Otherwise, we run the risk of conducting neuroimaging studies with limited or no behavioral correlates, and we may be enticed to draw inappropriate conclusions about the neural basis of cognition.

CONCLUSION

Although the effects of cannabis on cognition are nuanced, a few general trends emerge. With regard to acute effects among infrequent users, cannabis is associated with temporary disruptions in a range of cognitive domains, particularly learning and memory. Among frequent users, cannabis-related cognitive effects are more limited, although one consistent finding is a general slowing of performance. The major point here is that when investigating the effects of acute cannabis intoxication, it is crucial to take into account participants' drug-use histories, as frequent users may have developed tolerance to many cannabis-related cognitive effects.

The impact of long-term use of cannabis on cognitive performance seems mixed when the evidence is examined uncritically, with some studies showing disruptions in multiple cognitive domains and others reporting virtually no differences between cannabis users and nonusers. However, when appropriate measures are taken to control for potential confounds (e.g., inclusion of a sufficient washout period prior to initiating testing), regular cannabis use appears to have only limited effects on cognitive functioning. Finally, when considering the acute or long-term effects of cannabis on human cognition, it is critically important to bear in mind that cognitive performance is the primary behavior of interest, and neuroimaging and neurophysiological data should be used to supplement but not supplant cognitive data.

TABLE 12.1. SAMPLE OF STUDIES ASSESSING THE DIRECT EFFECTS OF CANNABIS ON COGNITIVE PERFORMANCE

Investigators	Drug investigated (dose)	Cannabis use history of participants	Outcome
INFREQUENT USERS			
Melges et al. 1970	Oral marijuana extract (0, 20, 40, 60 mg THC)	Unspecified ("normal male graduate students") [N=8, within-subjects design]	**Decreased performance:** immediate memory and temporal disintegration No effect: sustained attention and delayed memory
Tinklenberg et al. 1970	Oral marijuana extract (0, 20, 40, 60 mg THC)	Less than 1×/month [N=8, within-subjects design]	**Decreased performance:** immediate memory

Investigators	Drug investigated (dose)	Cannabis use history of participants	Outcome
Abel 1971	Smoked marijuana (undetermined THC content)	Unspecified (previous use, but not quantified) [N=20, between-subjects design, matched on performance on test of immediate free recall (prior to drug administration)]	Decreased performance: immediate memory No effect: delayed memory
Miller and Cornett 1978	Smoked marijuana (0, 5, 10, 15 mg delta-9-THC)	2–4x/week [N=16, within-subjects design]	Decreased performance: immediate and delayed memory
Curran et al. 2002	Oral marijuana extract (0, 7.5, 15 mg delta-9-THC)	Less than 1x/week [N=15, within-subjects design]	Decreased performance: delayed and immediate memory, complex reaction time, and attention No effect: reasoning, simple reaction time, implicit memory, verbal fluency, rapid visual information processing, and mental calculation
D'Souza et al. 2004	Intravenous 0, 2.5, 5 mg delta-9-THC	Median 21–50x/lifetime [N=22, within-subjects design]	Decreased performance: immediate and delayed memory, verbal fluency, working memory, distractibility, and reaction time No effect: learning and recognition and vigilance
Ilan, Smith, and Gevins 2004	Smoked marijuana (0, 3.45% delta-9-THC)	Between 1x/month and 1x/week [N=10, within-subjects design]	Decreased performance: immediate and working memory and reaction time

TABLE 12.1 (continued)

Investigators	Drug investigated (dose)	Cannabis use history of participants	Outcome
Ilan et al. 2005	Smoked marijuana (0, 1.8, 3.6% delta-9-THC)	Mean 15–17 cigarettes/month [N=24, mixed between- and within-subjects design]	**Decreased performance:** immediate and working memory and reaction time
Lane et al. 2005	Smoked marijuana (0, 0.89, 1.77, 3.58% delta-9-THC)	Between 2×/month and 12×/month [N=10, between-subjects design]	**Decreased performance:** decision making
Ramaekers et al. 2006	Smoked marijuana (0, 250, 500 µg/kg delta-9-THC)	Mean 3.4×/month [N=20, within-subjects design]	**Decreased performance:** problem solving, impulsivity, psychomotor control, and reaction time **No effect:** decision making
Hunault et al. 2009	Smoked marijuana [0, 29.3 (9.8%), 49.1 (16.4%), 69.4 mg (23.1%) delta-9-THC]; cigarettes containing 700 mg tobacco/300 mg cannabis	Mean 7.7 cigarettes/month [N=24, within-subjects design]	**Decreased performance:** immediate memory, sustained attention, psychomotor control, and reaction time **No effect:** selective attention and divided attention
FREQUENT USERS			
Meyer et al. 1971	Smoked marijuana (0, 250 mg marijuana leaf) and ad lib session (average): 420 mg (infrequent); 380 mg (frequent)	Frequent users: approximately every day [N=6] Infrequent users: ≤ 1×/week [N=6]	**Decreased performance:** sustained attention in infrequent users
Heishman, Arasteh, and Stitzer 1997	Smoked marijuana (0, 3.55% delta-9-THC)	Mean 4.4 cigarettes/week [N=5, within-subjects design]	**Decreased performance:** visuospatial processing **No effect:** immediate memory, time perception, and reaction time

Investigators	Drug investigated (dose)	Cannabis use history of participants	Outcome
Ward et al. 1997	Smoked marijuana (0, 1.8, 3.1% delta-9-THC)	Minimum 4 days/week [N=7, within-subjects design]	**No effect:** visuospatial processing, divided attention, immediate and delayed memory
Haney et al. 1999	Smoked marijuana (0, 1.8, 3.1% delta-9-THC)	Mean 5.8 days/week; 6.7 cigarettes/occasion [N=12, within-subjects design]	**Decreased performance:** visuospatial processing **Enhanced performance:** divided attention **No effect:** immediate and delayed memory
Hart et al. 2001	Smoked marijuana (0, 1,8, 3.9% delta-9-THC)	Mean 6.1 days/week, 4 cigarettes/day [N=18, within-subjects design]	**Decreased performance:** reaction time and inhibitory control **Enhanced performance:** sustained attention **No effect:** attention, immediate and delayed memory, visuospatial processing, reasoning, mental flexibility, and mental calculation
Vadhan et al. 2007	Smoked marijuana (0, 1.8, 3.9% delta-9-THC)	Mean 6 days/week; 3.9 cigarettes/day [N=36, within-subject design]	**Decreased performance:** reaction time **No effect:** decision making
Ramaekers et al. 2009	Smoked marijuana (0, 500 µg/kg delta-9-THC)	Infrequent users: 55×/year; 1.2 cigarettes/occasion [N=12] Frequent users: 340×/year; 2.3 cigarettes/occasion [N=12]	**Infrequent users: Decreased performance:** psychomotor control, divided attention, and inhibitory control **No effect:** problem solving **Frequent users: Decreased performance:** inhibitory control **No effect:** psychomotor control, divided attention, problem solving

TABLE 12.2.
SAMPLE OF STUDIES ASSESSING
THE EFFECTS OF CHRONIC CANNABIS USE
ON COGNITIVE PERFORMANCE

Investigators	Length of abstinence prior to testing	Cannabis use history of participants	Outcome
Block and Ghoneim 1993	24h	**Frequent users:** 7 or more times/week; 6.2 years; median use 20–39×/last thirty days [N=52] **Moderate users:** 5–6×/ week; 5.8 years [N=28] **Infrequent users:** 1–4×/ week; 5.5 years [N=64] **Nonusers:** [N=72]	**Decreased performance:** math and verbal expression and long-term retrieval **No effect:** vocabulary, interpreting literary works, short tests of educational ability, concept formation, learning, word associations, free associations, psychomotor tests
Solowij, Michie, and Fox 1995	Minimum 24h (range 1–30 days)	**Infrequent:** ≤ 2×/week [N=16] **Frequent:** ≥ 3×/week [N=16] **Controls:** mean 9×/ lifetime [N=16] **Short duration:** 3–4 years [N=16] **Long duration:** ≥ 5 years [N=16]	**Decreased performance:** selective attention and information processing
Fletcher et al. 1996	72h	**Older users:** median 5.2 cigarettes/day, 2–7 days/week, 34 years [N=17] **Older nonusers:** [N=30] **Younger users:** median 3.8 cigarettes/day, 2–7×/week, 8 years [N=37] **Younger nonusers:** [N=49]	**Decreased performance:** memory and learning (older users worse than older nonusers), selective and divided attention (older users worse than older nonusers) **No effect:** story recall, sorting task, response time, visual search, attention, mental flexibility No differences between younger users and younger nonusers on any measure

Investigators	Length of abstinence prior to testing	Cannabis use history of participants	Outcome
Pope and Yurgelun-Todd 1996	Minimum 19h (inpatient)	**Frequent users:** median 29 of the past thirty days, cannabinoids in urine [N=65] **Infrequent users:** median 1 in past thirty days, no cannabinoids in urine [N=64]	**Decreased performance:** mental flexibility, verbal fluency (only significant among lower-IQ users), delayed memory (figures), and learning **No effect:** immediate memory, delayed memory (words, prose), visuospatial processing
Pope et al. 2001	28 days (urine toxicology)	**Current frequent users:** at least 5,000×/lifetime [N=63] **Former frequent users:** 5,000×/lifetime, but fewer than 12 times in last 3 months [N=45] **Controls:** no more than 50 times [N=72]	**Decreased performance:** word recall, verbal learning and memory **No effect:** attention, visuospatial memory (except current users committed more errors at day 0), word association, mental flexibility, executive functioning, immediate and delayed memory (after 28 days)
Solowij et al. 2002	Median 17h	**Long-term users:** mean duration 23.9 years, near-daily use [N=51] **Shorter-term users:** mean duration 10.2 years, near-daily use [N=51] **Nonuser controls:** [N=33]	**Decreased performance:** learning and time estimation **No effect:** mental flexibility, attention
Block et al. 2002	26+ hours	**Frequent users:** 7 or more times/week; duration 2 or more years [N=18] **Controls:** no use or use 1–2×/lifetime [N=13]	**Decreased performance:** learning

TABLE 12.1 (continued)

Investigators	Length of abstinence prior to testing	Cannabis use history of participants	Outcome
Bolla et al. 2002	28 days (inpatient)	**Light users:** mean 11 joints/week [N=7] **Moderate:** mean 42 joints/week [N=8] **Heavy:** 94 joints/week [N=7]	**Decreased performance:** verbal memory, visual learning and memory, executive functioning, psychomotor speed, attention (only in lower-IQ subjects; enhanced performance in higher-IQ subjects) **No effect:** recognition, impulsivity
Eldreth et al. 2004	25 days (inpatient)	**Frequent users:** at least 4×/week, at least 2 years [N=11] **Controls:** no current/past use [N=11]	**No effect:** attention
Whitlow et al. 2004	12h	**Regular users:** 25 of 30 days, duration at least 5 years [N=10] **Controls:** <50×/lifetime, not in previous year [N=10]	**Decreased performance:** decision making **No effect:** pattern recognition, delayed matching
Bolla et al. 2005	25 days (inpatient)	**Frequent users:** 53–84 joints/week [N=5] **Moderate users:** 8–35 joints/wcck [N=6] **Controls:** less than 8 days/month [N=11]	**Decreased performance:** decision making

Investigators	Length of abstinence prior to testing	Cannabis use history of participants	Outcome
McHale and Hunt 2008	24h	Experiment 1: Regular users: at least 1×/month for past 6 months [Total N=37] a) Recent users—used within past week [N=12] b) Abstinent users—used within past month but not past week [N=25] Controls: nonusers [N=23] Experiments 2 & 3: Frequent users: at least 3×/week, 2 cigarettes/session, used within past seven days [N=18] Controls: [N=10] Heavy tobacco users: [N=20]	Decreased performance: verbal fluency, visual recognition, delayed visual recall, executive function No effect: prospective memory

13

Mental Health Risks Associated with Cannabis Use

Cheryl Corcoran, M.D.

Central to the current debate as to whether cannabis should be criminalized or legalized is the issue of whether it leads to harmful effects in some smokers, specifically psychiatric disorders of depression, anxiety, and psychosis. This debate is more muted in the United States, where states have experimented with legalizing "medical marijuana," or at least decriminalizing its use. By contrast, in Europe, there is a move toward greater restriction of cannabis; the famous "coffee shops" of the Netherlands are increasingly being shuttered as data emerges that supports an association of cannabis and psychosis. In the United Kingdom, the question of the safety of cannabis use, and hence its legal status, has become hotly contested.

Recently, *Lancet* published a systematic review (Moore et al. 2007), which concluded, "The evidence is consistent with the view that cannabis increases risk of psychotic outcomes . . . although the evidence for affective outcomes is less strong." The political heat and media attention in the U.K. has steadily increased; the Advisory Council on Misuse of Drugs first reversed its earlier determination that cannabis was benign and then announced it would review whether cannabis may be as harmful as other drugs of abuse (reviewed in Murray et al. 2007).

In the first part of this chapter, the evidence for an association between cannabis and psychosis will be detailed, with several caveats described that must be considered in evaluating the data. The reader is invited to draw his or her own conclusions as to whether cannabis use may indeed cause psychosis. A sober view of the data may lead to a consideration that lies between two opposite views, both often obvious to the people who hold them: (1) Cannabis is benign, also known as "I smoked weed all through the sixties and so did all my friends, and we are all just fine" vs. (2) a sort of modern medicalized "reefer madness," which concludes that of course cannabis causes psychosis and must be heavily restricted.

At the end of the chapter, we will briefly review the largely inconclusive studies regarding cannabis use and outcomes such as depression and suicidal ideation.

CAN CANNABIS USE CAUSE PSYCHOSIS?

Laboratory Studies

The paranoia-inducing effects of cannabis were observed as early as the nineteenth century, when a French psychiatrist, Moreau de Tours, took large doses of cannabis at the Club de Haschischins, giving cannabis also to students and patients (Murray et al. 2007). (Of note, other alleged patrons of this cannabis club included famous French writers such as Victor Hugo, Alexandre Dumas, and Charles Baudelaire and the French painter Eugene Delacroix.) In the twentieth century, studies showed that controlled administration of cannabis could lead not only to paranoia but to delusions and hallucinations as well (Murray et al. 2007). These studies were the precursors of the challenge paradigms whereby psychotic symptoms, anxiety, and cognitive deficits can be induced by the intravenous administration of delta-9-THC, an active ingredient of cannabis.

Real-World Studies

The fact that cannabis can induce transient psychotic symptoms is clear not only from such challenge studies in the laboratory, but also by experience sampling studies, which take place in the real world in real time. Essentially, in such studies participants are given a beeper and notepad and are asked to document at random times throughout the day (in response to a beep) whether (1) they had used cannabis or other drugs, and (2) if they had any experiences of feeling suspicious, or of having unusual thoughts or perceptual disturbances.

In one such study in Bordeaux, France, only psychosis-prone college students reported an increase in psychotic-like experiences—unusual perceptions and feelings that their thoughts were being influenced or controlled by others—in the context of smoking cannabis, an association that was not explained by concurrent use of amphetamines (Verdoux et al. 2003). While other students found cannabis use pleasurable and noted that it eased anxiety, these psychosis-prone students described cannabis as increasing their anxiety with less pleasurable effect (Verdoux et al. 2003). Time-lag analysis showed that cannabis use at one beep preceded but did not follow psychotic-like experiences at another beep, consistent with cannabis inducing transient psychotic symptoms.

Other support for the idea that cannabis can cause transient psychotic symptoms comes from surveys of people randomly selected from the general population. For example, among individuals ages eighteen to thirty-five in New Zealand, 14 percent of cannabis users reported "strange, unpleasant experiences such as hearing voices or becoming convinced that someone is trying to harm them" after smoking cannabis (Thomas 1996). Transient psychotic symptoms may not be benign, especially in young people, as they may be associated with a greater risk for more serious psychotic disorder later (Arseneault et al. 2004; Henquet et al. 2006).

Prospective Cohort Studies

The real question is not whether cannabis use can lead to transient psychotic symptoms, but whether it has a role in causing serious psychotic disorders such as schizophrenia. The time required for this type of epidemiological study—a prospective cohort study—is not on the order of minutes or hours, but years and even decades. In a prospective cohort study, large groups of people are followed over time to determine whether an earlier exposure, such as the use of cannabis, is associated with a later outcome, such as schizophrenia.

Even if there is an association, it may be false. One must always worry about potential confounders (other variables that are associated with both the exposure and outcome) and explain the apparent relationship between them. There are many possible confounders of an association of cannabis and psychosis. One is other drug use. That is, if cannabis is a gateway drug to the use of other drugs such as hallucinogens, then it may be the other drugs that are really contributing to schizophrenia, not the original cannabis use.

Also, causation cannot be definitively established short of doing what is called a randomized controlled trial, in which cannabis would be administered to healthy young people at random who would then be followed to see who developed psychosis. Clearly this alternative is unethical. But the problem with the prospective cohort study is that people may have characteristics that increase risk for both the exposure and the outcome. For instance, if young people destined to develop schizophrenia are themselves somewhat odd, this oddness might make them more likely to use cannabis. Emerging psychotic symptoms might induce a young person to use cannabis for relief. The cannabis use then would just be a marker of an evolving psychiatric disorder and might not play any role in causing it. This is among the strongest critiques of the claim that cannabis can lead to psychosis.

There are many prospective cohort studies that have examined the association of earlier cannabis use with later psychotic disorders such as schizophrenia, herein described. Keep in mind that although causation cannot be definitively established, there are factors that make a hypothesis of causation more believable. These include:

1. Temporal sequence (the exposure precedes the outcome);
2. Dose dependence (the greater the exposure, the more likely the outcome);
3. Biological plausibility (it makes sense in terms of what is known about the brain that the exposure could lead to the outcome).

Readers are also referred to the recent systematic review in *Lancet* (Moore et al. 2007), which concludes that the evidence supports that cannabis use increases risk of psychotic symptoms and disorders, even accounting for potential confounders.

The first of these prospective cohort studies was done in Sweden and evaluated approximately 45,000 young healthy men who were drafted for military service; these men were followed for fifteen years (Andreasson et al. 1987). Compared to the men who denied any history of using cannabis, those who endorsed use were about twice as likely to develop schizophrenia. Dose dependence was supported, as those who reported using cannabis more than fifty times were six times as likely to develop schizophrenia as those who denied any use.

A more detailed analysis of these original data was done a quarter of a century later (Zammit et al. 2002). A number of potential confounders were considered, including demographic characteristics, IQ, social function, and the use of tobacco, alcohol, or other drugs. Although low IQ, cigarette smoking, and poor social integration all predicted schizophrenia themselves, they could not account for the association of cannabis use at conscription and later schizophrenia. Again, dose dependence was demonstrated as in the earlier study, with the sixfold increase in schizophrenia among the heaviest users. The problem of other drug use was addressed not only by identifying this as a potential confounder, but by showing that men who endorsed cannabis use only and no other drug at the time of conscription were still more likely to develop schizophrenia.

The problem of whether subtle psychotic symptoms might induce cannabis use was addressed by repeating the analysis with the smaller subgroup of men who developed schizophrenia five years later and not earlier; they were less likely to have such subtle psychotic symptoms. Still, the association persisted.

In another study of drafted men, this one done in Israel, an association was also found for cannabis use and later schizophrenia, adjusting for the potential confounders of low IQ and poor social functioning (Weiser et al. 2002). As in the Swedish study, cigarette smoking also predicted later schizophrenia in this same Israeli cohort. However, Weiser and these same colleagues use their data to cast doubt on the idea that cannabis causes schizophrenia, as so many men who did smoke cannabis or cigarettes did not develop schizophrenia (Weiser, Davidson, and Noy 2005a).

The other major studies have followed a whole population over time, and most have occurred in New Zealand. Most well known is the Dunedin study, in which about a thousand children were assessed for any psychotic symptoms at age eleven, cannabis use at ages fifteen and eighteen, and diagnosis at age twenty-six of either depression or schizophreniform disorder (Arseneault et al. 2004). (Schizophreniform disorder is diagnosed when the full symptoms of schizophrenia are present, but the duration of illness has not clearly exceeded six months.)

This study found only a 50 percent increase in risk of schizophreniform disorder at age twenty-six associated with cannabis use by age eighteen, even adjusting for earlier psychotic symptoms at age eleven. However, cannabis use at the earlier age of fifteen was associated with a more than fourfold increase in diagnosis of schizophreniform disorder at age twenty-six, a risk that was reduced to threefold when psychotic symptoms at age eleven were accounted for in the analysis.

One in ten individuals who had used cannabis by age fifteen developed schizophreniform disorder! These data are consistent with a dose-dependent effect (which supports causation), as presumably the early users of cannabis would have a greater exposure to cannabis than those who started later. This study also addresses the question of potential confounding by evolving psychotic symptoms. Additionally, the use of other drugs by ages fifteen and eighteen did not explain the effect of cannabis use. Finally, teenaged cannabis use was specifically linked to later schizophreniform disorder, as it did not predict a later diagnosis of depression in adulthood.

Overall, these studies consistently show an association of teen cannabis use with adult schizophrenia, with a two- to threefold increase in risk (Andreasson et al. 1987; Zammit et al. 2002; Weiser et al. 2002; Arseneault et al. 2004). The temporal sequence of cannabis use and psychosis diagnosis in each of these studies, with a span of years between the exposure and outcome, is consistent with causation. Dose dependence has also been observed in multiple studies (Andreasson et al. 1987; Zammit et al. 2002; Arseneault et al. 2004), and is also supportive of causation. Potential confounders were addressed in these studies, including other drug use and the question of early psychotic symptoms (Zammit et al. 2002; Arseneault et al. 2004). However, as Weiser and others have pointed out, a two- to threefold increase in risk is not so sizable and could be explained by unrecognized confounding variables (Weiser and Noy 2005b). Finally, there is also the issue of potential publication bias; negative studies that find no association between an exposure and an outcome may be less likely to be published.

Biological Plausibility

Biological plausibility lends support to the hypothesis of a causal association. If there is a medical basis for the phenomenon in question, it makes more sense. Cannabinoid receptors are found throughout the brain, especially in regions implicated in schizophrenia, such as the limbic and prefrontal cortices, and also the striatum, where they co-localize with dopamine receptors (Reisine 1994). Cannabinoids promote dopamine synthesis and activity (Fernandez-Ruiz et al. 2004), inhibit dopamine uptake, and increase firing of dopamine neurons. This is quite relevant, as the dopamine hypothesis of psychosis and schizophrenia is well established, based on the observations that (1) antipsychotic medications work by blocking dopamine receptors; and (2) brain imaging shows that dopamine release is increased in the striatum in schizophrenia and is related to psychotic symptoms (Abi-Dargham et al. 2000).

Cannabis may also play a role in causing psychosis and schizophrenia through its interaction with other neurotransmitters, such as GABA and glutamate, and by reducing plasticity in the brain (the brain's ability to change in response to experience and learning) (Chevaleyre, Takahashi, and Castillo 2006).

However, biological data can also be marshaled against the theory that cannabis causes psychosis. As Weiser and colleagues point out, independent of cannabis use, there are more receptors for cannabinoids in the brains of patients with schizophrenia than in normal individuals. Also, genes for these receptors are associated with schizophrenia risk (Weiser and Noy 2005b). Therefore, it is possible that abnormalities in the cannabinoid system in the brain could lead independently to both cannabis use and schizophrenia. This would mean that cannabis use would be associated with schizophrenia, but this would be a false association and certainly not a causal one.

Biological data, specifically regarding genes, may be used to explain why only some individuals would develop psychotic symptoms and disorders as a consequence of cannabis use (Arseneault et al. 2004; Verdoux et al. 2003). COMT, or catechol-O-methyl-transferase, is an enzyme involved in breaking down dopamine. Individuals with a specific variation in this gene are more likely to develop psychotic symptoms and disorders after using cannabis, as seen in both both experience sampling (Henquet et al. 2006) and prospective cohort studies (Caspi et al. 2005).

CAN CANNABIS LEAD TO ANXIETY?

As with psychotic symptoms, an anxiety-inducing role for cannabis is supported by both challenge studies and experience sampling studies. The active ingredient of cannabis, specifically delta-9-THC when administered intravenously, induces not only psychotic symptoms but also anxiety in healthy individuals and stable schizophrenia patients. Increases at the same time in the stress hormone cortisol suggest anxiety may potentially mediate the psychosis-inducing effects of delta-9-THC. In real-world experience sampling studies, only highly psychosis-prone college students described cannabis as increasing their anxiety (Verdoux 2005), an effect not seen in a normal sample (Tournier et al. 2003).

By contrast, prospective cohort studies do not support a role for cannabis use in causing anxiety disorders, as reviewed in a meta-analysis (Moore et al. 2007); only two of seven studies found an association of anxiety disorder with previous cannabis use when potential confounding factors were adjusted for. Also, several studies had high dropout rates. If healthier individuals are more likely to drop out, whereas the anxious individuals are more likely to return, this could lead to an apparent association of cannabis use with anxiety that would be false.

CAN CANNABIS LEAD TO DEPRESSION?

Ten cohort studies of cannabis use and depression diagnosis were identified in the *Lancet* meta-analysis and review (Moore et al. 2007). Only half of these—five studies—reported a significant association after adjusting for a few potential confounders. In one study, the Dunedin cohort (described earlier), an association was found only for the subgroup of older adolescents; there was no correction for baseline depressive symptoms; and the association was only barely statistically significant.

Two other studies, which used standard diagnostic criteria for a major episode of depression, found an increase in depression risk of less than 20 percent associated with cannabis use, which might very well be accounted for by unidentified confounding variables. Another study also found just a marginal increase and only in a subgroup. The only study that found a robust increase in risk (fourfold!) evaluated the existence of depressive symptoms (which was not a diagnosis of depression) over only two weeks in individuals with clear abuse of or dependence on cannabis. In sum, the data are not strong for supporting a causal role for cannabis use in depressive disorder.

CONCLUSION

It is often asked why schizophrenia has not increased worldwide if cannabis use causes psychosis, since earlier use of more potent cannabis has increased and is now widespread (Smit, Bolier, and Cuijpers 2004). There are several responses to this important question. One is that an epidemic may be coming and simply hasn't arrived yet. In support of this is that in specific geographical areas like the Gambia (Rolfe et al. 1993) and parts of inner-city London (Boydell et al. 2006), an increase in psychosis has followed increases in cannabis use.

Another response is that cannabis use may simply lead to the earlier onset of an illness that was inevitable nonetheless. However, delaying psychosis onset is not a trivial endeavor, as it might allow individuals to consolidate social and vocational function before becoming ill, which may improve long-term course and functioning. Finally, another response, supported by many studies reviewed in this chapter, is that the psychosis-producing effects of cannabis are restricted to a subset of individuals who are vulnerable, in terms either of psychosis proneness or genetic vulnerability.

As schizophrenia is not so common, affecting about 1 percent of the population, a change of 0.01 percent or so will not look like an epidemic, even though this would mean that cannabis use accounts for 10 percent of schizophrenia. But compare this with the 5.5 percent of schizophrenia that is accounted for by family history (Mortensen et al. 1999), and consider that use of cannabis is a potentially modifiable behavior, whereas genetic susceptibility to schizophrenia is complex, and certainly cannot be changed at this time.

There are safe and effective treatments aimed at reducing the use of cannabis and other drugs in patients with schizophrenia, including first-episode patients (Addington and Addington 2001; Barrowclough et al. 2001). Such interventions may prove useful in young people at risk of psychosis who use cannabis, leading to prevention or delay of onset of psychosis, or at least a better course in those who develop psychosis and schizophrenia independent of cannabis use.

14

How Real Is the Risk of Addiction?

Ryan Vandrey, Ph.D., and
Margaret Haney, Ph.D.

Some may find a chapter on marijuana and addiction somewhat surprising as, historically, few consider marijuana to be an addictive drug, particularly in comparison with other drugs such as heroin, cocaine, and nicotine. While it is true that the majority of marijuana users do not develop significant problems related to their use, recent reports suggest that problems related to marijuana use can develop for a subset of users, and marijuana users are increasingly enrolling in drug treatment programs. It is uncertain whether this increase in treatment admissions solely reflects the recent change in criminal justice toward more court-ordered treatment, or whether other factors such as increased availability of services or marijuana potency also contribute.

The aim of this chapter is to review the current evidence regarding whether—and to what degree—marijuana users become addicted to marijuana or other drugs. We first describe the criteria that must be met for someone to be diagnosed as being "addicted." Second, these criteria are discussed with regard to marijuana, citing evidence from published scientific studies and large-scale surveys. Last, we comment briefly on the "gateway hypothesis," which suggests that the use of marijuana may alter brain function in a way that increases the likelihood of a user's addiction to other drugs of abuse (e.g., cocaine, heroin) compared to those who have never used marijuana.

While most people have a general idea of what addiction means, it is important to provide an operational definition so that it is clear what behaviors and characteristics the term refers to before addressing questions of addiction to marijuana and other drugs of abuse. The definition of addiction used here is that described as "substance dependence" in the *Diagnostic and Statistical Manual of the American Psychiatric Association* (American Psychiatric Association 2000). The *Diagnostic and Statistical Manual* (*DSM*) has been developed with the input of thousands of expert psychiatrists over several decades to carefully classify and characterize human mental health disorders, including drug-use disorders.

According to the *DSM*, addiction refers to use of a substance that causes the user significant impairment or distress, and is associated with at least three of the following effects within the same twelve-month period:

1. Tolerance develops (a need to use more of the drug to get the desired effect, or the same amount of drug has less of an effect than it used to).
2. Withdrawal symptoms occur when use of the drug is stopped and/or the drug or other drugs are used to avoid withdrawal symptoms.
3. Larger amounts of the drug are used or use persists for a longer period of time than was intended.
4. The user reports a persistent desire to reduce use of the drug or is unsuccessful in attempts to cut down or quit using the drug.
5. A great deal of time is spent in activities surrounding obtaining, using, and recovering from the effects of the drug.
6. Use of the drug interferes with engagement in important social, recreational, or work-related activities.
7. Use of the drug is continued despite knowledge that the drug is likely causing or worsening a health problem (American Psychiatric Association 2000).

The amount of scientific research conducted on marijuana addiction is far less than that related to dependence on alcohol, cocaine, and other major drugs of abuse. However, data from controlled laboratory studies, clinical trials, and surveys can help us better understand whether use of marijuana can result in the hallmark features of addiction described above.

The next section of this chapter reviews scientific publications and the outcomes of national surveys related to marijuana addiction, and, when possible, provides references for review articles that discuss the topic in more detail.

TOLERANCE

Tolerance refers to the phenomenon in which, following repeated exposures to a drug over time, larger doses of the drug are required to achieve a desired effect, or the same amount of drug has less of an effect than it used to for a particular user (for a review, see Stewart and Badiani 1993). Controlled scientific experiments have clearly demonstrated that tolerance develops to most effects of marijuana and THC (the primary active compound in smoked marijuana) following repeated exposure (Beardsley, Balster, and Harris 1986; Haney et al. 1997; Jones and Benowitz 1976; Kaymakcalan 1973; McMillan et al. 1970; Nowlan and Cohen 1977).

In these experiments, involving humans and several nonhuman species, tolerance was shown to develop reliably to the behavioral (e.g., general activity levels, task performance), subjective (e.g., feeling high), and physiological (e.g., increased heart rate) effects of marijuana. Preclinical studies suggest that tolerance likely develops due to a reduction in the number of cannabinoid receptors in the brain that occurs following repeated exposure to cannabinoids (Oviedo, Glowa, and Herkenham 1993; Fan et al. 1996). In recent large-scale surveys about drug use conducted in the United States and Australia, 21 percent and 22 percent of current marijuana users (used at least once in the past year) reported having developed tolerance to the subjective effects of marijuana (SAMHSA 2007; Teesson et al. 2002).

WITHDRAWAL

While early investigations into the occurrence of withdrawal symptoms following marijuana use in the 1970s showed mixed results, more recent research has demonstrated that a valid and reliable withdrawal syndrome can occur when regular marijuana use is abruptly stopped. Reports from controlled laboratory studies and surveys of people seeking treatment for marijuana-related problems indicate that anger and aggression, anxiety, depressed mood, irritability, restlessness, sleep difficulty and strange dreams, decreased appetite, and weight loss are the most common symptoms of the marijuana withdrawal syndrome (Budney, Novy, and Hughes 1999; Copersino et al. 2006; Haney et al. 1999; Hart 2002a; Vandrey et al. 2005a). Headaches, physical tension, sweating, chills, stomach pain, and general physical discomfort have also been observed during marijuana withdrawal, but are less common.

Most marijuana withdrawal symptoms occur within the first twenty-four hours of quitting, are most severe two to four days later, and last approximately one to two weeks (Budney et al. 2003; Kouri and Pope 2000). Of note, there is considerable overlap in marijuana withdrawal symptoms and symptoms of withdrawal from other abused drugs such as cocaine, alcohol, and nicotine (Hughes, Higgins, and Bickel 1994; Vandrey et al. 2005b, 2007). Because these withdrawal symptoms are time-limited, occur shortly after cannabis cessation, and are eliminated following a return to marijuana use or administration of THC, it appears that they represent a true withdrawal syndrome (for reviews, see Budney et al. 2004; Haney et al. 2005).

A large national survey conducted in Australia suggests that approximately 30 percent of current marijuana users report experiencing withdrawal symptoms when they stop using marijuana (Teesson et al. 2002). Further, a majority of those who seek treatment for marijuana-related problems or report using marijuana daily experience withdrawal symptoms when they stop using, and most report that the experience of withdrawal has directly resulted in failed attempts to quit (Coffey et al. 2002; Copeland, Swift, and Rees 2001a; Stephens, Roffman, and Simpson 1993; Copersino et al. 2006; Budney, Novy, and Hughes 1999).

UNCONTROLLED USE

Several of the diagnostic criteria for drug addiction in the *DSM* refer to circumstances in which someone is unable to control their use of the drug in question. In one instance, loss of control is characterized by decreased ability to limit use to planned occasions or amounts of the drug. It is not uncommon for people to set personal limits with regard to when (e.g., weekends or holidays only) and how much (e.g., three drinks or one joint) they use alcohol or other drugs.

Occasional deviations or exceptions to these limits are expected. It is when these personal limits are routinely violated that it is considered a loss of control and applied toward a diagnosis of drug addiction. It is important to mention that the *intent* of the user is what is important in judging this aspect of drug dependence. Recent surveys in the United States and Australia indicate that approximately 20 percent of current marijuana users report trouble restricting their use to intended personal limits (SAMHSA 2007; Teesson et al. 2002).

Another way in which loss of control is manifested is an inability to cut down or quit use of a drug despite the desire to do so. Recent national surveys indicate that, among active marijuana users, approximately 40 percent attempt to either reduce or quit use of marijuana each year. Of those, most try to quit on their own and are successful; however, approximately 16 percent are not (SAMHSA 2007; Teesson et al. 2002). Those who seek out and enter treatment for marijuana-related problems appear to have greater difficulty achieving abstinence. Relapse rates in clinical trials of marijuana users are comparable to those observed for people in treatment for other illegal drugs, including cocaine and heroin (Budney et al. 2000; Budney et al. 2006; Copeland et al. 2001b; Marijuana Treatment Project Research Group 2004; Stephens, Roffman, and Curtin 2000; Stephens, Roffman, and Simpson 1994). Currently, there are ongoing efforts to develop psychosocial and pharmacological therapies to assist the minority of marijuana users who have trouble quitting (for reviews, see Haney 2005; Hart 2005; McRae, Budney, and Brady 2003).

One more indication that control over drug use is lost is when a drug user spends an inordinate amount of time in activities surrounding obtaining, using, and recovering from the effects of a drug, whether intended or not. That intensive pattern of drug use can result in a host of maladaptive consequences for the user. Specifically, increased time spent engaging in drug-related activities can limit time spent with family, friends, and other social contacts that do not also use the drug, and can strain those relationships. Increased time spent on drug use can also result in decreased performance at school or work, or a failure to fulfill responsibilities at home, work, or elsewhere. Lastly, as time spent in activities surrounding drug use increases, time spent engaging in important social, occupational, or recreational activities likely decreases. These are particularly important consequences of drug use, because increased time spent with drug-using peers and poor social support has been associated with an increased likelihood of continuing to use drugs over time (Brewer et al. 1998).

With respect to current marijuana users, between 10 and 40 percent report that they spend a great deal of time obtaining, using, or recovering from the effects of marijuana (SAMHSA 2007; Teesson et al. 2002). Additionally, between 3 and 8 percent of all current marijuana users report that their marijuana use has caused problems at school, work, or home, strained interpersonal relationships, or caused a reduction in social, occupational, or recreational activities (SAMHSA 2007; Teesson et al. 2002). As would be expected, social or interpersonal problems associated with marijuana use are more common among those who use the drug more frequently and are prevalent in those who seek treatment (Coffey et al. 2002, Copeland, Swift, and Rees 2001a; Stephens et al. 2002).

Surveys indicate that the most commonly reported social or interpersonal problems related marijuana use are: "spending more time with smoking friends than other friends" (76 percent), "lowered self-esteem" (74 percent), "worried about feelings of personal isolation or detachment" (71 percent), "lacking self confidence" (68 percent), "worried about losing touch with friends or family" (67 percent), "difficulty getting same enjoyment from interests" (65 percent), "giving up hobbies because of smoking" (59 percent), and "problems between you and your partner" (58 percent) (Copeland, Swift, and Rees 2001a; Stephens et al. 2002). While these problems represent clinically important issues, it should be noted that more severe psychosocial problems such as job loss or child neglect that may coincide with addictions to cocaine or alcohol are infrequent among those who primarily use marijuana.

USE DESPITE PHYSICAL OR PSYCHOLOGICAL PROBLEMS

Another indicator of drug addiction is continuing use despite awareness that use of the drug is causing physical or psychological problems. Chronic use of marijuana has been associated with causing or worsening existing physical health problems, such as compromised respiratory function (persistent cough, bronchitis, or asthma) (Tashkin et al. 1975, 1987; Taylor et al. 2000; for a review, see Tetrault et al. 2007) and impaired cognitive functioning, particularly related to memory ability (for reviews, see Beardsley and Kelly 1999; Lundqvist 2005; Murray 1985).

Similarly, chronic cannabis use has the potential to contribute to the occurrence and severity of symptoms associated with mental health problems such as anxiety, depression, or schizophrenia (Deykin, Levy, and Wells 1986; Kandel et al. 1986; McGee et al. 2000). Continuation of marijuana use despite the recognition that it is causing such problems is clearly maladaptive. Among current marijuana users in the United States and Australia, between 4 and 11 percent report that they continue to use marijuana despite experiencing physical or psychological problems that they believed were either caused by or made worse by their marijuana use (SAHMSA 2007; Teesson et al. 2002).

Further, in two surveys of treatment seekers, a majority reported they had experienced the following effects as a result of heavy marijuana use:

"feeling paranoid or antisocial after smoking" (78 percent), "memory loss" (76 percent), "physical neglect" (68 percent), "pains in chest/lungs after a smoking session" (63 percent), "feeling depressed for more than a week" (59 percent), and "poorer than usual general health" (57 percent) (Copeland, Swift, and Rees 2001a; Stephens et al. 2002).

The evidence available from the laboratory studies and surveys described above clearly indicate that at least a subset of marijuana users endorse each of the criteria that compose the clinical description of drug addiction. As a reminder, however, a marijuana user must report impairment or distress and at least three of those criteria within the same twelve-month period to be considered addicted to marijuana. Using that criterion, survey studies conducted in the United States and New Zealand estimate that 4 to 5 percent of the total population has met the criteria for a diagnosis of addiction to marijuana at some point in their lives, a prevalence rate greater than any other illicit drug (cocaine 2.7 percent, heroin 0.4 percent) (Anthony, Warner, and Kessler 1994; Hall, Room, and Bondy 1999). In 2006, 2.6 million marijuana users in the United States met criteria for addiction to marijuana, more than for any other illicit drug (SAMHSA 2007).

That the rate of addiction to marijuana is greatest among all illicit drugs likely reflects the fact that marijuana is also the most widely used illicit drug in the developed world. When addiction rates are assessed only among those who have ever tried a certain drug, 9 percent of all those who reported having ever used marijuana met criteria for marijuana addiction at some point in their lives (Anthony, Warner, and Kessler 1994). While data indicating that approximately one out of every eleven people who try marijuana will meet criteria for addiction at some point in their lives is far from trivial, this rate of "conditional" addiction for marijuana is less than that observed for people who have ever used tobacco (32 percent), heroin (23 percent), cocaine (17 percent), or alcohol (15 percent) (Anthony, Warner, and Kessler 1994). Thus, although marijuana has lower addiction liability than many other drugs of abuse, the vast number of individuals who try it results in a large number of individuals who go on to develop problems related to their marijuana use.

A final topic to be discussed is the impact of marijuana use on other drug use. This is more commonly known as the marijuana gateway hypothesis, which proposes that use of marijuana increases the likelihood that other illicit drug use will be initiated (Kandel 2002). The next section briefly describes findings that support the hypothesis, potential explanations for variables that might mediate the relationship, and limitations of the data with regard to establishing causality between use of marijuana and other drugs.

Use of marijuana is clearly one of the strongest predictors of recreational and problematic use of "heavier" drugs such as heroin and cocaine. Moreover, it has been shown in multiple studies that those who use marijuana earlier in life and more frequently are more likely to use and develop problems with other drugs compared to those who start later and use less frequently (Fergusson, Boden, and Horwood 2006; Lynskey et al. 2003; SAMHSA 2001). For example, in a national survey in the United States, 62 percent of those who reported first using marijuana at age fourteen or younger had also used cocaine at some point in their lives. By contrast, among those who didn't smoke marijuana until age eighteen, only 29 percent had used cocaine, while fewer than 1 percent of those who never used marijuana used cocaine (SAMHSA 2001).

One explanation for why use of marijuana is such a high risk factor for later use of other drugs is that exposure to marijuana has direct biochemical effects that increase the likelihood of using other drugs. Several studies have been conducted in which cross-sectional or longitudinal surveys indicate that, after statistically controlling for alternative risk factors such as genetics (twin/sibling studies), socioeconomic factors, and co-occuring psychiatric problems, those who used marijuana were significantly more likely to have used and had problems with other illicit drugs (Fergusson, Boden, and Horwood 2006; Lynskey et al. 2003; Lessem et al. 2006).

While these studies make a compelling case, they cannot account for all potential confounding factors such as unshared environmental experiences among twins and siblings, differential peer influence, opportunities to use drugs, effects of tobacco or alcohol exposure (almost always used before marijuana), or some unmeasured underlying propensity to use drugs or engage in deviant behaviors that could account for rates of "hard" drug use independent of marijuana use (Morral, McCaffrey, and Paddock 2002; Tarter 2006).

An alternate interpretation of the progression from using marijuana to use of other illicit drugs focuses on the potential influence of sociological factors of acceptability, availability, and an interaction of the two. In this case, marijuana is the first illicit drug to be used, because culturally it is the most accepted and available of illicit drugs. Its use is promoted in the media, it is more likely to be used by parents of adolescents and thus found in the home, and there is less social stigma surrounding its use compared to other drugs.

After initiation, however, continued marijuana use usually involves an increasing level of interaction with deviant peers (drug dealers, other drug users) and new social settings, which also increase the availability of other drugs. Thus, the increased likelihood that individuals progress from using marijuana to other "hard" drugs is not a direct effect of marijuana, but rather is a result of a change in availability and environment. This hypothesis is supported by studies that indicate the drug first used by adolescents and young adults is significantly influenced by drug availability and cultural factors (Golub and Johnson 1994; Mackesy-Amiti, Fendrich, and Goldstein 1997; Tarter et al. 2006).

To identify clearly the role of marijuana in the progression to heroin and cocaine use and possibly addiction, controlled laboratory studies in non-humans will likely be needed. One such study demonstrated that rodents repeatedly exposed to THC prior to being exposed to morphine showed a greater behavioral response to the morphine compared with a control group that received morphine only (Cadoni et al. 2001).

This suggests that it is possible that repeated use of marijuana could make other drugs more rewarding, and thus increase the likelihood of developing problematic use patterns. However, much more controlled research would need to be conducted to demonstrate whether this or similar effects could account for the relationship observed between use of marijuana and other drugs, and to identify an exact neurobiological mechanism by which this occurs.

CONCLUSION

In summary, it appears clear that a subset of marijuana users meet the criteria required for a diagnosis of drug dependence (addiction) as described in the *Diagnostic and Statistical Manual of the American Psychiatric Association*. While heavy use of the drug does not necessarily indicate an addiction to marijuana, those who are addicted to marijuana likely use it on a daily or near-daily basis and report experiencing a range of emotional, social, and physiological problems that they feel are caused by their marijuana use.

These effects appear to be more prominent among those who seek treatment for problems associated with their marijuana use. Treatment seeking among marijuana users has increased considerably in recent years, and those who do seek treatment are no more likely than users of other drugs to be successful in quitting. More people meet criteria for addiction to marijuana than any other illicit drug, largely due to the fact that it is the most widely used illicit drug. Finally, there is a strong association between use of marijuana and later problematic use of other illicit drugs like cocaine and heroin, yet whether marijuana has a causal role in that relationship has not been established.

15
Driving Under the Influence

Paul Armentano,
Deputy Director of NORML

Policy debates regarding marijuana law reform invariably raise the question, How does society address concerns regarding pot use and driving? The subject is worthy of serious discussion. NORML's board of directors addressed this issue by ratifying a "no driving" clause to the organization's "Principles of Responsible Cannabis Use" (NORML 1996), stating, "Although cannabis is said by most experts to be safer with motorists than alcohol and many prescription drugs, responsible cannabis consumers never operate motor vehicles in an impaired condition."

Nevertheless, questions remain regarding the degree to which smoking cannabis impairs actual driving performance. Unlike alcohol, which is known to increase drivers' risk-taking behavior and is a primary contributor to motor vehicle accidents, marijuana's impact on psychomotor skills is subtle. Its real-world impact on automobile crashes is conflicting.

DRUGGED DRIVING: TRUE THREAT
OR FALSE PANIC?

Survey data indicates that approximately 112 million Americans (46 percent of the U.S. population) have experimented with the use of illicit substances

(U.S. Department of Health and Human Services, 2007). Of these, approximately 20 million (more than 8 percent of the population) self-identify as "current" or "monthly" users of illicit drugs (National Survey on Drug Use and Health 2007). More than 10 million Americans say that they've operated a motor vehicle while under the influence of an illicit substance in the past year. These totals, while far from negligible, suggest that the prevalence of illicit drug use among U.S. drivers is far less than the prevalence of alcohol among this same population (U.S. Department of Transportation 2003).

According to the U.S. Department of Transportation (2003), to date, "[The] role of drugs as a causal factor in traffic crashes involving drug-positive drivers is still not well understood." While some studies have indicated that illicit drug use is associated with an increased risk of accident, a relationship has not been established regarding the use of psychoactive substances and crash severity (Smink et al. 2005). Drivers under the influence of illicit drugs do experience an enhanced fatality risk compared to sober drivers. However, this risk is approximately three times lower than the fatality risk associated with drivers who operate a vehicle above or near the legal limit for alcohol intoxication (Grotenhermen 2007b). According to one recent review: "The risk of all drug-positive drivers compared to drug-free drivers is similar to drivers with a blood alcohol concentration of 0.05%. The risk is also similar to drivers above age 60 compared to younger drivers [around age 35]" (Grotenhermen et al. 2007a).

Marijuana is the most common illicit substance consumed by motorists who report driving after drug use (U.S. Department of Health and Human Services 1998). Epidemiological research also indicates that cannabis is the most prevalent illicit drug detected in fatally injured drivers and motor vehicle crash victims (U.S. Department of Transportation 2003). Reasons for this are twofold. One, pot is by far the most widely used illicit drug among the U.S. population, with nearly one out of two Americans admitting having tried it (CNN/*Time* poll 2002). Two, marijuana is the most readily detectable illicit drug in toxicological tests. Marijuana's primary psychoactive compound, THC, may be detected in blood for several hours, and in some extreme cases days after past use (Skopp and Potsche 2003), long after any impairing effects have worn off.

In addition, nonpsychoactive byproducts of cannabis, known as metabolites, may be detected in the urine of regular users for days or weeks after past use (Cary 2005). (Other common drugs of abuse, such as cocaine or methamphetamine, do not have such long half-lives.) Therefore, pot's prevalence in toxicological evaluations of U.S. drivers does not necessarily indicate that it is a frequent or significant causal factor in auto accidents. Rather, its prevalence affirms that cannabis remains far more popular and is far more easily detectable on drug screening tests than other controlled substances.

CRUISING ON CANNABIS:
CLARIFYING THE DEBATE

While it is well established that alcohol consumption increases accident risk, evidence of marijuana's culpability in on-road driving accidents and injury is far less clear. Although acute cannabis intoxication following smoking has been shown to mildly impair psychomotor skills, this impairment is seldom severe or long lasting (U.S. Department of Transportation 2003).

In closed-course and driving-simulator studies, marijuana's acute effects on psychomotor performance include minor impairments in tracking (eye movement control) and reaction time, as well as variation in lateral positioning (weaving), headway (drivers under the influence of cannabis tend to follow less closely to the vehicle in front of them), and speed (drivers tend to decrease speed following cannabis inhalation) (Grotenhermen 2007; U.S. Department of Transportation 2003; Ramaekers 2006 et al.; Hadorn 2004; Canadian Senate Special Committee on Illegal Drugs 2002; Smiley 1999). In general, these variations in driving behavior are noticeably less consistent or pronounced than the impairments exhibited by subjects under the influence of alcohol (Hadorn 2004). Also, unlike subjects impaired by alcohol, individuals under the influence of cannabis tend to be aware of their impairment and try to compensate for it accordingly, either by driving more cautiously (U.S. Department of Transportation 2003) or by expressing an unwillingness to drive altogether (Menetrey et al. 2005) .

According to a U. S. Department of Transportation review (2003) "The extensive studies by Robbe and O'Hanlon (1993), revealed that under the influence of marijuana, drivers are aware of their impairment, and when the experimental task allows it, they tend to actually decrease speed, avoid passing other cars, and reduce other risk-taking behaviors." Also stated clearly is the following, "experimental research on the effects of cannabis indicat[e] that any effects . . . dissipate quickly after one hour."

As a result, cannabis-induced variations in performance do not appear to play a significant role in on-road traffic accidents when THC levels in a driver's blood are low and/or cannabis is not consumed in combination with alcohol (U.K. Department of Environment; Chesher and Longo 2002). For example, a 1992 National Highway Traffic Safety Administration review of the role of drug use in fatal accidents reported, "There was no indication that cannabis itself was a cause of fatal crashes" among drivers who tested positive for the presence of the drug (U.S. Department of Transportation 2003). A more recent assessment by Blows and colleagues (2004) noted that self-reported recent use of cannabis (within three hours of driving) was not significantly associated with car crash injury after investigators controlled for specific confounders (e.g., seat-belt use, sleepiness).

A 2004 observational case-control study (Movig et al.) published in the journal *Accident Analysis and Prevention* reported that only drivers under the influence of alcohol or benzodiazepines experience an increased crash risk compared to drug-free controls. Investigators did observe increased risks—though they were not statistically significant—among drivers using amphetamines, cocaine, and opiates, but "no increased risk for road trauma was found for drivers exposed to cannabis."

A handful of more recent studies have noted a positive association between very recent cannabis exposure and a gradually increased risk of vehicle accident. Typically, these studies reveal that drivers whose THC/blood concentrations are 5 ng/ml—implying cannabis inhalation within the past one to three hours (Huestis, Henningfield, and Cone 1992; Mushoff and Madea 2006)—experience an elevated risk of accident compared to drug-free controls (Drummer et al. 2004; Grotenhermen 2007). Motorists who test positive for the presence of THC in the blood at concentrations below this threshold typically do not have an increased risk compared to controls (Grotenhermen 2007). However, this elevated risk is below the risk presented by drivers who have consumed even small quantities of alcohol.

Two recent case-control studies have assessed this risk in detail. A 2007 case-control study published in the *Canadian Journal of Public Health* reviewed ten years of U.S. auto fatality data. Investigators found that U.S. drivers with blood alcohol levels of 0.05 percent—a level well below the legal limit for intoxication—were three times as likely to have engaged in unsafe driving activities prior to a fatal crash as compared to individuals who tested positive for marijuana (Bedard, Dubois, and Weaver 2007).

A 2005 review of auto accident fatality data from France (Laumon) showed similar results, finding that drivers who tested positive for any amount of alcohol had a four times greater risk of having a fatal accident than did drivers who tested positive for marijuana in their blood. In the latter study, even drivers with low levels of alcohol present in their blood (below 0.05 percent) experienced a greater elevated risk as compared to drivers who tested positive for high concentrations of cannabis (above 5 ng/ml). Both studies noted that overall few traffic accidents appeared to be attributed to drivers operating a vehicle while impaired by cannabis.

DEFINING A RATIONAL "DRUGGED DRIVING POLICY"

The above review illustrates the need for further education and understanding regarding the effects of cannabis upon driving behavior. While pot's adverse impact on psychomotor skills is less severe than the effects of alcohol, driving under the acute influence of cannabis still may pose an elevated risk of accident in certain situations. However, because marijuana's psychomotor impairment is subtle and short-lived, consumers can greatly reduce this risk by refraining from driving for a period of several hours following their cannabis use.

By contrast, motorists should never be encouraged to operate a vehicle while smoking cannabis. Drivers should also be advised that engaging in the simultaneous use of both cannabis and alcohol can significantly increase their risk of accident compared to the consumption of either substance alone (Ramaekers et al. 2004; Williams et al. 1985). Past use of cannabis, as defined by the detection of inactive cannabis metabolites in the urine of drivers, is not associated with an increased accident risk (Ramaekers et al. 2004). Educational or public service campaigns targeting drugged driving behavior should particularly be aimed toward the younger driving population aged sixteen to twenty-five years, as this group is most likely to use cannabis (U.S. Department of Justice 2007; and to report having operated a motor vehicle shortly after consuming pot (U.S. Department of Health and Human Services 1998). In addition, this population may have less driving experience, may be more prone to engage in risk-taking behavior, and may be more naive to pot's psychoactive effects than older, more experienced populations. This population also reports a greater likelihood for having driven after using cannabis in combination with other illicit drugs or alcohol.

Such an educational campaign (Canadian Public Health Association, Pot and Driving Campaign, www.potanddriving.cpha.ca) was recently launched nationwide in Canada by the Canadian Public Health Association and could readily be replicated in the United States. Arguably, such a campaign would enjoy enhanced credibility if coordinated by a private public health association or traffic safety organization, such as the American Public

Health Association or the AAA Automobile Club, as opposed to the federal Office of National Drug Control Policy, whose previous public service campaigns have demonstrated limited influence among younger audiences (U.S. Government Accountability Office 2006).

Finally, increased efforts should be made within the law enforcement community to train officers and DREs (Drug Recognition Experts) to better identify drivers who may be operating a vehicle while impaired by marijuana. In Australia, efforts have been made to adapt elements of the roadside Standardized Field Sobriety Test (SFST) to make it sensitive to drivers who may be under the influence of cannabis. Scientific evaluations of these tests have shown that subjects' performance on the modified SFSTs may be positively associated with dose-related levels of marijuana impairment (Papafotiou, Carter, and Strough 2005). Similarly, clinical testing for cannabis impairment among suspected drugged drivers in Norway has been positively associated with identifying drivers with THC/blood concentrations above 3 ng/ml (Khiabani 2006).

Though the development of such cannabis-specific impairment testing is still in its infancy, an argument may be made for the provisional use of such tests by specially trained members of law enforcement. In addition, the development of cannabis-sensitive technology to rapidly identify the presence of THC in drivers, such as a roadside saliva test, would provide utility to law enforcement in its efforts to better identify intoxicated drivers.

The development of such technology would also increase public support for the taxation and regulation of cannabis by helping assuage concerns that liberalizing marijuana policies could potentially lead to an increase in incidences of drugged driving (Looby, Earleywine, and Gieringer 2007). Such concerns are a significant impediment to the enactment of marijuana law reform, and they must be sufficiently addressed before a majority of the public will embrace any public policy that proposes regulating adult cannabis use like alcohol.

16
Arrest Statistics and Racism

Harry G. Levine, Ph.D.

There are two things that need to be understood about marijuana arrests in New York City. First, possession of less than an ounce of marijuana is not a crime in New York State. Since 1977 and passage of the Marijuana Reform Act, state law has made simple possession of less than seventh-eighths of an ounce of pot a *violation,* like a traffic violation. One can be given a ticket and fined $100 for marijuana possession, but not fingerprinted and jailed. For over thirty years, New York State has formally, legally, decriminalized possession of marijuana.

Second, despite that law, from 1997 through 2008 the New York City Police Department (NYPD) arrested 430,000 people for possessing small amounts of marijuana, mostly teenagers and young people in their twenties. Most people arrested were not smoking pot. Usually they just carried a bit of it in a pocket. In 2008 alone, the NYPD arrested and jailed 40,300 people for possessing a small amount of marijuana. These extraordinary numbers of arrests and jailings, continuing for over twelve years, now make New York City the marijuana arrest capital of the world.

The arrests for marijuana possession first increased dramatically under Mayor Rudolph Giuliani. They have continued unabated under Mayor Michael Bloomberg. By 2008, Bloomberg had arrested more people for pot possession than Giuliani, and more than any other mayor in the world.

Why has the NYPD continued to order narcotics and patrol officers to make so many misdemeanor marijuana arrests? The reasons are many. The arrests are easy, safe, and provide training for new officers. The arrests gain overtime pay for patrol and narcotics police and their supervisors. The arrests allow officers to show productivity, which counts for promotions and choice assignments. Marijuana arrests enable the NYPD to obtain fingerprints, photographs, and other data on many young people they would not otherwise have in their criminal justice databases. And there is very little public criticism and thus far no political opposition to New York City's marijuana arrest crusade.

Do the pot arrests reduce serious and violent crimes? No, if anything they increase other crimes. Professors Bernard Harcourt and Jens Ludwig (Harcourt 2007) at the University of Chicago Law School analyzed NYPD data and concluded that the pot possession arrests took officers off the streets and distracted them from other crime-fighting activities. "New York City's marijuana policing strategy," they reported, "is having exactly the wrong effect on serious crime—increasing it, rather than decreasing it." Veteran police officers agree, terming the possession arrests "a waste of time." The arrests drain resources not just of police, but also of courts, jails, prosecutors, and public defenders.

Perhaps most appalling is the racial bias in the marijuana possession arrests. U.S. government studies have consistently found that young whites use marijuana at higher rates than do young blacks or Latinos. But the NYPD has long arrested young blacks and Latinos for pot possession at much higher rates than whites.

In 2008, blacks were about 26 percent of New York City's population, but over 54 percent of the people arrested for pot possession. Latinos were about 27 percent of New Yorkers, but 33 percent of the pot arrestees. Whites were over 35 percent of the city's population, but less than 10 percent of the people arrested for possessing marijuana. In 2008, police arrested Latinos for pot possession at four times the rate of whites, and blacks at seven times the rate of whites. Do the arrests violate New York State's decriminalization law? Yes and no. Yes, they certainly violate the spirit and intent of the 1977 law, which explicitly sought to eliminate the pot possession arrests and the stigma of criminal records, especially for young people. And yes, some police, in particular narcotics squads, do make some illegal searches and arrests.

But no, most of the arrests are probably technically legal. The NYPD has found easy ways to trick or intimidate young people so they allow a search,

TABLE 16.1. MARIJUANA POSSESSION ARRESTS OF WHITES, BLACKS, AND LATINOS IN NEW YORK CITY, 1987 TO 2008

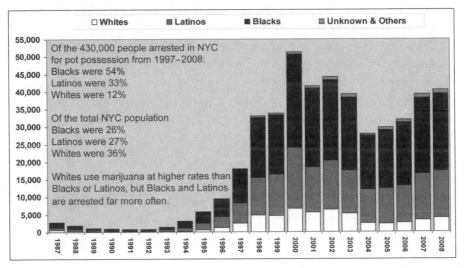

Source: New York State Division of Criminal Justice Services, Computerized Criminal History System (June 2009). Includes all fingerprintable misdemeanor arrests for NYS Penal Law Article 221.10 as the most serious charge in an arrest event. Ages 16 and older. This shows only the lowest-level misdemeanor arrests.

or even just take out their marijuana and hand it over to the officers.

Here's how the police do it: NYPD commanders direct officers to stop and question many young people and make arrests for possessing "contraband." In 2008, the NYPD made more than half a million recorded stop-and-frisks and an unknown number of unrecorded stops, disproportionately in black, Latino, and low-income neighborhoods. By far, the most common contraband young people might possess is a small amount of marijuana.

According to U.S. Supreme Court decisions, police are allowed to thoroughly pat down the outside of someone's clothing looking for a gun, which is bulky and easy to detect. But police cannot legally search inside a person's pockets and belongings without permission or probable cause.

However, police officers can legally make false statements to people they stop, and officers can trick people into revealing things. So in a stern, authoritative voice, NYPD officers will say to the young people they stop: "We're going to have to search you. If you have anything illegal you should show it to us now. If we find something when we search you, you'll have to spend the night in jail. But if you show us what you have now, maybe we can just give you a ticket. And if it's nothing but a little weed, maybe we can let you go. So if you've got anything you're not supposed to have, *take it out and show it now.*"

When police say this, the young people usually take out their small amount of marijuana and hand it over. Their marijuana is now "open to public view." And *that*—having a bit of pot out and open to be seen—technically makes it a crime, a fingerprintable offense. And for cooperating with the police, the young people are handcuffed and jailed.

Before Mayors Giuliani and Bloomberg, New York police rarely if ever did this to make marijuana arrests. Since 1997 the NYPD has used this procedure to make tens of thousands of marijuana arrests a year, averaging about a hundred a day, every day for over twelve years. This is more than ten times the average number of marijuana arrests the city made previously. As NYPD and New York Criminal Court data show, before 1997 marijuana arrests were less than 1 percent of all arrests. The lowest-level misdemeanor pot possession arrests are now over *10* percent of all arrests in New York City.

New York is extreme in the number of its marijuana arrests. But other cities are also making many pot possession arrests and jailings at high rates, often using the same techniques as the NYPD. As FBI arrest data shows, this includes Atlanta, Baltimore, Cincinnati, Cleveland, Denver, Houston, Indianapolis, Philadelphia, Phoenix, San Antonio, and other cities.

Since the 1990s, the U.S. "war on drugs" has emphasized making many low-level possession arrests, especially of marijuana. At least 40 percent of all drug arrests are now just for marijuana possession, and U.S. marijuana arrests are at an all-time high. In the last ten years, the United States has arrested more than 6 million people, mostly young people, for possessing marijuana. As in New York City, pot arrests in other cities are racially skewed, racially biased. Throughout the United States, young blacks and Latinos are stopped, searched, and arrested for pot possession at much higher rates than whites— even though young whites use marijuana at higher rates. Do the arrests harm the people arrested? Absolutely. They produce permanent criminal records that potential employers can easily find, often on the Internet. As even the New York City Health Department recognizes, "A marijuana conviction can keep you from getting a student loan, a job, a house or an apartment—even years later." In effect, the marijuana arrests provide the young, mostly low-income blacks, Latinos, and whites with a head start for unemployment and prison.

The arrests are expensive, but state and local governments do not have to pay for them all. Arrests for possessing even tiny amounts of marijuana and other drugs are subsidized by the U.S. government. Up to a billion dollars a year has been going to states, prosecutors, and police departments through the Byrne Grant Program to "fight" drugs and crime. Many Democrats in Congress have been strong supporters of Byrne Grants, including Senators Joe Biden and Barack Obama. In 2009, the economic stimulus package enacted by Congress added $2 billion to the Byrne Grant Program. This tripled Byrne Grant funding, raising it to the highest level ever. As a result, this epidemic of racially biased and stigmatizing marijuana possession arrests in New York City and elsewhere will grow even larger. The Obama administration's Department of Justice could alter Byrne Grant regulations so that police departments, prosecutors, and local governments cannot use the federal funds to subsidize arrests of people who possess only small amounts of marijuana. That alone could do a great deal to reduce the arrests, jailings, and stigmatizing criminal records. But police departments and prosecutors have enormous political clout in Washington. And other than a few civil liberties and drug policy reform groups, there is currently little organized opposition to the pot arrests.

Partly because of the economic crisis, some people, especially in California, have proposed that marijuana be legalized, taxed, and regulated like alcohol. Serious, broad-ranging debate about alternatives to marijuana prohibition would be a sensible, hopeful development. But marijuana legalization would constitute a huge change in U.S. drug law and is not likely anytime soon. Meanwhile, the great many damaging, expensive, racially biased marijuana possession arrests and jailings continue—even in places like New York that have legally decriminalized simple possession.

In the 1980s Barack Obama was a college student in New York City, living on the border of Harlem. He used marijuana, walked around the city a lot, and sometimes may have carried a bit of pot in his pocket. If the current policing policies of New York and other cities were in effect at that time, he might well have been arrested and jailed. If that had happened, Barack Obama would not be president today.

Is this what Americans want their police to be doing—arresting enormous numbers of young people, disproportionately black and Latino, and destroying their futures, for . . . *pot possession*?

17

Getting Busted Is Not So Funny

An Interview with Tommy Chong

Julie Holland, M.D.

JULIE HOLLAND: Can you recap what happened back in 2003?

TOMMY CHONG: Well, I was looking for some kind of gimmick to jump-start my career when the feds raided my house on February 23, at 5:00 a.m. They showed up at my doorstep with a twelve- to fifteen-member armed SWAT team, DEA agents, FBI—the Postal Service was even represented. There was a helicopter and Fox News out on the street.

JULIE: Fox News knew in advance? That's interesting.

TOMMY: Oh, yes. It was a big raid at the home of the infamous comedian Tommy Chong. And they were looking not for drugs, not for pot, but for water pipes, bongs. We'd been advertising Chong Glassware, different sizes and shapes of marijuana pipes, in *High Times* magazine. And Attorney General John Ashcroft and the boys and U.S. Attorney Mary Beth Buchanan decided that they'd take me down. Me and about fifty-five other companies. There were people in Pittsburgh who got time for having a head shop.

JULIE: But you got more jail time than anybody else.

TOMMY: More than everybody else *combined*.

JULIE: And not only were you in prison for nine months, but you had to pay a fine of $20,000, and you had to forfeit some assets, about $120,000, right?

TOMMY: Yes. It came down to costing me over half a million in cash.

JULIE: And now your company is defunct.

TOMMY: More than that, it was my ability to make money. I had to cancel all the movies we were going to do, and I was working on *That '70s Show,* so they stopped my income for nine months.

JULIE: So you lost acting gigs because of this?

TOMMY: I lost a couple million dollars in acting gigs, and I lost a good half a million in television gigs. It cost me a lot of money.

JULIE: I imagine you know that the estimated cost of Operation Pipe Dream* was over $12 million and included the resources of two thousand law enforcement officers.

TOMMY: I guess the government had something in mind. Personally, I think they were trying to defuse the antiwar movement.

JULIE: I saw your quote about how the only weapons of mass destruction they found were your bongs.

TOMMY: And then they accused me of saying that with a sneer. After I plead guilty, they talked to me to see if there was any remorse, and they said, "Do you have any comments?" and I said, "The charges speak for themselves." And it was written in my sentencing report that the prosecution noted that I said that with a sneer.

JULIE: So you plead guilty without a grand jury indictment, right?

TOMMY: It was so ridiculous.

JULIE: But I think I understand why you did it. It sounds like they were threatening to go after your son and your wife.

---

*Operation Pipe Dream was what the "feds" dubbed the investigation that led to the arrest of Mr. Chong.

TOMMY: That was the threat. They admitted that they had no evidence on me at all. There was no evidence that I owned the company. If it had gone to a jury, I wouldn't even have been charged. But they had evidence against my son and my wife. It was her signature on the check that started the business. And therefore they would have put my family in jail. So they knew I was going to plead guilty.

JULIE: These bongs are water pipes that could be used to smoke tobacco.

TOMMY: Or they could be an art collection. I've sold pieces to art collectors who don't even use them. And to pot smokers who don't even use them.

JULIE: The paraphernalia laws vary among states, so there are some states you can't ship to. What I still don't understand is why this wasn't entrapment. The DEA called your company and asked them to please ship some bongs to western Pennsylvania, and somebody in your company said, "No, sir, we cannot do that."

TOMMY: Right, we cannot do that because we would be breaking the law.

JULIE: So they just kept pestering, and calling the company and bugging whoever answered the phone until somebody finally took pity on this poor head-shop owner and sent the shipment.

TOMMY: It's in the documentary *AKA Tommy Chong*. We continually refused them, and then they personally flew to the factory. And I have a suspicion that they put an undercover guy in the factory before that, because we had hired a new guy, and then these guys came in and they ordered the bongs, and the new guy took the order, and somehow it slipped past everybody and got sent out.

JULIE: And so when it was sent out to western Pennsylvania, that was enough to trigger this whole thing.

TOMMY: Yes, the DEA shipping it to themselves.

JULIE: Now, if that's not entrapment, I don't know what is, especially if there's not someone on the inside. Their being so persistent and aggressive and finally getting it shipped seems like enough of an entrapment case. They're trying to persuade someone to break the law.

TOMMY: Yes, well, they were definitely out to get me, and they got me. And the truth is, they didn't have to go to all that trouble. If they didn't want me to sell bongs, all they had to do was make a phone call. If I had gotten a phone call from them, or my lawyer, or anybody, that said, You need to stop or you're going to jail, I would have stopped immediately, because it was my business, and it was my son's business.

JULIE: How's your relationship with Paris, your son, now?

TOMMY: Excellent. He quit the bong business and went back to school, and now he's acting as my manager with my wife and me.

JULIE: So, what do you make of Mary Beth Buchanan?

TOMMY: She is really on a vendetta. You know those kids in Texas, the Fundamentalist Church of Jesus Christ of Latter Day Saints (FDLS) group? I have a belief that Mary Beth was sort of raised like that, in a cult, like someone who's been brainwashed. She has absolutely no compassion whatsoever, and she seems to be like a robot, like a Stepford Wife or something.

JULIE: And did she get some sort of promotion after this all went down?

TOMMY: Actually, she got it before, but this put her on the map and brought her into prominence. And it led her to a position where she ended up firing all those U.S. attorneys for no reason.

JULIE: I didn't realize she was involved in that.

TOMMY: Yes. She and Attorney General Alberto Gonzales.

JULIE: And now this Operation True Test, a nationwide investigation targeting businesses that sell "masking products." There was a raid recently at Spectrum Labs; can you tell me about that? And this again is Mary Beth Buchanan?

TOMMY: She's the head of the task force that's taking down all the auxiliary pot providers like people that sell grow lights. She's busting hydroponic stores; she's busting detox laboratories.

JULIE: And masking products like Urine Luck?

TOMMY: Masking products help pot smokers pass drug tests, but when I was in custody, the feds told me that they test for the masking product, so in that way they don't really work. If you don't look for the masking product, though, you won't find it, so as a drug test, it works only when it's used by a company that doesn't want to lose its pot-smoking employees—like the FBI, for instance, which has had to lower its standards to attract recruits. Everybody has marijuana in their systems. So the masking substance helps employers like Home Depot keep their workers. The employees still smoke, and they can pass the test using the masking product. But it wouldn't work for the serious feds, or the Olympic athletes.

JULIE: Because they'll be testing for this masking product.

TOMMY: Which is also a detox product. It eliminates toxins from your system, so it works on other toxins too, not just marijuana. So there's a gray area there—if indeed taking stuff to help you pass the test is illegal. I don't know how that can be illegal.

JULIE: I still don't really understand how bongs can be illegal.

TOMMY: It's a technicality that they get you on. The law applies to everybody. They could have arrested me in California, but the DEA in California refused to consider water pipes illegal.

JULIE: So they had to do it through Pennsylvania?

TOMMY: Yes. There's only one state, Pennsylvania, and maybe Idaho, in which bongs are illegal.

JULIE: Now with the May 2008 raid at Spectrum Labs, there were nine search warrants issued, but none was within Mary Beth Buchanan's district.

TOMMY: Yes, but she's in charge of the law.

JULIE: So they not only raided Spectrum Labs, they confiscated 10,000 DVDs of *AKA Tommy Chong*? Is that all the copies there are?

TOMMY: Those were in the warehouse at the lab. We can have more made. They're being made and sold right now. But they weren't on the search warrant. No one was shown that search warrant; everything was sealed. It was a sealed indictment for future prosecution or something, and they said they can keep everything they seize for up to fifteen years.

JULIE: I watched *AKA Tommy Chong*, and it made me uncomfortable and paranoid. At one point someone asked you what prison was like, and you said, "Oh, you'll see." What are you getting at when you say that?

TOMMY: The way this country is going, anybody could be put in jail for any reason. People are in their own little bubbles, and that's how they divide and conquer. When they prosecuted me, all of a sudden my phone stopped ringing. I had one guy call me up before I went in, Pat Morita, the actor. Everybody else sort of took to the hills; they just put their heads down and ignored me. That's what happens when you get accused, not even convicted. You can even be innocent.

What the government's managed to do is take away all our freedoms. This government has trashed the Constitution. All the freedoms the founding fathers put in to ensure our right to the pursuit of happiness have been systematically eliminated. It's a totalitarian state now where anybody can be arrested. It's like how it was before the American Revolution—if England or its representatives felt like it, they could pass a law against anything. This government has no interest whatsoever in the medical aspects of marijuana. They just see pot as a way to imprison Americans who believe in the Constitution and the American way of life. I feel very strongly that George W. Bush and friends are owned and operated by the huge corporations; they're puppets who are controlled by the oil companies, and by alcohol and cigarette companies. They're taking apart the Constitution so they can profit. Global warming, insane oil prices, Middle East wars, all for the love of corporate profit and global power.

The marijuana laws are a perfect example, because here is a product that helps people, and yet people have gone to jail for years and died over this plant, because the government does not want its people to have this plant. So they have this law where only the government is allowed to own this plant.

JULIE: Next week I'm interviewing Dr. Mamoud ElSohly, who runs the grow farm in Mississippi. A lot of people complain that the government pot is of pretty poor quality.

TOMMY: Oh, yes, like everything government. It's not about the product, it's about the money you can make from the product. I had a conversation this morning with a radio guy who said, "Marijuana isn't legal because they can't tax it. It will be legal once they find a way to tax it." The whole tax idea is ridiculous anyway, because most of the tax money goes toward collecting the tax. It has nothing to do with where that tax is being used.

JULIE: I have talked to growers who would be perfectly happy to pay taxes. And people in the city who run distribution rings would be perfectly happy to pay taxes. At the Cannabis Cup festival in Amsterdam, I made a point of asking every grower I interviewed whether he or she would mind paying taxes, and not one person had a problem with it.

TOMMY: Absolutely. Because what's the difference? You pay sales tax, you pay income tax.

JULIE: Tell me what it was like to be in prison and to be a parolee. You were on probation for a year, which looked like a huge hassle in the documentary.

TOMMY: You know what I did, I treated everything like an assignment, like I was a reporter and I was in jail, and I'm here to get the story. And once I did that, then everything was fine. Because when you're in jail, the first thing they do is take away your pride. They humble you. But if you go in there humble, then you run the risk of being punked by the guards and by everybody else. So it's a tightrope you walk. You have to be humble, but you don't want to be a pussy. I've never felt so alone in my life. Normally, at least you have the thought of being free. You could be in a dead-end job, but the thought of being free keeps you sane. But when you lose your freedom, it's a dread, almost a panic, a claustrophobic feeling, and it just chokes you in your throat. It's the fear of losing control. But you have to get past that, and a lot of people don't, or it takes them awhile. But I did it. One night I just went inside myself and I found the strength, and I said, I'm here for a purpose. I had to invent a purpose for myself, and once I did that, then I was okay, then everything else was a learning experience.

Also, I used my "good vibe" method, which started with a writer named Emmett Fox. He's a spiritualist who's lectured around the world. He got so good at trusting the vibe, or the presence, that he never booked planes, he never booked hotels, he never prepared, because he had so much faith in his journey that he knew that everything was prepared for him. And so I used that theory. When your plane is canceled and you go up to the ticket office, there are a couple ways you can do it. You can go up there mad and make everything uncomfortable for everyone, or you can do what I do, which is smile. Once you "nice vibe" people, then all of a sudden doors open. You determine your own fate by your attitude. So that's what I did. I went into a nice-vibe mode, and I stayed in that mode right until I got out.

JULIE: But getting out meant going to a halfway house.

TOMMY: Yes. I was released, but I was only allowed to be home for an hour, and then I had to report to the halfway house for a month. I did eight months in prison and and one month in the halfway house on Western Avenue and Hollywood Boulevard in the Armenian area. I was allowed out during the day if I had a job, so I got one right away, at Gold's Gym, and I had to donate 30 percent of my earnings to the halfway house. Basically, I was getting paid to work out.

JULIE: I remember that part of the documentary. I seem to remember at the gym, there was a picture on the wall of Arnold Schwartzenegger, and there was an intimation that he had smoked pot at some point.

TOMMY: Oh, Arnold smoked pot regularly with everybody down there.

JULIE: I'd love to compile a list of all the politicians who've admitted to smoking. I imagine the list of people who've admitted it isn't as long as the list of the ones who have actually smoked.

TOMMY: Well, of course. The politicians aren't going to admit anything, which makes it interesting, because we're being run by a group of liars.

JULIE: I really would just love everybody to "out" themselves. If every American who smoked pot admitted it, I think that would help create the sea change necessary to change the laws.

TOMMY: As long as it's criminalized, everyone is afraid to admit it, though.

JULIE: And they're ashamed. The shame ends up compounding the compulsive behavior.

TOMMY: It's the only racist law left, if you think about it. It's the only Jim Crow law left. It discriminates against a group of people. That's why they call it marijuana. They could've called it cannabis or hemp, but they call it marijuana, because it has that Mexican, evil connotation to it.

JULIE: Is it true with probation that you violate it if you have a positive drug screen? You can go back to prison. Was that one of the requirements of your probation?

TOMMY: I got drug tested every week. And when I was in jail, there were snitches that would come up and offer me pot, but my buddy that I ran with would just shoo them away. I had to do pretrial probation, which means that I couldn't smoke pot before the trial, and that's when I found out about the masking product. They told me, Don't bother trying that stuff, because if you even have excess water in your urine, they'll violate your parole for that.

JULIE: These guys who violate their probation with positive urine tests, these are nonviolent crimes, and then they're being sent to prison for them.

TOMMY: Well, you know, Reagan's speechwriter was in jail with me. His name was Jay. He was straight as an arrow, and he told me all this crap about how he got in jail. So he was in there, real nice guy, and he gets out on something like a house arrest or something, then he was supposed to go to a halfway house. Anyway, the night he was home, he couldn't sleep, so he took a half a Valium, and they drug tested him and found Valium in his system and sent him back to jail.

JULIE: But that's not even an illegal drug.

TOMMY: And I know that was their plan, to get me in jail and then think I would violate. But I'm too smart for these guys.

JULIE: Tell me about the Marijuana Research Institute.

TOMMY: What I want to do is get a group of people involved with compiling statistics on the people who use marijuana, why they use it, how they use it, and what its effects are. The government's excuse is always "There's no studies showing it's therapeutic." But there have been studies, and the minute they show that it's good for you, or it's not as bad as they said it was, they stop the study. So I want to help support the research, because I really want to find out the good and the bad. Some people have had bad effects with pot. The saving grace is that it's not particularly addictive, so they don't have to keep doing it, they can quit. I also want to compile statistics of the chronic users. And whatever money we raise for that, I'd like to make sure that these researchers get paid well enough so that they can do their job.

JULIE: Part of the problem is, most drug research is funded by the pharmaceutical industry or by NIDA, neither of which is interested in spending any money to show any sort of beneficial or therapeutic effects from cannabis.

The other industry that's not interested in pot being legal is the petroleum industry, because of hemp. So between alcohol and pharmaceuticals and petroleum, that's a lot of power and lobbyists, and that's a lot of money.

TOMMY: That's a lot of money, and they're also managing to make sure that we don't have a planet to fight over.

JULIE: Well, it does seem like there's money to be made from cannabis, and I'm always asking, Haven't these guys crunched the numbers? Haven't they figured out that they could be making money from taxes instead of spending money on interdiction? I imagine they must know, but it's just not what it's about.

TOMMY: They do know. But they make more money from oil and the pharmaceutical people. Big Pharma and the government, they're the worst.

JULIE: In terms of lobbying?

TOMMY: For your health. They invent disease.

JULIE: That's absolutely true. I'm a psychiatrist, and I open up my medical journals and see ads for medicine, inventing diagnoses that don't exist, such as "excessive daytime sleepiness disorder," so they can market the use of stimulants. They are absolutely inflating symptoms into syndromes, making up new diagnoses, so they can sell us more medications.

TOMMY: And they give these doctors pockets full of free samples, so some of the doctors end up like drug pushers, to the point where it's disgusting.

JULIE: A large part of this book is about medical marijuana and using cannabis therapeutically. But another part of it is about our drug policy and how completely wrongheaded and antitherapeutic it is.

TOMMY: Well, tell me this: Why was acupuncture outlawed in America for so long? In California in the '70s, there was one acupuncturist when we started doing it. And in Canada it was totally outlawed. I had a brother-in-law who was an acupuncturist, and he faced criminal prosecution for practicing acupuncture. Finally they allowed it, the medical people started studying it themselves, learning how to heal themselves. But that's the power that the doctors have in this country.

JULIE: The American Medical Association is a huge lobbying presence in Congress, but I do feel like the tide is turning a little bit. There are physician groups that are getting behind medical marijuana, and fourteen states now have medical marijuana laws.

TOMMY: And Barack Obama says that he is against using federal DEA agents to raid dispensaries and arrest seriously ill people.

JULIE: Well, clearly, prosecuting patients is ridiculous. The government is inadvertently turning these patients into martyrs. Actually, they turned you into one too.

TOMMY: Well, the thing is with pot, it's such an eye-opening experience. You don't think in terms of violence or revolution, you mostly think in terms of just lying back and enjoying nature.

JULIE: Right. It can create an occasion for personal growth, psychospiritual exploration, and enlightenment. The problem, in the government's eyes, is that drugs *are* potentially subversive. I think people do pull back and see the "big picture," and sometimes they do think about revolution. I'm sure the government would prefer that we aren't so enlightened.

TOMMY: Of course they would prefer it, because that means there's no danger. I'm with Mahatma Gandhi on this issue. These guys are equipped with their SWAT teams to handle any kind of armed insurrection, but they're not really equipped to handle me on the radio talking crap about Mary Beth Buchanan. It's embarrassing to them.

JULIE: Speaking of SWAT teams, I heard with this May 7 raid, where they confiscated the DVDs of the documentary about you, there were thirty fully armed commandos raiding this office building in Cincinnati, with five overweight, middle-aged office workers being held hostage while they ransacked the place.

TOMMY: It's totally nuts. And what would stop it is if the news reports got out. But you'll notice Fox and all these other newscasters, they stayed away from that one.

JULIE: True. The only reason I heard about this raid at all was in an e-mail from Josh Gilbert, who directed *AKA Tommy Chong,* but it didn't really make it into the press.

TOMMY: But the way the Internet works, it gets a wider coverage because it was withheld like that.

JULIE: Right, today is May 12, and you can already read about the raid on Wikipedia.

Now, you were on *The Tonight Show with Jay Leno* when you got out of prison, and you're still being very visible in helping the fight against prohibition.

TOMMY: It's a good fight. In Toronto, they had a marijuana march, and they wanted me to come. And I told them I would rather be a behind-the-scenes guy. When I do a marijuana march, I want to have the people in wheelchairs and the people with MS, those are the people I want to march behind. Like Martin Luther King, I want to be up there with the cancer patients and the people that have a dire need to use marijuana as a medicine. And I'd like the Marijuana Research Institute to connect all these researchers who have the potential to help these patients.

18

The Collateral Consequences of Cannabis Convictions

Richard Glen Boire, J.D.

These are highlights from a longer chapter that also includes footnotes and references, available at ThePotBook.com.

EXECUTIVE SUMMARY

A conviction for a marijuana offense results in two different categories of punishment: the punishment directly imposed by the judge, and a range of collateral sanctions that are triggered by the conviction.

Current marijuana policy focuses almost entirely on the direct punishment imposed by the judge and has almost entirely ignored the collateral sanctions that result from a conviction. Yet the collateral sanctions associated with a marijuana conviction are significant and in many cases far exceed (in both severity and duration) the direct punishment.

In most cases, a felony marijuana conviction (for example, for growing marijuana) triggers the same collateral sanctions as those triggered by a conviction for murder, rape, or kidnapping. In many cases, the collateral sanctions for a marijuana-related conviction actually exceed those for a violent crime.

Collateral sanctions triggered by a marijuana conviction can include

219

revocation or suspension of professional licenses; barriers to employment or promotion; loss of educational aid; driver's license suspension; and bars on adoption, voting, and jury service. For people who depend upon public assistance, a marijuana conviction can trigger a bar on receiving food stamps and restrict access to public housing. In some states, these sanctions continue for life.

The ten states with the most severe collateral sanctions with regard to marijuana convictions are (in descending order of severity) Florida, Delaware, Alabama, Massachusetts, New Jersey, Oklahoma, Virginia, Utah, Arizona, and South Carolina.

The ten states with the least severe collateral sanctions (in ascending order) are New Mexico, New York, Rhode Island, Missouri, Maine, Vermont, District of Columbia, Pennsylvania, Kansas, and California.

In thirty-eight states, a misdemeanor marijuana conviction (for example, for personal possession of marijuana) can result in a bar on adopting a child. In seven of these states, this bar can operate for life.

In twelve states, a felony marijuana conviction (for example, for growing a marijuana plant) results in a lifetime bar on receiving food stamps or temporary assistance for needy families. In seven states, even a misdemeanor marijuana conviction can result in a bar or restriction on receiving food stamps or temporary aid for needy families. In three states, a misdemeanor marijuana conviction can result in a lifetime ban. Only felony drug offenses result in this ban—not robbery, not kidnapping, not even murder.

In twenty states, occupational licensing and certification agencies may deny, revoke, or suspend a professional license based on a misdemeanor marijuana conviction, even if the offense is completely unrelated to the person's duties.

In twenty-eight states, a student who is convicted of possessing any amount of marijuana will be denied federal financial aid for a year and may also be denied state educational aid for a year or longer.

In twenty-one states and the District of Columbia, a misdemeanor conviction for personal possession of marijuana can result in a driver's license suspension for at least six months.

In forty-seven states, a conviction for growing marijuana (or any other marijuana-related felony) results in at least some period of time during which the person is barred from voting. In six of these states, the bar on voting lasts for life.

In forty-six states, any marijuana conviction (and in some cases merely an arrest) can result in a bar from public housing, usually for at least three years.

These collateral sanctions should be recognized and included in a rational debate about marijuana policy and social justice and carefully considered when crafting or revising legislation.

CONCLUSION

In nearly every state, a person who commits a marijuana offense and fully serves his or her sentence (or successfully completes probation) is nonetheless subject to continuing and long-lasting professional debilitation, barriers to family life, and limits on civic participation. Across the United States, thousands of people convicted of marijuana offenses have lost their right to vote, to obtain professional licenses, to receive public assistance or public housing, or even to adopt a child. Further, under the laws of many states, employers may lawfully refuse to hire or promote a person because of a marijuana conviction (or, in some states, merely because of a marijuana arrest). Thousands of young people convicted of marijuana offenses have had their educations sidetracked or ended by being denied educational aid.

These are all collateral sanctions associated with a marijuana conviction, and for many people they can result in a lifetime of hardship—an unrecognized punishment that continues long after they have served their criminal sentence or completed probation.

POLICY RECOMMENDATIONS

States should enact the Uniform Collateral Sanctions and Disqualifications Act (UCSDA), which is currently being developed by the National Conference of Commissioners on Uniform State Laws (NCCUSL). Among other things, this act would collect all collateral sanctions in one title; require courts to advise defendants of the collateral sanctions triggered by a plea; define the judgments that qualify as "convictions"; limit the collateral sanctions applicable to employment, educational benefits, housing, occupational licensing, and voting; and provide for Certificates of Rehabilitation that would permit qualifying individuals to have their rights restored in whole or in part.

Like the NCCUSL, the American Bar Association recently completed four reports that examine collateral sanctions and culminate in six specific recommendations that the ABA urges federal, state, territorial, and local governments to develop or enact. All six of these recommendations would benefit persons convicted of marijuana-related offenses and should be adopted.

In some states, marijuana offenders can avoid a criminal conviction by successfully completing a "diversion" or "deferred entry of judgment" program. With respect to collateral sanctions, these programs are extremely important because nearly all collateral sanctions are triggered by a conviction. By avoiding a conviction, a person avoids the collateral sanctions. Thus, our study underscores the importance of diversion and deferred entry of judgment programs for marijuana offenses and instructs that legislators who are seeking to reduce the penalties associated with marijuana offenses would do well to focus on programs that not only reduce the direct penalties associated with conviction, but equally importantly, provide a method by which a period of probation results in no conviction. In most cases, this is the only way to avoid the collateral sanctions examined in our study.

States should consider enacting provisions that automatically expunge and/or seal some or all marijuana-related convictions after successful completion of the sentence or probation. Section 11361.5 of California's Health & Safety Code serves as a workable model for such a provision.

19
Harm Reduction Psychotherapy

Andrew Tatarsky, Ph.D.

Marijuana has been charged with the power to induce insanity and proposed as the gateway drug to all things evil: addiction, violence, sexual depravity. It's thought to be the most benign and least addictive psychoactive substance, able to ease the symptoms of a wide variety of illnesses. Is marijuana harmful or not? Who decides and how? What has your experience been? If you're concerned about your own use, this chapter will help answer these questions and create a healthy relationship to marijuana.*

I will discuss the potential harms associated with marijuana and offer some tips for minimizing them. Also described is a framework for creating a healthy relationship to marijuana. This approach has evolved from my work with patients and colleagues over the more than thirty years that informed my understanding of why substance use becomes problematic for some, and how others make positive changes in their use. Harm-reduction philosophy frames and influences the approach. An integration of strategies to deepen awareness and facilitate change provides a variety of tools to use in your own process. This chapter is written primarily for recreational and medical marijuana users and their families and friends, but others will find the framework useful for addressing other potentially problematic behaviors such as other substance

---

*I would like to thank Dr. Wendy Ellen Miller and Alexandra Pauline Tatarsky for their invaluable editorial comments and suggestions on the style, format, and content of this article.

use, eating problems, excessive working, computer games, and Internet use.

All substance users must discover for themselves what their healthiest, most self-affirming relationship is to substances. In part, this entails separating one's own experience from ideology about marijuana. Marijuana is a benign psychoactive substance for many people, but it can have serious negative consequences for others. The challenge for the user is to find a relationship to marijuana that maximizes the positive benefits while minimizing the negative consequences and potential risks. This may mean smoking less, using more safely, using for different reasons, instituting a different pattern of use, or stopping altogether. While stopping may be the best way to reduce the risk and negative consequences of using marijuana, it is not an answer for everyone; many concerned marijuana users are not ready, willing, or able to stop. They need an alternative approach that starts where they are: harm reduction.

HARM REDUCTION

Harm reduction is an alternative to the traditional abstinence-only approach to problem substance use. It began as a response to the failure of traditional treatment to address the explosion of serious drug and alcohol use in Amsterdam and Liverpool in the 1970s. The essence of harm-reduction philosophy is the acceptance of the fact that people use mind-altering substances. The focus is shifted from only trying to stop drug use to reducing the harms associated with substance use, acknowledging abstinence as one among many possible ways to accomplish this. Harm reduction seeks to support and empower users to make conscious, responsible, healthy choices regarding their drug use and other aspects of their lives. All positive changes, small and large, are considered successes.

The research on cannabis-related harm is generally in agreement—the public health risks are small. In my own practice over the years, the percentage of people I've seen who sought help for problems with marijuana is small relative to other drugs. However, marijuana can lead to serious consequences, and every user should know to reduce the chances of encountering them.

ACUTE HARMS

Acute harms are the most common negative outcomes associated with marijuana. They may occur while the user is intoxicated and generally don't last when the drug effect wears off.

Negative Psychological Reactions

Negative psychological reactions include anxiety, paranoia, a feeling of losing touch with reality, feeling "stupid," and being flooded by troubling thoughts. Some of these are more likely to occur for inexperienced users.

- Tip 1. If you experience overwhelming or terrifying feelings such as paranoia or intense disorientation, sit tight and remember that they will pass soon.
- Tip 2. The potency of marijuana varies widely. When you are unfamiliar with a certain strain of marijuana, it is always good to start with a very small amount and wait ten minutes to see how strong it is.
- Tip 3. Don't mix marijuana with other drugs that can intensify negative effects.
- Tip 4. Use in a safe place with trusted friends.
- Tip 5. People with severe mental illness should be aware that marijuana might cause psychotic episodes. A small percentage of people experience a loss of the normal sense of self or reality that can linger well beyond drug use. Some research has suggested that marijuana may cause schizophrenia to emerge in vulnerable people. The safest measure with this group of people is avoiding marijuana. If you are in this group and choose to use despite this risk, go to Tip 1 above.

Dysfunctional Thinking

Thinking can be disturbed, particularly in the areas of learning, attention, concentration, memory, and time sense. Activities that depend on these functions can be disrupted.

- Tip 1. Avoid using marijuana before activities that require intact cognitive functioning.

Impaired Motor Response

Motor impairment and slowed reaction time increase the risk of accidents while driving and using machinery.

- Tip 1. Do not drive or operate dangerous machinery while high. Also, be aware that there may be a hangover effect the day after heavy smoking.

CHRONIC HARMS

Chronic harms are the negative effects that result from long-term marijuana use. Cannabis dependence syndrome does occur with some users. Some research estimates that about 10 percent of people who have ever tried marijuana meet dependence criteria. The hallmarks of dependence are compulsion; craving; the sense of loss of control; continuing to use in spite of negative consequences; tolerance; and withdrawal. Common negative consequences I have seen are diminished effectiveness at work or school, problems with intimacy, social withdrawal, self-esteem problems (feeling like a "stoner"), disrupted creativity, and feeling bad about the sense of dependence itself.

These risks increase as frequency and length of use increase. People often wonder if one can become dependent on something that is reportedly not "physically addictive." If you consider that the effects of marijuana are caused in part by its impact on brain chemistry and functioning, and that dependence is related to biology, psychology, and social context, then it becomes easier to understand why chronic use of marijuana can lead to dependence. Any drug that is used for positive effects can come to be relied upon for these effects and so lead to the experience of dependence. The social and other external factors usually connected to using can become strong triggers for the urge to use. All these factors may combine in unique ways for each person to contribute to a growing sense of dependence. Identifying these factors can lead to steps you can take to develop a more controlled, moderate, or ritualistic relationship to marijuana or to determine if it is best to stop altogether.

- Tip 1. You might commit to breaking your current dependent relationship to marijuana and attempt to develop a different, less intense and harmful pattern of use. Some people find that they can, while others find that attempting a less harmful relationship is too difficult or practically impossible and decide to stop altogether.
- Tip 2. Be as clear and specific as you can with yourself about what changes you would like to make, in frequency and amount, as a goal to work toward.
- Tip 3. Decide on an approach to making this change. Many people find that it is easiest to take a thirty-day break from marijuana before attempting to institute a new pattern of using. This enables the system

to clear out the THC, reduce tolerance, and get over the discomfort of withdrawal that some people feel when stopping. Some prefer a weaning approach, that is, small steps toward the new pattern, while others prefer picking a date and making the change all at once. See what feels most appealing to you and give it a try.

- Tip 4. Monitor urges for using and try to sit with them ("urge surfing"). Putting time and space between the urge and what you choose to do about it, to smoke or not, cuts into the habitual aspect of dependence and supports a new, more conscious relationship to using.
- Tip 5. Dialogue with the urge. Ask yourself if this is a moment to use that is in accord with your new goals and relationship to using.
- Tip 6. Review your reasons for deciding to make a change; try to stay connected to your motivation.
- Tip 7. Identify what seems to be triggering the urge to use, and consider different strategies for addressing, managing, or expressing your triggers. Triggers can be internal, such as feelings and emotions, or external, such as particular people, things, or events. Possible alternatives are yoga as another way to relax and meditation as another way to let go of the world of responsibility.
- Tip 8. Behavior change requires "hanging in" with the process. Changing complex habitual ways of being (one way to think of dependence) is usually slow and gradual, happening in small steps, rarely in a straight line. As with any habit, you are working with the part of you that wants to hold on to the old way of being. Try to be patient, forgiving, persevering, and hopeful.

Abnormal Thought Patterns
Thinking can be disrupted, with a general decrease in attention, memory, learning, and organization that can be quite troubling.

- Tip 1. Try using smaller amounts and less often.
- Tip 2. Take days or weeks off to reduce the THC buildup in your system.
- Tip 3. Don't use the night or day before an important or new challenge.

Lung Problems

Problems such as lung congestion, coughing, chronic bronchitis, and precancerous changes are related to smoking. Water pipes may send higher concentrations of tar to the lungs because of the tendency to hold the smoke in longer. These effects are compounded when tobacco is mixed with marijuana.

- Tip 1. Eat cannabis products or drink cannabis tea to eliminate smoking-related harms. This will require patience, because effects come on slowly. It is also harder to gauge the amount you are taking this way, and the effects can last longer and be much more intense than with smoking. Exercise extreme caution with the amount you eat until you know how powerful the preparation is.
- Tip 2. If you must smoke, don't mix marijuana with tobacco.
- Tip 3. Don't inhale deeply or hold the smoke long. Deep inhalation won't get you significantly more stoned, but it will deliver much more carbon monoxide to your brain.
- Tip 4. Vaporizing is a good alternative to smoking marijuana. Vaporizers heat rather than burn the material. This process releases the THC and other cannabinoids without the toxic products of burning the plant material.
- Tip 5. Higher-potency pot can reduce the amount you smoke. Be careful to smoke a smaller amount to reduce the risk of negative psychological effects.

Infectious Diseases

Infectious diseases that are passed in saliva like spinal meningitis can also be spread through the sharing of smoking implements.

- Tip 1. Don't share joints and bongs.
- Tip 2. If sharing, don't let the joint touch your lips, and clean the bong before smoking from it.

FINDING YOUR HEALTHIEST RELATIONSHIP TO MARIJUANA

In this next section, I describe a framework for assessing the harm in your own use of marijuana, clarifying changes you'd like to make in your use and developing strategies to achieve these changes.

Setting the Stage for Positive Change with Self-acceptance

An attitude that is conducive to positive change embraces starting *where you are* with compassion, understanding, and acceptance as the first step. This creates a solid and safe foundation for the rest of the work and clears the way for learning to occur. Beginning a process of positive change does not require that we know the outcome of the journey; we just need to begin.

Internalized Stigma

Our culture stigmatizes drugs and drug users, overtly and covertly. We live with distorted messages in the popular media of drugs as bad and drug users as immoral, weak, degenerate, out of control, deceptive, hopeless, and so on. The stigma reflected in these negative images lives within all of us to some extent, in spite of our efforts to develop more realistic and enlightened views. When people have trouble with their substance use, these negative associations are likely to become activated, stimulating feelings of shame, guilt, anxiety, self-hate, and fear of other people's criticism and judgments. These reactions impede the ability to clearly look at what the problem is and consider the range of solutions that are available.

The disease concept of addiction, based on an assumption of powerlessness, is a myth that has been largely accepted and promoted by our culture. This concept holds that drug use that continues in spite of negative consequences reflects a loss of control and compulsiveness that are the hallmark symptoms of addictive disease. This hypothetical disease renders the user powerless over substances of all kinds, is chronic and progressive, and inevitably results in mental illness, incarceration, or death. A corollary of this presumption of powerlessness is that if you are unwilling to accept your disease, you are "in denial." The very belief or experience of having some control is an indication of your self-deception. In other words, if you try to take control, you are really in trouble.

This idea has also been internalized by all of us to some extent, and it can have a pernicious effect on users who develop problems. It goes something like this: "If I acknowledge that I am having trouble of some sort with my substance use, I will have to admit that I am an addict (an inherently shaming experience related to having to accept and publicly admit to a stigmatized identity), and then I will have to stop (the only acceptable or reasonable response to addiction). Since I neither want to stop using nor want to accept and admit to the shaming identity of addict, I will not admit to myself that I am having a problem." This way of thinking may also act as a self-fulfilling prophecy propelling the escalation of use and the loss of control it predicts.

Clarify What You Think of Yourself as a Drug User

You might begin working on your own harm-reduction process by spending some time trying to make explicit what you think and feel about yourself as a drug user, why you use drugs, and why you might be experiencing difficulties with your use. Think about how you are feeling about yourself for being in this predicament. Are you feeling any of the negative emotions that I mentioned above? Can you identify any of the stigmatizing ideas or tendencies to be overly self-critical, self-hating, or harsh for getting yourself into this bind? Have you unwittingly assumed that you are powerless to do anything about it short of stopping altogether?

You might do this work in self-reflection, journal about it, or find a trusted other to dialogue with. It is often in the attempt to articulate what we believe that we can make conscious and explicit what was previously unclear.

Determine What Is True for You

Try to separate your own desires and point of view from others' judgments and wishes for you; take them into consideration as important, but don't simply accept them. The tendency to take on others' points of view can interfere with the discovery of our own truth. I have seen this frequently become a setup for failure. Out of fear, shame, or guilt, problem drug users may agree with the assessment and wishes or demands of another only to find themselves rebelling in private. The private rebellion may give a sense of freedom from external control, but it obscures awareness of what the user truly desires for him- or herself.

Get in the Driver's Seat of Your Own Process of Change

You might counter the assumption of powerlessness by thinking of getting in the driver's seat of your own process of change. People pursuing any learning or change need to take charge of their process and realize that no one can do it for them. As with driving, you need to take charge of the process, have good skills (capacities for change), have a teacher or coach, and know where you want to go (goals) and the route that will get you there (techniques and strategies).

Cultivate Capacities for Changing: Curiosity, Awareness, and Tolerance of Feeling

To be a good driver of your own process of change, you must use certain mental skills or capacities. Particularly useful are self-acceptance, curiosity, self-reflective awareness, and the ability to sit with feelings. These capacities are ways of being with ourselves that help us focus on our experience and make more conscious choices.

Practice Self-acceptance

You didn't plan to have difficulties. You didn't choose to have the problems that you now suffer from. The choice to accept that you are here now is not giving yourself an excuse; it simply puts you in the best position to honestly assess what is happening and summon the self-support necessary to make positive change. Problems associated with drug use present opportunities to learn something about yourself. Try to challenge judgmental moralizing and shaming and blaming yourself. These reactions tend to close down exploration.

Compassionate, pragmatic self-acceptance of where you are, the essence of harm-reduction philosophy, is a powerful alternative to the self-condemning tendencies that are supported by internalized stigma. Recognize that your desire for change reflects positive motivation and awareness, two very important ingredients of the change process.

Curiosity

See what happens if you dialogue with the inner critic and try out some alternative ways to think about yourself and your drug use. Rather than condemnation, develop an attitude of curiosity, which brings openness to learning. Curiosity invites creative thought. Being curious about how your marijuana use interacts with other aspects of your self and your life, and whether there are self-defeating aspects of your use, provides a more positive attitude for reflecting on your use.

Self-reflective Awareness

This is the ability to observe your thoughts, feelings, perceptions, and behavior keenly and without judgment. Noticing the moment-to-moment flow of experience enables the discovery of event-thought-feeling-decision-action sequences that culminate in decisions about drug use. Self-reflection enables clarification of the meanings and functions that marijuana has for you.

Describe your experience here rather than judging it as good or bad, useful or not, stupid or smart.

Sitting with Your Feelings

Sitting with your feelings supports self-reflection. This capacity to reflect—to be still with yourself and your feelings—is central to stopping impulsive or compulsive marijuana use. We often react to intense feelings that we are unable to tolerate by using.

Our capacity to sit with feelings increases as we attempt it. We increase the intensity of feeling that we can tolerate in small increments, like strengthening a muscle. Slowing down the breath while attempting this can help you relax with what you're feeling. The relaxation helps us feel less uncomfortable, so we can try to name and describe our feelings in terms of the thoughts and sensations associated with them, helping demystify them, making them less vague and overwhelming.

These capacities can be cultivated simply by trying to remember to be curious, self-reflective, and tuned in to what you are feeling as you move through your day. Some people find it useful to have a time set aside each day to practice tuning in. Yoga and meditation are practices that support the strengthening of these capacities. Classes can provide a great deal of support for some who find group work to be inspiring.

Awareness/Relaxation Training Exercise

Set aside five to thirty minutes to do this exercise. Pick a comfortable, quiet place where you won't be disturbed. Put on some relaxing music or not as you choose. You can take turns trying this with a friend, one reading the instructions to the other. You can do this with eyes open, but many people find it easier to focus inward with eyes closed.

Step 1: Awareness

Imagine that you are like a scientist or a reporter interested in gathering information without judgment or interpretation. The data you'll observe is what's happening inside of your body. Bring your awareness into the present moment, the now. The future has not happened yet; the past is just a memory. Focus on the sensations you become aware of as you scan your body. Notice the sensations in your toes and slowly work your way up to the top of your head. Can you feel tightness? Coolness on the skin? Can you feel your heart beating? The pulse throughout your body? Shift your awareness to what you hear, see, smell, and taste. Become aware of memories, thoughts, and images that pass through your mind's eye. Notice all these experiences without judgment. If you find yourself moving away from this moment, getting hung up on a thought, gently move your awareness back to the present experience of sensation and perception.

Step 2: Stress/tension/anxiety reading

You can use this technique to explore any feeling. Here we will look at anxiety.

Imagine a scale that measures anxiety from ten, the most anxious you can be, to one, the most relaxed you have been. Notice signs of anxiety and tension that you feel in your body. Is there tightness in the jaw, shoulders, or chest? Do you feel trembling or tension in your muscles? Coolness in your fingers and toes? Notice your breathing. Is it fast and shallow, or slow and deep? If you get caught up in the story you have about why you are anxious (a story that might be creating the anxiety), try to let go of the thoughts and come back to the sensations of what is present in your body. Now estimate where you would place yourself on that scale. What number comes to you?

Step 3: Slow down the breath

Anxiety is related to an activated nervous system, triggered by conscious or unconscious thoughts of danger that stimulate the release of hormones. By taking your awareness off the threatening thoughts, focusing on the sensations of your breathing and slowing it down, a message is sent to the brain that it is safe and you can relax. Herb Benson of Harvard describes a natural relaxation response that is accessed by slow deep breathing.

Notice the sensations of breath going in and out of your mouth and nose. Notice the rising and falling of chest and stomach. On the next exhalation, exhale slowly and as completely as you can. Then slowly inhale a little more deeply than before. Hold the breath for a moment when you get to the top. Once again, exhale as slowly and as deeply as you can. Count to six as you exhale. Continue breathing like this for three minutes.

Step 4: Breathe out the tension

As you inhale, focus on your tensions or anxieties. Imagine you can breathe them away as you exhale. Inhale healing, cleansing breath to the tension spots and exhale what you don't want to carry with you. Imagine you can feel gravity pulling you down into the cushions under you. Give your muscles permission to stop working. Do this systematically from the bottom of your toes to the top of your head.

Step 5: Feeling recollection

As you breathe, think of a word or phrase that describes a feeling that you would like to recall. *Peaceful. Calm. Clear. Powerful. Grounded.* Can you remember feeling this way? Imagine you can inhale this feeling, carried by the breath to the areas in your body and mind that are carrying tension and anxiety. Inhale the feeling that you want, and exhale what you wish to let go.

Step 6: Visualization

Recall a moment in your life when you felt the way you want to feel. Get a picture of that place in your mind. Imagine you are there now. See the images of that place. Smell the smells and hear the sounds of that place. Let them all wash over you, reminding you of how you felt when you were there.

Step 7: Stress/tension/anxiety reading

Bring your awareness back into this room, back to the present, back to your body. Notice the signs of stress or anxiety in your body, and see where you would place yourself on the anxiety scale.

If you notice any change in how you are feeling, think about what techniques you found most useful in bringing about the change. Noticing, awareness of the breath, slow deep breathing, the word or phrase, the visualization.

You can use these techniques to strengthen your general awareness of yourself. Use them when you feel bad to clarify what you are feeling and why. Use them for relaxation when you are feeling tense, stressed, and anxious. Use them to sit with your urges to use marijuana. Explore where the urge is coming from and if using in that moment is the best choice for that situation. Identify what is happening around you and what you were thinking and feeling when you first had the thought about using.

Self-assessment

Ideally, your motivation to make specific changes in your relationship to marijuana is based on your own assessment of the place it has in your life. Before you can decide how to change your relationship with marijuana, you must be clear about how your current use is problematic. While you may ultimately decide that stopping is the best choice for you, a commitment to stop is not necessary to begin making positive changes in your use. As you identify negative aspects of your use, you can make small changes to reduce the harmful consequences. Assessment will help you become aware of negative consequences, how your pattern of use is causing them, and what other aspects of yourself or your life may be contributing to them. Your marijuana use may be intertwined with all the other aspects of your life. Understanding this relationship will provide clues to changes you might make in other life areas that have an impact on your relationship to marijuana.

Areas to look at are: How does use positively and negatively impact health, emotions, self-esteem, relationships, work, finances, social life, and identity? What roles and meaning does your use have for you? These need to be clarified to understand what anchors your current pattern of using. Marijuana may help people relax, promote introspection, feel more connected to their bodies, enhance sex or exercise, provide a sense of connection to a community, represent a rebellion against parental control, establish a sense of identity, access creativity, function as a form of self-soothing, connect with others, create a bridge or bond between people, engender a sense of being able to care for oneself without needing others, soothe emotional distress such as anxiety, intensify pleasurable experiences, and more. Despite these positive effects, many users feel conflicted about their relationship to marijuana because of the many problematic consequences of using that were discussed earlier.

Pot can help and hurt at the same time. Smoking to relax can make it difficult to learn other ways of relaxing or further inflame the causes of the tension such as work difficulties, relationship conflicts, or lack of exercise. Smoking to stop thinking about stressful life events may cause further anxiety and panic: the threatening events are still there, but one's ability to think them through rationally has been weakened by smoking. Dependency can be driven by the urgent wish to avoid dealing with challenging life events that don't go away and so give rise to a continual sense of needing to be high. Identifying the multiple meanings of the desire to smoke makes it possible to consider other solutions that may relieve some of the pressure to smoke.

Strategies

An analysis of your patterns of use helps clarify how you typically use marijuana, how it fits into your life, relates to your desire to use, and impacts on other aspects of your life. You might keep a journal noting and tracking your use over the course of a week.

- Describe the pattern. When, where, and how much do you use?
- Identify triggers and motives. What contributes to your desire to use? What were you feeling? What did you hope to get by using? What

were your justifications, reasons, and context, such as time of day, who
you were with, and what was happening around you?

- Evaluate the results and consequences. Describe the quality of the
high. Did it deliver what you wanted? How does it affect other aspects
of your life, such as your health, freedom, finances, relationships, intimacy, school or work, emotional life, self-esteem, social life, recreational life, and ambition?

- Consider whether your use comes from conscious choice or from
impulse and habit, when making judgments about excessive use, com-
pulsivity, impulsivity, and loss of control. Do you find yourself using
when you feel you shouldn't because of its potential harms? Is this
related to some clearly identifiable triggering feeling or event?

Embrace Ambivalence

Identifying ambivalence about using and changing deserves special attention. Ambivalence is always present when drug use becomes problematic,
and it must be embraced as a basis for considering alternative solutions. In
spite of some awareness about potential risks associated with using certain
substances, people still want to use them.

Changing habits is always hard. We creatures of habit like our habits! They are comfortable and predicable, serving important conscious and
unconscious functions. Like old shoes that we love, shoes that took us to so
many wonderful places and have so many meaningful memories connected
to them, we feel attached to our habits even if they come into conflict with
our current lives and interests. The investments we have in our old ways of
being contribute to our ambivalence about changing. This must be addressed
for us to move on. The parts of you that are threatened by your marijuana
use will feel at odds with the parts of you that are positively invested in it. If
both parts can be present in your experience at the same time, it will be possible to consider alternative ways of resolving the impasse or, at least, creating
a space within yourself for entertaining new possibilities.

Avoiding ambivalence by keeping the conflicting parts of your experience separate can cause a cycle to emerge: engaging in the problematic
behavior, committing to change, then engaging in the behavior and committing to change again, and on and on without confronting the fact that
these parts need to work together to create new solutions to the problem. A
battle between the opposing parts derails change, as each takes turns grab-
bing center stage rather than working out a new relationship to the other.

If these competing parts of us can stop fighting with one another, change becomes more possible. The way to resolve ambivalence is to be curious and open and respectful of both sides, embracing both simultaneously.

Set Goals

As self-assessment deepens, new goals can emerge. Goals can be quantum leaps or tiny forays into new territory, experiments with new ways of being. Every positive change, large or small, should be considered a success, as small changes add up to larger changes, giving us feedback about ourselves that contributes to a growing sense of confidence in our ability to change.

Once you've identified goals that you're curious about exploring, you'll feel motivated *from the inside* to work on this, rather than pressured to do it by someone else, a condition for change that is not very helpful in the long run. Choosing the goals that you're interested in dramatically increases the likelihood that you will stay with the process and achieve positive change.

The "Ideal Use Plan" is a strategy for clarifying what your healthiest relationship to marijuana might be. Based on your assessment of the risks and negative aspects of your current pattern of using, what changes might you make to minimize the risks and reduce the harm? When does marijuana play a positive role in your life, and when does it interfere with other important parts of your life? How might this new pattern of use look, as specifically as you can guess at this point, in terms of frequency, amount, and circumstances of use? What other changes might you make in your life that would support these goals? Bring a scientific, hypothesis-testing framework to your attempts to implement the new plan. What is the outcome of your attempt? Does it achieve the results you desire? Is it realistic? Are there challenges or obstacles that need to be considered in revising the plan?

Strategize for Positive Change

The final step in the process of change is to identify strategies that will help you reach your new goals. Strategies can include how you think and plan, what you will do differently, how you enlist support from others for your new goals, whom you spend time with or avoid, how you care for yourself in other ways, and how you address issues related to your use in other more effective ways. Rather than deprivation and simply trying to control yourself, this approach focuses on how you can care for yourself most effectively.

- Self-monitor this sequence: event-thought-feeling-urge to use-thought-choice
- Crave/urge surf. Notice the urge and sit with it. Take five seconds or three minutes or one hour. You can always choose to do the habitual thing anyway, but surfing the urge puts a little space between the craving and whatever you choose to do with that feeling. Describe the urge in terms of its feelings, sensations, wishes, and fantasies about what you want from using. While you are surfing the urge, you are not acting from impulse or habit. You are in charge.
- Playing with the habit rather than enforcing change can make the process easier and less of a setup for frustration. See what happens if you alter your rituals in some way.
- Dialogue with the urge. Speak to both sides of your ambivalence about giving in to the urge or not, and see if a decision to use at this point seems to be the best choice given all your interests.
- Identify your triggers. Turn your attention away from the urge and instead focus on what triggered it. Consider whether using is the best or only solution to that feeling, thought, or event. What else you might do to express, care for, or otherwise deal with the trigger?
- Eighteen alternatives. Brainstorm a list of eighteen alternative responses to the things that typically trigger your desire to use. (Eighteen is the number that a patient of mine came up with for himself.) Practicing alternatives reduces the risk of coming to depend on using as the only response to your triggers. Alternatives provide a range of ways to best care for yourself.
- Have a game plan. Plan in advance for each situation in which you will be using. Think about your intended goals for the event. Try to anticipate challenges to your plans, and prepare strategies to meet them. For example, what will you say when a friend questions you about your limited use? How will you respond when you know you have had enough and you feel the desire for more?

CONCLUSION

This chapter described many common acute and chronic harms associated with using marijuana, as well as tips for reducing the possibility of experiencing these problems. It introduced a framework based on harm-reduction philosophy that I've been using in counseling people grappling with substance use problems. This framework can be used as a guide for evaluating your own relationship to marijuana in an effort to develop the healthiest one possible. Important pieces of this process were detailed, including self-assessment of one's current relationship to marijuana, setting the internal stage for change, embracing ambivalence to change, and setting harm-reduction goals. A variety of strategies to evaluate and pursue harm-reduction goals was offered.

Change is a work in progress. As you develop new goals and strategies, see what works for you and what doesn't. Revise as you go, fine-tuning the plan to better suit your unique needs and interests. Following this path will lead you to your healthiest relationship to marijuana. I hope the ideas and strategies in the chapter enrich your journey!

PART THREE

The Clinical Use
of Cannabis

*Marijuana is one of the safest therapeutically active
substances known to man.*

JUDGE FRANCIS YOUNG,
THE DRUG ENFORCEMENT AGENCY

*Instead of taking five or six of the prescriptions, I decided
to go a natural route and smoke marijuana.*

MELISSA ETHERIDGE

That is not a drug. It's a leaf.

ARNOLD SCHWARZENEGGER

Introduction to Part Three

I have a private practice in psychiatry. Private. Why should the government dictate how I care for my patients, as long as it's safe? The safety profile of cannabis is peerless. "Marijuana, in its natural form, is one of the safest therapeutically active substances known to man. . . . In strict medical terms, marijuana is far safer than many of the foods we commonly consume," wrote Administrative Law Judge Francis Young in his recommendation to the Drug Enforcement Agency (DEA) concerning proper scheduling of cannabis. "By any measure of rational analysis," Young concluded, "marijuana can be safely used within a supervised routine of medical care." In 1988, Young ruled in NORML's favor and recommended placing cannabis in schedule III. The DEA's appeal was heard by John C. Lawn, then administrator of the DEA itself. Not surprisingly, in 1989, Lawn overturned all Young's findings. In 1994 the federal court of appeals for the District of Columbia upheld Lawn's decision, and these days, reform focuses on the state level instead of the federal.

What you will learn in the chapters that follow is that when behavioral restrictions are in place, with boundaries understood and adhered to, cannabis can be used as an effective medication to safely treat an abundance of symptoms and syndromes. And there are legions of patients—with muscle spasms, chronic pain, nausea, loss of appetite (the list goes on and on)—who will attest to its efficacy.

Alan Schuster, onetime director of NIDA (the National Institute on Drug Abuse), used to say, "The plural of anecdote is not data." Ironically, NIDA, which funds most of the world's drug studies, is also the institution putting up the most roadblocks in pursuit of this data. Until scientists and clinicians can prove the efficacy of cannabis, we are left with millions of anecdotes. Endorsements and pleas from the National Academy of Medicine, the Institute of Medicine, and even the American Medical Association to reconsider marijuana as a medicine haven't yet swayed the DEA to reschedule cannabis.

What's important to remember here is that cannabis started out not as a drug of abuse, but as an ancient medicine. When alcohol prohibition ended, and all the government officials needed a job, cannabis was taken out of the hands of prescribing physicians and reclassified as a black-market illicit drug, but making it illegal doesn't change the inherent medicinal properties of cannabis. The U.S. Pharmacopeia, a listing of remedies begun in 1820, first included cannabis in 1870. Throughout the second half of the 1800s, cannabis extracts were some of the most popular medications prescribed. The Pharmacopeia didn't delete cannabis until its 1942 edition, the first one published after cannabis was outlawed in 1937.

Since 1968, NIDA has been growing a supply of cannabis for research purposes under contract with the University of Mississippi's pharmacy school. In 1976, Bob Randall, a glaucoma sufferer, was arrested for marijuana possession, but he was acquitted due to a medical-necessity defense. He risked blindness if he couldn't control the pressure in his eyes. In 1978 Randall brought a civil suit against the government for access to his medicine and won. The government agreed to supply him with his medicine for the rest of his life. They considered it an Investigational New Drug (IND) and created a pretense that they would study this "new drug" with one research subject, Randall. The Compassionate Use IND Program, at its height in 1991, supplied thirteen patients. But when Randall explained to AIDS advocacy groups how to apply for compassionate use, and forty applications flooded the program, it was shut down in 1992. Those thirteen patients were "grandfathered in," and as the years went by, and the patients died, fewer remained in the program. Today there are four.

What is ironic, though, is that even though our government is dispensing medication to those four people, it still refuses to think of cannabis as a medication with any accepted medical use, and so it remains in Schedule I of the Controlled Substances Act, a category reserved for drugs with no accepted medical use. Yet the federal government holds a patent (#6630507) for medicinal use of cannabinoids as antioxidants and neuroprotectants. To further add to the irony, in 1999, DEA and FDA moved THC pills (Marinol and others) from Schedule II to Schedule III, a category for drugs with legitimate medical indications but some potential for abuse, alongside medications like Vicodin, codeine, anabolic steroids, and ketamine.

The problem with the oral THC pills is they get you higher than smoked cannabis and they last longer, while taking longer to "come on." Many physicians and patients have learned that dosages can be better titrated by using smoked or vaporized whole-plant preparations instead of orally ingested THC. To have the whole plant listed in Schedule I and its main psychoactive component listed in Schedule III is nonsensical, especially when you consider that THC is the chemical element in cannabis most thought to cause euphoria and the sense of an altered state. There are multiple chemical components of the whole plant that work together to bring about symptom relief; CBD (cannabidiol), for instance, is a constituent felt to modify some of the psychoactive effects of THC.

Oncologists and pain specialists readily agree that cannabinoids can reduce chronic pain, eliminate nausea, and stimulate appetite. A big problem in patients undergoing chemotherapy for cancer or AIDS is nausea induced by their life-saving medications. Nausea is difficult to treat and dreadful to live with; the medications available to treat nausea are quite expensive and often are not covered by prescription plans, while just a puff or two of cannabis will not only eliminate the patient's nausea for hours, but help build an appetite to maintain weight and nutrition.

These are key factors in maintaining some quality of life in patients with cancer, AIDS, and other debilitating illnesses. When patients begin to use cannabis to treat their pain, they are able to markedly decrease or stop their other pain medications, which can cause uncomfortable side effects like constipation (don't underestimate the impact of this one), nausea, vomiting, and sedation. There is mounting data that cannabinoids help enhance and complement response to opiate-based medications, allowing patients to significantly decrease their dosages (Cichewicz 2004).

Cannabis is also a potent and immediate-acting muscle relaxant, unclenching spasms and relaxing the smooth muscle of bladders of people suffering from spinal cord injuries, multiple sclerosis (MS), and amyotrophic lateral sclerosis. An interesting case report detailed that when an emergency room doctor allowed his patient to smoke some cannabis prior to having his dislocated shoulder repaired, the relaxed muscles allowed the physician to pop the joint back into place when prior attempts had been unsuccessful (Schweizer and Bircher 2009). Although inhaled smoke can act as an irritant to lung tissue, cannabis acts as a bronchodilator, helping open the airways in patients with asthma (Tashkin et al. 1975). In much the same way that the body will produce its own internal morphine when we're injured, we also produce our own internal cannabis, called anandamide (as further discussed in chapter 7, "Anandamide and More" by Mechoulam).

According to research at the University of Munich in Germany, patients with complex regional pain syndrome after traumatic injury have significantly higher blood concentrations of the endocannabinoid anandamide than healthy subjects. They concluded that the peripheral endocannabinoid system is activated in this syndrome (Kaufmann et al. 2009).

What many don't know is that cannabis is also an anti-inflammatory drug (Croxford and Yamamura 2005) and an immunomodulator (Lu et al. 2006). Because of the CB2 receptors on immune helper cells in the spleen and in the bloodstream, cannabis has the capacity to alter the course of autoimmune illnesses and inflammation responses. This means it can help reduce the damage done by strokes (please see chapter 25, "Cannabinoids and Neuroprotection" by Aggarwal and Carter for more on this), arthritis, MS, ulcerative colitis, and many other autoimmune diseases, as well as dampening the host-versus-graft syndrome in transplant recipients (O'Shaugnessy 2007).

According to researchers at the University of Barcelona in Spain, the endocannabinoid system is changed in the tissue of the colon of patients suffering from ulcerative colitis. They concluded from their studies that the "endocannabinoid signalling pathway, through CB2 receptor, may reduce colitis-associated inflammation suggesting a potential drug-able target for the treatment of inflammatory bowel diseases" (Marquéz et al. 2009).

There is also a growing number of journal articles attesting to the cancer-fighting properties of directly applied cannabinoids to cancer cells, including malignancies affecting the brain (gliomas), breast, prostate, lungs, pancreas, skin, and immune system (lymphomas) (Sarfarez et al. 2008). Cannabinoids can selectively kill tumor cells while leaving healthy cells unaffected (Guzman 2003). They can also inhibit new blood supply to tumors (angiogensis) (Blasquez 2003) and act as free radical scavengers (antioxidants) (Hampson 1998). In a large-scale study of chronic marijuana smokers, Tashkin's group found lower rates of cancer in the group that smoked versus the non-marijuana-smoking subjects. (Hashibe et al. 2006). The heaviest marijuana users in the study had smoked more than 22,000 joints, while moderately heavy smokers had smoked between 11,000 and 22,000 joints. While two-pack-a-day or more cigarette smokers were found to have a twenty-fold increase in lung cancer risk, no elevation in risk was seen for even the very heaviest marijuana smokers. In another study, ten to twenty years of marijuana use was associated with a significantly reduced risk (48 percent) of head and neck squamous cell carcinoma (Liang et al. 2009).

An interesting newer finding is that cannabis can help to treat and even to prevent the onset of diabetes; it exerts prometabolic effects in diabetic patients, helping normalize blood sugar, blood cholesterol, and lipid levels. What's more, the incidence of insulitis (the inflammation in the pancreas that can cause lowering of insulin) is reduced in these patients (Weiss et al. 2006, 2008).

Cannabidiol (CBD) is effective as an anticonvulsant, and many patients with epilepsy use cannabis to help control their seizures (Cunha et al. 1980). It should be noted that CBD is not "psychoactive" or euphorogenic. Also of interest to neurologists is that while most drugs, alcohol, and some medications suppress the growth of new brain cells, or neurons (called neurogenesis), when synthetic cannabinoids were applied to the hippocampus of rats, an area thought to be involved in memory formation, neurogenesis did, in fact, occur (Jiang et al. 2005).

Beyond the medical benefits of cannabis, one should not ignore the psychological and psychospiritual issues that are equally important. Using cannabis as an aid in relaxation, meditation, or just "being" can be an important component of self-care. Many stress-reduction therapies in medicine focus on meditation and being present and "in the moment" as a basis of health and mindfulness. Too many of our vices rely on distraction and escape, numbing our minds and bodies, but cannabis is a drug that, better than most, facilitates being in the moment and being mindful.

In the chapters that follow, clinicians and cannabis researchers outline the many potential benefits of medicinal cannabis. We all hope that physicians and scientists in America and abroad can further their understanding of this herbal medicine through continued clinical studies and patient care.

20

The Clinical Applications
of Medical Marijuana
An Interview with
Andrew Weil, M.D.

Julie Holland, M.D.

JULIE HOLLAND: I understand that you're co-editing a book with Donald Abrams that discusses using cannabis for treating cancer.

ANDREW WEIL: Yes. Actually, the book is on integrative oncology.* It includes a chapter by Donald on "Cannabinoids and Cancer."

JULIE: What's your take on the medical utility of using cannabis with cancer patients?

ANDREW: I think there is a potential in selected patients to use it as an appetite stimulant, for pain reduction, for the management of nausea and vomiting. But then there *are* possibilities that it may actually have immune-enhancing and anticancer activity. That's what we need to find out, but it looks promising.

JULIE: That was my next question. It seems as though cannabis is not just

---

Integrative Oncology, Abrams and Weil, Oxford University Press: 2008

for treating side effects of chemotherapy, but that it actually may have some role in prevention.

ANDREW: The trick is finding the right delivery system. I agree with Donald that vaporizers are much better than joints or pipes.

JULIE: There's a chapter in this book by Mitch Earleywine talking about harm reduction and the use of vaporizers,* which I think is really important.

ANDREW: It's a much better way to use it.

JULIE: And I wanted your take on Sativex. I know it's new, and I imagine you don't have a lot of experience with it yet, but what's your sense of it?

ANDREW: I'm very interested in the Sativex preparation. It looks more like a medical (as opposed to a recreational) product. So I think more doctors will be willing to use it.

JULIE: Because it's sublingual—under the tongue—or oral, as opposed to smoke-able?

ANDREW: Yes, and because it is manufactured and packaged as a pharmaceutical product.†

JULIE: I imagine we both have a sense that doctors, on some level, are never going to be fully comfortable recommending that their patients smoke.

ANDREW: That's one issue, and the other is that smoking doesn't cleanly separate it from recreational use, whereas the sublingual (under the tongue) spray does.

JULIE: Right, and the prescription would be for Sativex, specifically. Now, what is the law in Arizona? Can you prescribe? Can you recommend cannabis to your patients?

ANDREW: I can recommend by writing letters of recommendation, but I cannot prescribe, whereas in California, where I'm licensed, I can write prescriptions. There have been three initiatives here in Arizona that have all passed overwhelmingly, and then they've all been nullified by the governor or the legislature.

---

*See chapter 11, "Pulmonary Harm and Vaporizers."
†See chapter 29, "Sativex."

JULIE: And there's still this issue of the state law and the federal law not jibing.

ANDREW: Right. Here, the state law is not supportive.

JULIE: Are you comfortable recommending cannabis to patients? Is that something that you do? Or is it not really a big part of your practice?

ANDREW: I recommend it infrequently. One patient is a long-term patient with a spinal cord injury who has spasticity and pain. I have recommended it to a couple of other people with chronic pain and a couple of patients with multiple sclerosis, but this is not a significant part of my practice.

JULIE: So you have seen that in terms of an antispasmodic, it has some utility?

ANDREW: Yes. And I may suggest it to a few cancer patients, but Donald Abrams has really done the work there.

JULIE: Well, I'll be interviewing Donald for this book.* So, for cancer patients, a big part of the chemotherapy is that it induces this terrible nausea and vomiting and loss of appetite. My sense is that those side effects of the treatment, in particular, are hard to treat with conventional medication. Do you have alternative-medicine therapies that you think work as well as cannabis?

ANDREW: There are some Chinese herbal formulas that are used with chemotherapy and radiation that I have found to be helpful, but I think for appetite stimulation, we really don't have anything. For select patients, it (cannabis) is a good thing.

JULIE: I know for AIDS patients, with AIDS wasting, there seems to be a clear niche where it's useful.

ANDREW: I agree.

JULIE: Do you have an opinion about the indica versus sativa issue, in terms of which would be better for treating what?

ANDREW: No, I don't.

---

*Please see the following chapter for this interview.

JULIE: I was also wondering what your opinion is about synthetic cannabinoids like Marinol or Cesamet.

ANDREW: I think they're not as good as whole-cannabis preparations. They are more intoxicating, more sedating, and it's not so easy to titrate the dosage. I don't recommend them.

JULIE: Do you think that people are capable of titrating their own doses? A lot of people think that cannabis now is more potent.

ANDREW: They're perfectly capable of titrating their own dose, especially if they have some experience with it. If they have not used it, if they're novice users, they may have trouble and will need guidance. Anyone experienced with smoking cannabis can titrate the dose easily, regardless of potency.

JULIE: What's your opinion of the current system in place for physicians to recommend or prescribe cannabis to their patients? Is it adequate to meet the needs of patients? Should physicians be free to prescribe whatever they think works?

ANDREW: No. The system is dismal. It's a patchwork of state laws and the federal government working in opposition to each other. Yes, I believe physicians should have autonomy here and be able to prescribe what they think works, as long as they take note of evidence for safety and efficacy.

JULIE: Do you see a need for more clinical research to explore medical marijuana?

ANDREW: Of course. What Donald has done is great—we need much more.

JULIE: Are there any studies you're particularly interested in seeing happen?

ANDREW: Good ones on appetite stimulation, and basic research on the possibilities that cannabis protects against cancer and dementia.

JULIE: Do you have anything you'd like to say about hemp?

ANDREW: Hemp is a multipurpose, beneficial plant that has served human beings for thousands of years. It provides fiber, food, and medicine, as well as a psychoactive drug. I'm particularly enthusiastic about hemp foods such as whole seeds (delicious toasted) and oil (a source of healthy fatty acids).

JULIE: Any last thoughts on medical marijuana?

ANDREW: Its potential for harm is so low compared to most pharmaceutical drugs in common practice that we ought to be intensively exploring its medical benefits and the best way to realize them.

21
Medical Marijuana Research
An Interview with Donald Abrams, M.D.

Julie Holland, M.D.

JULIE HOLLAND: You have such a tremendous, impressive body of work. You've published so much in the field of therapeutic cannabis. I want to say thank you. Can you walk me through your history? Tell me about getting started, and how hard it was at the beginning. It took years to get the government to give you cannabis, right?

DONALD ABRAMS: I wrote a whole article about how hard it was (Abrams 1998). It all started when Rick Doblin* sent a little message to the director of research of the AIDS program at San Francisco General Hospital after Mary Rathbun was arrested in 1992, suggesting that a clinical trial showing the effectiveness of smoked marijuana should come from "Brownie Mary's"† institution, as if she were our dean! Somebody brought me the letter because they knew I did community-based clinical trials, and I was interested in investigating things that

---

*Rick Doblin is the founder and executive director of the Multidisciplinary Association for Psychedelic Studies (MAPS).
†Mary was an elderly woman who baked marijuana brownies for the AIDS clinic patients at SFGH, where she volunteered for many years.

people were using in the community. I picked up the gauntlet, but I knew Rick was not a physician, so I sent him the template for the University of California at San Francisco's Institutional Review Board (UCSF IRB) on how to design a clinical trial. I said, "Why don't you submit a proposal to me, and we'll see where we go from there." I thought that would keep him busy for a while, but within a week he had sent me back a nice protocol comparing three different dosages of smoked marijuana vs. Marinol.

JULIE: That must have surprised you. You think you're putting him off and you're never going to hear from him, and within a week you get the protocol.

DONALD: That was my introduction to Rick Doblin, you know?

JULIE: Right. Not a guy to be put off.

DONALD: At the time I was chairing a group called the Community Consortium, which was doing community-based clinical trials, and we all looked at his protocol, and everybody decided it would be an interesting thing to do. At the time, there had not been many antiretroviral drugs, and I had just done a study of the second and third generation of antiretrovirals, in patients who had failed the first. Having a new area to investigate was interesting. Plus, three years earlier, my own partner had died of AIDS. He had outlived three support groups at the hospital because, number one, he didn't take AZT, which was the only available antiretroviral at that time; and number two, he smoked a lot of marijuana. I wondered if there was maybe something to it, maybe it had some sort of benefit.

As I started to investigate what I needed to do to be able to do this, the challenges were stimulating. Every step of the way there was a little obstacle, and I just continued, trying to figure out how to get to the other side. A lot of the marijuana advocates and activists have a feeling there is a conspiracy going on, and the more I got into it, the more I realized they were right.

JULIE: So it's not just paranoia. I bet the government gave you a run for your money. If you like to be challenged, you're in the right field. Was the issue that the FDA approved the protocol but NIDA wouldn't release the cannabis?

DONALD: There was a roadblock at every step of the way. UCSF IRB made many comments, and we were able to cope with those, and they finally approved it. The FDA was very supportive and also approved it, and then I needed to get a Schedule I license from the DEA. To do that, I had to go to the Research Advisory Panel of California, and we needed to get marijuana from NIDA.

Rick had worked with someone in the Netherlands to import marijuana for the study, but the U.S. government wouldn't give us a letter saying it was okay to import it until they received a Dutch letter saying it was okay to export it. It became a catch-22, and it was impossible to figure out how to get out of that one. And then we were told we should seek a domestic source, which turns out to be NIDA. They're the only legal source of marijuana in the country. It took me two years to figure this out, but when I met with Alan Leshner, then head of NIDA, he reminded me they were the National Institute *on* Drug Abuse, not *for* Drug Abuse. And their congressional mandate is to study these drugs as substances of abuse, not as potential therapeutic agents.

JULIE: That's what the FDA is for, no?

DONALD: Right. So, in fact, our first studies, which were looking at the effectiveness of smoked marijuana in patients with the AIDS wasting syndrome, could not be done with NIDA marijuana in the mid-1990s, because there was no mechanism for them to supply marijuana for effectiveness studies. Subsequently, they developed a mechanism when the University of California Center for Medicinal Cannabis Research came into being, and they were funding efficacy studies.

When I applied for a DEA Schedule I license, the DEA didn't know who I was and were concerned about me, and both Tony Fauci from the National Institute of Allergy and Infectious Diseases (NIAID) and David Kessler from FDA wrote letters on my behalf. But it didn't much matter, because we couldn't get the marijuana from NIDA. And then in 1996, things changed when people voted for the California Compassionate Use Act (Proposition 215). And when protease inhibitors arrived, HIV wasting disappeared. The government threatened to take away privileges from physicians in California and Arizona who discussed the use of marijuana with their patients, and that was challenged by Marcus Conant (Ninth Circuit Court of Appeals Case No. 00-17222) in a lawsuit. This led to a number of government committees at the Institute of Medicine and the National Institutes of Health demanding more research on medical marijuana.

By that time, we had decided on a new approach, because a patient who also took Ecstasy had died on the new AIDS protease inhibitors. It was because of an interaction by way of the liver enzyme that metabolizes these drugs. I found out that was the same mechanism involved in the metabolism of cannabinoids. So we were invited to submit to NIH by Jag Khalsa at NIDA, who had funds available to study drug use in HIV patients. So, ultimately we got funded to do our study when it was altered from looking at the benefits of smoked marijuana to looking at the risks.

JULIE: Of mixing protease inhibitors and cannabis?

DONALD: Yes. So we did it as a safety study, thinking that would allow NIDA to supply us their cannabis, since their business is looking at these agents for their safety and toxicity. The NIH created a special study section to review this grant application because it was about HIV virology and immunology, and it was out of the purview of NIDA's area of expertise, so they called me and asked me to nominate a review committee. I did, and they scored us favorably, and we got funded, and we got NIDA marijuana, and we did our first study.

JULIE: And where did the research take you?

DONALD: Well, our first study was big. Each patient spent twenty-five days and nights in our inpatient unit. For twenty-one of those days, they either smoked NIDA marijuana cigarettes three times a day, or took dronabinol or placebo three times a day. We did a careful pharmacokinetic interaction study. We looked at the levels of HIV in the blood, and we looked at the immune system. We found that there was no significant pharmacokinetic interaction between cannabis and the protease inhibitors, that there was no damage to the immune system in patients using cannabis or dronabinol. Also, the viral load of the patients remained stable throughout the twenty-one days of exposure to the cannabinoids. We also found that patients gained weight smoking cannabis or even taking dronabinol. Previously, dronabinol hadn't been shown to be associated with weight gain, just an increase in appetite. But our study was too small to make that a primary endpoint.

But we showed that cannabis was safe in this relatively vulnerable patient population. We were fortunate to live in California and for the state to have a budget surplus at that time, so they could create the Center for Medicinal Cannabis Research. They appropriated $3 million a year for three years, which provided a mechanism to fund studies that were designed to evaluate the effectiveness of smoked marijuana in a number of clinical situations.

We were originally funded to do two studies: one in patients with HIV and peripheral neuropathy, and one in cancer patients with bone metastases who were on opioids. We started them at nearly the same time, two sixteen-patient pilot studies to determine if smoking marijuana had an effect on the pain. After evaluating sixteen patients, we were going to design randomized, placebo-controlled follow-on trials. We enrolled sixteen patients in the neuropathy study and about the first twenty on the randomized trial that followed it, but in that time, we enrolled only two cancer patients. Ultimately, the center took back our funds for that study, because it was clear we weren't going to be able to enroll it.

But for the neuropathy study, we were able to show that compared to the placebo cannabis, the smoked cannabis led to a decrease in the neuropathic pain. We also evaluated an experimental pain model in which we heated the skin and then applied capsaicin cream and measured the areas of "funny feelings" around that as another anchor for pain measurement. We knew we were going to get faulted by reviewers thinking we had pro-marijuana people enrolled in the study who were going to say "My pain is better." And maybe the blinding wouldn't be great, so maybe the placebo people wouldn't think their pain was better and the marijuana people would. So we did this much more objective experimental pain model to ground our findings.

In the meantime, we also got funded by the center to do a "double-dummy" study of cannabis and dronabinol in patients with delayed nausea secondary to cancer chemotherapy. It was going to be our first outpatient study, where people would get nine cigarettes and nine pills delivered to their homes and be instructed to take three a day for three days, and either one or both would be placebo. Some people got real marijuana and placebo dronabinol, some people got placebo marijuana and real dronabinol, and some people got two placebos.

It was an elegant design, but we enrolled only eight and we needed eighty-one, so again our funding was taken away.

JULIE: So it's much easier for you to recruit HIV patients than cancer patients into your studies? Because they don't live long enough to enroll in research?

DONALD: They sure do. The pain studies were in breast and prostate cancer patients with bone metastases, and those people may live for a long time.

JULIE: Then why?

DONALD: That's a good question that needs to be studied.

JULIE: Charlie Grob had a lot of trouble recruiting patients for his UCLA psilocybin cancer study also.

DONALD: So, Rick Doblin and Dale Gehringer, from NORML, brought to my attention that there is a vaporizer that may have some utility in delivery of cannabis through a nonsmoked method. I knew that smoking was something that people were not in favor of; people had said nobody smokes medicine and things like that. So after looking at some preliminary reports on the Volcano Vaporizer, we received funding again from the center to do a pilot study to compare the delivery of cannabinoids, smoked versus vaporized. This was an easy study to enroll for because we looked for healthy volunteers, ages twenty-five to forty, who were marijuana smokers.

We put them in our GCRC (outpatient clinical research center) for six days and gave them one of three different strengths of NIDA cannabis, either vaporized or smoked, each day, and $500 for completing the study. And with that, we demonstrated that the delivery system was effective, that we delivered similar amounts of cannabinoids with less expired carbon monoxide via vaporization compared to smoking. We found that the subjective highs were equivalent as well. In fact, most patients who participated preferred the vaporization delivery system to smoking. Now, that could be because NIDA marijuana is a bit harsh; it's been freeze-dried and has to rehydrated, but the majority favored the vaporization delivery system.

JULIE: So what came next?

DONALD: We thought that the question of opioids and cannabinoids being synergistic in relief of pain was a very important one that we wanted to answer. By this time, though, the center had run out of money and we were going to have to apply to NIDA again, so we used our prior model that we'd used with cannabinoids and protease inhibitors. We designed a study looking at the pharmacokinetic interaction of opioids and cannabinoids. And again, since I'm an oncologist, we chose to enroll cancer patients who had pain and were on MS Contin or Oxycontin twice a day. Although we received that funding three years ago, we were able to enroll only two cancer patients.

JULIE: So again you're having trouble finding cancer patients who want to participate in this kind of research.

DONALD: Now we've expanded the study to include any patient with any kind of pain, and we have enrolled ten. But they need to be taking the opioid medications twice a day, and we find that in the Bay Area, for whatever reason, many of these patients are taking these pain medicines every eight hours instead of every twelve hours, so that's been a problem for enrolling patients into the study.

JULIE: In terms of your patient population and what you see, what do you think are the differences between taking a synthetic oral cannabinoid versus the smoked whole plant?

DONALD: The plant has four hundred compounds and seventy additional cannabinoids compared to just delta-9-THC. I think some of those agents balance the potential adverse effects of the delta-9-THC, and you lose that when you just use the synthetic chemical by itself. In addition, there's low and variable oral bioavailability when it's taken by mouth. Also, there's a psychoactive metabolite, 11-hydroxy-THC, that is formed when THC is taken orally. When it's smoked, instead of waiting two and a half hours, the peak plasma concentration occurs in two and a half minutes, with a rapid decline over the next half hour, and there's much less of the sedating 11-hydroxy metabolite formed. So the kinetics are quite different. With the whole plant, you're getting a different product because it has so many other components in it.

JULIE: Which is more tolerable for the patient?

DONALD: When I did the study comparing dronabinol and marijuana and placebo, it was very clear to me that the dronabinol was very sedating. The dronabinol patients spent most of their time lying in bed, whereas the patients who were smoking marijuana seemed much more up and stimulated. We didn't ask about preference. In other studies where the patients are asked what they prefer, there is a preference for marijuana.

JULIE: Do you have a sense of the differences between THC, CBD, and CBN in terms of what seems to work better for what symptoms?

DONALD: I can't say. We use NIDA cannabis that has no CBD.

JULIE: Well, what do you think about that?

DONALD: It works, doesn't it? We were able to publish clinical trials showing it was beneficial in patients with neuropathy.

JULIE: People seem to have really strong opinions about indica versus sativa and different strains working better than others. I'm curious what you think about all that.

DONALD: I don't have enough information to really address this.

JULIE: When I was at the Cannabis Cup in Amsterdam,* some people were very opinionated about which components were more effective, or which strains were better for therapeutic use.

DONALD: Perhaps they have something to gain.

JULIE: You may be right. So, these days, are you not having as much trouble getting government approval for your studies?

DONALD: Well, certainly when we were working with the Center for Medicinal Cannabis Research, we had sort of greased the wheels with our first study, and I think there's really not much of a problem now. In fact, when people ask me to recount my difficulties early on, I have trouble doing so.

JULIE: This whole idea of politics trumping science, do you think things are changing?

DONALD: No, I don't think anybody bothers to really look at the research being done or make any policy changes on the basis of it.

JULIE: I still have the sense that the "party line" of our government is that

---

*The Cannabis Cup is a cannabis expo and competition held every Thanksgiving in Amsterdam and sponsored by *High Times* magazine.

there's no real medical advantage to using cannabis, that there's no clinical evidence to support medical marijuana, which is hard to believe. I was hoping you were going to say things have changed.

DONALD: No. You don't think that they have, and I don't either.

JULIE: What are your hopes for the future? What sort of things are you planning down the line?

DONALD: I don't have anything else planned at this point in time, to be honest. It's been so difficult to enroll patients; it's been a little frustrating. But I think we put together a very nice body of research. We first showed cannabis was safe, then we showed it was effective. We then showed that it can be delivered by a nonsmoked alternative delivery system, and now we're looking for synergism with other drugs and perhaps even being able to decrease some of the side effects of opioids. So it's sort of a nice progression or evolution of a research program. But what comes next . . . I don't have a plan.

JULIE: Well, you certainly do have this great body of work: HIV sensory neuropathy, neuropathy in general, AIDS wasting, pain control, the vaporizer studies. You've really done a lot to further the field. And you just finished editing a book* with Andrew Weil?

DONALD: Yes, I just finished writing my chapter on cannabinoids and cancer.

JULIE: That's great. Thank you, Donald, for all that you've done and are doing. Good work.

---

*Integrative Oncology, Abrams and Weil, Oxford University Press: 2008.

22

MAPS and the Federal Obstruction of Medical Marijuana Research

Rick Doblin, Ph.D.,
Executive Director of MAPS

A report on NPR, broadcast on February 18, 2010, and an associated article in the *LA Times* summarized ten years of work by the California State-funded Center for Medicinal Cannabis Research. The headline of the *LA Times* article was "UC Studies Find Promise in Medical Marijuana: As an $8.7-million state research effort comes to an end, investigators report that cannabis can significantly relieve neuropathic pain and reduce muscle spasms in MS patients. More research is urged."

The studies were funded with allocations from the state of California of $3 million a year for three years, generated as a result of the political work of State Senator John Vasconcellos. The FDA approved all the studies, and NIDA provided the marijuana. However, the charter for CMCR was to conduct some initial studies that would lead to the development of marijuana extracts and other nonsmoking delivery systems. NIDA was backed into a corner and couldn't refuse to provide marijuana for the state-funded research, but was reassured that the goal of CMCR was not to transform the marijuana plant itself into a prescription medicine (which is explicitly MAPS's goal).

One of the key CMCR studies of marijuana in neuropathic pain was conducted by Dr. Donald Abrams, UCSF (please see the previous chapter: an interview with Donald Abrams). MAPS provided him with funding for the travel expenses of subjects, which CMCR had not provided (Donald had initially assumed he would find enough subjects from the San Francisco area, which didn't happen). MAPS also worked with Donald by providing him with data from our marijuana/vaporizer research, which he used to obtain FDA permission and CMCR funding for the first study ever comparing smoked versus vaporized marijuana, looking at cannabinoid blood levels, carbon monoxide levels, and subjective effects.

This study showed that vaporization is a reliable way to deliver cannabinoids, and it's a nonsmoking delivery system that the FDA is more likely to approve than smoking. In this way, we had a key study funded by CMCR that helps with the development of the plant into an FDA-approved prescription medicine, since vaporization is the only nonsmoking delivery system that works with the plant itself rather than an extract.

I contacted Dr. Abrams in 1992 and got him involved in medical marijuana research initially, offering funding for a MAPS-sponsored study of marijuana in HIV-related wasting syndrome. That study was approved by the FDA and UCSF and several other review committees, but NIDA refused to provide the marijuana for the study. NIDA has a monopoly on the supply of marijuana that can be used in FDA-approved research. This is the key factor obstructing the development of marijuana into a legal prescription medicine.

After the 1996 California and Arizona medical marijuana initiatives, NIDA felt that it needed to support some research, otherwise the argument that FDA research was being stonewalled would generate support for further state-level reform efforts. NIDA then funded Dr. Abrams to study the risks of marijuana in HIV-postive subjects, in a protocol that excluded people who suffered from wasting syndrome. It was still a study worth conducting, so Donald went ahead with his study, which showed that there were no safety issues preventing marijuana use in HIV-positive subjects. Unfortunately for NIDA, its willingness to permit some marijuana research to move forward has been so limited, and NIDA and DEA's obstruction of marijuana drug development efforts so clear, that fourteen states have now approved medical marijuana laws, with more states to follow.

The FDA is definitely *not* the problem. In fact, the FDA has acted courageously, prioritizing science over politics when it comes to medical marijuana research. After Donald, MAPS worked with Dr. Ethan Russo on a marijuana/migraine study. This time, NIDA tried to get the FDA to refuse to review medical marijuana protocols before NIDA had decided whether to provide the marijuana. That would have deprived us of the persuasive argument that NIDA was refusing to provide marijuana to FDA-approved studies. After I took the matter to the FDA ombudsman, who reviewed NIDA's request with senior FDA management, the FDA decided that it should review marijuana the same way it reviews all other drugs.

The FDA practice is to review protocol designs even if the source of the drug is not certain. The protocol can be approved, but a "clinical hold" is placed on it until the source of the drug is resolved. Therefore, the FDA reviewed Ethan's protocol and approved it, as did an Institutional Review Board. This time, a NIDA/Public Health Service (PHS) review committee refused to provide the marijuana, and the study did not go forward.

After having two studies approved by FDA but blocked by NIDA's refusal to provide the marijuana, I realized that ending the NIDA monopoly on the supply of marijuana was the key step to opening the door to privately funded medical marijuana development. I searched for a year for the Rosa Parks of the medical marijuana production effort and found Dr. Lyle Craker, director of the Medicinal Plant Program at the University of Massachusetts at Amherst. Dr. Craker applied to the DEA in 2001 for a license to establish a MAPS-sponsored production facility. The DEA did its best to delay the process, "losing" the application for six months and then refusing to respond for over three years until we sued the DEA for unreasonable delay under the Administrative Procedures Act.

We eventually forced the DEA into an Administrative Law Judge (ALJ) hearing, which we won in February 2007, when ALJ Mary Ellen Bittner found that it would be in the public interest to end the NIDA monopoly and recommended that DEA should license Professor Craker. We benefited from excellent legal work provided pro-bono by Allen Hopper of the ACLU's Drug Law Reform Project and Julie Carpenter of the Washington, D.C., law firm Jenner & Block. State Senator John Vasconcellos, who arranged the funding for CMCR, testified for Professor Craker in our DEA ALJ hearing.

True to form, the DEA delayed responding to the ALJ recommendation for almost two years, finally rejecting the recommendation six days before President Obama was inaugurated.

The DEA made some sloppy procedural errors in its rejection, which we have taken advantage of, filing a Motion to Reconsider that halted the DEA's final ruling from going into effect. We've all been waiting for President Obama to appoint new leadership at the DEA to see whether it will grant our Motion to Reconsider or make its final order actually final.

To our deep disappointment, President Obama nominated Michele Leonhart, the DEA's current acting administrator, to be the next DEA administrator. She has been in a leadership position at the DEA since 2004 (appointed by President Bush) and has been a driving force behind the crackdown on medical marijuana. We're now trying to get senators on the Judiciary Committee who will have to vote on Leonhart's confirmation to raise the issue of DEA and NIDA obstruction of medical marijuana research.

MAPS is currently working on the protocol design and approval process for a marijuana/PTSD protocol. This protocol has several functions.

The first is to actually conduct the study, since many military veterans and other individuals with PTSD use marijuana to help control the symptoms of PTSD, and there has not yet been a single published study about this use of marijuana. The second function is to highlight the NIDA/DEA obstruction of medical marijuana research, since it will probably be the case that the NIDA/Public Health Service (PHS) review will reject the protocol, even after FDA has approved it.

We've designed the study to include marijuana of four potencies, limited to two grams per day. One group of subjects will receive 2 percent THC, one will receive 6 percent THC, the third group will receive 6 percent THC and 6 percent CBD, and the fourth will receive 12 percent THC. After growing marijuana for NIDA for over forty years, the University of Mississipi operation still doesn't have any strains with CBD, supposedly because nobody has ever asked for such strains. Our application will highlight NIDA's blundering approach to providing marijuana for research, since the anti-anxiety properties of CBD have been known for decades. It will probably take us about a year to determine how NIDA/PHS will respond (though the FDA will reply within thirty days!). Perhaps public support for helping these suffering veterans will generate enough pressure on NIDA/PHS for them to approve the protocol, or else the rejection of the protocol will help generate pressure on DEA to approve a license for Craker. We have obtained support for licensing Craker from forty-five congressional representatives and Senators Kerry and Kennedy, but that hasn't been enough yet to pressure the DEA to approve the license.*

---

*The DEA turned it down in January 2009, a week before Obama took office.

MAPS is also sponsoring research into MDMA-assisted psychotherapy (Ecstasy-assisted psychotherapy) for subjects with treatment-resistant PTSD. We have concluded two pilot studies, one in the United States and one in Switzerland, with a meta-analysis generating statistically and clinically significant reductions in PTSD symptoms in our full-dose MDMA group. We have just obtained FDA approval for a new MDMA/PTSD pilot study entirely comprised of U.S. veterans with chronic PTSD. We also have started an MDMA/PTSD pilot study in Israel and are close to starting additional MDMA/PTSD pilot studies in Jordan, Canada, and Spain.

MAPS's MDMA/PTSD research has taught us a great deal, and we're eager to try to conduct marijuana/PTSD research to compare and contrast with MDMA for PTSD. We can only hope that our marijuana/PTSD study will present NIDA/PHS with a dilemma: approve the study and provide marijuana so we can explore an important potential use of cannabis, or block the study and generate support for ending the NIDA monopoly itself.

23
The Government's Pot Farm

An Interview with
Mahmoud A. ElSohly, Ph.D.

Julie Holland, M.D.

JULIE HOLLAND: So you are a toxicologist, a forensic toxicologist?

MAHMOUD ELSOHLY: I'm a pharmacist by undergraduate original training, and a natural products chemist because that's what I have my Ph.D. in, pharmacognosy, which is the study of crude drugs like marijuana and opium. Currently my profession is that of forensic toxicologist.

JULIE: You published a book back in 2006 called *Marijuana and the Cannabinoids,* which I understand is a fairly technical book for a scientific audience.

MAHMOUD: That is correct.

JULIE: And you have a number of patents, some dealing with drug testing?

MAHMOUD: I have quite a number of patents, some dealing with drug testing, some dealing with product development activities, discovery issues, process patents, things of that nature.

JULIE: It sounds as though you have your hand in a lot of projects in Mississippi. One of the things your lab performs is drug testing. I understand that marijuana is the illicit drug with the highest percentage of positives in workplace drug testing?

MAHMOUD: That is correct.

JULIE: There's also a farm in Mississippi that you oversee. How involved are you in the actual growing of marijuana?

MAHMOUD: I am the director of that project, which is totally a university function. I am employed half the time at the university as a research professor and then the other half at my private lab doing the drug testing and the product development and the quality-control products and consulting. But as far as my function at the university is concerned, I am directing that particular project, which is a contract with the National Institute on Drug Abuse to provide standardized marijuana for research, along with a lot of other assigned activities that complement marijuana research in this country. So as part of that, we actually grow the plant cannabis and produce marijuana at different potencies so that cigarettes can be produced out of that material to go into the research activities that are required by different investigators across the country.

JULIE: So if someone has a NIDA-funded study looking at cannabis, they're going to get it from you, because there's pretty much nowhere else to get it in this country.

MAHMOUD: NIDA authorizes me to send this material to their investigators. The cannabis or marijuana is a Schedule I drug and therefore is only available to those on an IND (Investigational New Drug) for research. Because cannabis is a controlled substance, a Schedule I substance, only the government is authorized to distribute this material. We just happen to be under contract with the government to do that, so any material that goes out of our facility to another investigator has to be approved by the government, by NIDA.

JULIE: So it could be an FDA-approved study that isn't getting funding from NIDA, but it still needs NIDA's blessing, if NIDA is going to provide the study material.

MAHMOUD: That is correct.

JULIE: Are there times when FDA says yes and NIDA says no?

MAHMOUD: It appears that sometimes this might happen. A review board at NIH (National Institutes of Health) actually reviews protocols outside of FDA or NIDA. Somebody submits a protocol that might be approved by the FDA or not objected to by the FDA, but they send the same thing to NIDA. NIDA takes that protocol and gives it to the board that does the review. If the board sees no merit for doing the study, then NIDA would not give its approval.

JULIE: What I don't quite understand is that NIDA is not in the business of looking into therapeutic indications of drugs, right?

MAHMOUD: That's correct.

JULIE: So it seems as though they would have a hard time saying yes to some of the protocols that they're getting.

MAHMOUD: But NIDA is not the one to say yes or no; NIDA is just the agency that has the board that is looking at the merits of the protocol. If it makes sense in terms of its scientific merit, along with all the other factors that determine the merit of carrying out that study, then the board says yes. If the board says no, then it's not approved. But this has absolutely nothing to do with us, it's between NIDA and the FDA and the board and the investigators. I think maybe there was one protocol that I was aware of that did not get approved, but then later on there were some modifications that were made, and finally the investigators did get them to approve it.

JULIE: Is that the Donald Abrams study?

MAHMOUD: That is correct, and now he's finished with the study.

JULIE: Right. You also do potency monitoring on marijuana that's seized by the DEA?

MAHMOUD: We do monitoring of marijuana—physically confiscated material—that comes from different parts of the country. All the law enforcement agencies, the DEA in particular, send samples to us, to look at the potency of these materials, to assess what's out there.

JULIE: Do you think potency has changed over the years? You've probably been involved in this for a while.

MAHMOUD: Yes. Studies done in the '70s had marijuana potency somewhere around maybe half a percent or so, and today it's about 8 percent on average.

JULIE: And that's the percentage of THC? Because it's the predominant psychoactive chemical in cannabis, it makes sense to think of potency in terms of THC percentage?

MAHMOUD: Yes. The potency is how much THC is in the plant material by dry weight. If you look at the graph that shows this change, there was almost a continuous rise from the early '70s to about '83 or '84, where it leveled off at around 3 percent, dipped down a little bit, then started to come back up in '92 and was about 4 percent or so, and then it has been steadily going up with maybe plateaus two years in a row or something, and today it is right around 7 or 8 percent.

JULIE: When you do this testing for the DEA on the seized cannabis, is anyone looking for other things besides THC?

MAHMOUD: In our own analysis, we are looking for eleven different cannabinoids. The major ones that are significant enough to report are THC, CBD, CBC, CBN, CBG, and THCV. Some of the ones that would be there but in minute quantities are CBD-C3, CBL, CBT, and some other cannabinoids. But 99 percent of the samples don't have enough to be worth reporting about. So we typically report six cannabinoids on a regular basis.

JULIE: And what is a cannabis fingerprint?

MAHMOUD: The cannabis fingerprint is a program that I started back in the late '80s. We used to get a lot of questions about plant origin, such as, is there any way we can tell if these seizures are from the same place, where this material might be coming from? Is it domestic or is it foreign? If it's foreign, is it from Mexico or Colombia, Jamaica or Thailand? So I embarked on a study to look at the chemical composition of plant materials from different origins, and developed what is called the cannabis fingerprint, similar to what is already being used for heroin fingerprinting.

There is Turkish heroin and there is South Asian heroin. Their chemistry is different, the way they're processed is different—you can look at one and analyze it chemically and show where the material might be coming from. So, we applied that to cannabis, and of course there are different techniques and different chemistries, but the idea is about the same. We came to the conclusion back in 1991 or 1992, that, yes, you can actually analyze the chemical makeup of plant material of different origins, and there is enough difference between those that you can differentiate the source.

At that time, we had material from Mexico, Jamaica, Thailand, and Colombia, and we had some hashish from India, Pakistan, Lebanon, and different parts of the world. Then we had, of course, domestic material here in the United States from different states. We had material that was grown indoors and outdoors. We were able to show that, statistically speaking, we can determine with a reasonable degree of certainty, maybe 90–95 percent confidence, the origin of the cannabis.

The program was really not designed to put anybody in jail or to make a case that these two seizures come from the same source, or anything like that. It was basically for tracking—to tell where the material was coming from; it was basically for intelligence purposes. We had a whole database and everything, and then for some reason there were other drugs that were being pushed, so the program was basically dropped by the DEA. It's now coming back, and the Office of Drug Control Policy is interested in these fingerprints. So we are provided the samples, and now we have to start from scratch, because we lost all those years without keeping the database current. The materials available today are quite different than they were in 1992.

JULIE: So you have to build the whole database over again. When did you start rebuilding?

MAHMOUD: We started building the database by actually acquiring samples, actual material that we know is coming from a particular geographic location. We then analyze those materials, developing what we call a chemical fingerprint for that area. We're just beginning to work on this now, mainly looking at cannabis that is grown indoors versus outdoors. Then we are going to look further at the cannabis that is grown outdoors. Right now, we're focusing on domestic cannabis. The foreign we haven't even started, because we need cooperation from different countries.

JULIE: How can you tell the difference between indoor and outdoor? Does it have to do with the fertilizers used?

MAHMOUD: There are definitely differences in the chemistry of the plant, not necessarily on the cannabinoids, but on some of the other materials that are produced by the plant. It's the kind of lighting that they get, and the soil is not exactly the same. The difference is subtle and not easy to determine with the naked eye. The plant goes through a very intensive statistical analysis program called chemometrics to help us analyze the data and show these differences.

JULIE: Do you do any breeding down in Mississippi?

MAHMOUD: Not breeding per se, but we do genetic selection.

JULIE: How are breeding and genetic selection different?

MAHMOUD: For genetic selection, you take seeds coming from different plants. Each one of the seeds will actually produce a plant that is maybe a little bit different than the other. So within the same population of seeds, you can end up with quite a spectrum of potencies and genetic materials, simply because the cannabis plant is a highly variable species. You end up with different genetic materials out of the same thing.

We look at different individual plants and their makeup, and then pick the ones that have the chemical profile and the chemical makeup that suit what we are trying to do, and then we propagate that. This is opposed to breeding, where we start out by taking one male plant from a given source and a female plant from a given source, and then fertilize them and end up with seeds that have the genetic material of the mother and the father of that seed.

JULIE: It strikes me as very similar to humans mating.

MAHMOUD: That is true. That is because the cannabis plant is a dioecious plant, meaning you have male plants and female plants, so it depends on where the male plants come from and where the female plants come from. When these two get together, you have a possibility for hybridization that takes place, and you get something that may be similar to the mother or father, or maybe a hybrid in between.

JULIE: Do you grow both indica and sativa at the farm?

MAHMOUD: Yes, definitely we grow both.

JULIE: And hybrids too?

MAHMOUD: Well, yes, hybrids too. We look at the indica versus sativa in terms of the chemistry. The indica seems to have more CBD in it than the sativa. The majority of the plant material is available here in the United States; we analyze three or four thousand seizures every year. Ninty-nine percent of it is very high in THC and low in CBD.

JULIE: So are you saying that it's sativa, or just that they're hybrids?

MAHMOUD: It could be a hybrid, but nonetheless, it's more skewed toward the sativa end. Very few seizures have the indica-type chemistry.

JULIE: That seems to be the opposite of what I've been hearing.

MAHMOUD: Most of the material available in the program is sativa. What we see represents about 95 percent of what's out there, of what people are actually using, including those in California who are talking about the fact that the NIDA material doesn't have CBD. That's really not true, because we have samples coming out of California, and I could give you the statistics that show that the majority of the samples are sativa.

JULIE: With the Compassionate Program, those four patients who are still getting the canisters, are they getting indica or sativa from the farm?

MAHMOUD: All that is available right now on this particular investigator's request is a special makeup, which we are able to do. I communicated this to the people who talked to me about it; I told them that if they have a need, they should just request it. I think, most of the time, they're looking at what's available in the program, what's already made, and they just pick their material out of that. Maybe they don't believe that there are materials available that we can make on a small scale for a special study.

JULIE: You've been quoted as saying that you think that three hundred joints a month in the canister is too many, and I tend to agree with you, it seems like a huge number to me.

MAHMOUD: It is a huge number.

JULIE: Is it that it's not very potent? Wouldn't it make more sense to send out a higher-potency product so the patients could smoke less of it?

MAHMOUD: No. Let me clarify this, because I think this is a misconception of so many people. With the negative publicity that has been going on with the NIDA program, for political reasons, people are getting the wrong information. Let's go back to potency. The potency of cannabis, the material that is being used in the Compassionate Program, is probably between 3 and 4 percent. Those cigarettes weigh somewhere between 0.8 to 1 gram. So each cigarette will have somewhere between 24 and 40 mg of THC per cigarette. If you look at Marinol, which has been approved, it is either 2.5, 5, or 10 mg. It's very potent.

I can tell you that a few years ago I was approached to do a study for which they needed some material to do a dose-response study of 2 percent, 4 percent, and 8 percent. Of course the 2 percent and 4 percent are available in the current stock of material, but the 8 percent was not. So I got approval from NIDA to go ahead and make a small batch of 8 percent, which we did, and I provided it to the investigators. After they conducted the study, they called and talked to me about it, and said that the subjects who were actually experienced smokers could not tolerate this material, the 8 percent.

They then wanted do the dose-response study on 2 percent, 4 percent, and 6 percent. So we did; we got approval from NIDA, and we made a big batch of 6 percent. From the 8 percent material we made a small batch of hand-rolled cigarettes, but it had to be very similar to the other materials, it had to look the same, it had to be standardized. The important thing for people to know is that at the end of the study, the subjects were asked which session they liked the most in terms of the effect, and all these other things they score. What we found was that the majority of the subjects preferred the medium percent. Some preferred the 2 percent and some preferred the 6 percent, but the majority preferred the 4 percent. So this idea that the 4 percent is not potent enough is all just relative to what's on the market.

JULIE: The two complaints that I've heard about the marijuana cigarettes in the tin canisters is not so much about low potency, but that there were seeds and stems in them, or that it was old.

MAHMOUD: Yes, the fact is that some of the cigarettes are old.

JULIE: When did the program start?

MAHMOUD: I believe the program started back in 1968 or 1970, something like that. I don't know where the three hundred number came from or how it came about.

JULIE: Well, ten a day, no matter what the potency is . . .

MAHMOUD: That started from way back, and it just continued.

JULIE: It's funny, because the DEA is so worried about diversion. I don't understand how they think that one patient is going to smoke three hundred of anything a month.

MAHMOUD: It shouldn't be more than three cigarettes a day.

JULIE: I understand that you have a policy of first in, first out, whereby you ship what's older first, so these patients aren't getting very fresh pot.

MAHMOUD: Some of these materials have been around for five, seven, ten years, but this material has been stored under very appropriate storage conditions. They are in freezers at minus 20 degrees or lower, so they are preserved. There's no problem with the cigarettes. However, in response to that complaint, this year we're going to be making fresh new materials. We're also not going to make as much as we made before, so it won't be sitting too long.

We are not acknowledging that there is a problem with the age of the cigarettes. The difference might be in the flavor; the flavor might be better if it's not as old. But in terms of the efficacy or the pharmacological activity, the biological activity, it makes no difference.

JULIE: There's something odd about the government dispensing these joints to patients and saying, Here's your medicine, when they have placed cannabis in Schedule I, which says there's no medicinal value.

MAHMOUD: Cannabis is a Schedule 1 drug. When it is approved for these few patients or research subjects, it's not really approved as a medicine, it's approved as an investigational drug. So those cigarettes coming out to those subjects are supposed to be going to the physician—they don't go to the subjects—and the physician is supposed to be caretaker for this material and give it to the subjects as they need it.

JULIE: So it's almost like a research study with one person each, and there are four studies going on.

MAHMOUD: Exactly. That's how it's supposed to be.

JULIE: That makes sense. So what do you think about Marinol being a Schedule III and Sativex being approved in other countries? And why is nabilone Schedule II? What's the difference?

MAHMOUD: Nabilone is a much more addictive, much more highly psycho-logically active drug than THC.

JULIE: So it's a synthetic cannabinoid; it's not plant-based. But Marinol is plant-based?

MAHMOUD: The brand name Marinol is actually a synthetic THC. It's the exact same material as the material in the plants.

JULIE: I've heard that when Marinol goes generic, they may use plant-derived THC instead of synthetic.

MAHMOUD: What the DEA is proposing is that if they approve a generic Marinol, then any FDA-approved drug with the active ingredient of THC is going to be Schedule III, just like Marinol.

JULIE: And it wouldn't matter if it was plant-derived or synthetic?

MAHMOUD: That's right. To take plant-derived THC and make generic material out of it, you've got to go through the FDA and get approval. If it gets approved by the FDA, that means they are equivalent, that there's no difference, so it's going to be Schedule III. That means we can grow plant material to produce THC that could be used for generic Marinol or any other product that contains THC.

JULIE: I understand that the transdermal applications of THC don't get absorbed very well through the skin, and the problem with orally active THC is that the liver metabolizes it down to this chemical 11-hydroxy-THC. This is very potent, more potent than THC, and basically unde-sirable for the most part, which I think is the problem with oral delivery to some extent. What is your take on that?

MAHMOUD: There are two problems with the oral version. Number one is the fact that it is oral, and so it has to be absorbed; it's got to go through the liver and get metabolized and so on. But in addition to the metabo-lism part, absorption from the GI (gastrointestinal) tract is not consis-tent. Some people absorb quite a bit, some people don't absorb it at all, and some people absorb just a little bit.

JULIE: And if your stomach is full, you won't absorb as much.

MAHMOUD: So that erratic percent availability of THC from the oral ver-sion is a problem. Number two is the fact that it goes through the liver.

If you look at the blood levels of someone who is taking Marinol, you see there are almost equal amounts of THC and 11-hydroxy THC, which is a lot more psychoactive, a lot more potent than THC. Therefore you have a very psychologically active component circulating in the blood and causing the majority of the side effects.

So if you can avoid or bypass the first-pass effect of this liver metabolism, then you can deliver THC and have it as the circulating, active ingredient in the blood. That's the reason we thought about the suppository; it would be a good formulation to bypass that. We're working with this. It's an excellent preparation, a good product, but because it is a suppository, some people have a really hard time accepting it as a delivery system, although it is pharmaceutically acceptable and it's been around for years.

JULIE: Certainly for people who are vomiting or nauseated, it's a medically accepted option.

MAHMOUD: But it's still not out there yet. The pharmaceutical company has it, and hopefully they'll approve it before too long.

JULIE: Can you just review with me what the clinical indications of a THC suppository might be?

MAHMOUD: It would be for the exact same indications that THC is good for. Right now it's only approved for the nausea and vomiting of cancer patients and appetite stimulation in AIDS patients. But there are other indications that THC might be really useful for, things like glaucoma, pain—both neuropathy and arthritic pain—and in terms of a preoperative analgesic or antidepressant. There are just so many indications.

JULIE: I'm hearing a lot about muscle spasms too.

MAHMOUD: For any of those indications that THC is approved for right now, it would be easy to get the drug. For new indications, you'd have to go all the way through Phase 1, Phase 2, Phase 3 clinical trials, and so on. So it's more expensive to have a new indication than an already approved indication.

JULIE: What do you think about Sativex?

MAHMOUD: Sativex is a cannabis extract that has about equal amounts of CBD and THC. It's marketed as a product for sublingual use, but I am not 100 percent convinced. I believe that the majority of its effect is coming from oral.*

JULIE: They're saying that CBD matters.

MAHMOUD: Well, CBD might matter. People believe that CBD diminishes the negative effects of THC, the high that THC produces. In a way this is true, but not at that equal dose. You really need a lot more CBD than one-to-one to reduce the effects of THC. I think if CBD is helping this equation in any way, it's because CBD itself does actually have some type of biological activities of its own that are beginning to be shown now in the scientific literature. CBD is a nonpsychoactive cannabinoid that does have quite a number of effects that the psychoactive cannabinoids have. So it seems to me that CBD is going to be a very important drug in the future, but it's not there yet.

JULIE: People are saying that CBD has anti-inflammatory or even anticancer properties.

MAHMOUD: Yes, there are some effects like that, but THC has similar effects.

JULIE: Now, because the government has a hand in growing cannabis for clinical research, there may be a conflict of interest; they're not necessarily interested in creating the best product to show that it's therapeutic. Also, there's a potential conflict of interest with growing cannabis to use for generic Marinol, because smoked cannabis and Marinol are competitors for the same clinical indications or the same patients. So how do we know that the government's really growing good, effective cannabis for medical marijuana research?

MAHMOUD: This is a very subjective question, and the answer is going to depend on whom you're asking and why, but the bottom line is this: If you are talking about cannabis for a medical indication, what are you looking for? You're looking for THC, the active ingredient, so whether you grow material that's 4 percent or 6 percent, for instance, it only affects the amount of material you are going to smoke to get that dose

---

*People are supposed to put Sativex under their tongues so it gets drained from the neck veins to the heart to the brain, bypassing the liver. But in reality, some probably gets swallowed, which means the liver generates 11-OH-THC, which affects the "high."

of THC. I know you mentioned early on, "Why don't you make it with higher potency so that they don't need three hundred cigarettes?"

Well, it doesn't work like that. Maybe eventually it will, but the most important thing is the amount of THC that people are going to be getting. People make all kinds of claims about other components in there that might be affecting the overall activity of the drug, but nobody can really point to one single component that might be doing something that's helping a condition, aside from what THC is doing. And if there is such a component in there, why not develop that component? Let's say a component that has nothing to do with cannabinoids, no THC, no CBD, or any of those. Let's say, for example, that a flavonoid causes reduction in the inflammation. Why not develop that flavonoid as an anti-inflammatory?

Nobody has shown anything to indicate that if you take marijuana with the flavonoid versus marijuana without the flavonoid, you're going to get a difference in the final effect of the drug. They haven't shown that, but they talk about it as if it's a fact. So we have a whole range of different potencies, and if anybody wants to investigate that and show that you really need the 14 percent to get such-and-such effects, why not do the research with that? What difference does it make if I make it, or if some grower in California makes it? It makes no difference. The idea is to do the study, find the facts, and then come up and say that if the government is giving us material, we need this type of material. But nobody's doing that. They're just talking about it, complaining about it, but not really doing anything that's black and white to show that we need this.

JULIE: I think some people are just frustrated that the clinical research isn't going faster. It seems like the government needs proof that it's therapeutic so that it can move it from Schedule I to Schedule III. Now, as you know, there were hearings where the recommendation was Schedule III, but the DEA basically ignored the ruling. I don't know if there's a disconnect between the DEA and NIDA and the FDA, but where do you see this going?

There are fourteen states and Washington D.C. that have approved medical marijuana legislation and there's a push right now for passage of more state medical marijuana laws. But it seems like it has to go very slowly, state by state, instead of the federal government lifting the ban.

There is this Compassionate Program, and there are four patients in it, but why are there only four? Why was it closed down? The government's arresting some patients for using cannabis, but they're not arresting these four people. But the program's closed, right?

MAHMOUD: Well, there can still be a positive research program. There is all this research going on, Abrams and all the others, so people can participate in those studies. The Compassionate Program was closed, then it was reopened again to allow the clinical research with this material. So the program is not closed to having people participate in the clinical trials.

JULIE: You clearly think that there's some clinical indications for THC, at least.

MAHMOUD: THC, absolutely. My personal view is that smoking the drug is really not a good way to deliver THC. It's a totally unacceptable pharmaceutical way of delivering the drug.

JULIE: What about people using a vaporizer?

MAHMOUD: The vaporizer is not as bad as smoking, but it's the same idea, where you really don't know how much material you're getting. But definitely, I look at the vaporizer as a device that reduces the negative effects of smoking the material.

JULIE: Right, it's what I would call harm reduction.

MAHMOUD: The point is, all you really need to do is get the THC to go through and come out of the vaporizer so you can inhale it. Why not develop an inhaler that has THC in it?

JULIE: Like a metered-dose inhaler for asthma?

MAHMOUD: Yes.

JULIE: Well, has no one done that? It does seem like an obvious thing to do.

MAHMOUD: There are some people who are working on something like that, but it's like anything else, it takes time and money and clinical trials, and I think people just want to have a shortcut. Marijuana is a shortcut because it's available and easy to smoke, and the vaporizers were an offshoot of that. With a true pharmaceutical preparation, you know how much it's delivering, how much the subject is getting, and you know what kind of pharmacology you're going to get, and so on.

Remember with that vaporizer, if the subjects are like you and me and have never smoked marijuana, they are really going to have a hard time dealing with this. This vaporizer and the smoking material are not designed for the average subjects who are in need of a pharmaceutical preparation to deal with their ailments; it's for people who are used to smoking marijuana. They prefer to smoke marijuana; they don't want to use Marinol; they don't want to use a suppository, don't want to use a sublingual. They just want to smoke the material. So you're not going to provide them with any pharmaceutical preparation that's going to satisfy them, short of letting them smoke marijuana. I don't think the ones that really want to smoke marijuana even want the vaporizer.

JULIE: The bottom line is that there are millions of Americans who smoke marijuana, and some of them have AIDS or cancer or multiple sclerosis, and they would rather just use what they know works for them in a way that they are comfortable with. But the problem is that they risk prosecution, which is kind of crazy. I personally feel like my tax dollars could be put to better use than prosecuting patients.

MAHMOUD: That is something that I personally and my institution have nothing to do with. We are trying to provide a service to the government, and to the people, to the best of our ability, and some people are happy with what we're doing, others are not. I can't do much about that.

JULIE: What is your take on hemp and using hemp for industrial purposes? Do you know anything about hemp?

MAHMOUD: It's a good product, and it has good potential. The only problem with hemp that I see is from the standpoint of the DEA. Being able to grow hemp and other marijuana plants alongside of it makes it very difficult to tell the difference.

JULIE: They look very similar, but hemp is very low in THC. But it's not zero, right?

MAHMOUD: No, it's not zero. I think most hemp products have 0.2 percent or less THC.

JULIE: Basically not psychoactive?

MAHMOUD: Well, it would be. There is THC in there, and a layperson smoking hemp will actually get high. But it's not the same kind of material as marijuana. And also, hemp has higher amounts of CBD in it. The amounts are such that the CBD is more likely to subside the high of the THC, because it's five, six, ten times as much as the THC. Another thing about hemp is that because of the high amount of CBD, you can harvest the leaves of the hemp and extract it to make hash oil. You end up with a product that's very rich in CBD and is only one step away from THC.

JULIE: Do you think that's why it's illegal?

MAHMOUD: Well, it's illegal because it still has THC. Anything that has THC is illegal. But the reason hemp may be controlled and not open for production in the United States is those two issues. One, you can have regular marijuana growing with it and you wouldn't know the difference; and two, the hemp itself could be diverted to making hash oil from the plant leaves that have high CBD content, which could easily be converted to THC in just one step.

JULIE: It does seem to me that it could potentially be used as fuel, and with our current energy crisis, it's worth examining.

MAHMOUD: Well, I think you could get a lot more fuel out of cotton stalks.

24
Cannabinoids and Psychiatry

Julie Holland, M.D.

The study of cannabis and cannabinoids could be enormously beneficial to the field of psychiatry. Cannabis has been used as a treatment for depression, anxiety, inattention, malaise, and insomnia for thousands of years. Millions of people around the world are using marijuana to "self-medicate" these symptoms and others. For these two reasons alone, it would behoove us to have a better understanding of the medicinal properties of this plant.

Specific to the field of psychiatry, we have much to learn about the brain's endogenous cannabinoid system. To study THC, CBD, and other cannabinoids is to better understand ourselves, our brain chemistry, the brain's response to injury, and the underlying pharmacology of mind states such as paranoia and panic. Understanding the chemistry and physiology of the cannabinoid molecules could potentially help us create analogues and antagonists to treat other symptoms and diseases. (For example, the cannabinoid antagonist rimonabant can help curb appetite, or stop the "munchies," but, interestingly, it was rejected by the FDA due to concerns surrounding its ability to induce depression, anxiety, and suicidal thoughts.)

In my private practice, I see and treat many pot smokers. Some of them note that smoking marijuana helps them fall asleep or relax, and they tend to smoke at the end of their day. Others find it helps them focus, be creative, or become more meticulous and obsessive; these patients tend to use marijuana before starting a project. I have patients with attention deficit disorder (ADD) who feel it helps them pay attention to minute details. I also hear from a fair number of people with depression that it can reliably lift their spirits and create a much-longed-for sense of euphoria and hopefulness. Then there are my anxious or panicky patients who feel that pot makes their symptoms worse; they become more self-conscious and hyperaware, and they are not at all comfortable with marijuana's effects. On the other hand, I have some anxious patients who swear by it as an aid to relaxation. Any reasonable clinician should be intrigued by this phenomenon: Why are so many patients having such vastly different effects and experiences?

The joke I always make about cannabis with my patients is that it is a "mixed bag." Because there is such tremendous genetic diversity in cannabis, every strain is unique. Each time someone makes a purchase, they are getting a different medicine, so to speak. Hybrids abound in New York City as they do in the rest of the world, and it is nearly impossible to know just what the mix will be. If they buy an indica-predominant strain, they may become sleepier, more relaxed, and possibly less motivated. A sativa-predominant strain may help energize or focus their thoughts. Both strains seem to induce appetite, which may be a nuisance for some users, but a blessing for those patients made nauseated and anorectic by their medications or illnesses. Some strains might trigger paranoia, perhaps due to a high THC content, while another strain might have an opposite effect if it is CBD-heavy (see below).

Our brains, in particular the cortex where higher thinking and planning are performed, are full of receptors for cannabis. An interconnected network, the cannabinoid system, makes use of our own endogenously made cannabis-like molecules, which are called endocannabinoids. In much the same way as endorphins stimulate our opioid receptors, our bodies make anandamide to activate our cannabinoid receptors. Much like the human race and the opium poppy, we have been co-evolving on this planet with the cannabis plant since our beginnings. Cannabis was likely one of the first plants to be domestically cultivated.

It has been used as a medicine since the third century BCE, and it has a long history of being used to treat psychiatric complaints as well as physical ones (please see chapter 2 by Chris Bennett). The Atharva Veda (around 2000 BCE) tells of using *bhanga* to "release us from anxiety" (International Hemp Drugs Commission 1893). In ancient Assyrian medical texts, smoking is mentioned as a way to "dispel depression of spirits" (Thompson 1924).

People of the Dutch East Indies noted that cannabis "serves to drive away sorrow and bring them jollity" (Rumpf and Beekman 1981). In Burton's *Anatomy of Melancholy*, he describes the intoxication of cannabis as a "kind of ecstasy, an inclination gently to laugh." In England, in the mid-1800s, a tincture of hemp was used to treat morphine withdrawal, inducing "sleep; as an anodyne in lulling irritation . . . a nervine stimulant in removing languor and anxiety" (Clendinning 1843).

In France, the physician Jacques-Joseph Moreau de Tours first wrote of cannabis's potential for treating psychiatric patients in his book *Du hachisch et de l'alienation mentale: Etudes psychologiques* ("Of hashish and insanity: Psychological studies"), noting that hashish produced "manic excitement always accompanied by a feeling of gaiety and joy inconceivable to those who have never experienced it. I saw in it a means of effectively combating the fixed ideas of depressives, disrupting the chain of their ideas, un-focusing their attention on such and such a subject." And in America, an Ohio physician, reporting on a case he identified as "hysterical insanity," wrote of cannabis, "In those mixed and indefinable paroxysms of an hysterical nature, I have found no remedy to control or curtail them with equal promptness and permanency. . . . In sleeplessness, where opium is contraindicated, it is an excellent substitute. . . . Calmative and hypnotic, in all forms of nervous inquietude and cerebral excitement, it will be found an invaluable agent, as it produces none of those functional derangements or sequelae that render many of the more customary remedies objectionable" (McMeens 1860).

The English physician John Russel Reynolds, best known as the personal physician to Queen Victoria, had a long career of using and championing cannabis as medicine. Early reports of success treating depression, lassitude, and senile restlessness (Reynolds 1868) paved the way for forty years of successful practice. About the treatment of senile insomnia, he wrote, "I have found nothing comparable in utility to a moderate dose of hemp" (Reynolds 1890).

A British pharmacologist suggested, "In cases where an immediate effect is desired, [cannabis] should be smoked, the fumes being drawn through water, for fits of depression, mental fatigue, nervous headache, and exhaustion, a few inhalations produce an almost immediate effect, the sense of depression, headache, feelings of fatigue disappear and the subject is enabled to continue his work, feeling refreshed and soothed" (Dixon 1899).

Lewis, in 1900, described the effects of cannabis: "The mind seems wholly taken with thoughts of the moment. Very frequently a great inexplicable sense of relief is felt, the sensation being identical with that experienced by one who suddenly awakes from a horrible dream to the feeling of gratitude which is always felt at its unreality." In Southeast Asia, cannabis was used as a tonic in chronic illness, to induce sleep, and as a relaxant. In Vietnam, a preparation of cannabis seeds was used to "combat loss of memory and mental confusion" (Martin 1975).

Cannabis was used to treat delirium tremens (withdrawal from alcohol dependence) and addiction to cocaine and opiates. Mattison (1891) concluded, "In these, often, it has proven efficient substitute for the poppy. . . . My experience warrants this statement: cannabis indica is often a safe and successful anodyne and hypnotic." Cannabis has been used to treat opiate addiction (Mayor's Committee on Marijuana 1944) and alcoholism (Mikuriya 1970; O'Shaughnessy 2007) with good results. A study of THC in cancer patients reported positive psychological effects of "a tranquilizer and mild mood elevator, clearly without untoward effects on cognitive functioning and apparently without untoward effect on personality or emotional stability—at least as can be measured by psychological tests" (Regelson et al. 1976).

A survey of California clinicians working with cannabis revealed psychiatric symptoms to be a common indication for a prescription. (Nearly every patient coming to these clinicians had already been using cannabis to treat their symptoms, so a more appropriate term for what these physicians offer may be "approval," as opposed to "recommendation.") From Jeffrey Hergenrather: "In my opinion, there is no better drug for the treatment of anxiety disorders . . . ADHD, obsessive compulsive disorder, and Post Traumatic Stress Disorder" (O'Shaughnessy 2007).

Doctors responding to the survey reported that many of their patients were able to decrease their use of other psychiatric medications, like antidepressant, antianxiety, and sleeping medications, or else they used cannabis to treat their side effects of jitteriness or gastrointestinal problems in order to stay on their medications.

THE PSYCHOACTIVE EFFECTS OF CANNABIS

The psychoactive effects of cannabis are mediated primarily through the CB1 receptors (Pertwee 1997). (Please see chapter 12 on cognition for a review, as well as chapter 6 on the endocannabinoid system.)

The CB1 antagonist rimonabant has been shown to block the subjective effects of marijuana (Huestis et al. 2001) as well as induce depression. It is postulated that dysregulation of the endocannabinoid system is involved in the emotional processing of stressful events. In a study with mice, impaired CB1 receptor signaling interfered with stress-coping behavior (Steiner et al. 2008). In mice bred to have no CB1 receptors, many abnormalities were seen, taken as a whole to support an "increased susceptibility to develop an anhedonic state" (Martin et al. 2002).

As delineated in chapter 12 by Carl Hart, the subjective effects of cannabis depend on dosage, route of administration, and, most crucially, the set (expectations) and setting (environment). Also important is the person's familiarity with cannabis. Many of my patients have told me that they didn't get "high" the first time they smoked pot. Some theorize that this is because they didn't know what "high" was and couldn't recognize it when it was upon them. Others believe there is some sort of priming mechanism involved, the way one would have to prime the pump of a well. Not becoming intoxicated the first time one smokes cannabis is a curious, though not universal, phenomenon that deserves more study.

ANTI-PSYCHOTIC EFFECTS OF CBD: CANNABIS AND SCHIZOPHRENIA

While cannabis has frequently been implicated in causing or exacerbating psychosis, there are actually promising leads in using cannabidiol CBD as an antipsychotic medication. (Please see chapter 13 for more on this.) Unlike THC, CBD is a noneuphoriant, anti-inflammatory analgesic that does not bind well to the CB1 or CB2 receptors. Zuardi and colleagues (1997) have proposed that the ratio of THC to CBD is crucial in determining the effects of cannabis on psychosis, and these two components have been studied extensively. Currently, it is widely believed that cannabis strains that are higher in THC are more apt to produce paranoia and other symptoms reminiscent of psychosis, while those higher in CBD are less likely to do so. This is likely the problem with the strains known as "skunk," which have much higher ratios of THC to CBD. This may also end up being an issue with "Spice," a synthetic cannabinoid also known as K2 (made up of certain psychoactive chemicals such as JWH-018, JW-073, JWH-250, HU-210, and a homologue of CP-47, 497, that are, as of this writing, not yet scheduled; please check ThePotBook.com for more on this), which acts as a full, potent agonist at the CB1 receptor, as opposed to THC, which is a weak partial agonist.

While THC is responsible for the euphoric and anxiety-inducing effects of cannabis, CBD may modulate these effects, causing sedation and diminishing anxiety (Zuardi and Guimaraes 1997). Thus, strains with higher THC/CBD ratios may be more paranoia-inducing or anxiety-provoking, than those strains with higher levels of CBD. More importantly, CBD may actually diminish psychotic symptoms in patients who have them, such as those with schizophrenia (Zuardi et al. 1995). CBD was also found to reduce psychotic symptoms in a group of patients with Parkinson's disease (Zuardi et al. 2009).

In a 1994 study by Warner, psychotic patients who used marijuana had lower rates of hospitalization than those who abused other substances. They were also found to have lower activation symptoms such as psychomotor agitation. These patients reported beneficial effects on depression, anxiety, insomnia, and pain. In a review of twenty-three studies of schizophrenics using cannabis, fourteen studies reported that cannabis users had better cognitive performance than nonusers. Eight reported no difference, and only one study reported better cognitive performance in the schizophrenics who did not use cannabis. The authors say this meta-analysis confirmed their own experiences with cannabis-using patients (Løberg and Hugdahl 2009).

Negative symptoms of schizophrenia (thinking and talking less, having less motivation and activity) are particularly stubborn symptoms to ameliorate with antipsychotic medications. Bersani and colleagues (2002) noted a subgroup of schizophrenics who used cannabis to decrease their negative symptoms. On the other hand, Verdoux (2003) noted a significant association between cannabis use and the negative symptoms of schizophrenia. It is crucial that CBD be carefully studied to determine if it may have a place in psychiatry as an antipsychotic, potentially not only quieting the positive symptoms of schizophrenia (namely the paranoia and hallucinations), but also ameliorating the very difficult-to-treat negative symptoms of amotivation, depression or blunted affect, and talking and thinking less.

The prefrontal cortex is a particular area of interest in schizophrenia research. It is one of the parts of the brain known to be dysfunctional in people with schizophrenia, and many antipsychotics exert some of their beneficial effect there (Thierry et al. 1978). A high density of CB1 receptors can be found in the prefrontal cortex (Herkenham et al. 1990). The primary neurotransmitter abnormalities in schizophrenia involve dopamine, which interacts with the cannabinoid system. THC enhances the flow and utilization of dopamine in the prefrontal cortex (Chen et al. 1990) and, conversely, activation of dopamine receptors (D2) causes an increased outflow of anadamide (Giuffrida et al. 1999).

A 2009 study using receptor tracers and PET (positron emission tomography) scans showed that THC induces dopamine release in the human striatum. This implies that the endogenous cannabinoid system is involved in regulating striatal dopamine. This is important for two reasons. Not only is there dopamine dysfunction in this area in schizophrenia, but also drugs of abuse are often enhancers of dopamine levels, thus creating pleasure, excitement, and possibly an increased risk of addiction through this "reward pathway" (Bossong et al. 2009).

In a clinical case series, four chronic, treatment-refractory schizophrenic patients (who had reported improvement in their symptoms when they smoked cannabis) were administered oral THC (dronabinol). Three of the four showed significant improvement in core psychotic symptoms. The results would suggest "that the role of cannabinoids in psychosis may be more complex than previously thought. They open a possible new role for cannabinoids in the treatment of schizophrenia" (Schwarcz et al. 2009).

DEPRESSION

As reviewed above, there is abundant clinical lore, both ancient and recent, that cannabis can help lift one's mood. In my private practice, it comes up fairly often: my patients use marijuana to feel better. In an Internet survey of over 4,400 respondents (Denson and Earleywine 2006), those who use cannabis had lower levels of depressive symptoms than those who had never tried cannabis. Weekly and daily users of cannabis had less depressed mood and more positive affect than nonusers.

In an exquisitely complicated review paper (Hill 2005), melancholic depression was compared to an endogenous cannabinoid deficiency. Further, the author makes an excellent case for using the cannabinoid system as a target for future antidepressant development. In a follow-up paper, Hill and colleagues (2008) measured one of the endogenous cannabinoids, 2-AG, in depressed patients. Serum 2-AG content was significantly decreased in patients diagnosed with major depression, and the 2-AG content was progressively lower the longer the depressive episode.

In an overview by Mangieri and Piomelli (2007) of the cannabinoid system and depression, the authors state, "The overlap between the physiological functions altered by depression and those affected by cannabinoid receptor signaling is striking." They continue, "changes in levels of the cannabinoid CB1 receptor or the endogenous CB1 receptor ligands, anandamide and 2-AG, are observed both in humans suffering from depression and in animal models of depression, and experimental manipulation of CB1 receptor signaling has also been shown to affect emotional reactivity in rodents." CB1 receptors may be up-regulated in suicide victims suffering from depression, as was shown in a study of postmortem brains (Vinod and Hungund 2006). This may suggest a hypofunctioning cannabinoid system in depressed or suicidal patients.

BIPOLAR DISORDER

In a short review article (Ashton et al. 2005), several points were laid out. Though there are no placebo-controlled trials of cannabinoids in bipolar illness, there exist many anecdotal reports of patients experiencing relief of both the depressed and manic phases of their illness. CB receptors are plentiful in areas of the brain thought to be affected by bipolar illness. Patients may experience psychosis or a manic episode due to cannabis use, or they may be more sensitive to its effects than the general population. THC and CBD may have different effects on the various symptoms of bipolar illness.

The take-home message from this article is simple: more research needs to be performed so psychiatrists can ascertain whether cannabinoids, and CBD in particular, might have a role in the treatment of bipolar illness, although Zuardi did not see symptom improvement in two manic patients with trials of CBD (Zuardi et al. 2010). Some of my bipolar patients feel that cannabis destabilizes them, and one study by Strakowski and colleagues (2007) reported that cannabis use was associated with more time spent in affective episodes (depressed or manic phases of illness) and with rapid cycling.

Lester Grinspoon, in his 1998 article, gave multiple case reports of bipolar patients who had experienced marked relief from their symptoms with the use of cannabis, and who believed it to be more effective than standard medications. Others used cannabis to fight the side effects of their psychiatric medications, thus allowing them to remain on effective dosages. Dr. Grinspoon encourages clinical research to follow up on these convincing anecdotal histories and laments the "present social circumstances" that make "such studies almost impossible."

POST-TRAUMATIC STRESS DISORDER
AND OTHER ANXIETY DISORDERS

In many self-reports, relaxation and stress relief are benefits that cannabis consumers report. In animal and human studies, cannabinoids have been shown to reduce anxiety (Rubino et al. 2008; Musty 1984). The endocannabinoid system is found in many brain circuits believed to be involved in stress reactions, the extinction of fear, and emotional regulation (Jankord and Herman 2008; Akirav and Maroun 2007).

The endocannabinoid system is linked with the hormonal system known as the HPA (hypothalamic-pituitary-adrenal) axis and is thought to exert a basal level of inhibition. After someone has been emotionally stressed, it is possible that endocannabinoids help bring the HPA axis back to baseline (Viveros et al. 2007). The endocannabinoid system is also thought to be involved in the learned extinction of the conditioned fear response (Moreira and Lutz 2008). Because cannabis helps you forget, this has implications for the novel treatment of anxiety disorders as well as post-traumatic stress disorder.

CBD in particular seems to have antianxiety effects. In an experiment with college students in a public-speaking model of anxiety, CBD achieved significant improvement (compared with placebo) in subjective anxiety equivalent to diazepam (Valium) and ipsapirone, two medications (anxiolytics) known to decrease anxiety (Zuardi and Guimaraes 1997). Also, dronabinol (Marinol; THC) was found to relieve the symptoms of two patients with treatment-refractory obsessive-compulsive disorder (Schindler et al. 2008).

ADHD

Attention deficit hyperactivity disorder is characterized by impulsivity, difficulty sustaining attention, increased activity, and poor planning. The Internet is full of testimonials from doctors and patients alike suggesting that cannabis may have a legitimate place among other treatment options, the gold standard being stimulants such as amphetamine. A case report (Strohbeck-Kuehner, Kopp, and Mattern 2008) asserts that individuals suffering from ADHD may benefit from cannabis treatment in that "it appears to regulate activation to a level which may be considered optimum for performance. There was evidence that the consumption of cannabis had a positive impact on performance, behaviour and mental state of the subject."

In animal studies, Adriani and colleagues (2003) showed that a cannabinoid agonist reduced hyperactivity and normalized behavioral impulsivity in a spontaneously hypertensive rat strain, which is regarded as a validated animal model for ADHD. Also interesting in this animal model was the decreased density of cannabinoid receptors in the rats' prefrontal cortex (an area of the brain thought to be involved in executive functions such as planning and organizing). In another animal model of ADHD, Viggiano and colleagues (2003) showed that by enhancing endogenous cannabinoid levels in maternal rats, he could correct the chemical imbalance and improve the hyperactivity of the offspring in "high excitability rats."

It is not uncommon in patients with ADHD for them to "self-medicate" with caffeine, nicotine, cocaine, or speed. In one survey (O'Shaughnessy

2007), most clinicians who recommended cannabis for their patients agreed that it was preferable to the abuse of other illicit stimulants. In a study of cocaine-dependent patients with ADHD, there was significantly better treatment retention among moderate users of cannabis compared to abstainers or heavy users (Aharonovich et al. 2006).

MEMORY

The endocannabinoid system is involved in memory formation, consolidation, and modulation. Forgetting is an important part of natural brain functioning, and endogenous cannabinoids help to perform this function. Cannabinoids have been shown to interfere with long-term potentiation (the electrochemical basis for memory creation) in the hippocampus, one region of the brain felt to be crucial for memory formation (Riedel and Davies 2005). Animal studies with the CB1 antagonist rimonabant showed improved memory retention for social recognition involving olfactory cues (Terranova et al. 1996). Current theories on how cannabis interferes with memory function implicate the glutamate system and GABAergic axon terminals (see Mackie and Katona 2009 for a review). It is quite possible that cannabinoid antagonists could be a treatment for dementias such as Alzheimer's disease, and this is an area that deserves further study.

One particular aspect of memory that cannabis affects in animal and human studies is working memory. Rehearsing a phone number you've just heard before you dial it, or remembering your train of thought as you speak are two examples of working memory. A common stoner question: "Uh . . . what was I just saying?" Because disruptions in working memory are present in a cannabis-induced state and also in schizophrenia, cannabinoid antagonists may be helpful in ameliorating this symptom.

PRUNING AND LATE ADOLESCENCE

During my initial evaluation of a new patient, I always ask about prior experiences with psychoactive substances, and I have heard one story repeatedly: marijuana was enjoyable in the teen years, reliably causing giddiness or elation, but for many of my patients, when they smoked pot in their late teens or early twenties, they got more paranoid and self-conscious. Many of my patients, especially women, tell me that they simply gave up and stopped smoking at this time. But, in those who went back and tried it again after several years, this unpleasant reaction seemed to subside, and people found they could again enjoy getting high later in their twenties or thirties. (These patients have a wide array of ages, so I can't blame the quality of marijuana that was available in the eighties, for example.)

It is a curious coincidence that at the same time the brain is vulnerable to a first psychotic break—schizophrenia and manic episodes often begin in the late teens or early twenties, when the brain is undergoing pruning and reorganizing—is also when many people find they cannot tolerate cannabinoids. I would be delighted if there were more research into this particular phenomenon, or to learn if other clinicians are seeing this as well.

ADDICTION

Although the risk of becoming addicted to cannabis does exist (please see Vandrey and Haney's chapter 14), it is significantly lower than the risk associated with many other drugs, both legal and illegal. Compare the dependency risks in an Institute of Medicine report (1999): cigarettes (32 percent), heroin (23 percent), cocaine (17 percent), alcohol (15 percent), and marijuana (9 percent). It should also be noted that withdrawal from cannabis use is typically short-lived and mild, as opposed to potentially life-threatening (with alcohol) or nearly insurmountable (cigarettes). Although the numbers of people seeking treatment for marijuana dependence are higher than one might think, this may be due to changing drug laws and policies, where compulsory treatment instead of jail time requires enrolling in a rehab or drug program.

More clinically relevant to the field of psychiatry is the use of cannabis as a substitute for other drugs of abuse like cocaine, heroin, and alcohol. Multiple California clinicians responded to the O'Shaughnessy survey (2007) with tales of patients with prior out-of-control addictions who became stabilized on small amounts of cannabis. One physician reported more than 90 percent of his patients had reduced their alcohol consumption by using cannabis. From a medical and psychiatric perspective, the substitution of cannabis for other more toxic and addictive drugs is a good example of harm reduction.

A recent examination of postmortem brains of alcoholics showed alterations in endogenous cannabinoid levels in key brain areas thought to be implicated in alcoholism (Lehtonen et al. 2010). As more studies are performed, it is my belief that abnormalities in the endocannabinoid system will be found in many more patient populations.

TRUSTING PATIENTS TO ADJUST THEIR DOSE

We have all been warned repeatedly that the cannabis available today is more potent than what was available decades ago. While there is some debate about how crucial this is (some compare it to the difference between wine and beer, others to beer and whiskey), there is some uniformity about the pot-smoker's response: They smoke less of the good stuff. One of the advantages of smoking cannabis, as opposed to taking oral preparations, is that experienced smokers learn quickly how to adjust their dosages depending on how strong their marijuana is. Because the onset of action is minutes instead of hours, dosage can be easily regulated. Many clinical studies have shown that smokers are quite good at regulating their "high" with different types of cannabis (Heishman, Stitzer, and Yingling 1989; Herning, Hooker, and Jones 1986), using a mixture of more air and smaller or fewer "puffs" for a more potent strain of cannabis.

THE CANNABINOID AND OPIOID SYSTEMS

There seems to be some sort of synergy or overlap between the cannabinoid and opiod systems (Cichewicz 2004). Patients who use both opioids and cannabis notice a synergism between these two drugs (Welch and Eads 1999). More important, what I have heard repeatedly from caregivers is that patients who use cannabis to manage their pain typically require less opioid pain medications. The relative toxicity of these two medicines, as well as their side effect profiles, typically favors cannabis. Randomized, double-blind, placebo-controlled trials are needed to substantiate these claims.

Moderate cannabis use was associated with improved retention in a study of naltrexone treatment (an opioid antagonist) for opiate-dependence (Raby et al. 2009). Researchers noted that experimental studies are needed to directly test the hypothesis that cannabinoid receptor agonists exert a beneficial pharmacological effect on naltrexone maintenance, and to better understand the mechanism involved.

DEHABITUATION

Smoking cannabis often fills one with a sense of wonder, of childlike awe at one's surroundings. What is habitually seen and ignored suddenly becomes captivating, eliciting renewed attention and appreciation. This is especially evident when someone who is altered finds himself or herself out and about in nature. In talking about using cannabis to treat psychiatric complaints, it is worthwhile to consider the spiritual aspects of its use, the soul-feeding effects.

Many people who are depressed feel overwhelmed and defeated, their souls crushed as they "suffer the slings and arrows" of daily life. Certainly my patients in New York City are weighed down by a barrage of constant worries delivered around the clock via e-mail, voicemail, and to-do lists. If cannabis creates a sense of respite from all that, an oasis of sorts, might that be therapeutic in and of itself? Separating what is therapeutic from what is recreational can become quite murky with regard to treating depression. The euphoria or giddiness that may come from "recreational" use of cannabis may be just what the doctor ordered when the target symptoms are a depressed mood and a pessimistic outlook.

Think of the Dove bar commercial: "My moment. My Dove." Or the Starbuck's Frappuccino ad: "It's 'You' Time." What is being marketed here is the delineation of time, creating a marked boundary, a timeout, giving you permission to relax, perhaps to be alone, where no one can get to you, and there are no responsibilities or chores to be done. Meditation—sitting still, breathing deeply, and clearing the mind—is a therapeutic activity with myriad benefits for mental health and wellness. An herbal medicine to assist "going within," to facilitate psychospiritual exploration, to allow solitude, and, more importantly, comfort in that solitude may likewise have a positive impact on mental health.

CONCLUSION

Mental health disorders, like most physical ailments, are multifactorial. Psychiatric ailments have their basis in a triad of psychological, sociological, and biological underpinnings. If an herbal remedy can offer substantial relief, it makes sense to take advantage of that first and foremost, either as a substitute for other psychiatric medications, or as a complement to allow lower doses or enhanced compliance with a current regimen.

The bottom line is that we need to know more. More research needs to be performed so we can all adequately understand whether cannabis can be a useful adjunct to psychiatric healing and another "weapon in the armamentarium" of psychopharmacologists to combat psychiatric illnesses. This observation by Marian Fry, M.D. (quoted in O'Shaughnessy 2007), sums it up nicely: "Health is a state of mind, body, and spirit. By restoring their connection to nature, cannabis helps patients on all three levels."

25

Cannabinoids and Neuroprotection

Sunil K. Aggarwal, M.D., Ph.D., and Gregory T. Carter, M.D.

"Scientific" information disseminated by governmental organizations that promote and enforce cannabis prohibition laws would have you believe that consuming cannabis has no benefit for your brain and nervous system, and in fact has severely detrimental effects, with no exceptions. This must be the case, right? After all, how else can we account for the draconian penalties meted out for some violators of the cannabis prohibition laws? Clearly cannabis use must insidiously "rot" away one's brain, right? Wrong. Nothing could be further from the truth.

Although inhaling cannabis smoke may acutely stimulate the brain's natural "forgetting faculty," by no means does this imply that cannabis is causing "brain damage." Rigorous, peer-reviewed scientific work has consistently demonstrated that chemicals in marijuana, especially the cannabinoids, are actually neuroprotective and can be used to prevent and treat neurotoxicity and neuroinflammation. As your head begins to stop spinning, prepare to be startled by many other ground-shaking discoveries coming out of the emerging field of cannabinoid medicine.

In this chapter, we will review the importance of neuroprotection and the role that cannabinoids play in facilitating it. Let's begin by developing a basic understanding of the molecular signaling system in your body known as the endocannabinoid, or endogenous cannabinoid, system. The discovery of an endogenous cannabinoid system with specific receptors and ligands has taken our understanding of the actions of cannabis from folklore to valid science (Pacher, Batkai, and Kunos 2006). It now appears that the cannabinoid system evolved with our species and is intricately involved in normal human physiology, specifically in the control of movement, pain, appetite, memory, immunity, and inflammation, among others. The detection of widespread cannabinoid receptors in the brain and peripheral tissues suggests that the cannabinoid system represents a previously unrecognized ubiquitous network in the nervous system. Dense receptor concentrations have been found in the cerebellum, basal ganglia, and hippocampus, accounting for the effects of cannabis on motor tone, coordination, and mood state (Hollister 1986, 1988; IOM 1982). Low concentrations are found in the brainstem, accounting for the remarkably low toxicity of cannabis. Notably, lethal doses for cannabis in humans have not been described (Di Marzo, Bisogno, and De Petrocellis 2000; FDA 1992; Pertwee 2000).

One way to think of a drug that works via a receptor system is to think of a lock and key, where the receptor is the lock and the drug is the key. A perfect fit is required for the key (drug) to open the lock (receptor), which then triggers a cellular response when opened. So far we know of at least two molecular receptor proteins (CB1 and CB2) and two endogenously produced lipid cannabinoids, AEA and 2-AG (anadamide and 2-acylglycerol, respectively), found in numerous tissues throughout the body, including neural and immune tissues. The cannabinoid system helps regulate the function of other systems in the body, making it an integral part of the central homeostatic modulatory system, the check-and-balance molecular signaling network in our bodies that keeps us at a healthy "98.6."

However, as we all know, due to wear and tear, insult and injury, homeostasis can be thrown off-kilter by loads that the body's systems cannot rally from on its own. This is where cannabis botanical medicine is a boon. Modern medical science has confirmed the findings of millennia-old traditional healing systems—that dried cannabis flowers contain compounds that can treat and prevent disease. When cannabinoids found in the resin produced by flower glands of the cannabis plant are administered, they interact structurally and functionally with the body's cannabinoid system.

We will focus here on two well-studied phytocannabinoids (or plant-derived cannabinoids): tetrahydracannabinol (THC) and cannabidiol (CBD). Research has shown that what makes these molecules neuroprotective is their ability to influence brain and immune function at the molecular level, their powerful intrinsic antioxidant activity, and their actions on various other targets, known and unknown.

Why is neuroprotection important? Neuroprotection refers to mechanisms and strategies used to protect against neuronal injury, degeneration, or death in the central nervous system (CNS), especially following acute disorders such as stroke or traumatic brain injury or as a result of chronic neurodegenerative diseases such as amyotrophic lateral sclerosis (ALS), Alzheimer's disease (AD), and multiple sclerosis (MS) (Hill 2006). Neuroprotection has been proposed as a potential strategy to prevent the onset of neurodegenerative diseases (Carter and Weydt 2002; Carter et al. 2003). One common pathway of numerous neurodegenerative diseases is known as excitotoxicity.

Excitotoxicity refers to a process by which nerve cells are damaged and killed by glutamate, the major excitatory neurotransmitter in the mammalian brain, and other substances. Toxicity occurs due to overactivation of cellular glutamate receptors, leading to a pathological influx of calcium ions, which in turn activates cell-damaging enzymes. Another common mechanism of neurodegeneration that is often interlinked with excitotoxicity involves unchecked production of free radicals. Free radicals are atoms and molecules with unpaired electrons that are normally produced through oxidative processes in the body. When they are not scavenged and are allowed to accumulate, they can cause oxidative damage in cells through a process called oxidative stress. Cannabinoids can modulate both these processes and have been shown to be neuroprotective in several major human diseases, which we will now overview.

THE THERAPEUTIC ROLE OF CANNABIS IN NEURODEGENERATIVE DISORDERS

Amyotrophic Lateral Sclerosis

Amyotrophic lateral sclerosis (ALS), also known as Lou Gehrig's disease, is a rapidly progressive, usually fatal disorder characterized by the ongoing loss of motor neurons in the brain, spinal cord, and peripheral nervous system. The vast majority of ALS cases occur sporadically, with unknown etiology. ALS affects men more commonly than women, with a male-to-female ratio of approximately 1.5:1. ALS typically affects adults aged forty to sixty years, with a mean onset age of fifty-eight years (Krivickas and Carter 2005).

ALS is more common in urban areas, possibly due to environmental factors. Considerable geographic clustering has been seen in association with

ALS, most notably in the Western Pacific region of the world, but more recently in Gulf War veterans. Despite clustering, environmental or causal factors remain to be determined (Krivickas and Carter 2005). Young males with ALS have the best prognosis and may have a longer life expectancy.

A notable example of this is theoretical astrophysicist Stephen Hawking, who was diagnosed with ALS while in graduate school in his early twenties. He has now survived over four decades with the disease and continues to lecture all over the world, using a speech synthesizer activated by eye movement. Unfortunately, the typical prognosis for ALS is grim: about half of all ALS patients die within two-and-a-half years after the onset of symptoms (Krivickas and Carter 2005). Survival rates vary somewhat, depending on the patient's decision to use a feeding tube and assisted ventilation. Nonetheless, five years after being diagnosed, only 25 percent of ALS patients are still alive (Carter and Miller 1998).

An estimated 10 percent of all ALS cases are familial, usually inherited as an autosomal dominant trait. About 15 percent of these cases result from a gene defect on chromosome band 21q12.1, which leads to a mutation in the antioxidant enzyme Cu/Zn superoxide dismutase (SOD1) (Carter and Miller 1998). Emerging evidence suggests that this mutation results in increased oxidative stress for the motor neurons, which is presumably related to free radical toxicity, leading to cell death. ALS is not a rare condition; there are an estimated thirty thousand Americans living with it, and population studies indicate that the prevalence is increasing (Carter and Miller 1998; Krivickas and Carter 2005).

Studies suggest that excessive glutamate, an excitatory neurotransmitter in the CNS, is involved in the disease process. Serum, spinal fluid, and brain tissue of patients with ALS contain excessive levels of glutamate, which is apparently due to reduced clearance of glutamate from the motor cortex and decreased activity of glutamate transport proteins (Weiss 2004). Studies done in animal models of glutamate-induced neurotoxicity have shown that cannabinoids afford protection against oxidative damage induced by free radicals produced by glutamate (Hampson 2002; Hampson et al. 1998, 2000; Mechoulam and Shohami 2006; Raman et al. 2003; Van der Stelt et al. 2001). Administration of delta-9-THC both before and after the onset of ALS symptoms slowed disease progression and prolonged survival in animals compared to untreated controls (Abood et al. 2001).

Other trials in animal models of ALS have also shown that naturally occurring and synthetic cannabinoids slow down the progression of ALS (Bilsland et al. 2006; Weydt et al. 2005). Another recent study showed that blocking the CB1 cannabinoid receptor extended the lifespan of mice with ALS (Bilsland et al. 2006). This suggests that some abnormality within our internal cannabinoid system may be part of the underlying disease mechanisms in ALS. It is clear that cannabinoids are able to slow down the progression of ALS in mice, likely by acting as an antioxidant, among other mechanisms (Eshhar, Striem, and Biegon 1993; Hansen et al. 2001). This would limit the amount of damage done by free radicals produced by excess glutamate.

There are several other studies published using mice with a model of ALS that clearly show a significant benefit from cannabinoids, including delta-9-THC (Abood et al. 2001; Akinshola, Chakrabarti, and Onaivi 1999; Weydt et al. 2005). This same beneficial effect has also been shown in spinal neurons taken from these mice and cultured in nutrient gel (Weydt et al. 2002).

Based on these promising preclinical findings, some experts in this field are now recommending cannabis for their ALS patients (Greene 2007). In addition to the neuroprotective effect, patients also report that cannabis helps in treating symptoms of the disease, including alleviating pain and muscle spasms, improving appetite, diminishing depression, and helping manage sialorrhea (excessive drooling) by drying up saliva in the mouth (Amtmann et al. 2004). Indeed, in a large survey it was noted that ALS patients who were able to obtain cannabis found it preferable to prescription medication in managing their symptoms. However, this study also noted that the biggest reason ALS patients were not using cannabis was their inability to obtain it, due to either legal or financial reasons or lack of safe access (Amtmann et al. 2004).

In summary, there is strong scientific basis to support the use of marijuana in the pharmacological management of ALS. Moreover, further investigation both at the clinical and basic science level into the usefulness of cannabionoids in treating ALS is warranted.

Multiple Sclerosis

Multiple sclerosis (MS) is a chronic relapsing neuro-degenerative disease that produces widespread demyelination (loss of myelin, the insulative sheath that covers nerve cells to speed the transmission of signals) of nerve cells in the brain and spinal cord, leading to muscular weakness and a loss of coordination. In some cases the disease can be fatal. According to the U.S. National Multiple Sclerosis Society, about two hundred people are diagnosed every week with the disease, typically in the range of twenty to forty years of age.

Reports of the ability of cannabis to reduce MS-related symptoms including pain, muscle spasticity, depression, fatigue, and incontinence are now well established in the medical literature (Baker et al. 2000; Brady et al. 2004; Chong et al. 2006; Cosroe et al. 1997; DeSanty and Dar 2001; Greenberg, Weiness, and Pugh 1994; Meinck, Schonle, and Conrad 1989; Rog et al. 2005; Ungerleider et al. 1987; Wade et al. 2004a, 2003; Zajicek et al. 2003). This has led many MS patient organizations, including the MS Societies of Britain and Canada, to now stand in favor of the use of cannabis to treat MS (Page et al. 2003; Wade et al. 2004b).

Not only is MS-related symptomatology treatable with cannabis, but recent clinical and preclinical studies also suggest that cannabinoids may inhibit the disease progression. Investigators at the London Institute of Neurology reported that administration of the synthetic cannabinoid agonist WIN 55,212-2 provided significant neuroprotection in an animal model of multiple sclerosis (Pryce et al. 2003). The results of this study are important because they suggest that in addition to symptom management, cannabis may slow the progression of MS in a similar fashion to its reported effects in ALS. In both ALS and MS, cannabis and cannabinoid medicine may slow the neurodegenerative processes enough that it may ultimately limit the degree of chronic disability in these diseases.

Investigators at Vrije University Medical Center in the Netherlands reported in 2003 that administration of oral delta-9 THC boosts immune function in patients with MS (Killestein et al. 2003). These results suggest the possibility that cannabis may be a disease-modifying treatment for MS. More recently, clinical data from an extended open-label study (a study where there is no placebo, and the study participants know they're getting the active drug) of 167 multiple sclerosis patients reported that orally administered whole-plant cannabis extracts relieve pain, spasticity, and bladder incontinence, with effects lasting for an extended period of treatment (mean duration of treatment for study participants was 434 days) without requiring subjects to increase their dose (Vaney et al. 2004). These results demonstrate that cannabis, unlike other drugs to treat pain and spasticity, does not rapidly induce tolerance. Moreover, these results suggest that the cannabinoid therapy was actually slowing the disease progression, since the same dose remained equally effective over the course of this extended study.

The British government is now sponsoring a three-year clinical trial to assess the long-term effects of cannabinoids on MS-associated symptom management as well as disease progression. Moreover, Health Canada also recently approved the prescription use of a cannabis-based medicinal extract (Sativex, nabiximols) for the treatment of MS-associated neuropathic pain. Similar approval of cannabis extracts is pending or regionally approved in Britain and other European countries.

Alzheimer's Disease

Alzheimer's disease (AD) is also a progressive, neurodegenerative disorder of unknown etiology. However, beyond that, all similarity to ALS stops. AD is characterized by a progressive deterioration of memory and overall cognitive functioning. Other symptoms of AD include aggressive behavior and agitation, depression, appetite loss, and, occasionally, in advanced cases, difficulty walking. The disease is estimated to affect about 5 million Americans. In 2006 the worldwide prevalence was 26.6 million. By 2050, prevalence is expected to quadruple, by which time one in eighty-five persons worldwide will be living with the disease (Brookmeyer et al. 2007). Alzheimer's usually begins after age sixty, though some younger people may very rarely have early-onset Alzheimer's. The risk of developing Alzheimer's goes up with age. Around 5 percent of men and women ages sixty-five to seventy-four have Alzheimer's, and nearly half of those age eighty-five and older may have the disease, though Alzheimer's is not a normal part of aging.

There are a number of physiological and anatomical changes that occur in the brains of AD patients. Nerve cells die in parts of the brain that are vital to memory and other functions, and connections (synapses) between nerve cells are broken. This disruption in synaptic connections within the brain lead to impaired thinking and memory problems. Alzheimer's starts with mild memory problems and can end with severe brain damage. How fast the disease works and the course the disease takes vary from person to person. Average Alzheimer's patients live from eight to ten years after they are diagnosed, though they can live as long as twenty years. Biopsies of the brains of AD patients show numerous amyloid plaques—hardened protein deposits that are thought to directly cause most of the central nervous system dysfunction seen in AD.

Sometimes the term *dementia* is used to describe the symptoms caused by these changes in brain function. Some symptoms may include asking the same questions repeatedly; becoming lost in familiar places; being unable to follow directions; getting disoriented about time, people, and places; and neglecting personal safety, hygiene, and nutrition. There is no set schedule or rate at which people with dementia develop symptoms. While dementia is certainly part of AD, there are also many other conditions, reversible and permanent, that can cause dementia.

There are currently no Food and Drug Administration (FDA)–approved treatments or medications available that actually modify the disease course of AD. There are only a few drugs (Aricept [donepezil] and Namenda [memantine]) that have been FDA-approved to treat symptoms of the disease, but these drugs do not actually improve the long-term prognosis. None of these drugs halt the formation of plaques in the brains of AD patients.

There is now ample evidence in the medical literature to indicate that cannabis may provide not only symptomatic relief to patients afflicted with AD, but it also actually limits the formation of new plaques in the brain. Thus, it appears that cannabis may actually slow down the progression of the disease. In a study done at Scripps Research Institute in California, researchers reported that delta 9-THC, both in the test tube and in computer models, inhibited the enzyme responsible for the aggregation of amyloid plaque, which is the primary marker for AD, in a manner considerably superior to the FDA-approved AD drugs such as donepezil and tacrine (Cognex) (Eubanks et al. 2006).

This study identified a mechanism whereby cannabinoids can directly impact AD pathology. The researchers concluded that cannabinoids, including delta 9-THC, may provide an improved therapeutic treatment for AD that simultaneously treats both the symptoms and the progression of the disease. Other studies, both in vitro and in vivo, have shown that cannabidiol (CBD) and the synthetic cannabinoid WIN-55,212-2 can help prevent brain-cell death that results from exposure to the amyloid plaques and can also improve memory (Iuvone et al. 2004; Marchalant et al. 2008; Marchalant, Rosi, and Wenk 2007).

Other recent studies have shown that injecting the synthetic cannabinoid WIN 55,212-2 directly into the brain significantly decreased neurotoxicity and helped prevent cognitive impairment in rats injected with amyloid-beta peptide (a protein that induces AD in rats) (Ferraro et al. 2001; Ramirez et al. 2005). The cannabinoid appeared to reduce the neuroinflammation associated with AD. Previous preclinical studies have demonstrated that cannabinoids can prevent cell death by antioxidation (Hampson et al. 1998). In addition to potentially modifying the progression of AD, recent clinical trials also indicate that cannabinoid therapy reduces agitation and improves appetite and weight gain in patients with AD.

Daily administration of 2.5 mg of synthetic THC over a two-week period reduced nocturnal motor activity and agitation in AD patients in an open-label pilot study (Walther et al. 2006). Improved weight gain and mood state were also noted among AD patients administered cannabinoids in a separate study previously published (Volicer et al. 1997). Thus far, at least two chemicals in cannabis, THC and CBD, have been shown to be effective against AD-related pathology. Additional studies using cannabis to treat AD are clearly warranted, as we face a looming global epidemic of Alzheimer's disease as the population ages. Any advances in therapeutic and preventive strategies that lead to even small delays in Alzheimer's onset and progression can significantly reduce the global burden of the disease (Brookmeyer et al. 2007).

Tourette's Syndrome

Tourette's syndrome (TS) is a complex neurological disorder, the cause of which remains essentially unknown. The disease is characterized by tics, which are involuntary repeated movements or verbal expressions that occur spontaneously and without warning. The severity of this disease is variable, but in its worst expression, it can be quite disabling. As with ALS and MS, there is no cure for TS. However, unlike ALS and MS, the condition often improves with age.

TS is estimated to affect approximately 100,000 people in the United States (Tourette's Syndrome Association, www.tsa-usa.org). There have been numerous studies published investigating the use of cannabinoids for the treatment of TS. Starting in the late 1990s, Muller-Vahl and colleagues published a number of papers clearly showing the efficacy of cannabis in treating TS. Cannabis appears to decrease the tic severity score, or TSS. This is a reliable, reproducible, standardized rating scale to describe tic frequency and magnitude of the movements.

The patients also experienced an overall improvement in global functioning (Muller-Vahl 2003a; Muller-Vahl et al. 2001, 2002, 2003b, 2003c). In one case report, a single oral dose of 10 mg of delta-9-THC in a twenty-five-year-old man with severe, uncontrolled TS dropped the subject's total TSS from 41 to 7, an 84 percent improvement, within two hours following ingestion of the cannabinoid (Muller-Vahl 2003). The improvement was observed for a total of seven hours. A similar effect was also seen in patients following inhalation (smoking) of marijuana, confirmed again using the TSS rating scale.

The results continued to be positive even in a randomized, double-blind, placebo-controlled crossover single-dose trial of THC in twelve adult TS patients. The investigators reported a significant improvement in TSS as well as a decrease in obsessive-compulsive behavior (OCB) after treatment with delta-9-THC compared to placebo (Muller-Vahl et al. 2002). Investigators reported no cognitive impairment in subjects following THC administration, concluding, "THC is effective and safe in treating tics and OCB in TS" (Muller-Vahl et al. 2003b).

In a second randomized, double-blind, placebo-controlled trial (Muller-Vahl 2003a) involving twenty-four patients who were administered daily doses of up to 10 mg of THC over a six-week period, researchers reported that subjects experienced a significant reduction in TSS following long-term cannabinoid treatment with no impairment of learning, recall, or verbal memory. There was actually a statistically significant improvement in verbal memory span both during and after cannabinoid therapy.

Gliomas

Gliomas are rapidly growing malignant brain tumors that usually result in death within two years after diagnosis. Gliomas arise from glial cells, or glia, which are the major support structures of the brain and are the only non-neuronal cells of the CNS. In humans they outnumber actual nervous tissue (neurons) by a factor of about ten to one. However, because of their small size, they account for only about 50 percent of the cellular volume of the brain. Glia are ubiquitous in the nervous system and are critical in maintaining the extracellular environment. This includes supporting as well as coating (myelinating) the neurons.

Currently there are no known cures for gliomas. The best available standard treatments provide only minor symptom relief. However, there are numerous basic science studies and one pilot clinical trial demonstrating the ability of cannabis and cannabinoids to inhibit the growth of gliomas. One might wonder, why would cannabis inhibit the growth of a glioma? Here's a possible answer: glia are involved, actively or passively, in virtually all disorders or insults involving the brain. This makes them very important cells within the CNS, and we are now discovering that they are largely regulated by endogenous (internal) cannabinods.

We now know that there are at least two cannabinoid receptor subtypes. Subtype 1 (CB1) is expressed primarily in the brain, whereas subtype 2 (CB2) is expressed primarily in the periphery (Bouaboula et al. 1995; Di Marzo et al. 1994, 2000; Puffenbarger et al. 2000). Cannabinoid receptors constitute a major family of receptors within the central nervous system, similar to the receptors of other major neurotransmitters such as dopamine, serotonin, and norepinephrine (Di Marzo et al. 1994). There is considerable evidence that glial cells, from which gliomas form, are regulated through cannabinoid signaling systems. This provides further insight into understanding how the emerging therapeutic effects of cannabis actually work. Normally, glial cells express CB1 receptors, taking in and degrading the endogenous cannabinoid anandamide (Bouaboula et al. 1995). However, gliomas appear to express CB2 receptors. This may be an indicator of tumor malignancy (Sanchez et al. 1998, 2001).

The most recent therapeutic role for cannabinoids in the CNS evolved from the discovery that cannabinoids selectively induce cell death (apoptosis) in glioma cells in vitro and that THC and other cannabinoids lead to a spectacular regression of malignant gliomas in immune-compromised rats in vivo (Esposito et al. 2001; Galve-Roperh et al. 2000; Sanchez et al. 1998; Sinha et al. 1998). The mechanism underlying this is not yet clear, but it appears to involve both CB1 and CB2 receptor activation (Recht et al. 2001). A recent study comparing the antiproliferative effects of cannabinoids on C6 glioma cells suggests the involvement of vanilloid receptors (VRs) (Jacobsson, Wallin, and Fowler 2001), indicating that cannabinoids that stimulate both CB receptors and VR receptors would be better suited for glioma chemotherapy.

A nonpsychoactive cannabinoid found in cannabis, cannabidiol (CBD), inhibited the growth of various human glioma cell lines in vivo and in vitro in a dose-dependent manner. CBD produces significant antitumor activity both in the whole animal and in test tube cells, thus suggesting an application of CBD as an antineoplastic agent (Molina-Holgado, Lledo, and Guaza 1997). Another study showed that cannabinoids inhibited glioma tumor growth in animals and in human glioblastoma multiforme (GBM) tumor samples (Guzman 2003; Sanchez et al. 1998; Waksman et al. 1999).

More recently, the administration of THC to human glioblastoma multiforme cell lines decreased the proliferation of malignant cells and induced tumor cell death more rapidly than did the administration of WIN 55,212-2, a synthetic cannabinoid agonist (Guzman et al. 2006). Researchers also noted that THC selectively targeted malignant cells while ignoring healthy ones in a more profound manner than the synthetic alternative. A recent landmark human clinical trial demonstrated tumor volume shrinkage with intratumor THC injections in several patients with recurrent glioblastoma multiforme (Guzman 2006). It should be noted that a diagnosis of glioblastoma mulitforme is a virtual death sentence, with a five-year survival rate of fewer than 5 percent and with few treatment options; anything that slows its progression is extraordinary and should be vigorously pursued.

Compared to other traditional chemotherapeutic agents, the safety profile of THC is remarkably good. Taken together with its apparent antiproliferative action on tumor cells noted here, the basis is set for future trials aimed at evaluating the potential antitumor activity of cannabis. It is worth noting that, in addition to the ability of various cannabinoids to moderate glioma cells, there is an emerging body of evidence that demonstrates cannabinoids and endocannabinoids have the ability to inhibit the proliferation of other cancer cell lines, including breast, prostate, colorectal, lung, and uterine carcinomas, as well as gastric and pancreatic adenocarcinomas, leukemia, and various forms of lymphoma (Caffarel et al. 2006; Carracedo et al. 2006; Klein, Newton, and Friedman 1998; Ligresti et al. 2006). As a result, experts now believe that cannabinoids represent a new class of anticancer drugs that retard cancer growth, inhibit angiogenesis (the formation of new blood vessels that feed tumor growth), and the metastatic spread of cancer cells (Chen and Buck 2000; Guzman 2003; Kogan 2005).

Stroke, Alcoholic Damage, and Other Forms of Brain Injury

Recent studies have demonstrated the neuroprotective effects of synthetic, nonpsychotropic cannabinoids, which appear to protect neurons from chemically induced excitotoxicity (Hamelink et al. 2005; Hampson 2002; Hampson et al. 2000; Jiang et al. 2005; Nagayama et al. 1999; Mechoulam and Shohami 2002; Valjent, Pages, and Rogard 2001; Van der Stelt et al. 2001). Direct measurement of oxidative stress reveals that cannabinoids prevent cell death by antioxidation. The antioxidative property of cannabinoids is confirmed by their ability to antagonize oxidative stress and consequent cell death induced by the powerful oxidant retinoid anhydroretinol. Cannabinoids also modulate cell survival and growth of B-lymphocytes and fibroblasts, as demonstrated in these studies.

The neuroprotective actions of cannabidiol and other cannabinoids were examined in rat cortical neuron cultures exposed to toxic levels of the excitatory neurotransmitter glutamate. Glutamate toxicity was reduced by both CBD (nonpsychoactive) and THC (Eshhar, Striem, and Biegon 1993). The neuroprotection observed with CBD and THC was unaffected by a cannabinoid receptor antagonist, indicating it to be cannabinoid-receptor independent. CBD was more protective against glutamate neurotoxicity than either ascorbate (vitamin C) or alpha-tocopherol (vitamin E).

Cannabinoids have shown efficacy as immune modulators in animal models of neurological conditions such as experimental allergic encephalomyelitis (a common animal model for MS) and neuritis (El-Remessy et al. 2006; Friedman et al. 1995). These data suggest that cannabinoids might modify the presumed autoimmune causes of other neurological diseases, such as MS. Current data suggests that cannabidiol may have a potential role as a therapeutic agent for neurodegenerative disorders produced by excessive cellular oxidation, such as ALS, a disease characterized by excess glutamate activity in the spinal cord (Carter 1999; Panikashvili et al. 2001). This may have implications in treating pain in neuromuscular diseases (Jensen et al. 2005).

It is not yet known how excess glutamate affects cannabinoid homeostasis in the body, including endogenous levels of the endocannabinoids AEA (anadamide) and 2-AG (2-acylglycerol), as well as other constituents of their lipid families such as N-acylethanolamines (NAEs) and 2-monoacylglycerols (2-MAGs). Hansen and colleagues used three in vivo neonatal rat models characterized by widespread neurodegeneration as a consequence of altered glutamate neurotransmission and assessed changes in endocannabinoid homeostasis (Hansen et al. 2001). A forty-six-fold increase of cortical NAE concentrations (AEA, thirteen-fold) was noted twenty-four hours after intracerebral NMDA injection (a method for activating a class of glutamate receptors with the molecule N-methyl-D-aspartate), while less severe insults triggered by mild concussive head trauma or NMDA receptor blockade produced a less pronounced NAE accumulation.

By contrast, levels of 2-AG and other 2-MAGs were unaffected by the insults employed, rendering it likely that key enzymes in biosynthetic pathways of the two different endocannabinoid structures are not equally associated with intracellular events that cause neuronal damage in vivo. Cortical subfields in the brain exhibited an up-regulation of cannabinoid CB1 receptor mRNA expression and binding capacity following mild concussive head trauma and exposure to NMDA receptor blockade. This may suggest that mild to moderate brain injury may trigger elevated endocannabinoid activity via concomitant increase of anandamide levels, but not 2-AG, and CB1 receptor density.

Panikashvili and colleagues were able to show that 2-AG has an important neuroprotective role (Panikashvili et al. 2001). After closed-head injury (CHI) in mice, the level of endogenous 2-AG was significantly elevated. After administering synthetic 2-AG to mice after CHI, they found a significant reduction of brain edema, better clinical recovery, reduced infarct volume, and reduced hippocampal cell death compared with controls. When 2-AG was administered together with additional inactive 2-acyl-glycerols that are normally present in the brain, functional recovery was significantly enhanced. The beneficial effect of 2-AG was dose-dependently attenuated by SR-141761A, an antagonist of the CB1 receptor, implying a receptor-based mechanism of action for this neuroprotective effect.

Ferraro and colleagues looked at the effects of the synthetic cannabinoid receptor agonist WIN 55,212-2 on endogenous extracellular GABA levels in the cerebral cortex of an awake rat using microdialysis (Ferraro et al. 2001). GABA (gamma-aminobutyric acid) is a common inhibitory neurotransmitter in the mammalian brain. WIN 55,212-2 was associated with a concentration-dependent decrease in dialysate GABA levels. WIN 55,212-2-induced inhibition of GABAergic activity was counteracted by the CB1 receptor antagonist SR141716A, which by itself was without effect on cortical GABA levels. These findings suggest that cannabinoids decrease cortical GABA levels, an important neuromodulatory action, given that excessive GABAergic activity has been shown to be neurotoxic.

Cannabinoids may also be effective in post-stroke neuroprotective therapy. Sinor and colleagues showed that AEA and 2-AG increased cell viability in cerebral cortical neuron cultures subjected to eight hours of hypoxia and glucose deprivation, conditions that mimic ischemia, or inadequate blood supply, commonly associated with stroke. This effect was observed at nanomolar (very low) concentrations, was reproduced by a nonhydrolyzable analog of anandamide, and was unaltered by CB1 or CB2 receptor antagonists (Sinor, Irvin, and Greenberg 2000). These results imply that cannabinoids can have an important therapeutic role to play in preventing ischemia-induced brain tissue damage. Recently, cannabinoids have also been shown to actually stimulate the genesis of new neurons in the brain, specifically in the rat hippocampus (Jiang et al. 2005; Mishima et al. 2005). Further study is required to elucidate the scope of the neurogenic effects of cannabinoids.

A neuroprotective role for cannabinoids in staving off ethanol-induced neurotoxicity associated with heavy binge drinking has also been demonstrated. When cannabidiol is given concurrently with binge alcohol exposure in rats, they demonstrated a dose-dependent reduction in the normally substantial neurodegeneration observed in the hippocampus and entorhinal cortex (Hamelink et al. 2005). It is also likely that cannabinoids could play a beneficial role in preventing the glumatergic excitotoxcity seen in alcoholic withdrawal.

The leading cause of blindness in the United States occurs due to diabetes—a condition known as diabetic retinopathy. This is believed to be caused by ischemia in retinal tissues leading to excessive glutamate production, nitric oxide and superoxide production, and finally nerve-cell death. In addition, nearby microglia, sensing dysfunction, become activated and start an inflammatory process that often is cytotoxic. A recent study has shown that cannabidol may be used therapeutically to protect the retinal nerve cells that are essential for vision (El-Remessy et al. 2006). They showed that cannabidiol is able to function as an antioxidant that can neutralize toxic superoxides, inhibit the self-destructive process set in motion by the overactive microglia, and help increase the body's innate protective cannabinoid response by inhibiting the enzyme that destroys endocannabinoids.

Many more avenues await exploration in the field of cannabinoid medicine, and the future appears bright. Recently, cannabidiol was shown to be effective in treating neurodegenerative disorders caused by prions—the misfolded protinaceous infectious particles that cause bovine spongiform encephalopathy (mad cow disease), sheep scrapie, and, in humans, Creutzfeldt-Jakob disease, fatal familial insomnia, and other diseases. Russo first documented the possibility of cannabinoid medicine contributing to this area of therapy in 2003. Recently a team of French researchers (Dirikoc et al. 2007) reported that cannabidiol inhibited the accumulation of prion protein in both mouse and sheep cell culture, limited accumulation and resultant neurotoxicity of the aberrant protein in the brains of scrapie-infected mice, and significantly increased infected mouse survival time compared to untreated controls. They noted that cannabinoids' unique mechanism of action in treating tissue spongioform encephalopathies represent a new class of compounds for the treatment of these as yet uncurable diseases.

CONCLUSION

In this chapter we have attempted to summarize the recent research on cannabis with a primary focus on its emerging therapeutic role in treating neurodegenerative human diseases. We have reviewed many studies on cannabinoids that indicate important progress documenting the neruoprotective actions of cannabis in treating several major neurodegenerative disorders, including amyotrophic lateral sclerosis, multiple sclerosis, and Alzheimer's disease.

When cannabinoid receptors in the central nervous system are activated, this triggers signaling pathways in the brain that are linked to neuronal repair and cell maintenance, and the release of other compounds that further activate neuroprotective responses. Additionally, it is clear that our own internal marijuana, the endocannabinoids, are released in response to pathogenic events, thus representing a potential compensatory repair mechanism. Enhancing this "on demand" action of endocannabinoids is an important strategy the body uses to help prevent further brain injury as well as promote healing. The neuroprotective activities of both externally administered cannabinoids and the internal endocannabinoids are novel processes that can be effectively exploited to help promote and protect the nervous system in the face of disease or physical and chemical trauma.

26
Cannabis and HIV/AIDS

Mark A. Ware, M.D., and Lynne Belle-Isle

Human immunodeficiency virus (HIV) and/or acquired immune deficiency syndrome (AIDS) affects more than 33 million people worldwide (UNAIDS 2009). In the debate surrounding the medical use of cannabis, one does not need to look far to find the contributions of people living with HIV/AIDS (PHAs). Whether as political activists advocating for greater access to medical marijuana, as participants in surveys of medical cannabis use, or as research subjects in clinical trials evaluating the safety and efficacy of medical cannabis, PHAs have contributed significantly to the ideology of cannabis as medicine as well as the evidence base on which clinical and political decisions are made.

The Canadian AIDS Society was the first national nongovernmental organization to officially adopt a position on HIV/AIDS and the therapeutic use of cannabis (Canadian AIDS Society 2004). This chapter explores the main medical reasons why the HIV/AIDS community is invested in the cannabis debate and illustrates how converging evidence from anecdote to clinical trials have paralleled developments in cannabinoid physiology; the cumulative experience of PHAs with cannabis cannot be ignored.

Despite great advances in the development of pharmacological agents to reduce the impact and severity of HIV infection, the clinical picture of HIV/AIDS is still dominated by debilitating symptoms such as pain, nausea, and loss of appetite. We will review each of these symptoms in turn and consider the evidence for cannabis in each. Cannabis, for the purposes of this chapter, refers to the herbal plant material "marijuana." Drugs derived from cannabis are called cannabinoids and include tetrahydrocannabinol (THC, also known as dronabinol and sold as Marinol), cannabidiol (CBD, prepared with THC and available as Sativex), and the synthetic cannabinoid nabilone (Cesamet).

PREVALENCE OF CANNABIS USE BY PATIENTS WITH HIV/AIDS

One of the unique aspects about cannabis in medicine is that it is a drug with which the population has had considerable experience in both recreational and medical use. Worldwide, cannabis is used by 3 to 9 percent of the general population. It is therefore important to ask how cannabis is used among PHAs and why. This information may help determine what areas need most research and where research data are lacking. It may also be useful in understanding why cannabis is used and help with doctor-patient discussions.

Several papers have attempted to estimate the proportion of PHAs who use cannabis for medical purposes; these are summarized in Table 26.1. One Canadian study found that 37.3 percent of 160 HIV clinic patients reported current use of cannabis (Ware et al. 2003). These results are consistent with American studies that have shown that prevalence rates ranged from 23 to 37 percent (Woolridge et al. 2005). It has been estimated that between 15 and 33 percent of PHAs use cannabis for medical purposes in North America (Braitstein et al. 2001; Dansak 1997). In a Canadian AIDS Society survey of PHAs, more than 90 percent of those who reported using cannabis for medical purposes did so to stimulate their appetite, while 68.7 percent used it to reduce pain and 67 percent to reduce nausea and vomiting. Perhaps not surprisingly (and somewhat reassuringly!), these are the areas that have received most research attention.

PAIN: THE EPIDEMIOLOGY OF PAIN IN HIV

The prevalence of pain in patients living with HIV/AIDS has been estimated at 60 percent (Breitbart et al. 1996a; Hewitt et al. 1997; Larue, Fontaine, and Colleau 1997; Lebovits et al. 1989). Pain interferes with daily living and is a marker for reduced survival (Frich and Borgbjerg 2000). While pain associated with HIV/AIDS is well documented, it is often underrecognized and undertreated in clinical practice (Breitbart et al. 1996b; Hewitt et al. 1997; Larue, Fontaine, and Colleau 1997; Lebovits et al. 1989; McCormack, Li, and Zarowny 1993; Morley-Forster 2006; Rosenfeld 1996).

TABLE 26.1. PREVALENCE SURVEYS OF CANNABIS IN PHAs

Author	Year	Prevalence	Reason for use	Associations
Dansak	1997	32%	nausea vomiting indigestion appetite improvement	
Braitstein et al.	2001			
Furler et al.	2004	29%	appetite stimulation weight gain	household income
Prentiss	2004	23%	anxiety +/- depression improved appetite increased pleasure relief of pain	severe nausea recent use of alcohol
Woolridge et al.	2005	27%	improved appetite muscle pain nausea anxiety nerve pain depression paresthesia	
Fogarty et al.	2007	44%		complementary or alternative therapies HIV/AIDS-related illness or other illnesses in the past 12 months higher CD4/T-cell counts lower incomes young age fewer casual partners in the prior six months

Painful conditions associated with HIV infection include pain due to headache, herpes simplex, peripheral neuropathy, back pain, herpes zoster, throat pain, and arthralgia (Hewitt et al. 1997; Singer et al. 1993). In addition, clinical experience suggests an increasing incidence of pain due to malignancies (e.g., lymphoma, anorectal carcinomas) and associated treatments (e.g., radiation therapy, chemotherapy). Of these conditions, the pain syndrome that has been most widely studied is HIV-associated neuropathy. Neuropathy is a disease of the nerves, caused by the HIV virus or the medications used to treat HIV. The pain arises from the damaged nerves being exquisitely sensitive to normally non-painful stimuli. They can also send pain messages to the brain in the absence of any stimulus at all.

The annual incidence of symptomatic peripheral neuropathy associated with HIV/AIDS has been estimated at 36 percent (Schifitto et al. 2002), with estimates of the prevalence of neuropathy of 30 to 55 percent, rising with severity of disease (Husstedt et al. 2000).

CANNABIS AND HIV-ASSOCIATED PAIN

The treatment of pain is an important reason why many persons living with HIV use cannabis. To date, no randomized, controlled trials of prescription cannabinoid products for HIV-associated pain have been conducted, but there have been several studies of the safety and efficacy of smoked cannabis for HIV-associated peripheral neuropathy.

Donald Abrams and his team pioneered the studies of cannabis and HIV/AIDS with a safety study evaluating the effects of oral THC and smoked cannabis on plasma levels of antiretroviral medications. They found no clinical evidence of drug–drug interaction or changes in the cytochrome P450 enzymatic metabolism of antiretroviral medications (indinavir and ritonavir) (Abrams et al. 2003). A second study by the same team found that smoked cannabis was effective at reducing painful HIV-associated neuropathy, as well as effective at reducing pain from a heat-capsaicin model of peripheral neuropathy (Abrams et al. 2007; Ellis 2008). (Please see chapter 28, "Pain Management," by Mark Wallace and Ben Platt; and chapter 37, "Prescribing Cannabis in California," by Jeffrey Hergenrather, for more information on treating pain with cannabis.)

NAUSEA

Nausea is one of the main reasons for cannabis use by persons with HIV/AIDS, based on the surveys described earlier. Nausea may be caused by illnesses associated with HIV infection or by the antiretroviral drugs used to reduce the viral load. It may even be triggered by just thinking about the medication (so-called anticipatory nausea).

The ability of cannabinoids to treat nausea has been recognized for a long time; the oldest prescription cannabinoids (dronabinol and nabilone) were approved for the treatment of nausea and vomiting following chemotherapy (Tramer et al. 2001). Newer antiemetic drugs such as ondansetron have mostly replaced cannabinoids in routine clinical practice, but they remain available for patients who do not respond to the conventional agents.

There are no specific data on the use of cannabis to treat nausea in HIV patients. Nabilone has been suggested in two reports to be effective for nausea in AIDS patients (Flynn and Hanif 1992; Green et al. 1989). These reports from 1989 and 1992 have not been replicated, despite nabilone being available.

APPETITE

The effects of cannabis on increasing appetite have been known to recreational cannabis users for a long time (the so-called munchies). This has been reproduced in trials and has led to the approval of oral THC as a treatment for loss of appetite (anorexia) associated with HIV/AIDS.

The effects of THC on appetite and weight were evaluated in eighty-eight patients with AIDS-related anorexia and weight loss. In this trial, the PHAs were randomized to receive either 2.5 mg dronabinol twice daily or placebo. THC was associated with increased appetite, improvement in mood, and decreased nausea. Weight was stable in dronabinol patients, while placebo recipients had a mean loss of 0.4 kg. Side effects were mostly mild to moderate in severity (euphoria, dizziness, thinking abnormalities) (Beal et al. 1995).

The authors went on to study the effects of long-term (twelve months) THC administration in ninety-four PHAs who were given dronabinol orally-2.5 mg once or twice daily. THC was associated with consistent improvement in mean appetite. Patients tended toward stable body weight for at least seven months (Beal et al. 1997).

FOOD INTAKE

In addition to showing the effects of canabinoids on appetite, retrospective reviews of hospital charts have shown that oral THC improves appetite and reverses weight loss among hospitalized PHAs (Dejesus et al. 2007). Haney and colleagues found that smoked cannabis (1.8 and 3.9 percent THC) and THC (5 and 10 mg) given four times daily in a randomized, placebo-controlled trial of PHAs resulted in equal effects on food intake (Haney et al. 2007), with smoked cannabis at 3.9 percent, THC also having a positive effect on sleep.

ADHERENCE TO DRUG THERAPY

In addition to possible symptom control, cannabis use has been shown to be associated with improved compliance or adherence with antiretroviral therapy (ART) through improved treatment of nausea or improved overall self-care (de Jong et al. 2005; Wilson, Doxanakis, and Fairley 2004). This raises the intriguing possibility that cannabis use, if it does help patients tolerate their ART, may improve survival rates (Garcia de Olalla et al. 2002).

CANNABIS DOSAGE

The lack of standardization of cannabis used by patients in surveys makes estimating cannabis dosage very difficult. PHAs appear to use one or fewer joints at each dosing point, but frequency of dosing ranges from weekly to more than once daily. Important questions such as what constitutes a "joint" are not easy to address, but data can be gathered from other sources. Compassion club patients in San Francisco report using approximately one ounce (27 g) of herbal cannabis per month (Harris, Jones, and Shank 2000). A Canadian AIDS Society survey revealed that the average amount of cannabis used per month was 65.9 g (2.35 ounces), ranging from 0.25 to 300 g per month. The amounts of cannabis used may vary between individuals depending on characteristics such as delivery system (joint versus pipe), admixture with tobacco, THC content of cannabis used, and smoking characteristics such as length of inhalation and breath-holding time.

RISKS OF CANNABIS USE

Few areas of the debate around cannabis use are as controversial as the issue of safety. The key point here is that most of our knowledge of the adverse health effects of cannabis are based on studies of recreational use, and even such data have been collected during a time in human history when recreational cannabis use has been illegal, so the unwanted effects cannot really be put into context. We do not know what this effect has had on the true analysis of benefit and risks. It is widely accepted that cannabis is safe in overdose; a lethal maximum dose is not known. Here we briefly address one of the specific issues of cannabis use in HIV: immune function.

EFFECTS ON IMMUNE SYSTEM

Abrams and colleagues studied the effects of oral THC and smoked cannabis on viral loads and CD4/CD8 T-cell levels among PHAs and found that smoking three cannabis cigarettes (3.95 percent THC) or THC 2.5 mg three times daily over twenty-one days did not have significant effects of these parameters (Abrams et al. 2003). Moreover, patients who were treated with cannabinoids actually gained more weight than those who were on placebo. In concomitant studies, this team also found no effects of cannabinoids on plasma levels of ART (Kosel et al. 2002).

CONCLUSION

Ultimately, the use of cannabis by PHAs poses many challenges, including access and quality control, but it is clear that the evidence base is supportive of a therapeutic role for cannabis and cannabinoids in this population. The main caution is that the studies are small. However, large-scale trials will probably never be conducted in this area, so we have to make do with the data we have. Suffice it to say that for most of the claims that PHAs have made for medical use of cannabis, there have now been research studies to support these effects.

A final consideration comes from reflecting on consultations regarding medical cannabis use. It is sometimes hard to determine what is medical use and what is social (or "recreational") use, and indeed it is well known that some cannabis use is "mixed" (Belle-Isle and Hathaway 2007; Fogarty et al. 2007; Furler et al. 2004). This question goes beyond use in HIV/AIDS and touches on all areas of medical cannabis use. There is little doubt that someone smoking cannabis to alleviate nausea to allow them to tolerate their medications is medical; but should we consider smoking cannabis in the evening to relax as medical use for stress management?

Ultimately these questions should be brought up between patient and doctor in an open and honest way. There may be important issues at stake that may need other treatment approaches; no matter how "natural" or "herbal" cannabis is considered to be, it can still be considered a medication or drug, and nonmedical ways to manage stress (e.g., meditation and/or exercise) may need to be considered. Few people, if given the choice, would take medications when nonmedical approaches may be as effective, and such approaches deserve to be given as much chance as possible. As well as being safe, they may get patients constructively engaged in their own self-care and less reliant on medications and drugs. That said, there is no longer any reason why doctors and patients should not be able to have rational discussions about the possible role of cannabis and cannabinoids as part of a holistic approach to the treatment of persons living with HIV/AIDS.

27

Multiple Sclerosis and Spasticity

Denis J. Petro, M.D.

This chapter is provided as a guide for patients with multiple sclerosis (MS) considering cannabis as a treatment in cases where "conventional" medical management has failed. Particular attention is directed to individual symptoms and their response to cannabis based on published scientific research. Since symptom severity and disability can be highly variable, no simple recommendation concerning cannabis use can be made in isolation from the specifics of an individual patient.

Multiple sclerosis is the most common cause of chronic neurological disability in young adults (Rusk and Plum 1998) and is more likely seen in women and in those who grew up in northern latitudes. In the United States, an estimated 350,000 people are affected; worldwide, more than 1 million people have the diagnosis of MS. As a chronic nervous system disorder, MS is a progressive illness in which the body breaks down its own myelin, the protective sheath on neurons that allows more effective neurotransmission. It is treated with drugs intended to alter the clinical progression of the ongoing assault on central nervous system myelin. These drugs are designed to decrease symptoms such as pain, muscle spasms, weakness, and other functional disabilities. Cannabis has been used to treat some symptoms of MS. It is the intent of this chapter to provide some guidance for patients considering using this treatment.

While the medical literature documents the collected observations of physicians and patients throughout the ages, nothing surpasses the impact of personal observation of a clinical response in an individual patient. For this author, seeing my patients—in the neurology clinic and on the wards in the 1970s—respond to cannabis piqued my interest in its therapeutic potential.

A twenty-seven-year-old man was referred for evaluation and treatment of his severe spasticity (Petro 1980). In addition to weakness and fatigue in his legs, he experienced frequent severe nocturnal leg spasms while resting in bed. His symptoms were not improved by conventional medications, including muscle relaxants. At the suggestion of a friend, the patient tried cannabis, with immediate beneficial effect. When asked to refrain from cannabis use for the six weeks between clinic visits, he returned with more prominent spasticity, leg pain, and uncontrolled muscle spasms. In addition, he now complained of several episodes of urinary incontinence.

At the insistence of the patient, he left the clinic and returned one hour later. On his return, the findings on examination of the nervous system were remarkable, with normal deep tendon reflexes and a negative Babinski sign (a reflex associated with impairment of CNS motor function). The patient admitted to smoking marijuana in the interval between examinations. Since cannabis provided much better control of symptoms when compared to conventional drugs, the patient continued his pattern of therapeutic cannabis use for control of his spasticity without adverse effects. This single patient observation provided the rationale for the first clinical trial of a cannabinoid drug, delta-9-THC, in the scientific literature (Petro and Ellenberger 1981).

Recognizing that current MS treatment is less than optimal, the use of cannabis offers an opportunity to demonstrate the therapeutic potential of cannabinoids on a number of neurological symptoms. In a survey of 471 people with MS in the United Kingdom, use of cannabis was acknowledged by 8 percent (Somerset et al. 2001). Based on the MS incidence in the United States, one can estimate that as many as 28,000 MS patients in the United States may be using cannabis at any one time.

A representative example of cannabis use in South Africa (James 1994) reported the experiences of a female MS patient:

A few years ago I had started to eat small quantities of marijuana . . . the effects were immediate and remarkable. Control of bladder functioning, which was a humiliating problem, is restored to normal and has been a liberating influence in my life-style. I can now go out shopping, to the theater, and various other places, without anticipation of dread and panic. Painful and disturbing attacks of spasticity are relieved and now restful patterns of sleep are ensured where previously sleep was disturbed by urinary frequency or pain and discomfort. Not least, I can laugh and giggle, have marvelous sex and forget that I have this awful, incurable, intractable disease.

The challenge for physicians is to evaluate patient observations using scientific methodology. Beginning with the first publication of the beneficial effects by Petro (1980), research with cannabis in MS now includes over two dozen studies evaluating safety and efficacy. Since the cannabis plant contains at least sixty cannabinoid compounds, the scientific literature must be evaluated carefully due to the variability in absorption and metabolism of individual cannabinoids. In addition to extensive human trials, research involving an animal model of MS has demonstrated the site of action of cannabis at receptor sites in the brain, thus strengthening the rationale for using cannabis in the treatment of MS.

In the period from 1988 to 2006, more than one hundred peer-reviewed scientific articles on cannabis and MS were published. Yet on April 20, 2006, the FDA said that "no sound scientific studies" supported the medical use of marijuana. This was despite the overwhelming body of peer-reviewed research in support of the therapeutic effects of marijuana in conditions such as chemotherapy-induced nausea and vomiting, AIDS wasting, neuropathic pain, and spasticity.

The challenge for patients with MS is to assess the information presented in the media with attention to two basic questions: Is cannabis effective, and is it safe?

TREATMENT OPTIONS: DISEASE MODIFICATION AND SYMPTOM MANAGEMENT

In patients with MS, disease activity can be modified by appropriate drug therapy. Management of an acute episode of demyelination is sometimes achieved to a limited extent with corticosteroids. Disease modification is difficult to assess because MS is a chronic, unpredictable disorder in which the burden of white matter involvement (how many axons have been demyelinated) is highly variable, and the clinical response to any drug treatment may be modest at best. Six drugs have been approved to modify the clinical course of MS: Avonex (interferon-beta-1a), Betaseron (interferon-beta-1b), Copaxone (glatiramer acetate/copolymer 1), Rebif (interferon-beta-1a),

Novantrone (mitoxantrone), and Tysabri (natalizumab). In addition, immunosuppressants such as corticosteroids, methotrexate, and cyclophosphamide have been used to alter the natural history of MS with some success.

CANNABIS TREATMENT: DISEASE MODIFICATION

While patients may claim that cannabis can alter the natural history of MS, no prospective clinical trials have been conducted to prove this. Data from animal research supports cannabis as a possible disease-modifying therapy. The immune-mediated disease created by scientists, experimental autoimmune encephalomyelitis (EAE), is considered an animal model of MS. Lyman and colleagues (1989) demonstrated that the oral administration of delta-9-tetrahydrocannabinol (THC) was effective in the prevention and suppression of EAE.

This research suggested that delta-9-THC might prove to be a new and relatively innocuous agent for the treatment of MS. In animal studies, cannabinoids have been shown to be neuroprotective for toxic insults as well as in the EAE animal model. In the clinical trial of Zajicek and colleagues (2003) in patients with MS, exacerbation rates were lower in cannabinoid-treated patients compared with placebo ($p < 0.05$). This observation is consistent with the preclinical observation of the neuroprotective effect of cannabis. It remains remarkable that cannabis may slow neurodegeneration, which ultimately causes chronic disability in MS, yet no clinical trials are underway to test this hypothesis.

CANNABIS IN SYMPTOM MANAGEMENT

Manifestations of MS are many and depend on the location of CNS lesions. Since MS lesions have a predilection for certain anatomic locations, recognizable clinical syndromes are common in MS. Surveys of symptoms in MS have shown the most common symptoms to be fatigue, balance impairment, muscle disturbances (weakness, stiffness, pain, and spasm), and bowel and bladder impairment. In chronic MS, signs and symptoms of motor dysfunction are found in at least 75 percent of patients; sensory impairment is noted in 50 percent. Cerebellar abnormalities such as difficulty with balance are found in at least a third of MS patients. Autonomic symptoms including bowel, bladder, or sexual dysfunction are found in at least 50 percent of patients. Cognitive impairment is seen in 40 to 55 percent of chronic MS patients.

A survey of cannabis-using MS patients in the United States and United

Kingdom by Consroe and colleagues (1997) reported improvements after cannabis use in spasticity, chronic pain, emotional dysfunction, anorexia/weight loss, fatigue, double vision, sexual dysfunction, bowel and bladder dysfunction, visual dimness, impairment in walking and balance, and memory loss (in descending order). This report suggests that cannabis may significantly relieve signs and symptoms of MS such as spasticity and pain along with a number of other complaints.

Since clinical trials using cannabis in plant form have been difficult to conduct, a number of oral cannabinoid preparations have been developed. The cannabis extracts used in treating the symptoms of MS contain both the psychoactive cannabinoid delta-9-THC and cannabidiol (CBD), which antagonizes some of the negative effects associated with delta-9-THC, including sedation, tachycardia, and mood alteration.

A list of MS symptoms that can be influenced by cannabis use is shown in Table 27.1 below. The clinical data regarding cannabis in symptom management is divided into three groups: symptoms in which clinical data supports the use of cannabis (spasticity, pain, bladder dysfunction, and nystagmus); symptoms in which very little clinical data is published, yet the potential for clinical benefit exists (fatigue, sexual dysfunction, and sleep disturbance); and symptoms that are made worse with cannabis (tremor, postural regulation, and cognitive impairment).

TABLE 27.1. MULTIPLE SCLEROSIS SYMPTOMS AFFECTED BY CANNABIS USE

Improved	Possibly improved	Made worse
Spasticity	Fatigue	Tremor
Neuropathic pain	Sexual dysfunction	Postural impairment
Bladder dysfunction	Sleep disturbance	Cognitive impairment
Nystagmus		

SPASTICITY

In the nineteenth century, O'Shaughnessy (1842) used hemp extract in treating muscle spasms associated with tetanus and rabies. Reynolds (1890) reported using cannabis to treat muscle spasms, epilepsy, migraine, and other conditions. While medicinal cannabis use continued through the 1900s, little was published concerning cannabis and spasticity until the 1970s. Spasticity is caused by impaired conduction in myelinated nerve fibers, manifested as spasms, pain, and muscle stiffness. A survey of ten males with spinal cord injuries was published in 1974. Five patients using cannabis reported reduced spasticity, three patients noted no effect, and two patients did not have significant spasticity (Dunn and Davis 1974).

The use of cannabis to treat spasticity associated with MS has been reported by a number of investigators over the subsequent years. Petro (1980) reported one MS patient who used cannabis to treat nocturnal leg spasms and the fatigue associated with spasticity. Petro and Ellenberger (1981) conducted a double-blind clinical trial that demonstrated statistically significant reduction in spasticity following the oral administration of delta-9-THC in doses of 5 and 10 mg. Investigators have confirmed this observation using delta-9-THC, whole-plant cannabis, and the synthetic cannabinoid Cesamet (nabilone).

In an animal study by Baker et al. (2000), cannabinoids improved spasticity and tremor in mice with chronic relapsing experimental allergic encephalomyelitis (CREAE) and indicated that the cannabinoid system may be active in control of spasticity and tremor. The first large randomized, placebo-controlled trial in MS (CAMS study by Zajicek et al. 2003) failed to demonstrate a significant treatment effect of Marinol or a cannabis extract containing delta-9-THC and cannabidiol.

Unfortunately, the investigators limited the cannabinoid dose to 25 mg daily, well below the 30 mg daily dose predicted by Petro and Ellenberger in their clinical trial conducted over twenty years prior to this study. However, some measures of function, such as walk time and spasticity symptom scores, were improved significantly. This trial (along with most other studies using cannabis derivatives) is limited, since oral administration of cannabinoids leads to unpredictable blood cannabinoid levels and demonstrates lower bioavailability than smoked cannabis. With mixed results from clinical trials in MS-related spasticity (not unlike FDA-approved drugs for this indication), cannabis should be reserved for patients when other therapy has failed.

Since a considerable body of scientific evidence supports the efficacy of a number of different cannabinoids in spasticity, review articles (Gracies, Nance, and Elovic 1997; Consroe 1999) and medical texts (Compston 2001) include cannabis as a treatment option in spasticity. In *Brain's Diseases of the Nervous System, Eleventh Edition* (Compston 2001), among the treatments for spasticity associated with MS, cannabinoids are listed along with baclofen, dantrium, benzodiazepines, and tizanidine. Since the potency of differing cannabis preparations varies, and absorption is dependent on the route of administration, no information comparing the risks and benefits of cannabis with standard antispasticity drugs is available.

NEUROPATHIC PAIN

Because of the nature of MS as a disruption of transmission of nerve impulses, symptoms commonly seen include brainstem seizures, facial pain, and spasticity. Central pain syndrome is a neurological condition due to damage or dysfunction of the central nervous system (CNS), which includes the brain, brainstem, and spinal cord. The syndrome is caused by stroke, MS, tumors, seizure disorders, brain or spinal cord trauma, or Parkinson's disease, and in MS is often difficult to treat.

Anticonvulsants and antidepressants are commonly used in MS pain syndromes, with limited benefit. Based on small studies, which demonstrated positive effects on neurogenic symptoms, Rog et al. (2005) conducted a trial of Sativex in sixty-six patients with MS and central pain syndromes. Sativex was found to provide beneficial effects in relief of central pain as well as pain-related sleep disturbance. Inhaled cannabis might be expected to be more effective in neuropathic pain due to the rapid onset of action and ability to titrate the dose to receive effective control of pain. Inhaled cannabis delivers biologically active cannabinoids to the brain almost instantaneously (seconds to a few minutes), whereas oral preparations require fifteen minutes to as much as one hour to achieve adequate pain relief. With inhaled cannabis, if adequate analgesia is not achieved with an initial dose, the need for a second dose can be determined within a few minutes. Also, inhalation avoids rapid metabolism in the liver and cannabinoid metabolites play a smaller role in drug action.

BLADDER DYSFUNCTION

Bladder impairment in MS is seen in up to 80 percent of patients at some time during the course of the disease. It can vary from slightly inconvenient to potentially life-threatening when renal function is compromised. Bladder function is disrupted due to spinal cord lesions in MS. Drugs used in the treatment of spasticity, such as baclofen and diazepam, are often effective in treating bladder symptoms in many MS patients. MS patients also report improvements in bladder function after cannabinoid use.

Based on the observations of improved urinary tract function, an open-label pilot study of cannabis-based medicinal extract (CBME) has been reported by Brady and colleagues (2001). In this study sublingual CBME improved lower urinary tract function in ten of ten patients with advanced MS and refractory urinary tract dysfunction over eight weeks of treatment. The authors suggested that cannabis is a safe and effective treatment for urinary problems in advanced MS. Investigators in the CAMS study (Zajicek et al. 2003) conducted an analysis of MS patients with urge incontinence found cannabis showed statistically significant benefits versus placebo.

NYSTAGMUS

Nystagmus is an eye-muscle abnormality often associated with MS. These uncontrolled eye movements are distressing to patients and impair vision during attacks. In a single-patient clinical trial, a fifty-two-year-old man with MS and disabling nystagmus was studied in the United Kingdom over three months before and after cannabis use in the form of cigarettes, nabilone, and cannabis-oil-containing capsules (Schon 1999). The investigators demonstrated improved visual acuity and balance after inhaled cannabis and were able to correlate the therapeutic effect with changes in serum cannabinoid level.

Responding to this, Dell'Osso (2000) reported an individual with congenital nystagmus whose oscillations dampened after smoking cannabis. The patient was able to read small print on a poster across the room, which was not possible before smoking cannabis. Dell'Osso commented that while he had seen similar reports from patients, cannabis research is discouraged in the United States, making further studies impossible. Researchers in the United States have not been able to conduct scientific studies in MS-related nystagmus due to the obstruction by regulatory authorities, much to the detriment of patients with this distressing disability.

FATIGUE

Fatigue is one of the most frequently reported symptoms in MS and is clearly distinct from fatigue experienced in an otherwise healthy individual. The mechanism for fatigue in MS is unknown. In the only study addressing the effect of cannabis on fatigue, Consroe and colleagues (1997) reported survey data showing that 60 to 70 percent of subjects reported cannabis reduced fatigue states (tiredness and leg weakness). No controlled clinical trials have investigated the possible use of cannabis in MS-related fatigue.

SEXUAL DYSFUNCTION

Treatment of sexual dysfunction in male MS patients includes a range of options including pharmacological treatments such as Viagra. No treatment other than local administration of artificial lubrication is available for treatment of sexual dysfunction in females. In the Consroe and colleagues survey of cannabis effects on MS signs and symptoms (1997), fifty-one subjects reported sexual dysfunction, with 62.7 percent claiming improvement in sexual function after cannabis. Aside from this survey data, no objective clinical trial data has been reported concerning cannabis treatment of sexual dysfunction in MS patients. The use of cannabis in patients using Viagra is contraindicated due to the potential for drug interaction with vascular consequences such as dilation or constriction (McLeod, McKenna, and Northridge 2002).

SLEEP DISTURBANCE

Sleep disturbance can include a number of afflictions such as insomnia, snoring, and sleep apnea. A significant cause of sleep disruption is seen in MS-related pain syndromes. Here, cannabis may represent an effective treatment option. In a recent paper, Russo (2007) presents a comprehensive review of the cannabis-based medicine Sativex in treating pain and sleep-related syndromes. Since cannabis can clearly improve symptoms associated with sleep disturbance, use of cannabis to improve sleep quality is rational and worthy of further clinical study.

TREMOR

Tremor in MS is treated with beta-blockers, anticonvulsants, or, in rare cases, surgical procedures. In a survey of patients with MS by Consroe and colleagues (1997), 90 percent of subjects with tremor reported improvement after cannabis. In a study of eight MS patients with tremor and disturbed balance, oral THC was effective in two subjects, with subjective and objective improvement (Clifford 1983).

In an effort to resolve the issue, Fox and colleagues (2004) conducted a randomized, double-blind, placebo-controlled crossover trial of oral cannabis extract in fourteen MS patients with upper-limb tremors. Analysis of the results showed no significant improvement in any objective measures of upper-limb tremor with cannabis extract compared to placebo. However, there was a nonsignificant trend for patients to report improvement in their tremors, with five patients noting improved tremor on cannabis extract compared to only one on placebo. It is possible that cannabis causes a subjective effect on tremor, perhaps an effect on mood or mental function, or a small objective effect below what the study was powered to detect.

POSTURAL REGULATION

The complex integration of sensory and motor function required for regulating posture is impaired in many MS patients. Impairment of posture is most disabling for patients, distressing for caregivers, and frustrating for physicians. In a study of ten MS patients, inhaled cannabis increased postural tracking error both in MS patients and in normal control subjects. Some authors have reported incorrectly that this is a negative study of spasticity. Since postural dysfunction is a common finding in MS and is seen in 30 to 80 percent of patients, many patients have both motor and postural symptoms. Cannabis should be used with extreme caution in patients with spasticity and postural deficits.

COGNITIVE IMPAIRMENT

Cognitive impairment is seen in approximately one-half of MS patients and is characterized by mild memory loss and increased difficulty with complex tasks. The disease-modifying drugs may limit cognitive impairment by decreasing white matter lesions over time. Clinical cannabis studies have not addressed the effects of cannabis in MS patients, but data from other clinical research in normal healthy subjects has demonstrated consistent impairment in memory and cognitive function after cannabis.

CONCLUSION

In the past twenty years, the scientific basis for cannabis-related benefits in MS has advanced significantly. The description of specific CNS receptors for cannabinoids lends credence to previously reported improvements seen in spasticity and neuropathic pain. Clinical trials have shown some positive effects in symptom management in MS regarding spasticity, pain, bladder dysfunction, and sleep. Compared with conventional treatments, cannabis is at least as safe as current therapy. Since clinical trials comparing cannabis with other drugs have yet to be conducted, absolute determination of the place of cannabis in MS therapeutics has yet to be determined.

Unfortunately, critics of medicinal cannabis continue to argue that approval of cannabis to treat serious symptoms in an incurable disease would somehow "send the wrong message" with regard to the issue of drug abuse in general. Opponents of a rational cannabis policy apparently would prefer patients to suffer pain and disability in their quest for a victory in the war on drugs.

28
Pain Management

Mark S. Wallace, M.D., and Ben Platt, M.D.

Cannabis has been utilized as an analgesic for centuries. As information regarding its therapeutic potential entered the medical literature in the mid-1800s, its use became more widespread (Iversen and Snyder 2000). In the early twentieth century, it became increasingly scrutinized for its psychoactive effects and recreational use and was removed from the U.S. Pharmacopoeia in 1942 (Amar 2006). However, preclinical studies (as opposed to human studies) continued, and numerous neurobehavioral tests confirmed marijuana's analgesic effects (Bicher and Mechoulam 1968; Sofia et al. 1973; Kosersky, Dewey, and Harris 1973; Bloom et al. 1977). In the 1980s, more research focused on cannabinoid receptors; in the 1990s, the two G-protein-coupled cannabinoid receptors CB1 and CB2 were discovered (Howlett et al. 2002). This led to a surge in preclinical and clinical studies to assess the therapeutic potential of cannabis. Preclinical studies elucidated the sites of action of cannabinoids and showed that the brain, spinal cord, and peripheral nervous system were all involved (Hohmann, Briley, and Herkenham 1999; Welch and Stevens 1992; Martin et al. 1995; Richardson, Kilo, and Hargreaves 1998). Many of these studies were performed using animal models that also confirmed the analgesic effects of cannabinoids.

CLINICAL STUDIES ON CANNABINOID ANALGESIA
Human studies must be interpreted carefully, as there are several variables that can affect the outcomes: the route of administration (oral or inhaled),

the drugs studied (synthetic delta-9-THC, other synthetic cannabinoids, or inhaled cannabis), and the dosages used. Other factors include the study design and whether it involves experimentally induced pain or clinical pain (Walker and Huang 2002).

Studies in Healthy Volunteers

Experimental studies have produced mixed results. Several studies have shown that cannabis increases the pain threshold, suggesting it has an analgesic effect (Greenwald and Stitzer 2000; Milstein et al. 1975). Other studies have found either no effect on pain or an increase in pain perception (Naef et al. 2003; Zeidenberg et al. 1973; Hill et al. 1974; Clark et al. 1981). One study showed a dose-dependent effect of smoked cannabis on experimental pain (Wallace et al. 2007). Cannabis cigarettes with 2 percent THC produced no effect on pain, 4 percent THC significantly decreased pain, and 8 percent THC significantly increased pain. This emphasizes the above point that dosage and route of administration are likely to have a substantial effect on the results of any study.

Studies in Clinical Pain

Well-designed clinical studies are limited. A comprehensive literature review identified only fourteen studies that used a randomized, double-blind, placebo-controlled design. They vary in cannabinoid studied, dosages used, and routes of administration; they will be discussed below grouped according to the type of pain that was studied.

Cancer Pain

Patients with cancer pain were the first to be studied and have also been studied the most. One study administered oral THC at 5, 10, 15, and 20 mg dosages to ten patients with various cancer diagnoses (Noyes et al. 1975a). The results showed pain relief significantly better than placebo at dosages of 15 and 20 mg, but also noted that these dosages produced substantial confusion and sedation. Another study by the same authors examined thirty-six patients with various cancers and compared oral THC at 10 and 20 mg dosages to codeine (Noyes et al. 1975b). THC at 10 and 20 mg was found to be equally analgesic to 60 and 120 mg codeine, respectively. Again, 20 mg THC produced unpleasant drowsiness and mental cloudiness, but 10 mg THC was relatively well tolerated.

Similarly, two studies were done on patients with cancer pain looking at the effects of 4 mg of benzopyranoperidine, a synthetic analog of THC (Staquet, Gantt, and Machin 1978). The first found it superior to placebo and equivalent to 50 mg codeine, while the second found it superior to placebo and to secobarbital. Again, sedation was the major side effect, but it occurred with similar frequency for both the study drug and the comparison drugs. Opposite results were obtained when another group performed a similar study of benzopyranoperidine on patients with cancer pain and compared it to codeine and placebo (Jochimsen et al. 1978).

At doses of 2 and 4 mg, benzopyranoperidine was less effective than 60 and 120 mg codeine and was not more effective than placebo. The researchers reported that pain was actually augmented by benzopyranoperidine and found an incidence of sedation similar to codeine. It is difficult to draw conclusions from these studies as the patient population was heterogenous, with many different types of cancer pain.

Neuropathic Pain

Neuropathic pain is a type of chronic pain that is caused by abnormal nerve function in the peripheral or central nervous system. Common causes include diabetes, shingles, alcoholism, and HIV, among others. Four studies have been performed on patients with various types of neuropathic pain.

The effects of oral cannabidiol were studied on ten patients with various painful neuropathies (Lindstrom, Lindbolm, and Boreus 1987). They were given a total of 450 mg/day in divided doses for one week; no analgesic effect was demonstrated. The synthetic cannabinoid CT-3 was studied on twenty-one patients with chronic neuropathic pain and was compared to placebo (Karst et al. 2003). Patients received 40 mg for four days and then 80 mg for three days. CT-3 provided significant pain relief at three hours compared to placebo, with less of a response at eight hours. Side effects included mild dry mouth and sedation.

A sublingual spray of either 2.7 mg THC alone or mixed with 2.5 mg cannabidiol was evaluated on forty-eight patients with neuropathic pain due to brachial plexus root avulsion, usually the result of a trauma in which the nerves that supply the arm are torn away from the spinal cord, resulting in severe arm pain (Berman, Symonds, and Birch 2004). Both resulted in small but significant improvements in pain as well as quality of sleep. Side effects were reported as mild to moderate and included sleepiness and dizziness. Despite small reductions of pain, most patients said it was enough that they would like to continue to use the study drugs.

The only clinical study on inhaled cannabis evaluated its effect on neuropathic pain attributed to HIV (Abrams et al. 2007). Fifty patients smoked either 3.56 percent THC cannabis cigarettes or placebo cigarettes three times a day for five days. Smoked cannabis significantly reduced pain by 34 percent, compared to 17 percent with placebo. Side effects were mild and included sedation and anxiety.

Acute Pain

Acute pain, called nocioceptive pain, is a normal neural response to some sort of painful stimulus, generally either an injury or surgery. Three studies have evaluated the effects of cannabinoids on acute pain.

The first was done on people who were otherwise healthy and scheduled to receive four tooth extractions (Raft et al. 1977). THC was administered intravenously in doses of 0.22 and 0.44 mg/kg and compared to diazepam (Valium) and placebo. Analgesia from the low dose of THC was better than placebo but less than diazepam, whereas the high dose of THC provided less analgesia than both placebo and diazepam. Anxiety and dysphoria were the biggest side effects. This effect is consistent with healthy volunteer studies that show an increase in pain with higher doses of the cannabinoids.

Another synthetic cannabinoid, levonantradol, was compared to placebo on fifty-six patients with acute pain (Jain et al. 1981). Four different intramuscular injections (doses of 1.5, 2, 2.5, and 3 mg) all provided significant analgesia, but the authors were unable to produce a significant dose-response curve. Side effects were mild, with drowsiness being the most frequent.

The effect of oral THC on postoperative pain was evaluated on forty women after hysterectomy (Buggy et al. 2003). On the second day after surgery, the patients were given either 5 mg oral THC or placebo. No statistically significant analgesic effect was reported, and side effects were minimal.

Chronic Pain

Chronic pain can be due to either neuropathic causes as discussed above, or nociceptive causes such as arthritis. The effects of Sativex, an oromucosal (sublingual) spray containing THC 2.7 mg and cannabidiol 2.5 mg, were compared to placebo on fifty-eight patients with chronic pain due to rheumatoid arthritis (Blake 2006). Sativex produced significant pain relief with movement and at rest and improved quality of sleep, but did not decrease morning stiffness. Side effects were mostly mild to moderate, with dizziness being the most common.

Another chronic pain study evaluated the effects of a sublingual spray containing either 2.5 mg THC alone, 2.5 mg cannabidiol alone, or a combination of the two, and compared them to placebo in thirty-four patients with chronic pain due to various causes (Notcutt 2004). The sprays containing THC alone, and THC with cannabidiol, were shown to be significantly better than placebo for relieving pain. All three sprays were significantly better than placebo for improving quality of sleep. The most frequent side effects were dry mouth, dysphoria, and sedation.

TABLE 28.1. SUMMARY OF PUBLISHED STUDIES ON CANNABINOID ANALGESIC EFFICACY

Study population	Agent	Delivery method	Outcome	Reference
Healthy volunteers	Marijuana	Smoked	+	Greenwald and Stitzer 2000
Healthy volunteers	Marijuana	Smoked	+	Milstein et al. 1975
Healthy volunteers	Marijuana	Smoked	+ moderate doses − high doses	Wallace et al. 2007
Healthy volunteers	THC	Oral	0	Naef et al. 2003
Healthy volunteers	THC	Oral	0	Zeidenberg et al. 1973
Healthy volunteers	Marijuana	Smoked	−	Hill et al. 1974
Healthy volunteers	Marijuana	Smoked	−	Clark et al. 1981
Cancer pain	THC	Oral	+	Noyes et al. 1975a
Cancer pain	THC	Oral	+	Noyes et al. 1975b
Cancer pain	benzopyranoperidine	Oral	+	Staquet, Gantt, and Machin 1978

Study population	Agent	Delivery method	Outcome	Reference
Cancer pain	benzopyranoperidine	Oral	−	Jochimsen et al. 1978
Neuropathic pain	Cannabidiol	Oral	0	Lindstrom, Lindbolm, and Boreus 1987
Neuropathic pain	CT-3	Oral	+	Karst, 2003
Neuropathic pain	THC	Sublingual spray	+	Berman, Symonds, and Birch 2004
Neuropathic pain	THC/cannabidiol	Sublingual spray	+	Berman, Symonds, and Birch 2004
Neuropathic pain	Marijuana	Smoked	+	Abrams et al. 2007
Acute pain	THC	Intravenous	+ low doses 0 high doses	Raft et al. 1977
Acute pain	Levonantradol	Intramuscular	+	Jain et al. 1981
Acute pain	THC	Oral	0	Buggy et al. 2003
Arthritis	THC/cannabidiol	Sublingual spray	+	Blake et al. 2005
Chronic pain	THC	Sublingual spray	+	Notcutt et al. 2004
Chronic pain	THC/cannabidiol	Sublingual spray	+	Notcutt et al. 2004
Chronic pain	Cannabidiol	Sublingual spray	0	Notcutt et al. 2004

+ = decrease pain, 0 = no effect, − = increase pain

Headaches

References on the use of cannabis for the treatment of headache date as far back as the sixth and seventh centuries. Between this time and up to the nineteenth century, there continued to be citations attesting the efficacy of cannabis for the treatment of migraine. However, after cannabis was dropped from the U.S. Pharmacopeia, the reports largely disappeared (Russo 1998).

Preclinical research has suggested that cannabis may have a role in the treatment of migraine through inhibitory effects on serotonin type 3 receptors and by blockade of serotonin release from platelets (Fan 1995; Volfe, Dvilansky, and Nathan 1985). In addition, the cannabinoids bind to areas of the periaquaductal gray matter, (an area of the brain that modulates pain transmission where the opioids work to relieve pain), which has been implicated in migraine generation (Lichtman, Cook, and Martin 1996).

There are only two references to the use of the cannabinoids for the treatment of headache in the twentieth century. Noyes and Baram reported on five patients who used cannabis to treat painful conditions, of whom three had chronic headaches. All three subjects reported relief that was comparable or superior to ergotamine tartrate and aspirin (Noyes and Baram 1974). A second article presented three cases in which abrupt cessation of frequent, prolonged daily marijuana smoking resulted in severe migraine attacks (El-Mallakh 1987). This suggests a rebound headache, which usually results from abrupt cessation of frequent use of abortive treatments for migraines.

Reports on Smoked Cannibis

Several case series have been published discussing patients who self-medicate with cannabis. One study interviewed fifteen patients who smoked cannabis for therapeutic reasons and noted that twelve of them reported improvements in pain and mood, and eleven of them reported improvement in sleep (Ware et al. 2002). Another study performed a cross-sectional analysis of 209 chronic noncancer-pain patients and found that 15 percent of them reported using cannabis to treat pain (Ware et al. 2003). They reported improvements in pain, mood, and sleep, and stated side effects were primarily dry mouth and euphoria.

A study of thirty patients who use medical marijuana at a pain center in Canada found that 93 percent of patients reported moderate or greater pain relief (Lynch, Young, and Clark 2006). Side effects were reported by 76 percent of patients; they included increased appetite, weight gain, and slowed thoughts. In the Netherlands, a questionnaire was sent to 300 patients who received medical marijuana for various reasons (Gorter et al. 2005). Of the 107 patients who responded, 8.6 percent reported they used it primarily for pain.

CONCLUSION

The Institute of Medicine report on the medical use of marijuana in 1999 acknowledges that cannabis can produce an analgesic effect (Joy, Benson, and Watson 1999). It further recommends that additional research be done to assess how beneficial this effect can be. As has been shown here, eight years later, only a limited amount of research has been performed. The quality of this research is quite variable and, as stated earlier, is influenced by many factors that can affect the outcomes and preclude generalizations about the effects of cannabis on pain.

When one analyzes pain medicine from an evidence-based approach, it becomes apparent that there is not a lot of literature to support many practices that are commonly used. Pain is difficult to study because it is a subjective experience that is affected by many aspects of patients' lives. Physicians' clinical experience is potentially more likely than clinical studies to detect a beneficial analgesic effect from cannabis.

Preclincial studies have demonstrated that the cannabinoids have analgesic activity similar to other analgesics such as the opioids. However, the clinical studies are inconclusive and suggest that there may be a therapeutic window of analgesia. Doses above this therapeutic window might actually increase pain. This stresses the need for further research on the analgesic effects of the cannabinoids. As long as the medicinal use of marijuana remains illegal at a federal level, the true analgesic potential of cannabis may never be known.

29

Sativex

William Notcutt, M.D., F.R.C.A., F.F.P.M.R.C.A.

The use of cannabis as a medicine was widely studied in the United Kingdom for fifty years, from the 1830s on. The emergence of purified opiates and aspirin eclipsed these studies. It was over one hundred years later that the possibility of cannabis as a medicine finally reemerged as being worthy of clinical study. The discovery of the endocannabinoid system (still barely acknowledged within mainstream medicine) provided the scientific basis for this. In 1997, the British Medical Association produced a book weighing the current evidence and strongly encouraged further research. In 1998 and 1999, the Institute of Health in the United States and a scientific subcommittee of the House of Lords in the United Kingdom produced reports coming to similar conclusions (Morgan 1997; Iverson and Snyder 2000; House of Lords 1998).

Within society, too, there were changes in attitudes to the therapeutic use of cannabis in the late 1990s in the United Kingdom. People suffering from multiple sclerosis (MS) and other diseases were prepared to talk about the subject publicly without universal scorn.

In the 1970s the treatment of chronic pain as a recognized specialty was starting to emerge, but it was still based within anesthesia, where performing "nerve blocks" to eliminate the pain was most common. Palliative care was in its infancy, but, with the use of drugs like morphine, was beginning to improve. After the discovery of endorphins (the body's own morphine-like chemicals), there were huge developments in neurochemistry, leading to an explosion in potential treatments for pain. Furthermore, the psychology of pain became better understood. However, our understanding of pain has become far more complex than expected.

Since the 1970s, small-scale clinical studies on cannabis were carried out, but with great limitations to their application. The biggest problems have been the regulatory restrictions on cannabis, the lack of basic science, the absence of suitable standardized drug formulations to study, and the lack of a perceived need to develop the drug. Further, it is worth noting that until the last ten years, clinicians had not begun to take seriously the pain problems of patients with MS.

For many years, the only cannabinoid available in the United Kingdom was nabilone, but this was licensed only for the treatment of intractable nausea and vomiting associated with cancer chemotherapy. However, it often caused significant side effects, probably associated with its metabolism and route of delivery.

In the mid-1990s I treated more than sixty patients with nabilone for chronic intractable pain for whom other measures had not been successful. There was no doubt that it was effective and helpful for roughly 50 percent of patients, but side effects (dizziness, sedation, and dysphoria) were common, and many patients could not continue. It proved difficult to get the correct dose, and many patients who had used both nabilone and plant cannabis preferred the latter.

As the weight of evidence grew, it became increasingly convincing that the plant cannabis could be a useful, safe, and interesting medicine. If the plant extracts could be standardized to medicinal grade and delivered accurately, then the dosing could be controlled and effective doses precisely established.

Therefore, there was a need to move away completely from smoking cannabis. Smoking is unacceptable to most patients, and it is impossible to standardize the dose given by this method. It is thus almost impossible to undertake the classical types of clinical research necessary to explore the many possible uses. Finally, it would prove very difficult to regulate the use of smoked cannabis and to define clearly medicinal versus recreational use. Providing patients with a recognizable medicine would allow a clear distinction to be drawn from recreational cannabis, which would satisfy regulatory authorities and politicians. The difference between opium (smoked) and morphine (a purified extract of opium) is a useful comparison.

In 1998, GW Pharmaceuticals was established in the United Kingdom to develop a cannabis-based medicine (CBM). The British government gave its support to this project. The two main problems were the production of a standardized formulation of cannabis and the development of appropriate method(s) of drug delivery.

STANDARDIZED DRUG EXTRACT

Most basic research on cannabis has been done looking at either delta-9-tetrahydrocannabinol (THC) or cannabidiol (CBD). However, any extract contains approximately sixty-six cannabinoids in varying concentrations and includes other chemicals such as terpenes and flavonoids. In the past, tinctures of cannabis were prepared by using alcohol to extract cannabinoids derived from plant material of unknown cannabinoid content. This posed problems not only for clinicians wanting to know the dose, but also for researchers wanting to identify exactly what was producing the observed clinical effects. Regulators who are used to dealing with standardized single-chemical drugs have great problems in defining and understanding complex plant extracts.

There were two solutions to these problems. The first was to use cloned plants that would have a reproducible "fingerprint" of cannabinoids and other chemicals, in a steady ratio within any specific extract. Second, by selective breeding, plant lines could be established with a very high ratio of a specific cannabinoid (e.g., THC, CBD). By creating plants with a greater than 95 percent content of a specific cannabinoid, it would become possible to study the effects of both individual chemicals and also standardized blends of extracts of different composition. The first two extracts that GW Pharmaceuticals produced were Tetranadex and Nabidiolex, both containing greater than 95 percent of cannabinoid as THC and cannabidiol respectively.

DELIVERY ROUTE

While the extracts of cannabis were being developed, the problem of how to deliver them was addressed. Taking cannabis by inhaling it into the lungs is a rapid method of drug delivery. Mimicking smoking by inhaling a nebulized spray was considered, but the oily nature of cannabis makes it very difficult to administer in this form. It would be possible to heat it and convert it into a vapor (as occurs in a cannabis cigarette). However, there are great difficulties in producing a device that delivers a vapor cool enough for the patient, while at the same time satisfying the safety concerns of regulatory authorities.

The oral route was an obvious second choice. However, the absorption is variable and slow, taking an hour or more and making titration to an exact dose effect difficult. Furthermore, THC undergoes a different metabolism when it is absorbed through this route, which may lead to greater psychoactive side effects. The rectal route (suppository) would have similar problems and is not a preferred route of taking medicines in most countries.

The possibility of sublingual administration (under the tongue) was considered. A description of the administration by this route was described as early as 1897 (Marshall 1897). The extract would be sprayed onto the lining of the mouth and absorbed directly into the bloodstream. This also gave the possibility of a faster effect than seen by other routes, except inhalation into the lungs (smoking) or intravenous. Preclinical trials carried out on healthy human volunteers showed that absorption occurred within fifteen to twenty minutes.

The way was now open for high-quality clinical studies using standardized extracts delivered sublingually. Anecdotal evidence gathered from those using illicit plant cannabis as a medicine showed a preference for using types of cannabis with a substantial CBD content. Earlier work in the 1980s had suggested that CBD ameliorates some of the psychoactive side effects of THC, although the other clinical effects of CBD were unclear (Zuardi et al. 1982).

The first clinical (Phase II) trials of the new extracts were carried out both in Great Yarmouth and Oxford in the United Kingdom in 2000 using three different preparations. These were THC, CBD, and a 1:1 mixture of THC and CBD. From the initial crossover studies in patients (mostly with MS), it appeared that the mixture of the two cannabinoids was optimal. There was little difference in clinical effectiveness between this and THC by itself. However, the side effect profile was better using the mixture.

CBD alone did not seem to be nearly as beneficial. It was therefore decided to focus the next cohort of studies on the 1:1 mixture of THC and CBD. This mixture of cannabinoids (with ethanol and propylene glycol 1:1, to aid spray delivery, and peppermint flavoring) came to be known as Sativex (sativa extract). In producing Sativex, ethanol (alcohol) is not used to extract cannabinoids from the plant material, unlike with previous tinctures.

From the initial studies, it emerged that this method of dosing (under the tongue) enabled patients to rapidly, reliably, and conveniently find the appropriate level of medication without, for the most part, suffering unacceptable side effects. The only drawback has been the unpleasant taste.

Thus, patients became able to administer the drug safely, allowing them to get on with their lives. A fundamental difference between patients and recreational users is the level to which they will administer the drug. For the patient who is immobilized because of pain or other unpleasant symptoms, the objective is a more comfortable state and an ability to do more. Therefore psychoactive effects have to be kept to a minimum. Furthermore, for many patients, the ability to continue employment and other activities was critical, including for those who required a high level of cognitive functioning (accountants, lawyers, etc.).

One great advantage that patients noticed early in the studies was the ability to carry their medicine with them and to administer it when they were away from the privacy of their own home without undue comment (or worse).

STUDIES IN MULTIPLE SCLEROSIS AND BEYOND

The next cohort of studies on MS focused on two main symptoms, pain and spasticity (tightness in the muscles). The U.K. government encouraged the study of Sativex for the symptoms of MS, as this group of patients had spoken out loudest about the therapeutic potential of cannabis. MS is an extremely complex disease, with each patient having individual patterns of damage to the nervous system and subsequent symptoms. It quickly became evident that patients were often getting more than one benefit from the drug. In particular, improvement in sleep, which allows patients to better cope with pain and other unpleasant symptoms, was frequently reported. General improvements in mood and reductions in depression and anxiety were commonly seen.

Further complexities with the studies emerged. The patients undergoing the studies were selected on the basis of their unresponsiveness to conventional treatments for their pain or spasticity. These were "worst-case scenarios." As a result, benefits were predictably likely to be lower than one would expect to see in patients who were less severely disabled. Also, the inclusion of such patients in clinical trials like these generated great expectations in what the new drug might do. These expectations could cause an exaggerated response (the so-called placebo effect). The classical style of a double-blind, randomized, placebo-controlled trial is notoriously difficult to undertake in patients with chronic pain, unlike with other diseases such as diabetes or high blood pressure, and there are many fewer studies.

Results are now emerging from a number of studies demonstrating the effectiveness of Sativex in neuropathic pain, rheumatoid arthritis, and cancer-related pain (Rog et al. 2005; Blake et al. 2006). The common side effects of Sativex during the clinical trials were lightheadedness, dizziness, and somnolence, all of which were predictable and occur with almost every psychoactive drug used in pain management.

Since the start of the studies in 2000, there have been many patients who have continued to use Sativex after the end of the studies. No psychiatric or psychological symptoms have emerged that are attributable to Sativex. In particular, no significant dependency has been shown, and patients have been able to discontinue Sativex without significant problem.

Sativex has also been used as an unlicensed medicine in a group of patients who were not part of any clinical trial. This has shown that it can be used successfully by patients who are not as disabled as those taking part in clinical trials, but who are continuing in full- or part-time occupations.

The slowness of the regulatory authorities in providing a license for Sativex in the United Kingdom reflects a number of factors. There has been a substantial increase in the bureaucracy associated with the clinical trials, extending the time that it takes to achieve completion; the methodology required by the regulators (double-blind, placebo-controlled) does not work well with this group of patients; the patients treated have generally been those who have no other options available; and there is probably still a political unwillingness to facilitate the therapeutic use of cannabis while the debate on recreational use rages on. Ya think?!,

From our clinical experiences over the last seven-and-a-half years, Sativex has proved to be an easy drug to use. Furthermore, the side effects have been limited and easy to manage. The mortality rate from NSAIDs (anti-inflammatory drugs) is significant (approximately two thousand deaths per year in the United Kingdom). Opiates are effective analgesics but pose a number of major problems when used for chronic pain. Cannabis extracts may be emerging as a safe, simple, and effective alternative in comparison with most other medicines used in the treatment of pain and spasticity.

PART FOUR

Cannabis Culture

I think people need to be educated to the fact that marijuana is not a drug. Marijuana is an herb and a flower. God put it here. If He put it here and He wants it to grow, what gives the government the right to say that God is wrong?

WILLIE NELSON

If someone wants to do drugs . . . as long as he or she isn't corrupting minors or driving under the influence or endangering others, shouldn't a person have that right?

BRAD PITT

Why is marijuana against the law? It grows naturally upon our planet. Doesn't the idea of making nature against the law seem to you a bit . . . unnatural?

BILL HICKS

Introduction to Part Four

As a parent, I recognize that one of the important lessons to teach my children is about moderation: Not too loud. Not too rough. Not too much. You can do it, but be careful about this and don't forget about that. Most kids learn that growing up means tempering your behavior in order to fit in and succeed. This sort of upward mobility is what it's all about in America. We can all agree that some altered states greatly impede that kind of progress if they are practiced in excess. Sometimes being altered means being incapacitated to some extent; that is a near-truism. But acutely altered does not necessarily mean chronically impaired. There are times when an altered state is useful, when drug experiences can be life-affirming or life-changing. Some drugs help provide a glimpse of the "macro," a larger map of where things stand and where one is heading. Good ideas can come from "stepping outside the box" and seeing the bigger picture. Psychospiritual exploration, soul-searching, communing with the self—these are normal and important components of the human experience.

Adolescence is a prime time for this sort of exploration, and for questioning, testing limits, and defying both death and authority. The chances that your kids aren't going to have to tangle with cigarettes, alcohol, or drugs are virtually nil. Drugs are a bit like power tools. As parents, it is our job to teach kids the difference between a toy and a tool. ("Don't touch that! It's daddy's tool, it's dangerous!") What we really should be saying is: "You need to learn how to use this first." We are obligated to equip our children with knowledge about drug and alcohol safety. Us. Not the police. Not the government. We, as parents, need to teach our own children. And so we need to learn all we can. Most importantly, we should model responsible behavior.

Many families are struggling with their loved ones as they discover drugs. I think if kids have enough good things in their lives, they'll be able to navigate these waters, but they will surely need help from their parents.

When children have emptiness in their lives and in themselves, if their families are torn apart, they may well be left with a hole they'll try to fill for the rest of their lives. We are afraid for our children's futures when they start using drugs, but most American kids are going to experiment. Most teens say marijuana is easy for them to get, in many cases easier to obtain than alcohol and tobacco (where they are required to proffer ID), and nearly a quarter of those surveyed estimated they could "score" within an hour or less (CASA 2008). Recent Monitoring the Future Study* results (Johnston et al. 2008) show that teen marijuana use is on the rise again after a slight dip, and, more importantly, the perceived risk of its use is down.

We're going to have to figure out what to say to our kids that will actually keep the lines of communication open. (Please see Rosenbaum's chapter 30 for much more on this.) Our children need to be advised and guided throughout their childhood. Optimally, we can speak openly about learning to use drugs as tools, to note ill-desired effects, to modify behavior, and to balance risks and benefits, and we can teach kids to make that analysis themselves.

Modeling healthy behavior is the smartest thing we can do, to show our children how to healthfully integrate altered states into their lives. Think of how we teach kids about alcohol, how we allow them sips of wine at the dinner table. This way, they get to see altered states successfully navigated. The problem is, when we make it illegal to smoke cannabis, we prevent all that communication. Everyone is forced to hide drug use, which then defines the behavior as shameful. This aura of shame forces kids to lie to their parents, and parents to hide their use from their kids. I'm reminded of a scene in the movie *Sideways* in which Sandra Oh's character hides the joint, but not the wine glass, when her daughter comes out of her bedroom to see what the adults are up to. We don't talk about smoking pot because not everyone does it, and most importantly, because it is a crime. And there have been cases of kids taught and coached by DARE programs who turn in their parents, resulting in asset forfeiture of their house, or in parents losing custody of their children.

And so I want to applaud Neal Pollack's bravery in his piece, and support him with a quote from Marian Fry, M.D., in a survey of California

---

*Monitoring the Future is an ongoing study of the behaviors, attitudes, and values of American secondary school students. Each year, a total of approximately 50,000 eighth-, tenth-, and twelfth-grade students are surveyed.

clinicians who provide cannabis approvals. Fry noted in her response that pot-smoking patients with parenting problems saw an "enhanced flexibility and an ability to identify the child's needs as those of a separate and unique individual. . . . Improved communication leads to shared experience. The parent becomes *present* and the child benefits from the increased positive attention. . . . Patients say cannabis makes them less self-centered and egocentric and more aware of the needs of other people. It makes them aware of how their own behavior affects other people and how they may be contributing to a negative interaction" (O'Shaughnessy 2007; emphasis added).

One interesting way to view our current drug policy is this: the American government is like an overcontrolling parent, and the American populace is like a rebellious toddler. You can't have these cookies, so I'm going to put them on a high shelf where you can't reach them. So the toddler climbs up on the counter, steals the cookies, and eats them in a closet. Making the cookies taboo just makes them more enticing. A policy of total forbiddance drives the behavior underground, where it becomes clandestine, unsupervised, and infused with guilt. The hiding and shame that result from the illegality then lace the behavior with an adrenaline charge, making the experience more salient, and potentially reinforcing, adding to its addictive quality. The enhanced shame and fear at being discovered (or prosecuted) also may require more self-soothing actions, fueling repeated drug-taking behaviors. Our drug policy is making us act like addicts!

We, as primates, are naturally social beings. We crave connection and community. Because we have to hide our behavior, the illegality necessitates social isolation, secrecy, and negativity where there needn't be any. On the other hand, when we are lucky enough to find friends and family who share our predilection for cannabis, we bond with them vehemently, hiding together, happy to have a partner in crime. Any pot smoker will tell you how heavenly it is to spend time in Amsterdam, where a popular saying, "*Vrijheid, blijheid,*" literally means "Freedom, joy" but is meant as something like, "Do your own thing," or "Live and let live." There, people smoke openly, chatting with strangers, uniting lovingly over nothing more than a shared pastime, relieved to be free of the shackles of clandestine, furtive puffing characteristic of much of America.

Guilt exacerbates our national problematic drug use. Perhaps if we were to honor the practice, to normalize it and destigmatize it, we, like the Dutch, would find that we had less of a national drug problem. Parents know that when you make cookies less of a big deal, the desire for a steady supply of cookies wanes. Geneen Roth, a great writer on food and appetite issues for women, has shown me that cutting out the idea of forbidden foods (and making peace with my own appetite) was the key to my weight loss. Women's magazines have embraced the theory that restrictive diets aren't as smart as healthy eating that occasionally honors our cravings.

Being an adult means being responsible, understanding that there are consequences to our actions, and learning to anticipate and take ownership of those consequences when they do occur. Being treated like a child will not foster growth. Perhaps we should take a page from the Book of Rasta. The Rastafari way, in which God is said to reside within each of us, teaches personal responsibility. Faith and inspiration are found within the self. There is no "Thou shalt not," there is only "I and I." The self and the higher self (the Holy Spirit) reside as one within the body, not in heaven or a church. For Rastas, cannabis is a sacrament, and smoking it becomes a spiritual act, bringing them closer to Jah. Ganja is seen as a way to cleanse the body and mind, heal the soul, and elevate the consciousness.

The answer for our culture, ideally, lies in cultivating a healthier approach toward altered states, and to integrate cannabis use into our lives, much as we have social drinking. Normalizing the behavior removes the adrenaline charge, subtracting the guilt and therefore the compulsion to medicate away the shame. We must recognize and accept that we all need down time, a Sabbath. McDonald's reminds us that we "deserve a break today." Coca-Cola portrays itself as "the pause that refreshes." (Caffeine is probably America's most socially sanctioned drug. Roughly 90 percent of adults have a daily cup of coffee or tea. Headaches caused by caffeine withdrawal, occurring when the habit is abruptly discontinued, are a widespread, well-understood phenomenon.) Even the alcohol industry has a slogan that embraces moderation: "Enjoy responsibly." Alcohol use by adults is permitted, but dangerous behaviors associated with drunkenness (such as driving while under the influence) are punished. It makes sense to treat cannabis the same way.

More Americans are coming to this conclusion. A Gallup Poll in October 2009 showed that support for legalization, at 44 percent, is at a forty-year high (up from just 27 percent in 1979). A nationwide Zogby Poll in 2009 put support at 52 percent. A Field Poll in April 2009 found 56 percent of Californians surveyed were in favor of legalizing, regulating, and taxing marijuana like alcohol and cigarettes. Among likely voters on the East Coast, 48 percent endorse legalizing marijuana.

Outing ourselves as otherwise law-abiding and responsible employees and employers, parents, citizens, and, most of all, taxpayers is a good first step. Many of us are tired of being outlaws. We'd like to pay our "sin taxes" and stop hiding.

30
What to Tell the Children

Marsha Rosenbaum, Ph.D.

The 2008 Monitoring the Future survey states that more than 47 percent of high school seniors have tried illegal drugs at some point in their lifetimes; 36 percent used a drug during the past year; and 22 percent profess to have used drugs in the past month.

To understand teenage drug use, it is imperative to recognize the context in which today's teens have grown up. Alcohol, tobacco, caffeine, over-the-counter, and prescription drugs are everywhere. Though we urge our young people to be "drug free," Americans are constantly bombarded with messages encouraging us to celebrate, relax, and medicate with a variety of substances. Drugs are an integral part of American life. The *Journal of the American Medical Association* reported that eight out of ten adults in the United States use at least one medication every week, and half take a prescription drug (Kaufman et al. 2002). One in two adults in this country uses alcohol regularly; and more than 97 million Americans over the age of twelve have tried marijuana at some time in their lives—a fact not lost on their children (Substance Abuse and Mental Health Administration 2006).

While "peer pressure" is often blamed for teenage drug use, the 2008 State of Our Nation's Youth survey found that, contrary to popular belief, most are not pressured to use drugs. Instead, teenage drug use seems to mirror modern American drug-taking tendencies (Peter D. Hart Associates 2008). Some psychologists argue that given the nature of our culture, teenage experimentation with legal and illegal mind-altering substances should not be considered abnormal or deviant behavior (Newcomb and Bentler 1988; Shedler and Block 1990).

PROBLEMS WITH CURRENT PREVENTION STRATEGIES

Americans have been trying to prevent teenage drug use for over a century—from the nineteenth-century Temperance campaigns against alcohol to Nancy Reagan's "Just Say No" mandate. A variety of methods, from scare tactics, to resistance techniques, to zero-tolerance policies and random drug testing have been used to try to persuade young people to abstain.

The effectiveness of these conventional approaches has been compromised by:

- the unwillingness to distinguish between drug use and abuse by proclaiming "all use is abuse";
- the use of misinformation as a scare tactic; and
- the failure to provide comprehensive information that would help users reduce the harms that can result from drug use.

In the effort to stop teenage experimentation, prevention messages often pretend there is no difference between use and abuse. These hypocritical messages are often dismissed by teens who observe their parents and other adults using alcohol without abusing it. They know there is a big difference between having a glass of wine with dinner versus with breakfast. Many also know that their parents have tried an illegal drug (likely marijuana) at some point in their lives without significant untoward effects.

Few things are more frightening to a parent than a teenager whose use of alcohol and/or other drugs gets out of hand. Yet virtually all studies have found that the vast majority of students who try legal and/or illegal drugs do not become drug abusers (US GAO 1993; Duncan 1991). We need to talk about alcohol and other drugs in a sophisticated manner and distinguish between use and abuse. If not, we lose credibility. Furthermore, by acknowledging distinctions, we can more effectively recognize problems if and when they occur.

SCARE TACTICS AND MISINFORMATION:
MARIJUANA AS A CASE IN POINT

A common belief held by many educators, policy makers, and parents is that if young people believe drug use is risky, they will abstain (Bachman, Johnson, and O'Malley 1990). In this effort, marijuana (the most popular illegal drug among U.S. teens) is consistently mischaracterized by prevention programs, books, ads, and websites, including those managed by the federal government. Exaggerated claims of marijuana's dangers are routinely published, bolstered with assertions of scientific evidence, but the most serious of these allegations falter when critically evaluated.

I am a medical sociologist. In my workshops, parents regularly question claims they have heard about marijuana:

- Is it true that marijuana is significantly more potent and dangerous today than in the past?
- Is today's marijuana really more addictive than ever before?
- Does marijuana really cause users to seek out "harder" drugs?
- Is it true that smoking marijuana causes lung cancer?

Two books can help answer these questions, *Marijuana Myths, Marijuana Facts* (1997) and *Marijuana: A New Look at the Scientific Evidence* (2005). Each found that claims of marijuana's risks had been exaggerated, even in some instances fabricated (Zimmer and Morgan, 1997; Earleywine 2005). These same conclusions have been reached by numerous official commissions, including the La Guardia Commission in 1944, the National Commission on Marijuana and Drug Abuse in 1972, the National Academy of Sciences in 1982, and the federally chartered Institute of Medicine in 1999.

Using these resources, as well as many others, here is how I have tried to answer parents' questions:

POTENCY

Many people believe that the marijuana available today is significantly more potent than in decades past: as marijuana-growing techniques have become more advanced and refined, there has been a corresponding increase in the plant's average psychoactive potency, otherwise known as its THC (delta-9 tetrahydrocannabinol) content level. (Please see chapter 23 for more on this point.)

The federally funded University of Mississippi's Marijuana Potency Project estimates that average THC levels have increased since 1988 from approximately 3.7 percent to over 8 percent. However, the National Drug Intelligence Center reports that "most of the marijuana available in the domestic drug markets is lower potency, commercial grade marijuana" (University of Mississippi Marijuana Potency Monitoring Project 2007; National Drug Intelligence Center 2007); and the Drug Enforcement Administration (DEA) affirms that of the thousands of pounds of marijuana seized by law enforcement annually, fewer than 2 percent of samples test positive for extremely high (above 20 percent) THC levels (US DEA 2005).*

In short, it appears that marijuana now is, on average, somewhat stronger than in the past, though variation has always been the norm. Essentially, marijuana's increased strength is akin to the difference between beer (at 6 percent alcohol) and wine (at 10–14 percent alcohol), or between a cup of tea and an espresso.

Furthermore, even with higher potency, no studies demonstrate that increased THC content is associated with greater harm to the user (Earleywine 2005). In fact, among those who report experiencing the effects of unusually strong marijuana, many complain of dysphoria and subsequently avoid it altogether. Others adjust their use accordingly, consuming very small amounts to achieve the desired effect (Herning, Hooker, and Jones 1986; Abrams et al. 2007).

ADDICTION[†]

Although marijuana does not create the physical dependence associated with drugs such as alcohol and heroin, a minority of users find it psychologically difficult to moderate their use or quit. The vast majority of those who experience difficulty with marijuana also have preexisting mental health problems that can be exacerbated by cannabis (Tims et al. 2002). According to the National Academy of Sciences, 9 percent of marijuana users exhibit symptoms of dependence, as defined by the American Psychiatric Association's DSM-IV criteria (Joy, Benson, and Watson 1999).

---

*Marijuana Potency Project data in May 2009 showing seized marijuana averaging 10 percent THC included samples of seized hashish and hash oil, which naturally has double the THC percent of cannabis.

†Please also see chapter 14 for a broader discussion of addiction.

Those who argue that marijuana is addictive often point to increasing numbers of individuals entering treatment for cannabis. While some of these individuals are in rehab because they (or their families) believed their marijuana use was adversely impacting their lives, most were arrested for possession and referred to treatment by the courts as a requirement of their probation.

Over the past decade, voluntary admissions for cannabis have actually dropped, while criminal justice referrals to drug treatment have risen dramatically. Two thirds of all individuals in treatment for marijuana are "legally coerced" into treatment (Office of Applied Studies 2005, 2002; Copeland and Maxwell 2007).

THE GATEWAY THEORY*

The "gateway" theory suggests that marijuana use inevitably leads to the use of harder drugs, such as cocaine and heroin (Kandel 1975; Gabany and Plummer 1990). However, population data compiled by the National Survey on Drug Use and Health et al. demonstrate that the vast majority of marijuana users do not progress to more dangerous drugs (Zimmer and Morgan 1997; Brown and Horowitz 1993; SAMHA 2006; RAND Corporation 2002). The gateway theory was also refuted by the Institute of Medicine and in a study published in the *American Journal of Public Health* (Joy, Benson, and Watson 1999; Golub and Johnson 2001).

The overwhelming majority of marijuana users never try any other illicit substance (Advisory Council on the Misuse of Drugs 2002). Furthermore, those populations who do report using marijuana in early adulthood typically report voluntarily ceasing their cannabis use by the time they reach age thirty (Kandel and Yamaguchi 1984; Bachman et al. 1992; Joy, Benson, and Watson 1999). Consequently, for most who use it, marijuana is a "terminus" rather than a "gateway."

Today's research also reveals that the vast majority of teens who try marijuana do not go on to become dependent or even use it on a regular basis (SAMHA 2006; Tarter et al. 2006).

LUNG CANCER

Although inhaling cannabis can irritate the pulmonary system, research has yet to demonstrate that smoking marijuana, even long term, causes diseases

---

*For more on the Gateway Theory, please see chapter 14 on addiction.

of the lung, including cancer. Most recently, in the largest study of its kind ever conducted, National Institute on Drug Abuse researcher Dr. Donald Tashkin and his colleagues at the University of California at Los Angeles compared 1,212 head, lung, or neck cancer patients to 1,040 demographically matched individuals without cancer and reported, "Contrary to our expectations, we found no positive associations between marijuana use and lung cancers . . . even among subjects who reported smoking more than 22,000 joints over their lifetime" (Kaufman 2006; Hashibe et al. 2005; Zimm 2007).

JUST SAY NO OR SAY NOTHING AT ALL

Most drug education programs are aimed solely at preventing drug use. After instructions to abstain, the lesson ends. There is no information on how to avoid problems or prevent abuse for those who do experiment.

Abstinence is treated as the sole measure of success and the only acceptable teaching option. This approach is clearly not enough. It is unrealistic to believe that at a time in their lives when they are most prone to risk-taking, teenagers—who find it exciting to push the envelope—will completely refrain from trying alcohol and/or other drugs (US GAO 1993). The abstinence-only mandate puts adults in the unenviable position of having nothing to say to the young people we need to reach the most—those who insist on saying "Maybe," or "Sometimes," or even "Yes" to drugs (Botvin and Resnicow 1993).

Teenagers will make their own choices about alcohol and other drugs, just as we did. Like us, their mistakes will sometimes be foolish. To help prevent drug abuse and drug problems among teenagers who do experiment, we need a fallback strategy that includes comprehensive education, and one that puts safety first.

SAFETY FIRST: A REALITY-BASED APPROACH

Keeping teenagers safe should be our highest priority. To protect them, a reality-based approach enables teenagers to make responsible decisions by:

- providing honest, science-based information;
- encouraging moderation if youthful experimentation persists;
- promoting an understanding of the legal and social consequences of drug use; and
- prioritizing safety through personal responsibility and knowledge.

In the same way that we encourage a designated driver for teens who drink alcohol, or condom use to prevent HIV, other STDs, and teen pregnancy, we should focus on reducing the harm associated with risky behaviors. Reality-based sex education strongly encourages abstinence, but it also provides accurate "safe sex" information. According to the Centers for Disease Control and Prevention (CDC), this approach has resulted not just in the increased use of condoms among sexually active teenagers, but has also served to decrease overall rates of sexual activity (Kann et al. 2000).

This effective, comprehensive prevention strategy presents a strong case and provides a model for restructuring our drug education and abuse prevention efforts. Teens need an honest, comprehensive drug education.

HONEST, SCIENCE-BASED EDUCATION

Young people are capable of rational thinking. Although their decision-making skills will improve as they mature, most teenagers are learning responsibility and do not want to destroy their lives or their health (Moshman 1999; Quadrel, Fischoff, and Davis 1993). In our workshops with students, they consistently request the "real" facts about drugs so they can make responsible decisions—and the vast majority actually do. According to the 2008 National Survey on Drug Use and Health, although experimentation is widespread, 90 percent of twelve- to seventeen-year-olds choose to refrain from regular use.

Effective drug education should be based on sound science and acknowledge teenagers' ability to understand, analyze, and evaluate. The subject of drugs can be integrated into a variety of high school courses and curricula, including physiology and biology (how drugs affect the body), psychology (how drugs affect the mind), chemistry (what's contained in drugs), social studies (who uses which drugs, and why), and history and civics (how drugs have been handled by various governments).

Fortunately, today's educators have a new resource and should consider the innovative approach devised by Rodney Skager. His 2007 booklet, "Beyond Zero Tolerance: A Reality-Based Approach to Drug Education and School Discipline" (available at www.safety1st.org), takes educators step by step through a pragmatic and cost-effective drug education and school discipline program for secondary schools.

As Dr. Skager suggests, through family experience, peer exposure, and the media, teenagers often know more about alcohol and other drugs than we assume. If drug education is to be credible, formal curricula should incorporate the observations and experiences of young people themselves. Classes should use interaction rather than rote lecturing (Martin, Duncan, and Zunich 1983; Austin and Skager 2006). If drug education is to be effective, it should be deemed truthful and valuable by the students. Countless studies have shown that D.A.R.E., the largest drug education program in America, is ineffective in preventing drug experimentation in its recipients, and this may well be due to its content.

THE IMPORTANCE OF MODERATION

The vast majority of teenage drug use (with the exception of nicotine) does not lead to dependence or abusive habits (Nicholson 1992; Winick 1991; Goode 2004). Teens who do use alcohol, marijuana, and/or other drugs should know how to recognize irresponsible behavior when it comes to place, time, dose levels, and frequency of use. They must control their use by practicing moderation and limiting use. It should be made clear that it is impossible to do well academically or meet one's responsibilities at work while intoxicated. It is never appropriate to use alcohol and/or other drugs at school, at work, while participating in sports, or while driving or engaging in any serious activity.

UNDERSTANDING CONSEQUENCES

Young people must understand the consequences of violating school rules and local and state laws against the use, possession, and sale of alcohol and other drugs—whether or not they agree with such policies.

With increasing methods of detection such as school-based drug testing and zero-tolerance policies, illegality is a risk in and of itself that dwarfs the physical effects of drug use. There are real, lasting consequences of using drugs and being caught, including expulsion from school, a criminal record, and social stigma. The Higher Education Act has resulted in the denial of college loans for 200,000 U.S. students convicted of any drug offense while they are enrolled in school (Students for Sensible Drug Policy 2006).

Fortunately, zero-tolerance policies—which have contributed to a high-school dropout rate of 30 percent in this country—have come under serious attack. The American Psychological Association concluded in 2006 that such policies are "backfiring," making students feel less safe and undermining academic performance (Reynolds 2006). Support is now growing for "restorative practices" that attempt to bring students closer to their communities, sports teams, and schools rather than suspending or expelling those who are troublesome or truant. Young people need to know that if they are caught in possession of drugs, they will find themselves at the mercy of the juvenile and criminal justice systems.

More than half a million Americans, almost a quarter of our total incarcerated population, are behind bars today for drug violations. As soon as teenagers turn eighteen, they are prosecuted as adults and run the risk of serving long mandatory sentences, even for something they believe to be a minor offense. In Illinois, for example, an individual caught in possession of fifteen Ecstasy pills will serve a minimum of four years in state prison.

WHAT'S A PARENT TO DO?

There are no easy answers, but for parents who have requested specifics, here are the steps I suggest:

Step 1: Listen

The first step is to "get real" about drug use by listening to what teens have to tell us about their lives and their feelings. This will guide us toward intelligent, thoughtful action.

A useful venue is the dinner table, but there are many other natural openings for conversation, such as the portrayal of drug use in movies, television, and music. If we can remain as nonjudgmental as possible, teenagers will seek our opinions and guidance. Let them know they can talk freely. Our greatest challenge is to listen and try to help without excessive admonishment. If we become indignant and punitive, teenagers will simply stop talking to us.

Remember that advice is most likely to be heard when it is requested. Realize that teens bring their own experiences to the table, some of which you may not want to hear. But breathe deeply and be grateful when they share these experiences, because this means you have established trust.

Step 2: Learn

Parents and teachers need to take responsibility for learning about the physiological, psychological, and sociological effects of alcohol and other drugs. This involves reading and asking questions.

Familiarize yourself with teenage culture through print and electronic media, especially the Internet. Watch MTV. Learn about the array of drugs available to young people, but be sure your sources are scientifically grounded and balanced. Any source that fails to describe both risks and benefits should be considered suspect.

The Safety First Project website, www.safety1st.org, contains balanced information with a "Drug Facts" section about the effects of today's most prevalent drugs (including abused prescription medication) and alcohol. These easy-to-read fact sheets are in PDF format and available for download anytime. You may order a hard copy by going to www.safety1st.org. There is a list of recommended books on the site as well.

Step 3: Act

It is important to keep teens engaged and busy, especially from 3:00 to 6:00 p.m., when the use of drugs by bored, unsupervised teens is highest. Extracurricular programs such as sports, arts, drama, and other creative activities should be available to all secondary school students, at low or no cost to parents. Become an advocate for such programs in your community and teens' school.

Prevention is fundamentally about creating caring, connected relationships and an open exchange of information. There are no easy answers, just thoughtful conversations. When it comes to opening the ongoing "drug talk," some parents don't know where to begin, but teens often respond better to a "just say know" approach than to the one-sided "just say no" messages they've been hearing all their lives. Many parents today are baby boomers who themselves experimented with drugs in the 1970s and 1980s. The question, "What should I tell my child about my own past drug use?" comes up in every workshop I facilitate. Many parents are uneasy about revealing their own experience, fearing such admissions might open the door to their own teen's experimentation. While you do not need to rehash every detail, it can be very helpful to share your own experiences with your teen because it makes you a more credible confidant. Honesty is usually the best policy in the long run. Just as parents often know or eventually find out when their child is lying, teenagers have a knack for seeing through adults' evasions, half-truths, and hypocrisy. (And eventually one of your siblings or close friends will delight in recounting your "youthful indiscretions" to your eager child.)

Relationships built on trust are key in preventing and countering drug use. While it is tempting to cut through difficult conversations and utilize detection technologies such as urine testing, think long and hard before you demand that your child submit to a drug test. Random, suspicionless school-based drug testing has been shown to be ineffective and often counterproductive. Regarding in-home test kits, researchers at Children's Hospital in

Boston, who studied home drug-testing products, warn that most people are not appropriately educated about the limitations and technical challenges of drug tests (including collection procedures, the potential for misinterpretation, and false-positive/-negative results). They also note unanticipated consequences and the negative effect on parent-child relationships of collecting a urine sample to ascertain drug use (Levy, VanHook, and Knight 2004).

The reality is that a trusting, open relationship with a parent or other respected adult can be the most powerful element in deterring abusive patterns. And trust, once lost, can be hard to regain.

Teenagers need to know that the important adults in their lives are concerned primarily with their safety and that they have someone to turn to when they need help. If they find themselves in a compromising or uncomfortable situation, they need to know we will come to their aid immediately.

Step 4: Lead

PTA leaders and other parent groups often request Safety First speakers for their meetings. Outside "experts" are not necessary. Parent workshops are fundamentally about opening a discussion to share science-based information and to connect with others in the community. Training resources and information about such workshops (such as our DVD, *Safety First: The Workshop*) are available on our website, www.safety1st.org.

The emphasis on safety-oriented strategies does not mean we are giving teens permission to use drugs. It simply affirms that their welfare is our top priority.

Step 5: Help

If you believe a teenager (or anyone else) is having a negative reaction to alcohol and/or other drugs: Do not allow a person who has consumed too much alcohol and has passed out to lie on their back. Many people in this situation have choked on their own vomit and asphyxiated. If you fear something is seriously wrong—if a person is unconscious or having trouble breathing— do not hesitate to phone 911 immediately. The lives of many young people could have been saved if paramedics had been called—or called sooner.

Even when it's not an emergency, there is little more disturbing to a parent than a teenager who is obviously intoxicated, stoned, or high. Many parents want to know how to identify problem use, what to do about it, and when to seek professional help. Concerned parents should start by visiting the Get Help section at www.safety1st.org for a discussion of counseling, treatment, and a list of references and resources. Also, psychologist Stanton Peele, Ph.D., lays out criteria for deciding whether your child needs treatment, and your role as a parent, in his new book, *Addiction Proof Your Child*. For parents concerned that their teen may have a marijuana problem, I also recommend Timmen Cermak's book, *Marijuana: What's a Parent to Believe?* (Peele 2007; Cermak 2003).

Keep in mind there is no one-size-fits-all method for dealing with troubled teens that have alcohol and/or other drug problems. Many of today's well-meaning programs are still unevaluated and inflexible. Be especially leery of boot camp–style programs that can do more harm than good, such as those studied by journalist Maia Szalavitz in her book, *Help at Any Cost: How the Troubled-Teen Industry Cons Parents and Hurts Kids.*

In the end, the healthiest kids, whether or not they experiment with drugs, have parents who are present, loving, and involved. Carla Niño, past president of the California State PTA, gives the following advice: "Trust your instincts, which are to love your kids enough to give them the space to explore and grow, to forgive their mistakes and to accept them for who they are. Kids go through tough times, sometimes seemingly prolonged. Those who make it do so because they're embraced and loved by their families."

31

Pot, Parenting, and Outing Myself

Neal Pollack

When my son was eighteen months old, my best friend from high school came through town on his way to California. He's a respected physician and my most trusted medical counselor. We went back to my office and looked over my stash.

"Dude," he said. "You've got to stop smoking this shit."

"I know," I said. "With the kid around . . ."

"You need to buy a vaporizer."

"Oh."

"You get really high, and you don't mess up your lungs. Also, there's no odor. It's awesome."

My thirty-fifth birthday was approaching, and I needed to get myself a present. So I went vaporizer shopping online. I found a website that sold a sleek, gorgeous ceramic contraption called the Silver Surfer. New terms entered my stoner lexicon: *heat source, mouthpiece, whip, wand*. It would be the greatest present I'd ever give myself. No more apple bongs for me. I had to consume my THC wisely. I was a dad now.

Five years have passed since I bought my Silver Surfer, and I'm still a stoner. In fact, I'm more of a stoner than ever. We now live in Los Angeles, where if you have 100 bucks and an hour of free time on a weekday afternoon, you can get a prescription. According to shocking recent news reports,

361

L.A. has more medical-marijuana dispensaries than Starbuck's franchises. I pass a half-dozen walking from my car on the way to get my hair cut, and a half-dozen more on my way to the grocery store. My arrival in California coincided with the golden age of marijuana culture. The state may be broke, filthy, horribly overpriced, and perpetually on fire, but at least the weed is good and plentiful.

In addition to being a stoner, I'm also still a dad. Actually, I'm kind of a professional dad. I wrote a book about the topic and have been keeping blogs about my son, and about the infinite trials of parenthood, for far too long. Yet I'm rarely allowed to discuss my two favorite pastimes in the same paragraph.

When I did a blog for Parents.com, they explicitly said that I wasn't allowed to discuss drug use. A modified version of this piece, published for an online magazine, brought out comments like, "You are not being there 100 percent for your kid and your family. Even after sundown, the parents have a responsibility to be baseline in case there is an emergency like a fire or a robbery or the kid has an asthma attack."

Well, first of all, my kid doesn't have asthma. Also, do you really expect me to not suck on the vaporizer because I *might get robbed*? Robbers have no idea whether you're stoned or not, and even if they did, they wouldn't care. They'd probably just steal your weed. As for the dangers of fire, we had a fire of sorts in the house once. My wife started something in the fireplace, but it was raining and there was something wrong with the flue. Then she went to fetch the kid from his after-school program purgatory, and the living room started filling up with smoke. Things were getting pretty hot and ashy in there. When I opened the window, a huge gust blew some paintings off the wall and some vases off the fireplace. I ended up putting out the logs with a fire extinguisher and making a huge fucking mess all over the place. My wife came home to find the living room soaked with foam and water and strewn with broken glass. And I wasn't stoned. I can't imagine the outcome would have been any worse if I had been.

It never really occurred to me to give up weed just because I'd become a parent. If anything, parenthood meant that marijuana became a larger part of my life. Whereas before the boy's arrival I'd often leave the house after 9:00 p.m. for a party, or a bar, or a movie, now my social life has contracted. I have no money and all my friends are either parents, and therefore have no time for socializing, or they are single, and therefore have no time for socializing with parents. I rarely leave the house except to sit in a baseball stadium full of drunken *cholos*. A hit off the Silver Surfer and a night of

Turner Classic Movies often seems like an acceptable compromise.

Then the morning comes, and responsibilities rise concurrently. I don't Silver Surf when I have to drive Elijah somewhere, I don't do it when I'm going to be alone with him for any extended period of time, and I'm very rarely baked before sundown. Since all that put together accounts for 97 percent of my parenting time, there's very little crossover with the weed. When crossover time does occur, it's often during a session of what Elijah calls "playing rough." As far as I know, being slightly baked doesn't prevent a guy from wrestling with his son on the bed, or engaging in pretend swordfighting as a character named Alexander the Donut or Genghis Cheeseburger. In fact, one could argue that the pot, while not necessary for these activities, definitely enhances them. Kids don't mind when you say something weird and incongruent while playing. They *prefer* it.

Anyone who says it's impossible to be a stoner and a parent has either never been a stoner, or never been a parent. Weed doesn't prevent me from being a good dad. I never forget anything. Play dates and birthday parties and swim lessons get arranged. Stuff gets bought. The kid takes his vitamins, and I comb the dead skin out of his hair. I'm never neglectful. I'm always attentive and supportive. Sometimes I'm a little grumpy in the mornings, but I've always been a little grumpy in the mornings.

Occasionally, I'll be stoned at the wrong moment, which will lead me to misjudge children's entertainment, like the time I told my wife, "Dude, *64 Zoo Lane* is so *trippy.*" Or I'll try to watch *Best in Show* with my kid because he likes dogs, forgetting that the opening scene has Campbell Scott and Parker Posey in therapy because their dog saw them having sex. I left that scene very quickly, especially when my kid chimed in by saying, "Can I just watch *The Land Before Time?*"

The dominant attitude among stoner dads—and moms—goes like this: Consuming pot is something like watching college football or masturbating, that you used to do all the time, but now will do only if it's convenient and appropriate to the moment. Still, there's a kind of secret, unspoken society. I've been to many backyard family barbecues where another dad and I will discover that pot is a shared habit. The discussion will quickly veer into the familiar. We discuss our favorite varietals. We recount great pot-smoking moments of our past. Someone tells a story about a dude he knows who's got a medical marijuana prescription. Then things invariably wind down the same way:

Random Dad: "So do you have any?"

Me: "No. Do you?"

Random Dad: "Nah. I had some a few weeks ago."

Other Random Dad: "I've got a bunch at home. Give me a call when you want some."

Random Dad: "Cool."

Me: "Cool."

We have these conversations in hushed tones. One night, I posted a tweet that I was going to get high so I could tolerate the school fundraiser, and all night the other dads winked at me in the hallways, asking me how I was feeling. The answer: I'm feeling the same as I would otherwise, except that I'm a little bit stoned. It all starts to feel a little silly. I wish that stoner parents would out themselves. The stoner parents I know are no better or worse than other parents. It makes no difference. It means nothing. And we should stand tall.

Once, pot-smoking parents weren't so controversial. My parents never consumed anything stronger than box wine; my dad was the only soldier in Vietnam, other than maybe John McCain, who didn't do drugs. But even if my parents had stashed a half-ounce of Maui Wowie in the underwear drawer, I can't imagine it would have been a big deal around the house. The country was loose about weed then. No one gave it much of a thought.

When I was a kid, a *Time* magazine cover like the one on December 9, 1996, would never have been possible. An aging Michael Doonesbury sits on his daughter's bed, while Garry Trudeau's talking joint character stands in the background. The text reads, "You tried pot when you were young. Maybe you even inhaled. So now what do you say to your kids?"

Even though I wasn't to be a dad for six years, and hadn't even met my wife yet, I knew then that the culture had turned. Parenting, rather than just being a natural, if challenging, by-product of biology, had somehow become a sacred act. And smoking pot was a violation of its sanctity. Well, I never bought into that, and I'm not alone. Society is right to demand that parents treat their kids with respect and love, and provide them with food, clothing, and shelter. Sainthood, or the perception of sainthood, shouldn't be a requirement.

But I guess this is a good time to answer the question: How *do* I tell my kid about pot? And I can honestly answer: I don't know. I'll probably just be up front about it and say, "Yes, I use it, and I can do that because I'm a grownup." Also, I'll tell him about my prescription, and then I'll explain to him why there are prescriptions, and how cannabis is a great drug for sick people. If he's interested, I can give a brief and entertaining lesson including the history of marijuana laws, and then we can talk about alcohol prohibition, too, and how that relates to the current legal status of marijuana. If nothing else, it'll give me a good excuse to watch *The Untouchables* with my son.

Since I more or less consider weed legal, and suspect that it will be totally legal within my son's lifetime, at least in certain states, I'll tell him that when he's a grownup, he can decide whether he wants to use it, just like he gets to decide about alcohol and prescription drugs. I may even tell him that I only tried it once as a teenager, and ended up trying to tear a phone book in half and then coming home and sobbing in my mother's arms. Clearly, my mind wasn't ready then. It really should be an adult recreation. "But if you do consume marijuana," I'll say, "never, ever drive afterward, preferably not until the next day, and never get into a car with a stoned driver."

I may give him more information than that, or slightly less. But I don't see why I should hide it from him. Do you really think he's not going to find out some other way?

But that's for his teenage years. In the meantime, I'm downplaying my marijuana use. Mostly, it doesn't come up, though there are occasional situations, like when I get a bag of the strong stuff and there's a stench in the house, my wife and I refer to the smell as "Daddy's stinky tea," or, alternatively, we tell him that the dog got sprayed by a skunk.

Then there was the time Elijah found a little pipe on the stairs one day and asked about it. I told him it was for a snowman. When he pointed out that there's no snow where we live, ever, I told him, "I'm mailing it to a friend so he can build a snowman with his kids."

I have a bathroom off my office that I use as a peccadillo repository of sorts. The other day, Elijah used my bathroom because the other one was occupied. He spotted the Silver Surfer on the floor.

"What's that, daddy?" he asked.

"Nothing," I said. "Just something daddy uses to help him with his breath."

"Good," he said. "Your breath stinks sometimes."

"Yeah, well, so does yours," I said.

And so goes the thrilling life of a stoner dad. It all gets done. The kid's in bed by 8:30, his teeth clean, his hair washed, his belly full of nutritious fish oil. He does his homework, we read to him, and the next day's schedule gets planned. Then my boy climbs into his bunk bed and pretends that his stuffed guinea pig is Genghis Khan. I go upstairs to my vaporizer for a little nightcap. And when, twenty minutes or so later, the kid calls out for some fresh water and a little backrub before sleep, I go to him gladly, in a very good mood.

32

Cannabis
Stealth Goddess

Doug Rushkoff

Back around the time he was dying, Timothy Leary kept returning to an odd little game where he'd ask people to rank their drugs. Most of us assumed it was the illness (or the morphine) getting the best of him, because he just kept doing it with everyone.

"Come on, sit down on the bed," he'd say to whoever happened to be visiting that day. "Get a pen, and list the drugs in order."

And most people put them in order of least to most intoxicating, addictive, intense, or dangerous. You know—sugar, caffeine, nicotine, pot, alcohol, coke, speed, acid, heroin, DMT . . . or something along those lines, depending on a person's individual predilections. There was no "right" answer; some people even created multiple axes, with hallucinogens along one line and opiates on another.

It's an interesting little thought experiment, and it would be as foolish to underestimate its depth as to underestimate the depth of Leary's own impact on drug culture. For once you get over the official medically or socially acceptable understanding of how all these drugs should be ranked, you come down to your own. For the bulimic, I imagine glucose would seem a more devastating opponent than opium. Many an alcoholic can still drop acid with less personal risk than taking a single sip of vodka. Others might put any opiate in front of a psychedelic, amphetamine over an opiate, or nitrous oxide and crack at precisely the same level.

Once I had a good year or two to think about it, I realized that for me the drug that would go on top of the list—the "most" whatever-it-is-we-think-of-as-most—is pot. Yes, the pot of my youth as much as the hydroponic subspeciated pot of today's generation. Pot is the most demanding of drug mistresses—more than even LSD or DMT, whose own voices, though stronger in the moment, tend to wear off once the drug has done its thing. True, if you take acid you'll never be the same; you'll simply get used to the fact that your worldview is arbitrary. But LSD doesn't call for you. LSD doesn't get pissed off if you spend too long away from it. LSD may change your life, but it doesn't *ask* you to.

Pot is different. It's subtle and seemingly innocuous, but it forces a broadly critical examination of who one is, where one is going, and why. Like no other chemical, it stops time, forcing the question of why one is in motion in the first place. In this sense, pot is the most powerful drug on the block.

Sure, smoking crack can be as permanently devastating as getting whacked in the head by one of its addicts. But smoking pot is more like confronting famed reggae toker Bob Marley who, while singing peacefully about "three little birds," also means to foment a "movement of ja people" more devastating to the way you live than a mere mugging. *Exodus,* his landmark album, evokes the biblical delivery from slavery. For Marley, this is both the literal release of the repressed from their bondage, and the mental release of the repressors from the exploitation to which they have become addicted.

This is the truest sense in which marijuana serves as a gateway drug. It's not (just) the entry point to a world of more potent plants and chemicals; it is the gateway to a mind-set liberated from arbitrarily repressive constructs. For the poor, destitute, or exploited, pot offers the temporary experience of grace, as well as a vision of another, more just society. The quest for immediate relief or revenge gives way to the knowledge that repression itself is a dance that the repressor must ultimately lose. The world goes around, the sun will come up another day.

For members of the repressive society—and this means most of the people with access to or interest in an essay like this—pot serves as a gateway to this same knowledge. The job, money, security, or success to which one has been aspiring is, itself, delusional and based on the exploitation of someone else. Straight life is dualism: the zero-sum game of scarce resources, winners and losers, college admissions, test scores, job applications, and making "something" of oneself. Stoned life is the knowledge that none of this really matters, and that any effort expended in the pursuit of these false goals usually involves some amount of bearing down, forcing oneself, or even resorting to treachery.

For a white kid, getting stoned means seeing the world as the Native Americans did. The Earth isn't just something you pave over for cars to move faster. Animals aren't made of "meat." And the guy who mops up after you at the high school cafeteria wasn't born a janitor. You live in the same world he does. The longer you're unable to see it, the uglier it's going to be for you when you do. Dig?

I had always assumed there was only one possible response to pot's message, and that was to give up. Either panic, completely quit smoking, and choose the straight man's hallucination of progress and purpose, or maintain a relationship with marijuana with the understanding that certain activities and attitudes will have to change. Yes, marijuana is a relationship drug. I don't mean that it's a medium through which we relate to others, but that it's a drug with which one ends up having a relationship.

Like a girlfriend or boyfriend who sees the "real" you, marijuana desperately wants you to shed the artifacts of the Western European colonialists among whom you live, and just stop where you are. Every action has a reaction. Assess the impact. What happens when you throw that plastic bottle in the trash? Where and under what conditions was this videogame cartridge assembled? Which side of what equations am I on?

And even if you make it through those moments of self-questioning and engagement, the next time you're stoned, they'll come back. The longer you wait to toke up again, the more surprisingly hard pot will come down on you once you're fully stoned. If you haven't made the adjustments she's requested from you, she'll want to know why. Yes, pot will give you the greatest gifts she has to offer—but she wants something in return. She wants your soul

Just as Marley's music forces listeners to decide whose side they're on, marijuana forces a kind of duality on its users: live straight, or live stoned. You're either with me or against me. Oppressor or oppressed. Even if the place the stoner goes is delightfully nondual, this nondual place is decidedly different from the duality in which he or she is living the rest of the time. Stoned vs. nonstoned is about as dual as it gets. Even the folks who take a bong hit first thing in the morning know what it's like to wake up straight. That's why they're taking the hit. They've agreed to stay with her—and chances are they're no longer capable of oppressing anybody.

In short, pot raises consciousness, creates a relationship, and—

immediately after its peak—forces a self-evaluation. That's the step that really can't be avoided. Looking outward merely changes the critical inventory from things *intended* to persons *impacted*. Only another hit can delay the inevitable look within, and the higher you go, the more intense a self-examination will be demanded once you crest.

None of this has to be painful or paranoid, of course. If you're living a virtuous life, if you don't have slaughterhouse meat sitting on the counter or Mexicans in the backyard blowing leaves into piles for three bucks an hour, you may not have to confront anything awful at all. If you're a permaculture farmer, a massage therapist, or a folk musician, you're already operating in a pretty hemp-compatible way. Most kids and students are so hardwired by media and adolescence to think of themselves as the repressed that they don't even have room to consider their own complicity in maintaining class structure or injustice. For them, peaking simply means the discussion will turn from how good the pot is to how they're going to go about finding some more.

Paranoia is reserved for the elder, more experienced users—and at that, only the ones who both hear pot's messages and repeatedly refuse to comply. Who in their right minds would *change their lives* to conform to what they were thinking when they were *stoned*? The only time it really seems to matter is when one is stoned, and, well—it's probably just because pot is so much stronger these days, or because I'm older now and really shouldn't be taking drugs anyway.

After a few hundred conversations on precisely this subject with pot users and ex-users alike, I've come to a conclusion about the mechanism behind pot's ability to raise and question conscience—particularly in older, more experienced users. To put it most simply, *pot stops time*. Or at least it creates the illusion that time has ceased to move forward. When you are stoned, you are no longer in motion. Even if you are moving, you are no longer moving *toward* something—but simply *moving*.

The lean-forward of your directed, intentional life ceases. You are still doing what you are doing, but the goal no longer exists. The simplest effect of this time-stoppage is to bring focus to the task at hand. There is no goal; there is only process. The stoned farmer isn't growing pumpkins; he is planting a seed—or, better, clearing dirt with his finger, placing the seed in the impression left behind, and covering it with fresh soil. Then doing it again, with Zenlike attention to detail, texture, and grace. The act in this moment is all there is.

Likewise, however, once time is removed from the equation, goals can no longer be used to rationalize your tactics. Without ends, no "means" can be justified. They must be judged on their own merit. So what are you doing?

For those accustomed to avoiding life's more existential dilemmas by busying themselves with activity, this slipping out of sequential time can be enough to induce some serious psychic trauma. For them, to just *be* is hard enough. Especially if they've been avoiding who they are for a long while. (Interestingly, I don't see this happening often in first-time users, however old or even tragically unethical in their daily pursuits. It's as if pot will induce this set of reactions only in a person with whom she has had a long-term relationship or extended series of flings. Only the people she really cares about.)

Kids are immune to this effect. Like baby turtles on the beach hatching from their eggs and running instinctually toward the water, kids have a forward momentum intrinsic to their very being. A sixteen-year-old is leaning forward just for the very fact that he's not full-grown. Adults, however, make their own momentum. If adults are moving toward anything other than death (or maybe childbirth), it's by their own design and a product of their active will. Stoned, however, time stops. The self-generated momentum ceases, and whatever that motion was helping hide comes to the surface.

Most users experience this on a simple, literal level. They think of it as if marijuana is a little angry that they've been working so hard and taking so little time to enjoy her offerings. They feel that marijuana is letting them know that they need to balance the work/play ratio a bit better; they've become too serious. Some who get this message decide pot is a "bad influence," urging them to be more decadent, earn less money, or make some other irresponsible decision. It's enough to make many adults quit.

People who think of themselves as committed artists, activists, or intellectuals often have a more layered experience of this same phenomenon. The marijuana session becomes an invitation to stop and evaluate the integrity of their work or its consistency with purported intentions. It's the moment that the upcoming gallery show means less than the paint on the canvas or the sensory quality of the image. And it's a dangerous moment for any artists already struggling with their motives or even just plain motivation. In fact, in my own informal polling, the impact of marijuana on motivation was second only to "paranoid effects" as a reason for quitting the drug altogether.

Given all this, what I had most trouble understanding were the kinds of people—old friends from my college days, for instance—who could work as stockbrokers or corporate lawyers all day for months on end, and then charter a jet out to a rock concert or the Burning Man festival and smoke pot for a week. Not only did they seem capable of surviving pot's introspective zone with nary a guilty flush, they could go back to work Monday morning and continue to push "interest free" mortgages or other shamelessly predatory financial instruments.

I finally decided to spend a weekend with them to figure out their formula for maintaining such a decidedly arm's-length relationship with a drug that so many others experience as all-or-nothing. And the answer turned out to be a second drug, cocaine (actually coke mixed with methamphetamine—"speed"), that they were using along with the pot. No big wonder, then, how they avoided the timelessness and purposelessness of pot: just create some fake time with speed and synthetic purpose with cocaine. They wrestled pot to the ground and turned her into an unwilling party drug. I can only hope she gets a few of these people alone some day.

But for me and countless others who've taken the time to think about it, pot is a drug that requires a level of respect, trepidation, and devotion that most people aren't prepared or expecting to give her. And while regular use can dampen the immediately felt impact of pot's invitation to exchange promise for process, this doesn't mean the drug isn't making its very presence known.

Take the work of two of Hollywood's most famous daily pot smokers, the late Robert Altman and Oliver Stone. Altman's movies imitate the stoned mind wandering from synchronicity to synchronicity, contenting themselves with pattern recognition and requiring their narrative-bound audiences to do the same. Stone's, on the other hand, bring us with him into the paranoid scenarios of the stoned mind daring itself into increasingly nightmarish territory—as if the ability to play in these regions somehow purges them of their power. Given his almost obsessive return to this dark side, the paranoid vision seems only to be gaining more hold over his awareness. Then again, it's hard to spend tens of millions of dollars on a piece of violent entertainment without the spirit of weed objecting on some level.

Which all goes back to my initial sense that marijuana is the stealth queen of all drugs. Any user knows how big a wallop LSD or DMT is going to deliver and typically prepares accordingly. A difficult trip may not be expected, but it's not completely unexpected, either. Marijuana, on the other hand, presents a peculiarly deep set of contradictions for its users—particularly for adults, and particularly for those who have the privilege of living with a disproportionate share of the world's riches. By stopping time, pot offers, just like an orgasm, a little preview of death—and you know what they say about a rich man, a camel, and the eye of a needle.

Is it coincidence that this same genus very likely holds answers to our energy and environmental challenges? Hemp agriculture could likely solve both the energy and CO_2 crises at the same time, with an astoundingly good biomass-to-fuel ratio, excellent carbon absorption, and the *opposite* of topsoil depletion.

At the very least, we should render unto marijuana the respect this plant drug deserves. Cannabis, in both its function on the psyche and its potential uses on the planet, offers us a new relationship to the death and decay so many of us spend so much time avoiding. Maybe a few more people need to have some harrowing experiences with her to realize this.

33

Gardener's Rights, Forgetting, and Co-Evolution

An Interview with Michael Pollan

Julie Holland, M.D.

JULIE HOLLAND: Can we start with the catnip story?

MICHAEL POLLAN: I always kept a little patch of catnip in my garden for my old tomcat, Frank, who really liked it. It's not a very difficult plant to grow. The patch was hard to miss, because it was so shrubby. But every evening around five or six o'clock, just around the time that I was going to the garden to harvest something for dinner, Frank would come down there and look at me. What he wanted to know was where that catnip was, because he managed to forget every single night. And I would point it out to him or sometimes bring him over to it, and then he would pull some leaves off, sniff them, eat them, and start rolling in the grass. He was clearly having a powerful drug experience. Then he would sneak away and sleep it off somewhere.

But the interesting thing was, as much as this became part of his daily routine, he could not remember where the catnip was. And it occurred to me that this might be a kind of evolutionary strategy on the part of the plant: instead of killing the pest, it would just really confuse it. Killing pests can be counterproductive, because they breed or select for resistance very quickly. This happens with a lot of poisonous types of plants, as it does with pesticides. But if the plant merely confuses the pests or disables their memory, it can defend itself against them overindulging. Pure speculation, as I say in the book. It occurred to me that it might help explain what's happening with cannabis, which of course also disables memory.

JULIE: So THC could potentially protect the plant from pests by discombobulating them so they forget where they found it?

MICHAEL: It potentially is doing that. The big question is why plants would evolve very specific chemical compounds that have this strange effect on the mental processes of mammals, and that's one theory that I came up with to explain it. There is also, of course, the pure-chance theory. Maybe the THC is doing something else entirely, like protecting the plant from UV rays or performing some other function for the plant, or maybe it does indeed kill insects. But it just so happens that THC also unlocks this particular receptor network in humans.

JULIE: I am very interested in the idea that we co-evolved with cannabis on the Earth for ten thousand years and that we've got receptors for this plant substance inside our brains, that we've got cannabinoids and anandamide inside us. You've written about cannabis helping you forget as sort of a helpful strategy or adaptation, and there's a line in *Botany of Desire* about forgetting as a prerequisite to human happiness and mental health. I guess anandamide is our brain's own drug for coping and enduring. It's not just the benefits of forgetting—what's that line, "Do you really want to remember every face you saw on the subway this morning?"

MICHAEL: Yes, Raphael Mechoulam keyed me in to that idea. We understand the evolutionary utility of memory, but we don't often think about the utility of forgetting. And it was that comment by him that made me realize that it's almost as important to be able to forget as it is to remember. Forgetting, in this case, isn't just a fading of the memory, but an active process for editing, because we take in far more information than it would be useful to retain. There's just so much detail in our visual field (not to mention the other senses) at any given moment that a lot of what our brains are doing is figuring out what is worth remembering, what can be shucked, and what should just be remembered for a little while and then let go. So we need some sort of mechanism for doing it, and Mechoulam's speculation was that one of the functions of anandamide would be to help us prune the sensory data of everyday life, short-term memory in particular. I found that a very persuasive theory, and it certainly gels with the experience of a brain on marijuana, because things that happened just minutes ago are gone, and I think that has a lot to do with the texture of the experience.

JULIE: There's no doubt that short-term working memory is temporarily diminished when somebody gets high. But what I think is enjoyable to people is this idea of dehabituation, that they're seeing things with fresh eyes. Memory is the enemy of wonder. When people get high, everything is new and intense because of this forgetting, because it's dehabituated.

MICHAEL: It's a childlike way of looking at the world—Wordsworth's child. The child sees everything for the first time; and, of course, to see things for the first time, you have to have forgotten that you've seen them before. So forgetting is very important to the experience of awe or wonder.

JULIE: It aesthetisizes commonplace things. When something is sort of distanced or estranged, it somehow becomes more beautiful.

MICHAEL: It italicizes it, in a way. You set it apart, and you actually see it. It gives a freshness to things that we take for granted all the time. I think it's definitely a part of all drug experiences in one way or another, but marijuana seems to have the ability to do this with ordinary things, putting them up on a pedestal.

JULIE: That sort of perception provides breaks in your mental habits, provides the power to alter mental constructs, and offers new ways of looking at things, so drugs can then function as "cultural mutagens," a phrase you use.

MICHAEL: Looking at the whole history of drugs and culture—whether you're talking about music, or art, or writing—there's this very rich tradition of artists who have availed themselves of various drugs and have attributed great insight or creativity to their experience with those drugs. And one of the mechanisms that might explain this is that the drugs shift ordinary perception, allowing you to see things from a new perspective, and that is kind of mutagenic; it triggers change.

I used that metaphor with some care because, obviously, 99.9 percent of the time, drug experiences are not making any contribution to culture whatsoever, and they're usually a complete waste of time and can also lead to all sorts of problems. So I liken them to mutations: you put out enough novelty in the world in the form of insider experience, and some of it is bound to be really productive, in the same way that if you put enough mutations into a gene or an organism, some of them are going to produce incredible advances, but most of them will be maladaptive. That's the other reason why I thought *mutagenicity* was the right term. It's not as if there's a one-to-one relationship—you try this, and you're going to have an amazing artistic experience. I think the odds are probably the other way.

JULIE: So speaking of metaphors, you describe cannabis buds as perpetually sexually frustrated, ever-lengthening flowers. I feel like our culture is so separated from nature now that it's a big part of our problem. This striving flower is a great metaphor for our reaching out, wanting more—more meaning, searching for spirituality, though half the time we settle for materialism or consumerism. What do you think we can do to reconnect more with nature? Do you see plant-based medicines being helpful?

MICHAEL: I think they are. We have this inbred idea of nature and culture as opposed to each other, with mind and body on opposite sides of the big divide. One of the things that's really striking to me about all plant mood-changing substances is that idea. If things out in the natural world can change the content of your thoughts, can you really say that matter is on one side and this thing called spirit on the other? It really suggests that the categories are messier and more intertwined than we'd like to think.

There's a whole tradition in the West of suppressing plant-based drugs and plant-based knowledge. That's what the story of the Garden of Eden is all about. It wasn't the content of the knowledge that Eve got in the garden that was the problem; it was that she got it from a plant. A big part of earlier religions, which often had a drug component to them, was that there was wisdom in nature, and consuming natural substances was how you acquired wisdom. That was a very threatening idea to monotheism, which wanted to have this one God up in the sky; it wanted to take our eyes off of nature as a place where we might find wisdom, comfort, and so forth.

The whole Judeo-Christian tradition has a history of a strong anti-nature component. Nature is to be subdued, nature is what we are different from: we distinguish ourselves from animals. It's always about inserting that distance between us and the other animals, or us and the trees, because people used to worship trees. So, to the extent that you wanted to establish this new kind of God, you had to reject nature and natural experiences of all different kinds. So I do think there is potential in returning to this appreciation of the fact that our consciousnesses can be affected by the plant world, not to mention the fungal world.

JULIE: I love the idea of a garden being a place of sacraments. In *Botany of Desire,* you wrote, "Letting nature have her way with us now and again brings our upward gaze back down to earth." This idea of nature as teacher and as healer, of a plant as medicine, is so basic to our culture, but we've gotten away from that to a large extent.

MICHAEL: Yes, and there are many reasons for that. One is the religious tradition and another is the patent laws.

JULIE: You can't help but blame Big Pharma to some extent.

MICHAEL: Well, the fact is that the drugs that are nearest at hand and most common, the plant drugs, can't get past Big Pharma. There is an investment that goes into studying their value, and it is always the same—the synthetic drug is better, newer, and fresher. People forget that LSD is synthesized from a mold that grows on rye, and a great many drugs have been created in that way. Opium is another great example. So we denigrate those drugs by saying they're not as pure; we don't know exactly what's in them. There's a profit motive in belittling what the plant world gives us.

JULIE: It reminds me of *In Defense of Food,* where you talk about food being reduced to its building blocks.

MICHAEL: It's a reductive approach.

JULIE: And Big Pharma chooses to be reductive over something more complex and whole, like a plant.

MICHAEL: That's the real issue with THC and cannabinol, and there are others too.

JULIE: Well, anybody who has taken a pharmaceutical THC pill will tell you, it doesn't really feel like that experience is similar to smoking pot.

MICHAEL: Yes, that's right, and it's different in important ways. It probably has to do with various energies between the different compounds or just simply various combinations, but our science has trouble embracing that kind of complexity. It really needs to break things down into molecules for the purpose of a study, but plants really are more than the sum of their chemical parts. And our efforts to tease out the single active ingredient, whether it's a vitamin in carrots, or a drug in leaves, usually don't work out, because these things are really complicated. Reductiveness also has a negative effect when you look at the white-powder drugs. Cultures in South America have a very healthy relationship to the cocoa leaves.

JULIE: They will just chew a whole leaf.

MICHAEL: Or they will make tea. From the reductive perspective, that is the same thing as smoking crack, but, of course, it isn't. There are other things going on in the leaves: the psychoactive compounds are diluted in various ways with other compounds. It's a very different thing, and to say we're talking about the same molecule in all instances is probably false.

JULIE: I can think of one example where just giving a single molecule did seem to create a good experience: in the Johns Hopkins study, where they administered psilocybin, as opposed to whole mushrooms, to healthy subjects who had rich spiritual lives. They were able to show that they could engender a mystical state with psilocybin.

When you mentioned fungus before, there are certainly plenty of plants that are able to change our consciousness, like mushrooms or cannabis.

Many people think of plants as spiritual teachers, and as healers, which naturally leads us into the whole medical marijuana issue.

MICHAEL: I think in a metaphorical way, they do teach us, but I don't think they set out to teach us. There's a lot we can learn from them, and whether it's spiritual, again that goes to the separation of spirit and matter, which I don't buy. People mean many different things when they talk about spirit. I get really uncomfortable around terms like *spiritual*, because I'm not sure what it means.

JULIE: Well, one aspect of spirituality is to be present, to focus on the here and now, which I think cannabis can help people do. So this idea of "here and now" taking us away from the "then and there" of Christian salvation, the transcendence and the Power of Now—I don't know if you are interested in any of that.

MICHAEL: I've written about that idea of "here and now" a lot, and, in fact, in my architecture book I did that too. I wrote a book called *A Place of My Own,* and there was a chapter about foundations in which I talked a lot about that idea of here and now, and how there's a tension between those two sets of values. Both of them are present, usually.

JULIE: Do you think it's safe to say that cannabis can sometimes help place you in the "now"?

MICHAEL: Yes, I think it has the effect of absorbing you in the here and now—partly by increasing this forgetting function we were talking about, and also by creating a really single-minded focus on whatever is in front of you. I think that is a very powerful thing. Also, it's not a desiring drug, it's a satisfying drug, and I really believe in that distinction. Have you ever read David Lenson's books?

JULIE: Sure, *On Drugs.*

MICHAEL: I think it's just full of brilliant ideas. It's a terrific book and really has never gotten the recognition it deserved. He compares marijuana to cocaine. Cocaine is a desiring drug, always about the next high; it really is the consumer-culture drug, where satisfaction is just over the next horizon. One more purchase, one more snort. And marijuana is like, "Hey, whatever's here is fine."

JULIE: And also, "No, thanks, I'm good. I've had enough."

MICHAEL: Exactly. And it's part of the reason why the go-getter culture frowns on potheads: they don't want enough, they don't buy enough.

JULIE: Pot ends up being subversive because it doesn't move that agenda forward.

So, what do you think of the California medical marijuana situation?

MICHAEL: It's a mixed bag. It's wonderful to see it normalized and regularized for a lot of people. I know many people who have their couple of plants, and it's not a big deal. It gives you a taste of what a sane drug policy might look like. On the other hand, there is incredible abuse. A great number of people are pretending to be medical marijuana growers or sellers when they're not. And they're abusing the system in a way that I think may lead to the collapse of this whole regime, and the blame will be on them. It won't be on the DEA.

JULIE: I totally agree. I hope that California understands that the rest of the country is watching them to see how they do. This is a big experiment, and they're bushwhacking and leading the way, and I really don't want them to screw up.

MICHAEL: There's so much money in this, and the temptation is so great. I just worry that they're going to ruin this experiment, and California's failure will be used to keep it from happening anywhere else.*

JULIE: I want to talk to you about the politics of gardening. You wrote about victory gardens in the October 9, 2008, issue of the *New York Times* magazine. There's a real grow revolution happening now, with people growing their own pot, partly because these hybrids are so easy to grow indoors. I think it helps people feel self-sufficient and self-determined.

MICHAEL: And it's safer in various ways. They aren't having to transport things in public conveyances. In a way, this is how it should work. It also takes cannabis out of commerce in very healthy manner, given the drug laws we have. So I do think there's something very satisfactory about growing it yourself, growing your own drugs and enlisting yourself in your care and not depending on other people.

JULIE: When I'm weeding my garden, it makes me feel powerful: this plant can stay, this weed has to go. I'm in charge, like a bouncer. And when the government steps in and tells us what we can grow in our gardens and

---

*In November of 2010 California will vote on whether to legalize marijuana for recreational use.

what we can put in our bodies, it just seems to me that it's out of their jurisdiction. And having our own gardens helps us take some responsibility for the climate crisis.

MICHAEL: There is a literal value in terms of helping the climate. But part of this situation is the specialist mindset, depending on others to take care of your problems. To the extent that gardens teach that you can do things on your own, that the real prerequisite for solving this climate problem is figuring out a different way to live, taking up gardening is a valuable skill we're going to need when things get bad.

JULIE: Where do you see hemp fitting into this? Not only is hemp-seed oil good for your body, but hemp as fuel could be very good for the environment.

MICHAEL: I don't know that much about it, but I think it's a shame that we haven't researched what this very unusual and useful fiber can do. I think for paper it's got good potential. I have no idea if there is a potential for ethanol.

JULIE: It seems that it does have the potential to be used as fuel. We are using corn now as an energy source for everything; hemp could be an upgrade from corn.

MICHAEL: Yes and no. You still need agricultural land to do it, and I think one of the issues with ethanol is that we are using some of our best agricultural land to feed our cars rather than our people. It may be that hemp could grow in places where corn can't grow, in marshy lands. But in general, it has the same problems: it needs tilled land to grow in. It's not like grass, which can grow anywhere.

JULIE: Where do you see cannabis and hemp fitting into "going green"? Doesn't it fit an organic model more than an industrial model?

MICHAEL: There's nothing inherently green about it; look at all the technology and fertilizers used to grow it right now in a lot of places. So I don't see it fitting one model more than the other. I'm sure there are contributions that hemp could make, and I think the universities should be paying attention, studying and analyzing it. I think the lack of research on both hemp and marijuana, given their potential, is criminal.

JULIE: When you tried sativa in Amsterdam, you said that you felt "neither stupid nor paranoid."

MICHAEL: Yes, but I don't know how much of that was due to the chemistry versus the context. You're smoking in a place where it's legal, so if there were any paranoia, it would likely be diminished. Research has talked about setting, and I think people underestimate just how important it is. But it also seems likely to me that there are real differences in the nature of the experience between the two strains, indica and sativa, and depending on the kind of work people do, they tend to like one more than the other. They may have physical aches and pains that they are trying to relieve. And indica, I think, has more CBD in it, and maybe that would explain why it helps. But of course, expectation plays a part in this too, because when people come to expect something from a drug, they're going to get it.

JULIE: Can you talk a little bit about our government's drug policy, especially in terms of intervening with our gardening?

MICHAEL: I think as an adult, you should be free to grow anything you want on your own property as long as you're not taking it other places. The idea that the government can tell you what you can grow in your garden, strikes me in a visceral way as wrong. Our right to privacy should include that.

JULIE: I wanted to thank you for mentioning asset forfeiture and the prisoners of the drug war in *Botany of Desire*. I know it was an aside, but it's an important issue. If you grow cannabis, can you lose your house?

MICHAEL: Yes, you can, and people don't realize that. The kind of seeds that you choose to plant in your garden could result in the complete loss of your house and your property. And you don't even have to plant it; someone else could plant it on your property. They don't even have to tie the plant to you to seek forfeiture of the asset. So a stranger could plant it, or your kid could plant it, and you could lose your house.

JULIE: You talked about Frank waiting until five o'clock to find the catnip. There's something ritualized in that. He could control himself and wait. He could keep it in check.

MICHAEL: Well, yes. He had other work to do during the day. He wasn't getting high at breakfast.

34
Cannabis, Business, and Philanthropy
An Interview with Peter Lewis

Julie Holland, M.D.

JULIE Holland: You're a well-known philanthropist. You're a major supporter of the Guggenheim Museum and of Princeton and Case Western Reserve Universities. But you've also given very generous donations to the ACLU and the Marijuana Policy Project. Why?

PETER Lewis: Well, I have thought for a long time that prohibition of marijuana is absurd, and the manifestations of that prohibition are bad for our society at almost every level. Therefore, if I can do something to help have marijuana regulated similarly to alcohol, which is my objective, then I will be making an enormous contribution to the quality of life in my country.

JULIE: What do you think about the amount of money we're spending to enforce marijuana prohibition?

PETER: On its face, based on examination of any set of facts, it is a gross waste of money. Its only practical rationale is to imprison certain segments of the population so the jailers can make a living.

JULIE: What do you think about the possibility of our country making money from cannabis, and taxing it, instead of spending billions to enforce the drug laws?

PETER: It takes an idiot not to do it.

JULIE: I know! Haven't these guys crunched the numbers?

PETER: Perhaps they don't really understand what they're doing. Actually, I think that prosecutors, jailers, and jail-builders are very influential in the process of keeping prohibition in place.

JULIE: The prison-industrial complex needs to keep itself going?

PETER: Yes. And then there is all this religious crap that goes on, which I don't relate to. There is no logical rationale. One has to dream up illogical rationalizations.

JULIE: Right. Certainly, from a financial point of view it makes no sense.

PETER: From any point of view it makes no sense! When you outlaw behaviors that people engage in whether they're outlawed or not, it just makes liars out of everyone—whether it's prostitution or gambling, whatever. It's insanity, but it goes on. It's just terrible.

JULIE: I'm afraid it's our puritanical roots showing. Now, you have sort of "outed" yourself to some degree as a pot smoker, true?

PETER: Yes.

JULIE: Why did you do that?

PETER: Well, it happened in two phases. First there was an article about me in *Fortune* magazine. The reporter found out from a former employee that I smoked, and she put it into the article, so that was the first time. It said that I was a functioning pothead, but it was complimentary about my business skills. That was fifteen years ago, maybe. And then nine years ago, I was going to New Zealand on holiday, and I was arrested at the Aukland airport with some marijuana in my briefcase. That got a lot of publicity.

JULIE: Have you continued to be open about your pot smoking, or are you not comfortable talking about it?

PETER: I can talk about my experience of smoking pot; I don't know if I'd say when I did it.

JULIE: I guess I'm just wondering how you feel it's helped you or hurt you in terms of running a business.

PETER: It helped me a lot. Running a business turns out to be a pretty lonely thing to do. Marijuana would help me commune with myself. It would turn my daily collection of information into some kind of understanding of what was really going on—what the key components were, what the emotional components were. It made me better at my job. Except for activities that require physical dexterity like playing tennis, I think it basically helped me be better at almost anything I ever did.

JULIE: I don't want to put words in your mouth, and I hate to use the expression "outside the box," but I am wondering if your pot smoking helped you run Progressive Insurance Company, to come up with new ways to do things, perhaps that other people hadn't thought of?

PETER: Well, Progressive made its success by operating a car insurance business differently from anyone else who operated a car insurance business. And the ideas that went into making it different . . . I'll say this: marijuana kept me open to craziness and to new ideas, to stuff that no one ever thought about before. It kept me open to doing things that everybody else said you shouldn't do.

JULIE: Did it hurt you in business at all? Did it hurt you interpersonally, or in how you ran the business?

PETER: Oh, I don't think so at all. I think it helped me interpersonally, in a major way. I think it made me a much better manager. I didn't begin using pot until my mid-forties. I was introduced to it by my children. And I changed . . . It was a bad time. I had separated from my wife, gotten divorced, and I started in psychotherapy, so I can't attribute everything to pot, but I became much more sensitive to the importance of emotions, to considering and managing around the way people feel. And we built a company that was one hundred people when I took it over that is now twenty-seven thousand people.

JULIE: Wow . . . Do you still smoke?

PETER: From time to time. I am like millions of other marijuana smokers for whom it is a joyful, life-enhancing substance. That is why, more than thirty years later, I continue to use marijuana occasionally, privately and responsibly.

For me, marijuana relaxes, lessens anxiety, connects feelings to thoughts, enhances sensuality, stimulates appetites, and makes me enjoy being by myself. Smoking marijuana has helped me accomplish what I set out to do, made me easier to be with and easier on myself. It allows me to be more accepting of, and caring for, other people.

Marijuana being illegal is a tragedy I want to correct. Most people at least occasionally use some substance to alter their consciousness, of which marijuana may be the most benign. Alcohol is more disorienting to the mind and damaging to the body, and more likely to provoke violence. The enforcement of marijuana prohibition is racially discriminatory, expensive, and ineffective.

Marijuana is excellent medicine for appetite enhancement, glaucoma, multiple sclerosis, and much, much more. I advocate and support efforts to legalize marijuana, and to regulate and tax it in the same way that alcohol is. I feel deeply that helping achieve this objective is one of the best contributions I can make to the well-being of our great country.

JULIE: Can you put a price tag on your philanthropy? How much have you spent?

PETER: I've probably given away about $400 million. And I was instrumental in forming the Center for American Progress four years ago. I've been supporting politically progressive efforts for a long while now.

JULIE: Well, I truly appreciate all your efforts, and I want to thank you for all you've done. I hope that your altruism will inspire others to get more politically involved.

35
Thots on Pot

Jeremy Wolff

The simplest answer to the complex question of what pot does is dishabitu-ation. It delinks the habits of mind. This change takes place at a profound and basic level, and its effects are thus multifarious and unlimited. Different pot at different times can, as a drug experience, feel like acid, booze, speed, or smack. And the range of its psychological effects is mirrored by its mate-rial usefulness: the practical uses of hemp, as fiber, food, and pharmacy, are in seamless parallel with human needs.

Hemp and reefer: material and spiritual, physical and psychological, male and female: everywhere you look, cannabis's intersection with humans is about dualities in unity. Oppositions basic to the human psyche are appar-ent, by analogy or actual function, in this single plant. How we view pot and its powers reveals how we choose to see: in wholeness or in separation.

Dishabituation is the blurring of paths, which, like habits, are places you have been before, routes you can follow without thinking, according to unreflected sense cues and existing neural patterns. These paths exist if we follow unconsciously; search for them and they scatter, unrecognizable and meaningless. Stoned, you see the woods and the world differently. The path is not apparent; you discover things you have passed by, but you are lost.

We are creatures of habit: literally, of clothing, costume, custom. Pot removes the clothing of the mind, the literal habits of thought. The panic when we resist is like holding on to the last garment being pulled off us. We are naked before pot, and what we see first is ourselves. Primary social inhibitions are revealed by mindless munchies and tension-releasing laughter. In the body, pot can relax and release held energy, or heighten tension and contraction due to overawareness of everything, including breathing. In the mind, perception becomes fresh, new seeming, profound. Thoughts, too, are bound or released in an excess of meaning, from paranoia to enthusiasm.

Pot facilitates intuition, the dishabituation of thought. But the thing about insights from pot is, you're always stoned when you get them. A stoned thought, no matter how majestic, is subject to self-ridicule. What you see, and learn, you have to hold with faith. This is the uncertainty principle.

Dishabituation changes polarity, the direction of the prevailing winds. This altered brain-state has a synchronous relation to human countercultural styles. Pot could never be an opiate of the masses. Unlike the numbness of rum or the work-uses of coffee, Coke, and cigarettes, it won't keep the machines running. Nomadic cultures revered pot because it was a tool for change—for making it and for dealing with it: an unsettler. China was first the Land of Hemp and Mulberry, but as its civilization crystallized, cannabis use was discouraged in favor of opium, more likely to keep the kids down on the farm. Pot won't change you physically—there is almost no physical response, no lethal dose. But in its revelation of the habitual and the cultural, it can change your social identity and your self-perception, which are the origins of its subversion.

Pot was the Be Here Now and Back to Nature drug: in cannabis's dishabituation of the senses is the reenchantment of our perceptions of nature. For the beats and hippies, pot was a release into acoustic space from the visual conformity of the straight culture of the 1950s: the primal pot experience was closing your eyes to hear and feel the music. Enchantment is literally "singing into"—adding depth and resonance to insights, making them felt, physical, and moving. At the dawn of the TV Age, as most information comes in via eyeballs closely focused on screens, pot reminds us of the surrounding senses of sound and touch and space. In the space age, pot reveals the depth of space and not just its distance, and the spaciousness of the present, stilling the reel of unrolling time.

In these current testosterone times (SUVs, Timberlands, mountain bikes, shooter games, pitbulls, pro wrestling, Kalashnikovs), pot's dishabituation appears essentially feminine or yin in style. The rocket-shaped technologies to leave the planet and to destroy the planet have evolved simultaneously, in an instant of geologic time. This is the millennial, macrocosmic dilemma we are currently balanced upon. Our connection with cannabis is one of the few things acting as a balance to the current cancer of yang: marijuana is the Earth, *mater,* matter heard from.

This isn't to say that pot is inherently feminine—it appears so as a reflection of the zeitgeist, in contrast to a country, culture, and cosmos on an epochal yang jag. It is inherently *altering;* it will change whatever consciousness you are in, just as likely to bum out a hippie as turn on a square. Cannabis is a reminder of the mutability of consciousness, a challenge to the ego's hubris and materialism. There is spirituality inherent in confronting a reality that is only relative.

These ideas are not new. Hemp and humans co-evolved on Earth. Perhaps no aboriginal strains of hemp exist; only cannabis strains showing cultivation have survived to the present. As cannabis is defined by its relationship to humans, so the oldest human artifacts (both material and mental) contain traces of cannabis. Hemp gave us the tools to be human—the ideas as well as the materials. Clothing, woven of hemp, is among the technologies that allowed our survival. Canvas, from cannabis, powered human exploration via the sails of ships and the media of artworks.

Cannabis is one of the oldest words to survive unchanged to the present—from the ancient Babylonian: *cane* + *two.* One plant with two parts, male and female, and two opposite functions: a stong fiber, and a psychoactive drug. Physical and mental, material and spiritual, these ideas are expressed so clearly in one plant. A paradox of unity and duality that demanded a language of signs rise to the level of poetry. The Chinese character for hemp, *ma,* depicts two different plants, male and female, under the roof of a drying hut: nature under the shelter of human culture. This idea of "cultivation" is the biological essence of culture—a refinement of the contact between nature and humanity for the benefit of both. The ancient written image of pot is a depiction of agriculture, of post–hunter/gatherer civilization, as a relation between plants and humans. Pot was the plant from which the idea of the Garden grew—the word made flesh.

The Chinese word for "grind" is formed from *hemp* + *stone. Hemp* + *hand* is *"rub."* "Numb" is *hemp* + *wooden.* And hemp plus the sign of negation is "waste." In these examples, hemp is both a material and mental tool for creating concepts—which arise from and are abstracted from a physical image. Cannabis is the building block of poetic thought and language. The concept is a higher resolution of a material duality: *hemp* + *stone* = "grind." Literally and figuratively, materially and mentally, cannabis is a source of meaning.

What is now figurative in language was once literal. Things could be understood, handled, or grasped; people had inclinations or attitudes. Primates reached this figurative place by an evolutionary move, a literal change of posture: we stood up, putting our heads over our hearts, because our survival depended on it. In physical terms, this meant balancing, reaching, and climbing. The insight of climbing—borrowed from the effects and structures of cannabis—is the dynamic of grasp and release: habit is to hold, dishabituation is to release. In the trees, the creative leap was literal—it required dexterity, grasping and letting go.

Evolved from the acoustic depths of the sea, our fear of the void is the fear of visual exposure, of open spaces where we were the prey of cats and raptors. In the safety of the trees, released from the grip of fear, we had perspective, and leisure to contemplate, away from the constant demands of survival—philosophers in the trees. With the evolution of awareness came the possibility that existence could be more than survival, or that survival could be more than a response to fear, and could include the encompassing of joy.

For primates, *above* was not only improved survival but new power. *Superior*—which describes a physical relation to gravity—came to mean better. In this case, the concept allowed left-brain thought (and the right hand) to perceive itself as above the right brain. What was originally positional—right—became dominant: Right. Left, from roots meaning weak or useless, became conflated with wrong, and the feminine, yin, right-brain world, was judged as not just positionally different, but inferior. Relatively different became absolutely wrong.

The gravity of the Earth—the weight of the world—is all that gives "being above" its superiority. This abstraction only makes sense from the viewpoint of land mammals, less so for human beings with a sense of infinite space. Copernicus recalled this in 1532, and Galileo seconded the motion. It didn't go over too well then, and today, we still don't really believe it. There is no Right Side Up, but *superior* as absolute, not relative, is ingrained in our language and thus in our thought.

This schism in the brain and body and community is apparent in Western history, and everywhere today. Natural dualities or paradoxes do not fit comfortably in this scheme and are forced out of balance by physical power or abstract judgment: right makes might. These are the root myths of monotheism: God is a man and removed from nature, men are superior to women, the brother on the right fights the brother on the left. Mankind is banished from the Garden, and heaven is separate from and superior to Earth.

Issues of gravity justify points of view. Arabs and Jews—pork-shunning, circumcised tribal Semites—are brothers first and enemies second, from the same dysfunctional family. The challenge to the human family is in how we see our superiority, and our physical and psychological reflex toward *up:* a position of power and dominance, or a platform for consciousness and perspective.

The location of our selves in our heads may seem natural, but the move is likely recent. In all Asian languages, the word for mind is the also the word for heart. The Egyptians, my daughter tells me, took the brains out of mummified bodies because they considered it waste; the heart was the seat of consciousness. Heart-consciousness is another victim of the move to the right, from yin to yang, from the acoustic to the visual. The heart, like love, is blind; It is the difference between resonance, which can be felt, and insight, which is just an idea. We have separated the mental from the physical, like a glob in an electroplasmic lava lamp. Adrift, we are dependent upon the mind's eye, and under this visual stress, we are always looking ahead, and are disembodied.

Literal rightism is a real force and can be mapped in the movement of "the West" from Babylon to Jerusalem, Istanbul, Athens, Rome, Vienna, Paris, London, and New York. Manifest destiny culminated on our West (left) Coast via the railroad, the gold rush, and the massacre of Native Americans, who were the dead opposite: a people compelled eastward from the edge of Asia. California was the end of the line: nowhere to go but up, or out. Psychedelic culture, the Jet Propulsion Lab, silicon chips, and proto-legal cannabis are among the signs the break-boundary was reached. Now California is pushing back, its culture and rediscovered Eastern spiritual practices spreading eastward.

We were born into the sea. Our ancestors moved to land and arose to the temporary unreality of a flat and straight-line world perpendicular to inexorable gravity. We are slowly stepping back into the ocean of space— the psychic space of screens and psychedelics, and also the reality of rising rockets and orbiting satellites. The biological imperatives to build, to climb, to rise, are still with us, and may, consciously or not, drive us to destroy and abandon Earth. The evolutionary destiny of our species may be elsewhere, and this could just be the route by which we prepare to leave the planet. God left Earth, and we may follow.

For those still here, the pot plant is a reminder of what successful survival requires: a leftness and a rightness of things. Cannabis has a duality in its basic strains—indica and sativa, which are primarily physical and mental in their effects respectively: stoned and high. Being high suggests a possible resolution of the yang superiority complex. "High," as a way of being above, is quite different from superior: above in awareness but not in power. It implies a perspective that is good for the organism, not a position of dominance over another part of the organism. Higher awareness raises the species above a life ruled by fear and gives us a reason for living, for the work of learning and building.

The arts were not extraneous or merely aesthetic—they were acquired technologies of successful survival. Rituals of art, dance, and chant, facilitated by cannabis and other plants, were created, developed, and continued because they worked. As much as practical-seeming technologies like climbing, clothing, and talking,/the arts were techniques for using beauty and ecstasy to convey wisdom, to create social unity and the psycho-organic bond and quantum technology sometimes called love./Love is a technology. It creates life biologically, and as a consciousness tool it expands the organism—it is a link of communication and cooperation that functions to reveal and make accessible otherwise imperceptable dimensions. A simple structural analog is the learned co-operation and stereoscopic benefits of two eyes working together—a higher connection that reveals a dimension invisible to separate organs operating alone.

An ancient word for this heart of humanity was *yos,* Sanskrit for wellbeing and health. *Yos,* in its movement west, mutated into *jus,* right, the root of all judgment. Under this cosmic shift, the yang conspiracy, a felt *reason* became the abstract Reason. Love was removed from sex, and male priests put on the habits of witches and shamans—literally put on the goddess's clothing—to usurp the feminine or nature-based orders. Alcohol culture moved in, and the alternatives were demonized. Pot was replaced with wine and incense. Clothing as a tool of power and identity survives in the literal meanings of habits and vestments. The pope still wears a dress.

What we lose as all forms of the feminine are devalued is, in a word, beauty. This is the loss of ethics in the loss of aesthetics: without the experience of beauty, conscious human life loses its reason. We deny that we were born with the aesthetic perfection of babies (the perception of acute life force, now just "cute"), and conceived at the peak of female sexual power.

The female orgasm is the basic unit, the quantum, of survival, since it connects directly the joy of life with the perfect ground for conception. Male orgasm is easy, and rape will make babies, but to maximize the life—the health of infants and the species—a positive balance of male and female, starting with love and orgasm and ending with domestic cooperation, is ideal. The reproductive system does not require, but works best with, female orgasm. What works is love. Jesus said this, but that doesn't mean that it isn't technically accurate.

Female sexual power, the terror of the patriarchy, resides with smells of funk and skunk—the same primal odors, fecund and deep, as the best-bred female buds. Pot's smells are essential, and pot culture is essentially olfactory: what gives away a stoner first is his smell. The smoker, after the first toke, cannot smell his own pot. These odors become natural or neutral in the place you go to when you are stoned. Smokers are united by this olfactory neutrality, sharing something at a level they can no longer consciously sense.

Smell is the most profound and least mediated sense: not abstracted into form or color, smell is the brain's direct cellular link and response to the outside world. Like sexual attraction, it unites the duality of the aesthetic and the technical: what smells bad *is* bad.

The experience of beauty, in the present and not as an abstraction, is a door that pot can reopen. For men particularly, this joy can be hard to sit with, the intensity hard to take. The male-female duality is about more than external genitalia; yin is in everyone and includes, among other things, the not particularly girlish ability to observe, to "take things in." Being able to stand still and reflect with passive, unfocused attention doesn't make you gay. Hunting and fishing, with their implicit virility, are two activities that still allow men to sit at ease in nature. Learning to live without beauty, men lose their roles as protectors and companions of beauty.

Not observing is also called denial. Just as closing your eyes helps you hear in depth, so you need silence to see more clearly. The racket sound of the gaming arcade we now live in makes it very easy not to see. The audio-visual bombardment of television screens is the equivalent of constant noise, and you literally can't hear yourself think, or see what's really there.

Screens are like pot in that they are both dishabituating. Screens (everything from phones to flatscreens) are entrancing not because of their content, but because of their glowing technical novelty. The loss of nature means that more of what we perceive around us is aesthetically ugly. In this context, the electric re-creation of the senses via screens is a blissful escape, and a reminder of the wonder of perception itself. But this is experience as entertainment, two senses masquerading as five, two dimensions masquerading as three, reality as a business. A generation of kids is disappearing into their Xboxes, and we don't know yet what they do. Addiction, probably; ADD, for sure.

Pot is not a cure for all this. You may experience the reenchantment of nature, if there is nature to be found around you. Alternatively, pot can promote a self-perpetuating, nihilistic avoidance, and you may fall further into a screen or other forms of elsewhere: "couch-lock" is a favored and apt term to describe the strongest indica strains.

Pot is an everyday organic, like coffee and beer. (Hops, used in making beer, is the only other member of the family *Cannabinaceae,* and is also cultivated for the resin of its female flowers. Decades before it revolutionized pot-growing, hops were propogated from female cuttings: references to "hop-clones" can be found as far back as 1915.) Weed is in the world and of the world: the people's psychedelic, the grounded mind-drug. It grew out of the field, not out of the laboratory. It is the elephant in the room of psychedelic studies, much of which does not consider it psychedelic.

As Terry Southern explained in his story "Red Dirt Marijuana" back in 1960, "workin'-hour gage" made work fun, made it swing, and you could still talk to the boss. You can operate in the straight world on pot, and it is more subversive for this. As the kid in the story learns, alterable consciousness is part of the adult terrain, a challenge you can learn to handle and enjoy, like swimming. It is a rite of passage, if not for adolescents per se, then for the adolescent mind: it shows that how you think can be changed.

The effects of cannabis are an intensification or compression of the effects of life, of experience, the extremes of which are risky, especially to the naive or unprepared, the mentally ill or otherwise weak. Ancient cultures no doubt had rules about cannabis use, and its power was controlled. This knowledge was part of the cultural environment, as the plant was part of the natural environment. Proscription and demonization add an unnecessary allure and diminish a necessary and worthy respect for its power. This is especially important for adolescents, who are most longing for its proffered feelings of maturity and meaning and are also most likely to be injured by its real psychological effects.

Humans have used pot forever and for everything; it is of practical use to artists and others. It will show you what you're doing wrong, whether you want to see or not. This can inspire new understanding or drive you deeper into denial. It can get you out of a rut, like travel or taking two weeks off, or put you into a new, brain-big rut. Change is the promise of every puff, and this eternal temptation is also its biggest risk. Dishabituation is a tool; habitual use defeats the purpose.

PART FIVE

Steps in the Right Direction

The illegality of cannabis is outrageous, an impediment to full utilization of a drug which helps produce the serenity and insight, sensitivity and fellowship so desperately needed in this increasingly mad and dangerous world.

CARL SAGAN

The War on Drugs was never, ever about drugs, it's about bigotry. You can change the law, but changing the prejudice and fear of bigots who hide behind drug war rhetoric is a far more challenging task. It's time to expose the Drug War and the bigots who promote the ideology of "Zero Tolerance."

STEVE KUBBY

If the words "life, liberty and the pursuit of happiness" don't include the right to experiment with your own consciousness, then the Declaration of Independence isn't worth the hemp it was written on.

TERENCE MCKENNA

Introduction to Part Five

It doesn't take an expert to see that things are very wrong with the current legal status of cannabis. Our government says there is no accepted medical use for it, yet it holds a patent (#6630507) for medicinal use of cannabinoids as antioxidants and neuroprotectants, and it distributes canisters of rolled joints to a few select patients in the Compassionate Use Program. Sativex, a whole plant extract that is administered sublingually, is being approved in other countries as a prescription drug, but not in the United States. Our government says it needs proof that marijuana is in fact therapeutic, though it makes this impossible to prove, with its monopoly on substandard plant material from the one FDA-approved farm in Mississippi, and the maze of federal approval required for research to proceed. FDA requires NIDA to sign off on cannabis studies, a hoop that no other drug researchers need jump through.

Ironically, while cannabis contains multiple components, it is believed that only the THC causes euphoria, yet only synthetic THC is legal in our country, while all the other nonpsychoactive compounds are illegal. Prescription oral THC pills are listed in Schedule III, which means any doctor can call them in to a pharmacy, while smoked cannabis (which contains THC as its primary psychoactive component but has many other compounds that modify and mitigate some of THC's effects) is listed in Schedule I, in the same category as heroin.

"Oral THC is slow in onset of action but produces more pronounced, and often unfavorable, psychoactive effects that last much longer than those experienced with smoking," according to a 2008 report published by the American College of Physicians, calling for legal protection for medical marijuana patients, reconsideration of marijuana's federal classification as a Schedule I drug, and expanded research. In December 2009, the American Medical Association likewise called for a reconsideration of the scheduling.

Cigarettes and alcohol, drugs that are harmful and addictive (meaning they meet criteria for schedule I status), remain unscheduled while causing half a million deaths annually. In America, 1,200 people die every day from diseases associated with cigarette smoking while 35,000 die yearly from alcohol-related illnesses. A full 20 percent of deaths in America are caused by cigarettes and alcohol every year. The FDA finally realized, in 2008, that it had to step in and try to regulate a drug that kills half its users, cigarettes.

In the United Kingdom in October 2009, Professor David Nutt, chairman of the British Advisory Council on the Misuse of Drugs, was forced to resign after saying that cannabis was a safer drug than cigarettes and alcohol. This happens to be true. Cannabis kills no one. It is impossible to overdose. It does not cause cancer like cigarettes, and it is basically nontoxic to the brain and liver, unlike alcohol. Also, it does not lead to violence the way alcohol can. Alcohol is involved in the majority of assaults, rapes, domestic abuse cases, and car accidents. Cannabis has no association with these crimes.

But there is tremendous lobbying by the pharmaceutical industry, alcohol distilleries (the beverage industry—beer—has a lobbyist in each state in the country), the textile industries, and petroleum interests to keep the status quo in the prohibition of cannabis and hemp. There are millions of Americans who believe that our government has no right to dictate how we alter our consciousness in the privacy of our own homes, or which medications we choose to take. There are many of us who are responsible adults, hardworking, otherwise law-abiding taxpayers, who are able to healthfully integrate cannabis into our lives much the way that others are "social drinkers." (Perhaps the best road to take here is to "out" ourselves, displaying the bumper sticker Bill Maher spoke about: I'm a Stoner and I Vote.)

I am a physician who advocates medical marijuana use and research, as well as a tax-and-regulate framework for legalization, because I am a harm reductionist. We need to look at which drugs and drug policies create the least damage, what carries the least risk. People are going to alter themselves with drugs and alcohol. This is a basic tenet of being human. Altered states are often an integral part of our gatherings, whether we toast the bride and groom at their wedding or have tailgate parties before the big game. Our drug policy needs to dispassionately and apolitically examine the risks and benefits of all drugs, including cigarettes and alcohol. Which are toxic to our bodies, our minds, and our societies? When comparing cannabis with alcohol and tobacco, head to head, Professor Nutt was absolutely correct.

As of this writing, fifteen states and Washington, D.C., have some medical marijuana law in place, with more states pending. Two states are voting on decriminalizing cannabis use soon, with more to follow. There is a sea change afoot, a momentum to the movement to tax, regulate, and provide patients with this herbal medicine. Those of us who are involved in the reformation of our country's drug laws are buoyed by the turning tides. (It may well be that the "Great Recession" was the greatest thing ever to happen to cannabis prohibition, much like the Great Depression helped repeal alcohol prohibition.) It is with this optimism that we present the last section of this book, signs of hope, things moving in the right direction, a healthier, more sane social policy for dealing with this medicinal plant.

Interviews with Patients Out of Time founders and an ACLU lawyer, and essays from a California physician who makes cannabis recommendations and a Canadian drug researcher involved with compassion clubs, all help give us a feel for how things *could* work, how patients who need this medicine can receive it with the compassion and dignity they deserve. A financial analysis of prohibition's costs vs. the potential windfall from a policy of taxation, and an examination of Dutch drug policy vs. America's, drives home the point that, quite simply, we're doing it wrong over here. There are better ways of dictating health care that don't involve sticking our heads in the sand and hoping this demon weed will go away. Groups like the Marijuana Policy Project, Drug Policy Alliance, Students for Sensible Drug Policy, and National Organization for the Reform of Marijuana Laws are helping mobilize Americans to stand up, be counted, and vote for change. I encourage you all to get involved in this important social movement.

36
Patients Out of Time

An Interview with
Al Byrne, L.CDR. (retired), and
Mary Lynn Mathre, R.N., C.A.R.N.

Julie Holland, M.D.

JULIE HOLLAND: Can you tell me how Patients Out of Time started?

AL BYRNE: In 1990 Mary Lynn, who is a nurse, and I, a medical marijuana patient, were on the board of directors of NORML and had
been for years. We wanted to stress the issue of medical marijuana for
personal reasons, and we convinced the board to hold a conference in
Washington, D.C., to discuss these issues. Mary Lynn got together the
first five Investigational New Drug (IND) patients from the federal government's compassionate use program, led by Bob Randall. The conference had a debate that was fortunately carried by C-SPAN, which ran
the whole conference and debate live, but then they ran it over and over
again. NORML received an extraordinary amount of phone calls, from
people we've never heard of to big-time celebrities. We decided we had
something there. So we worked as a group for a number of years. The
group comprised those five patients, a couple of other people, and Mary
Lynn and me. Then in April 1995 we actually incorporated in the state

of Virginia as Patients Out of Time. We filed as a 501(c)(3) nonprofit, and we now operate as an educational charity.

JULIE: And why did you choose that name?

AL: I actually made it up. I was looking for an acronym that we could use, and POT came to mind. For the *P* it was pretty easy to get "patients." We are patient-oriented; we advocate for patients. Many of the people I had known or interviewed over the years were sick or dying. They were running out of time.

JULIE: So you are primarily a patient advocacy group? What sorts of things do you do?

AL: We had formed the organization as an educational entity. The first thing we did was to take those five patients and make an eighteen-minute video called "Marijuana as Medicine." I believe it was the first video ever made on the subject. It won awards all over the country and overseas; it's been shown ten to twenty thousand times by now. It's sort of an icon. And what we did simply was to interview these five patients, ask them a few questions, and they answered on camera. They indicated that they were getting government pot, and it had done a number of things. It allowed them to see, it kept them alive, it kept them off pharmaceuticals, it gave them a better life. We began to show it to health care professionals. We started off with the Virginia Nurses Association (we live in Virginia). Mary Lynn went to their leadership, and there was a unanimous positive vote from the district presidents, followed by delegate approval at the state convention in 1994.

   That gave us an idea: as eight or ten people in the wilderness, we were nobody. Even if we were medical patients who were getting our cannabis from the government, we were still nothing. But if we had the Virginia Nurses Association behind us and then others of equal credibility, maybe we had an argument, maybe then somebody would really listen to us. And that list grew and grew.

   Mary Lynn drafted a resolution and presented it to the American Public Health Association at the open forum meeting in San Diego in 1995, and the assembled delegates voted to support the use of medical cannabis. Fourteen other state nursing associations have now joined the cause. Mary Lynn's presentation then helped convince the American Nurses Association (ANA) to support our issue. And just recently we added to our list the American College of Physicians, another distinctive and well-respected organization that understands and supports this complex issue. So, we thought, with all these professional medical organizations agreeing with us, certainly the government would understand that this is not a joke, and this is not a legalization effort. But they continue to run with blinders on.

The conference that we held here in April 2008 was an accredited conference where people in the health care profession received continuing medical education credits, and it was blessed by the American Nurses Association and the American Medical Association.

JULIE: So the American Medical Association (AMA) is now also behind Patients Out of Time.

AL: I think the AMA has blessed our work since we had our first conference in this series back in April or May 2000 at the University of Iowa, sponsored by its medical school and nursing school. In essence, those two organizations, the AMA and the ANA, have been the backbone of our accreditation since the year 2000, and they continue to support our mission, continually accrediting POT's conference series. At our 2008 conference, the AMA director of ethics and legal issues spoke to address this issue: Why is it that the American medical establishment can think that medical marijuana is a good idea, and yet the politicians still think that they have more knowledge about this than the doctors and the nurses? The whole thing is preposterous.

JULIE: Well, that seems to be a question on many minds.

AL: That question must be asked repeatedly to point out the government's ignorance on this issue.

So, after the video, we wrote a book with seventeen different authors contributing from around the world, called *Cannabis in Medical Practice: A Legal, Historical and Pharmacological Overview of the Medical Use of Marijuana*. The book tackles the issue of medical marijuana from the point of view of medicine, science, and research. It was the only book referenced by Dr. Janet Joy's commission on the Institute of Medicine report of 1999.

Then we organized an accredited conference in 2000, with the help of Dr. Melanie Dreher, a nurse Ph.D., and, at that time, dean of the Nursing School at the University of Iowa. She's on our board of directors. She was the leader of the effort to get this first conference accredited; she gets all the glory, as far as I'm concerned. It was televised at seven remote locations in the United States and Canada, and just like the C-SPAN broadcast in the 1990s with the calls to NORML, a diverse group of people saw this, including the Oregon Department of Health and Human Services, which co-sponsored and helped accredit our 2002 conference. Our third conference was sponsored by the Virginia Nurses Association. The University of Virginia's law school, medical school, and nursing school were all co-sponsors, among other people. Our fourth conference was co-sponsored by the California Nurses Association and the School of Medicine at the University of California–San Francisco. UCSF was so thrilled with what we did and the quality of our conference that it asked us to do it again.

But the problem here, for us, is that we still might as well be those five lone patients who don't mean anything to anybody, because no one in our government is willing to acknowledge that we are even here. No one hears the voices of these respected medical and nursing associations.

JULIE: Cannabis is still a Schedule I drug, which by definition says it has no legitimate medical use.

AL: Right. The Petition to Reschedule Cannabis was submitted in October 2002 to the Drug Enforcement Agency (DEA) by a coalition led by Dr. Jon Gettman. In that petition we ask the basic question, "Is marijuana a medicine or not?" We submitted references that accompany fifty thousand pages of documentation from around the world. (The petition and the fifty thousand pages can be found at the website www.drugscience .org.)

The United States has been reluctant-to-resistant about having meaningful research done here, so there's much less data coming out of America, yet Dr. Joy's group had very few references from outside the United States.

The DEA had three years to make their decision. They took three years to the day, and their decision was to pass the petition to the Department of Health and Human Services (HHS), with merit. The time frame for HHS's decision passed in the summer of 2008. So our legal people called up HHS and said, "You have not met the requirements of the law." HHS said, "Well, the response to the petition has to be signed by the surgeon general, and we don't have one right now." We said, "Yes, but there's an acting surgeon general." But they said, "No, it's not the same, so when we get a surgeon general we'll get back to you." Finally in March of 2010, the DHHS sent their recommendations back to the DEA, and at present we are waiting once again for the DEA to make their final decision.

Now, this is while people die. Totally unacceptable. So we're suing them. But they don't care, because by the time our lawsuit works its way into the Washington court system, they will be gone.

JULIE: First of all, it amazes me that the DEA was allowed three years to make a decision. That seems like an insane amount of time when the Food and Drug Administration (FDA) makes their decisions in thirty days.

AL: Well, I agree. When Dr. Gettman submitted this document to the DEA, they had to go out and hire a Ph.D. to study it, because they really don't have qualified people on their staff for this level of medical inquiry. So then this newly hired DEA Ph.D. called up Jon one day and said, "I can't find a couple of these references. I don't know how to get hold of them." Well, seventeen pages of references, maybe a couple of them might be obscure or hard to get hold of. "Which ones are giving you trouble?" "*Nature* magazine, how do I get that?"

JULIE: Oh, come on. Were they putting you on?

AL: This is true. They couldn't even find something from the Department of Justice. At one point, the DEA told us that they couldn't handle our request because they didn't have anybody to interpret all these different languages (we had submitted references in German and French). These guys in the DEA and HHS, they seem to think that even if there's a marvelous medical system that's well developed in France, it doesn't count. So that's the petition study. Everyone else is learning about medical marijuana except the DEA!

Many medical professionals, medical schools, nursing schools, state nursing organizations, the ANA, and the AMA have assisted us either overtly or quietly to get this information out to other doctors and nurses. The 2006 and 2008 conference proceedings are now available through the UCSF School of Medicine's continuing medical education website where doctors and nurses from anywhere in the United States can view these videos online, take an exam, pay a fee, and receive online accreditation for Clinical Cannabis Therapeutics. All these conferences, including the 2010 one in Rhode Island, can be accessed through a link on our website at www.medicalcannabis.com. A large portion of our conference consists of patients telling their stories, how cannabis helped them, and then having their primary physician come on after them to say, "Yes, what that patient just told you is the truth, I watched it happen." These conferences deal with real human beings with real medical problems, and the medicine that has helped them.

A guy wrote me just a couple of weeks ago from France, I didn't know him from anywhere, but he found out about us. He has attention deficit disorder (ADD). He said, "Mr. Byrne, I've been looking all over the world for real-life information about ADD and cannabis. Can you help me?" I said, "Yes, go to Google, search for 'Patients Out of Time,' look up Dr. David Bearman and a video called 'Mothers Know Best.' You'll get everything you need to know and all the references you ever wanted from those two sources." He e-mailed me back two days later, and he was just so grateful. He was passing this information on to his French doctors and his French colleagues that this information really does exist. "See?" he said to his physician. "I didn't make it up."

The government really shouldn't deny it any longer. Dr. Gettman has put in front of them the scientific information that is there. I believe Patients Out of Time, as a principal petitioner, has done its job and has accomplished its mission in this regard, which is education. All I'm waiting for now is the politicians to be able to learn how to read.

JULIE: I'm remembering when the court cases went on in the '80s for the DEA to reschedule marijuana, and the recommendation by Frances Young was to put it in Schedule II, I believe. Remember this quote? "One of the safest therapeutically active substances known to man."

AL: That's correct, and actually Mary Lynn and I were involved in that. It was like a twenty-one- or twenty-two-year-long lawsuit, that's how long they dragged that one out. We were sitting on the board of NORML, and we kept voting to allocate money to continue that fight, along with some other organizations.

JULIE: I'm sure you remember that even though the administrative law judge made that recommendation, the DEA just completely ignored the ruling and kept cannabis in Schedule I.

AL: The administrative law judge was clear as a bell: This is medicine, and you ought to declare it medicine and perform more clinical research to refine it. And they totally blew him off for political reasons. John Lawn (then current head of the DEA, a political appointee) made the political decision; he resigned two weeks later and went to work for the New York Yankees. They set up some doctor, and they made him make the announcement that they were killing the IND Compassionate Use Program. All these bureaucrats are making political decisions, not medical decisions, for millions of people. How ludicrous is that? And somebody like Lawn, of course, has no medical training at all. Anybody want to call up Dr. Lawn and see if he can diagnose or treat them? It's absolutely absurd.

One thing I'd like to reiterate about Patients Out of Time is that we are patient-oriented, patient-led, doctor- and nurse-led. Our president, Mary Lynn, is a nurse. Our board of directors is composed of patients or medical professionals. The other people in the advocacy/activist world are not like us. The Marijuana Policy Project (MPP) is run by a marketing specialist. NORML is run by administrators. The Drug Policy Alliance (DPA) is run by a lawyer. I'm not knocking any of these professions, but when a lawyer comes out talking medicine, I'm not sure a lot of doctors and nurses will pay attention to that information.

JULIE: My sense is that everybody is sort of working for the common cause, they have very similar goals, and everyone's sort of chipping at it from different angles. I don't necessarily think it's a bad thing.

AL: We disagree with you. As patients and medical professionals, we do not think that lawyers are the people who should talk about medical diagnoses and their treatments as though they know what they're talking about. If the press or anyone else has a question about the medical use of marijuana, it should be answered by a medical professional. We think that's logical, and we hold that position as an organization. We welcome the MPP, and we welcome the DPA. All we say is, Ethan Nadelmann, if you get a medical question, how about having that press guy call up Dr. Petro or Dr. Sanchez-Ramos or Dr. Abrams?

We're in the education business. We hold this biennial conference series, and we're heavily committed to the continuing effort to reschedule cannabis.

JULIE: So you are not only educating patients, nurses, and doctors, but you're also attempting to educate the government. Good luck with that!

AL: I don't want to make it sound like we're not a cooperative group. For instance, we joined with Rick Doblin and the Multidisciplinary Association for Psychedelic Studies (MAPS) in Professor Lyle Craker's attempt to grow cannabis at the University of Massachusetts back in 2002. I testified, describing how poor the quality of the medical cannabis is. Dr. Mahmoud ElSohly, who runs the University of Mississippi Marijuana Project, testified that the Missoula studies of 2001—the work that Dr. Ethan Russo, Mary Lynn and I, and the four medical patients did—was falsified.

JULIE: What do you mean it was falsified?

AL: He lied under oath in a DEA courtroom, in which sat Rick Doblin. In the Missoula study, which examines the health of four of the federally supplied medical marijuana patients, there are photographs, some of which show the seeds and stems that are wrapped up in the federal patient's cannabis cigarettes that they receive from the government. As any fifteen-year-old knows, you don't want seeds and stems in your marijuana cigarettes. So the first thing these guys have to do when they get their cigarettes is to unroll them, take out all the seeds and stems, take what's left (and of course their amount has been significantly diminished because the dosage is issued by weight), throw away the seeds and stems—or keep them for demonstration purposes, which is what we did—then smoke their cannabis, which the government agrees is their medicine. So, we took pictures of the seeds and stems from two cigarettes that we unrolled in Dr. Russo's kitchen in the presence of about fifteen people. We put the pictures in the book, in the study, and we published it.

When ElSohly was under oath, he was asked how those seeds and stems could possibly be there, and he said, "They're not. They've doctored the photographs. There is no way those seeds and stems were ever put in a cigarette that I issued."

That's a lie. Under oath, a lie. So, Rick Doblin was in the courtroom, and he actually used the DEA's hotspot wireless, and I happened to be sitting at my computer, and he wrote me asked, "Can you under oath refute that?" I wrote back and said, "Absolutely." He made a motion to his attorney, and I was given two days to submit a document to the

DEA to refute that. When the document was presented to the DEA attorney, Rick will tell you he froze; he was speechless for two minutes. His entire case had just been trashed. And shown the documents, the judge allowed all of it. This destroyed the government's case that they had a viable product, and of course Rick is still waiting for the decision. That is the length that these government employees, including a Ph.D., will go to. They will lie in a court of law, and the lie was not considered perjury by the government.

JULIE: I wonder why it wasn't considered perjury.

AL: The judge and the government lawyers never followed up on it.

JULIE: Well, that's not right, obviously. Now, what about ElSohly having a conflict of interest with his farm? He plans to make money growing cannabis for Marinol.

AL: He's also been trying to create a cannabis suppository.

JULIE: Right. So it's in ElSohly's best interest for the government pot to be lousy. I guess it's in the government's interest also. If they're doing research on really lousy pot, it's harder to show its medical effectiveness.

AL: The federal government probably hopes these guys in the Compassionate Use Program die. And there's only four left, so they're getting their wish. There's no telling how much better shape these people would have been in, or if they would have lived longer, if the product they had gotten was better. We have no idea. If you're dealing with a marginal-to-inferior prod uct that a teenager wouldn't give you $100 an ounce for in downtown Cleveland, why are you giving it to a patient and saying that it's a com- passionate program? It's exactly the opposite. And the age of this stuff is incredible. Back in 2007, the canisters of joints were often marked 1988 or 1992 or something.

JULIE: So they're giving out fifteen-year-old dried-out seedy, stemmy pot?

AL: Anybody want to take a fifteen-year-old dried-out aspirin? This whole program, put under investigation by anybody with any sense of ethics at all, it's a travesty. A sham.

JULIE: Mary Lynn, I wanted to hear from you, as a nurse, about the kind of patients that you've been meeting over the years.

MARY LYNN MATHRE: Oh, all kinds of patients. One interesting thing: so many patients come forward to let us know how many medications they have gotten off of because of marijuana. For example, chronic pain patients need an opiate (like morphine, Oxycontin, or Dilaudid), some kind of strong, habit-forming opiate, to help with the pain. Beside that, they need a stool softener, because the opiates cause tremendous constipation. Then they'll need an antidepressant, either because of the effects of the opiates, which are depressants, or because of living with chronic pain that's never removed. All the drugs that they get turn them into zombies, to some extent.

JULIE: And they also get nauseated or dizzy from the opiates.

MARY LYNN: Right, and then they need to take a medication to fight the nausea. But then, along comes the cannabis. They take cannabis, their bowels seem to move just fine. And very quickly, their opiate use drops off to nothing or to much lower doses. So the constipation's no longer a problem, and if they had nausea, that's no longer a problem. And the depression's no longer a problem. So now, instead of all those medications, they just need smaller opiate doses and the cannabis.

JULIE: That's it. They do seem to synergize each other's effects.

MARY LYNN: The sad thing is that today's physicians are so afraid that everybody's going to become addicted, and in their fear, they make patients sign a contract saying, Yes, I will abide by random drug-testing, and should I take any illicit drugs, you can break my contract and not give me any opiates any more.

JULIE: And that would include cannabis, unfortunately?

MARY LYNN: It does. I've given talks at the University of Virginia to the pain center, and very often I think some doctors hear me, but they'll still go along with it. If the patient uses cannabis, then they take them off their pain meds. That just does not make sense, logically or medically. It is clearly not the safest or best thing for the patient, to deny them treatment.

I think the pharmaceutical industry as a lobby is one of the biggest fighters against marijuana as medicine. They see that a lot of their pharmaceuticals might not be as necessary if people have access to cannabis.

JULIE: Another potential lobbying group is the whole prison-industrial complex. The jails are filled with cannabis "offenders."

MARY LYNN: Al would say it's a jobs program. There are so many people whose livelihood now depends on the drug war, and the most popular drug out there is cannabis. What would they do if this went away? All the prisons we built!

JULIE: Well, one idea is, we could turn them into indoor grow houses!

MARY LYNN: There's an idea! But the saddest thing is the people who have already been suffering—these patients—it is just so criminal to put them in jail. A classic example would be Todd McCormick. His mother made a brief presentation at one of our conferences. He was a cancer patient; he knew cannabis worked. He got caught in a grow operation and landed in jail. While Todd was imprisoned, that young man had his share, like other patients, of being traumatized by his environment, by violent criminals or prison guards . . . for growing a medicinal plant. To grow it for other patients, to be put in jail, and to have that trauma—he came out with a very serious case of post-traumatic stress syndrome. And that goes for many patients who are put in jail: they're not big, strong, healthy people who are ready to fight and fend for themselves. This is one of the atrocities that nobody wants to talk about.

JULIE: There are so many drug arrests in America, but no one's really talking about the fact that patients themselves are being arrested and prosecuted.

MARY LYNN: But there are many, many patients who are in jails and not getting their medicine. There was a terrible case in Oklahoma; a paraplegic man was put in prison in 1992. That was a time and state where asset forfeiture was a big thing. He happened to have a nice big corner lot, with an auto repair shop which was all seized by the government, but he was really sick. So he was put in prison, sentenced to life plus sixteen years, all for possessing two ounces and having two Colt revolvers under his pillow. He ended up needing to be hospitalized because he just wasn't doing well without his medicine. And it took a governor's pardon to get him out of there, but it was delayed because of the Oklahoma bombing in 1995.

The author Peter McWilliams, another medical marijuana patient, was also charged with growing. His mother put up her house as a bond to get him out of jail. Out of respect for his mother, he did not use cannabis, which was treating his nausea and vomiting. He ended up choking to death on his own vomit, because he didn't have his medicine.

Day in and day out, many patients who want it and need it actually won't come forward to get it, because they don't dare break the law. Health care professionals can advise that marijuana might be helpful, but then how do they help protect the patient to make sure they get something that's okay, that hasn't been sprayed with chemicals, that doesn't have mold on it? And in the states where patients are allowed to grow it, how many have a green thumb? It's been an ongoing dilemma. Some people can look the other way and say, "Well, it's okay. It's legal in California." But it's like yes and no.

The biggest thing for patients is that they can use cannabis and stop many of their other medications. It helps them like nothing else. They actually live a better quality of life. Montel Williams is a perfect example. In his book he talks about how he was literally in a closet with a gun to his head. He could not stand the fact that with the narcotics to help his pain from his multiple sclerosis, he was a zombie and just couldn't function. And somehow, he didn't go through with pulling the trigger on the gun, but he did find out about cannabis. And he told his audience on the air, "I take this medicine, and because I take it, I am here able to do this show. If I were on the opiates, I would be home like a zombie and have no life." He's careful, though, because something could happen, and people would want to exploit his popularity to bring him down, but at the same time, do the police really want to risk arresting him? It would create the wrong kind of publicity, because the public is for it. The American people, for the most part, get it. Any poll will show that.

Patients Out of Time is trying to push the health care professionals to go beyond the excuse that it's against the law, and to quit putting their heads in the sand. The law is wrong. There is plenty of science to back up the medical claims. Not only can you say that it has therapeutic value, it also has an extremely wide margin of safety. It is a very safe medication that can make all the difference in the world for certain patients. It can increase their productivity and enhance their quality of life. From a health care perspective, it is unethical not to fight for the patient, not to try and get that medicine. Why not put them on the least harmful medication to see if it works, rather than start something that could hurt their kidneys, their heart, or their liver? So we really try to push health care professionals, saying that the public expects you to base your decisions on science, not on the law. And if the law is wrong, then as a patient advocate, you should be helping change the law; you can't just sit there quietly. You've got to go out there and tell somebody, tell your congressman.

We're saying to the DEA, you cannot keep cannabis in Schedule I; it does not belong there. This is a safe medicine. You know how certain medicines get taken off the market because they find out something about the side effects? Maybe the pharmaceutical companies hid some of the data, or they didn't have enough people using the medicine to see the potential risk in their studies. But any researcher can look at cannabis and marvel at its safety. It's been out there for so many years and has never killed anybody.

The government's big argument is, "We don't want people smoking medicine." But in the early days, back in the 1920s, they actually did have an inhaled form of cannabis. We have a box of a medicine called Cannadonna. It was belladonna and cannabis, designed for asthma, and it was smoked.

In today's world, people smoke cannabis because that's the most effective way to get the right dose. It works immediately, you won't throw it up, and you can tell how much you need. But smoking can be harmful to the lungs, so the new answer to that is, use a vaporizer. Our drug laws are so crazy: You shouldn't smoke, it's bad for your lungs. Oh, there's a less harmful way to ingest it? Then we'll make it illegal; we'll call a vaporizer "paraphernalia."

The safer, better way to use cannabis, to get it into your system right away, is to vaporize it as we do other medications. You see people at the hospital with masks stuck to their oxygen machines that vaporizes their medications.

JULIE: Do you mean the nebulizers for asthma treatment?

MARY LYNN: Right. It's the same idea.

JULIE: Well, I've got some information in this book about vaporizers, but I'm also wondering about sublingual applications or transdermal applications, or even rectal applications. (Please see chaper 11 on vaporizers.) There are plenty of other ways to get cannabis into your system besides smoking it.

MARY LYNN: You're exactly right. There are Canasol eye drops from Jamaica for glaucoma; there are salves that people can use. There's the sublingual spray Sativex that's now available in Canada through GW Pharmaceuticals. Patients don't want to have to grow their own medicine, and they don't want to have to depend on somebody else to do it either. What they're not guaranteed is the same stuff, or the same quality. One day they'll take it in a better form and need this much, and later they get another batch and they find out they need more.

JULIE: As long as it's illegal, there's going to be no quality control at all, and no standardization of doses.

MARY LYNN: Right. These patients don't always know what they're getting. Health-care professionals are uncomfortable with it because they feel like they don't know how to prescribe it, and yet the physicians who come to know it learn that it's no big deal if the patients take a little too much or too little. It's got a wide margin of safety.

GW Pharmaceuticals, with their clinical trials of Sativex, actually had patients that were taking too much, so they encouraged them to wait at least fifteen minutes before deciding if they needed more. Take a little, see how it is, and then eventually you'll know what the right dose is for you, and you'll get it right. They understood that the patients could figure out what their correct dose was.

JULIE: I interviewed Andrew Weil, and that was one of the things I really appreciated him saying, that people are capable of titrating their own doses.

MARY LYNN: They absolutely are. It would be interesting to hear what Geoffrey Guy of GW Pharmaceuticals has to say about Sativex.

JULIE: Willie Notcutt has written a chapter on Sativex for this book.

MARY LYNN: I heard him speak about the clinical trials at a conference. He had one patient with multiple sclerosis who was bedridden, and after the use of cannabis she was actually able to get back up on a horse. The illness had tightened her up so much that she couldn't move around very well, and the Sativex loosened her up and relaxed her muscles. It helped her to the point that she could get up on a horse and ride.

Something Al alluded to was about the name Patients Out of Time. As soon as it came out of his mouth, we said, "That's it!" When we incorporated in '95, many people we knew had died. There were two amazing people, a young couple from Florida, Kenny and Barbara Jenks. Kenny was a hemophiliac, and he had AIDS and didn't know it. He got it, of course, because of all the blood products he needed for transfusions. Clotting factors for hemophiliacs come from hundreds of donors. Hemophiliacs were a high-risk population when it came to HIV/AIDS. So in the days before anybody knew much about it, he got bad blood. He got infected, didn't know it, and infected his wife. So you've got this kid and his wife. And they're both very, very sick, and they're poor, living in Florida in their trailer. Most of their days were spent in bed with a garbage can at the side of the bed to throw up in. Their support group suggested they try cannabis. "No, no, it's illegal. We don't do that," they said. Kenny got brave enough, and he tried the cannabis. Then he was up and out of bed, able to eat breakfast, do whatever. He eventually talked Barbara into trying it, and then she started functioning.

Next comes the usual thing, they got caught, arrested, prosecuted. But luckily, the judge was lenient; he sentenced them to community service to each other. The judge was kind of at a loss, but he was obligated to create some penalty, and yet he didn't want to do it because he recognized they were innocent people. Kenny and Barbara eventually got to Bob Randall with the Alliance for Cannabis Therapeutics (ACT), and they ended up being among the first patients who got therapeutic cannabis. ACT was really the first organization to start things off at the very beginning of the patient movement; it was the first medical marijuana advocacy group.

JULIE: Bob Randall started that, right?

MARY LYNN: Yes, Bob and his partner, Alice O'Leary. And upon his death, they turned it all over to us, because they felt Patients Out of Time was a continuation of what they had been trying to do. Once Bob gained access to medical marijuana, he formed the Alliance for Cannabis Therapeutics, wondering, How come I can get this from the government for my glaucoma and it works, but the rest of America can't have access to this? Anyway, he found out about Kenny and Barbara Jenks, and he helped them apply for the compassionate use IND. This was before they closed the program. So, after Barb and Kenny both had access to marijuana, Kenny became quite the activist. He would go to these conferences and he'd be out there at a table, with the paperwork that the patient would need for the compassionate IND program.

JULIE: Here's what I don't get. Why were there only five patients in this compassionate program?

MARY LYNN: At the time when we first met, there were five. After our panel at the NORML conference that aired on C-SPAN, as the numbers started growing, Barb and Kenny were two of the people who were included in that. So here he is going to these conferences, and the DEA comes up to him and says, "You've got to cut this out." They tried to scare the heck out of him, but he knew he had a death sentence with his AIDS, and he'd just say, "What are you going to do? Kill me?" And he wouldn't stop. Anyway, both Kenny and Bob died before '95.

When the compassionate use program closed in 1992, it was after we had that presentation, and hundreds of applications started coming in to the FDA; most of them were for AIDS patients. The federal government realized, "Uh-oh, people are finding out about this," so they shut the program down. When they did, the five had grown into fifteen patients who were getting medicine. I don't know for sure, but thirty-three or thirty-five patients had been approved but had not yet gotten their medication. Hundreds of applications were waiting to be approved, and that's when the first Bush administration said, "We're closing it down. You'll continue to get your medicine; nobody else will." That was in 1992. By 1995 there were only seven or eight patients. As we speak today, there are only four left alive.

JULIE: Is it fair to say that the government shut down the program because it started to get a lot of applications?

MARY LYNN: I think it's very fair to say that. When Louis Sullivan was the secretary of Health and Human Services, he made a statement that, because of the AIDS patients, we can't have this program. There'll be rampant sex if they get hold of this cannabis.

JULIE: You're kidding me! How puritanical can our government get?

MARY LYNN: These people are taking this medicine to stay alive!

The four that are left alive are the ones in the Missoula study,* where we performed many tests, as thorough a physical exam as you can get and then some. We did neuropsychological testing, which is very involved. We did CT scans and pulmonary function tests to look at the

---

*The Missoula study can be found on Drugscience.org and MedicalCannabis.com.

lung function; we really fully assessed how people were doing. I think Barbara or somebody might have had a little mild bronchitis, which supports the idea that the dry, old cannabis, which burns a little hotter, is rougher on the lungs.

JULIE: Right. They were smoking joints, too. They weren't smoking through water, and they certainly weren't vaporizing.

MARY LYNN: Exactly, and they had gotten rid of so many other medications; their health was so much better with the marijuana. George McMahon with his nail-patella syndrome, which is a very rare disease, is in his fifties now, and they usually don't live that long. Medical marijuana is like a medication for survival.

37
Prescribing Cannabis in California

Jeffrey Hergenrather, M.D.

My interest in marijuana began in the mid-'60s when I went off to college. I wasn't the first among my peers to try it; as a premedical student and an athlete, I was very cautious about the possibility of doing mental or physical harm to myself. My premedical education was so demanding that my experimentation with cannabis was occasional to infrequent, though my interest in the manifold uses of the plant—both medicinal and spiritual—and cannabis science grew steadily. I remember searching my medical school library in 1970 for scholarly books and reviews, only to find generally polarized reports with very little modern scientific investigation.

I discussed this fact with the dean of my medical school at Brown University in hopes of recruiting his support for my interest in cannabis research. All this occurred just prior to Nixon turning against the recommendation of the Shafer Commission, which favored President modification of the Controlled Substances Act of 1970 by decriminalizing cannabis. This effectively removed any opportunity for studying cannabis outside of the government's control.

After residency in 1977, my family moved to The Farm, an intentional community in Tennessee, where cannabis was used as a sacrament among its several hundred residents, despite the fact that this was in violation of state and federal laws. For the next five years, I served as a general practitioner in the community. Time after time, I learned of cannabis helping people with all kinds of maladies. I observed both young adults and people in old age using cannabis with no significant adverse effects or dependence. I witnessed its use in childbirth as a helpful tool that not only didn't impair the progression of childbirth, but would, in fact, often facilitate the process of labor and delivery. In backing up hundreds of deliveries where cannabis was used, I never observed adverse effects in the mothers or their babies. In due course I began recommending cannabis for a number of conditions for which I had found it to be an effective medication.

Over twenty years have passed, and I am now a cannabis specialist in California, with a practice of over 1,600 patients who use cannabis for a wide range of conditions. Such a practice was made possible by the passage of the ballot initiative Proposition 215, the Compassionate Use Act of 1996, stating that Californians have a right to use cannabis if approved by their physician.

In 1997 my twenty-four-year-old son was dealing with the consequences of a high cervical spinal cord injury, which included pain and muscle spasms. He had tried various medications to control his symptoms, but none worked as well as cannabis. It was fast and effective without adverse effects, and—like nothing else—it eased his mind. Despite a discussion about his findings with his internist, and the fact that he clearly had a qualifying condition, he was turned down in his request for an approval to use cannabis. He came back to me to ask for my approval.

I granted it, and thereafter found it increasingly difficult to say no to other disabled people with similar conditions. My discomfort about the decision had nothing to do with the ethics of helping my adult son, or the safety of the plant. It had everything to do with the law. With respect for my son's doctor and the many other good physicians like him, their discomfort about recommending cannabis is understandable; they don't have reliable information or training, or, worse, hear threats from the federal government and the state licensing board about possible sanctions, probation, or loss of license. In this hostile environment, it's easy to say no to making cannabis approvals. Nonetheless, I had opened the door, and by 1999, I'd made my transition from a twenty-six-year career in emergency medicine to that of cannabis consultant.

Who self-medicates with cannabis? Cannabis users come from all walks of life—they are indistinguishable from the population as a whole. I'm continually amazed to find elderly people and older health professionals coming to my office to legalize their use of cannabis for a variety of serious medical conditions. These people do not fit the profile of users that the media fixates on: the young, healthy-looking person. I do have healthy-looking young patients in my practice, but appearances don't always reveal the whole story. People with migraines, seizure disorders, inflammatory bowel disease, and multiple back surgeries don't hobble to the office because they try their best to be seen as healthy people, not patients with disabilities.

Except for those with rare malignancies and other very serious conditions, cannabis is not appropriate for children. Young adolescents start using cannabis at a younger age when they are troubled. They complain of anxiety, depression, and a variety of painful ailments. Most physicians who make cannabis approvals don't recommend cannabis to these teenagers unless they are accompanied by parents and have a very serious medical problem. The most common cannabis users are between twenty-five and seventy-five years old. They include carpenters, plumbers, construction workers, equipment operators, blue-collar workers of all kinds, nurses, doctors, lawyers, judges, county and federal employees, law enforcement officers, counselors, teachers, health care workers, professional drivers—persons from virtually every occupational field.

In California hundreds of thousands of people have consulted a doctor for approval of their use of cannabis. There is no state requirement to register these people, so the numbers can only be estimated; they probably exceeded 400,000 people by the end of 2007. The process is entirely private, between the patient and the physician, as it should be. In my private practice, the mean age for all patients is forty-seven years old, slightly younger for men than for women. This is a bell-shaped curve of distribution that is truncated after sixty years of age, probably because the older generation lacks familiarity with the use of cannabis, given that it was less commonly used prior to the 1960s. About 98 percent of adult patients seeking a cannabis recommendation have already tried cannabis in the past. In many cases they had either abstained from cannabis use for years or had been using it "recreationally" at the time they discovered that cannabis was the best choice for a new medical problem.

CHRONIC PAIN

Chronic pain is the presenting complaint for about 60 percent of patients seeking cannabis approvals in my practice. Injuries and degenerative diseases account for the majority of these painful conditions. When chronic pain is associated with muscle spasms, cannabis is particularly effective. Most muscle spasms are relieved within minutes by inhaled vapors or smoke. I am currently treating about one thousand patients for chronic pain, about 10 percent of whom had been dependent on opiate pain medication. They needed to maintain a regular schedule for pain control and to avoid opiate withdrawal symptoms. Typically, within a year of legally using cannabis as an adjunct for pain control, about half of these patients discontinue regular use of opiates and nonsteroidal anti-inflammatory drugs (NSAIDS).

The reason for choosing cannabis over other medications is that cannabis has a variety of pleasant allied effects, whereas opiates, NSAIDs, and antidepressants have a long list of serious, very troublesome, and even lethal adverse effects.* For cannabis, the allied beneficial effects include mental ease, muscle relaxation, and a change of focus from pain-induced stress and mental anguish to happy, funny, and creative thoughts.

Another allied benefit is found by many parents suffering from chronic pain: They report that their child-rearing skills are far superior after using cannabis. None report that their parenting skills are compromised. Most people prefer to avoid driving within an hour or two of use, but studies have found that drivers who use cannabis are safe drivers.

NAUSEA AND ANOREXIA

About 10 percent of my patients have nausea and anorexia associated with AIDS-related illness,† cancer, cancer treatments, and various gastrointestinal problems. The wasting syndrome of AIDS has been effectively treated for years with a combination of cannabis and HIV drugs. AIDS patients will tell you that cannabis has saved their lives. The use of cannabis readily controls nausea and vomiting and helps restore appetite, thus combating the side effects of the regular administration of HIV medications.

Patients give compelling reports of cannabis relief for a variety of other conditions including ADD, ADHD, asthma, autoimmune diseases, brain trauma, cerebral palsy, diabetes types 1 and 2, dystonia (muscle spasm), severe menstrual pain, epilepsy, harm-reduction management of addictions and substance abuse (including alcohol, tobacco, cocaine, benzodiazapines, amphetamines, heroin, etc.), inflammatory bowel diseases, mental disorders (including post-traumatic stress disorder, anxiety disorder, depression,

---

*Please see chapter 28 on pain management for a more in-depth discussion of this topic.
†Please see chapter 26 for a more in-depth discussion of cannabis in relation to AIDS.

bipolar disorder, obsessive-compulsive disorder, schizoaffective disorder, and schizophrenia), migraine, morbid obesity, multiple sclerosis, muscular dystrophy, neurologic and other neurodegenerative diseases, organ failure and transplants, persistent insomnia, psoriasis and eczema, rheumatic diseases (including rheumatoid arthritis, lupus, ankylosing spondylitis, Sjögren's syndrome, scleroderma, Reiter's syndrome, and Behcet's syndrome), spastic disorders, spinal cord injury, and Tourette's syndrome.

CANCER

To maintain standards of professionalism consistent with my training, I cannot claim that cannabis cures cancer, but the benefits are clear and compelling. Cannabis has anticancer properties in addition to the well-publicized improvement of appetite and control of nausea and vomiting associated with chemotherapy. In some cancers, it has an even greater treatment role.

Recent studies have shown that/activation of the CB1 and CB2 cannabinoid receptors results in increased tumor-cell death and reduced tumor-cell growth in multiple types of cancer. Cannabinoid compounds can reduce growth of cancer indirectly by inhibiting angiogenesis—the process of forming new blood vessels. One constituent, cannabidiol (CBD), is the most effective inhibitor of a cancer gene and protein Id-1, which is expressed in aggressive hormone-independent breast cancer cells/Cannabidiol is the first nontoxic exogenous agent that can significantly decrease Id-1 expression in breast cancer cells, leading to down-regulation of tumor aggressiveness, thus inhibiting the metastasis of aggressive human breast cancers in vivo (in living beings). We also know that abnormally high levels of Id-1 have been found in other forms of cancer. Especially promising about this new research by McAllister and colleagues is that if CBD can inhibit Id-1 in breast cancer cells, then it may also prove effective at stopping the spread of cancer cells in ovarian, colon, brain, melanoma, and prostate cancer where these genes and proteins are found.

What follows are my clinical observations—a few heartening reports of the clinical courses of some of my patients with a confirmed diagnosis of metastatic cancer.

Case 1, CA, Glioblastoma Multiforme

PJ, a fifty-year-old man, was still enjoying riding motorcycles and surfing when he began having right-sided headaches with increasing frequency and severity in the spring of 2003. Within three weeks he saw his primary physician, but when he began dropping things from his hands and slurring his speech, his doctor sent him to the emergency room (ER) for a brain scan. PJ was found to have a large stage 4 brain tumor in his parietal area, subsequently diagnosed as a glioblastoma multiforme. PJ underwent brain surgery in July 2003, followed by radiation therapy. He was also referred to a clinical study at a major teaching hospital.

Now over four years since his surgery, PJ continues to improve, despite the ominous prognosis of glioblastoma multiforme. Untreated patients are found to live one to three months from diagnosis. Treated patients have a median survival of ten to twelve months. In the best-case scenario, people are alive at eighteen months; very few are still alive after five years. What's different in PJ's case is that every day he takes at least five cannabis capsules that he prepares for himself. The cannabis helps PJ with his appetite and sense of well-being. Of great interest is the fact that he has been seizure free and without recurrence of the tumor on all his follow-up brain scans and MRI and PET scans (three or four times per year since 2003).

Back from his road trip to visit family, PJ is out riding his bicycle with increasing confidence, and he has applied to get his driver's license back again.

Case 2, CA, Neuroblastoma

Nick was six years old when he was diagnosed with stage 3 neuroblastoma, later diagnosed as stage 4 relapsing refractory neuroblastoma. Supposedly nobody beats this cancer. His parents had made the choice to allow their son to use cannabis at the age of nine after he became the only survivor of his metastatic neuroblastoma study group in San Francisco. He began using cannabis to reduce his pain, anxiety, and insomnia and to increase his appetite. Nick reported that none of the conventional medications worked as well as cannabis for all these symptoms. First supporting his cannabis use was Dr. Tod Mikuriya, a California pioneer in cannabis therapeutics. Mikuriya then referred eleven-year-old Nick to me when his family moved to my town. After extensive treatments at several medical centers for many years, he went into remission when he was thirteen years old.

On his sixteenth birthday, Nick and his mother were invited to speak at a neuroblastoma conference. When asked what Nick did differently to be in remission, Nick's mother asked if this was a good time to talk about medical marijuana. Silence was followed by a change in the topic of discussion, as the oncologists and researchers did not want to deal with the truth of the matter.

Even though he was a rare survivor of this cancer, his use of cannabis would not be permitted by the cancer treatment protocol. Nick was three years and three months into his remission from cancer when he died of sepsis from a perforated bowel, a complication of the extensive scarring and organ damage from his many radiation, surgery, and chemotherapy treatments. Nick's mother said that his oncologist recognized that Nick "bought many years of life" by using cannabis. She believes that she may be invited back to the conference in the future to tell the rest of the story. In his memory, his mother has created a website, www.nicksnow.com, to tell his story.

Case 3, CA, Metastatic Melanoma

DS is a fifty-three-year-old woman who received a diagnosis of stage 3 melanoma when a lesion was removed from her left arm over twenty-seven years ago. Reportedly, her doctor had misdiagnosed the mole for over a year, assuring her that she could treat it with ointment. Seven years passed before a metastatic melanoma tumor was found in her stomach and esophagus. Eighty percent of her stomach was removed in an effort to contain the melanoma. Just eight months later, another metastasis was found in her left ovary, followed by another tumor on the right ovary and fallopian tube. Despite bacillus Calmette-Guerin (BCG) at UCLA and interleukin-2 therapy at the City of Hope, tumors came back in her thigh and several other bone sites. Several surgeries, radiation therapies, and chemotherapies followed as the metastases continued. An epilepsy disorder began with the discovery of a dermoid tumor in her brain.

Ten years have elapsed since DS and her fourteen-year-old son moved to my community. What changed in her case is the near-daily use of cannabis that did not begin until after her move to northern California. She subsequently discontinued cancer and seizure medications. She has been stable for the past ten years with no additional conventional therapies.

In all these cases, the use of cannabis is associated with reducing the aggressiveness of highly malignant, difficult-to-treat cancers. Some of my other cancer patients who passed away were able to achieve comfort and peace of mind with cannabis use before they died.

Donald P. Tashkin, M.D., professor of medicine and medical director of pulmonary function at UCLA, has published results of extensive federally funded studies on the risk of cannabis smokers developing cancer. Despite the fact that cannabis smokers are inhaling known carcinogens, and cellular damage is occurring in bronchial epithelial tissue, Tashkin found no association between cannabis smoking and lung or airway cancers. In fact, there appears to be a reduced incidence of cancers in those tobacco smokers who also smoke cannabis. What is the mechanism that prevents damaged cells from becoming malignant in cannabis smokers? This question deserves further investigation.

AUTOIMMUNE AND RHEUMATIC DISEASE

Many patients with rheumatic disease experience a reduction in the frequency and severity of flare-ups. For those continuing to use immune-modulating medications, such as methotrexate, or prednisone, the quantity and frequency of use is markedly reduced. The picture is similar whether patients have rheumatoid arthritis or systemic lupus erythematosus. Lupus patients have been in remission for years thanks to cannabis, and the rheumatoid arthritis patients, though their cases are not completely quiescent, are manageable with much less intervention than before cannabis.

INFLAMMATORY BOWEL DISEASE

Another condition that I have followed with interest is Crohn's colitis, a form of inflammatory bowel disease. Over thirty years ago, while I was a medical student in my surgical rotation, my first patient was an unfortunate woman in her early thirties who was emaciated and dying from Crohn's disease. Now, in my cannabis consultation practice, I am finding that Crohn's patients seek cannabis approvals because they have already found that it changes the course of their disease.

After the first several patients reported marked improvement in their conditions with the use of cannabis, I approached the other physicians in the Society of Cannabis Clinicians about these findings. They reported similar experiences with their Crohn's patients. Subsequently, I circulated a questionnaire to these doctors for their inflammatory bowel disease patients to report on their experience with cannabis. I'm now working on publishing the findings on the first thirty patients who have completed the survey.

All surveyed patients with Crohn's disease report statistically significant improvement in signs and symptoms in all categories explored: pain in the gut, anorexia, nausea, vomiting, fatigue, depressed mood, and activity level. The number of stools per day was reduced, the body weight increased, and all patients reported that the frequency and severity of flare-ups were reduced.

I reported this information in an (in vitro) pilot study of twelve patients to the International Association for Cannabis as Medicine (IACM) in 2005. There was a nearly simultaneous report in the journal *Gastroenterology* that diseased bowel tissue taken as biopsy specimens from Crohn's patients had large quantities of cannabinoid receptors. Activating these receptors with cannabinoids promoted healing of the gastrointestinal membrane. This could offer therapeutic relief to patients suffering from inflammatory disorders such as Crohn's disease and ulcerative colitis. This laboratory evidence from Wright and colleagues in 2005 represented the first research in the scientific literature that supported the anecdotal evidence of our patients that cannabis was a useful treatment in Crohn's disease.

ATTENTION DEFICIT DISORDER (ADD)

TT is a sixteen-year-old boy who seriously damaged his knee in a motorcycle accident. I might not have approved cannabis for this young man for his pain, but I found that he also had a problem with attention deficit disorder (ADD). His parents were struggling in their effort to manage his condition. He had already failed in a private school, where he could only manage a D average.

TT was referred to a pediatrician who prescribed a commonly used ADD amphetamine drug. His parents gave this a trial for several weeks until they witnessed bizarre mood swings and suicidal comments. For the first time their son said that he thought about killing himself. With her back to the wall, his mother stopped the prescribed amphetamine and allowed her son to try cannabis after school in an effort to alter the course of his illness. His attitude and ability to focus immediately improved. With afternoon and evening use of cannabis at home, TT is now getting As and Bs in the public school system. He uses cannabis after school and at bedtime with excellent results and no adverse effects. He tells his parents that—finally—he can focus his attention.

The reports of benefits with cannabis use occur in countless seemingly unrelated conditions. As you look at the location and role of the cannabinoid receptors and the endocannabinoid system in human physiology, it is easier to understand the vast and disparate medicinal uses of cannabis, the uncommon safety of natural plant cannabinoids, and the potential target for many new pharmacologic agents. Those people with maladies for which cannabis provides relief or is purported to provide relief may be asking their doctor, "Is cannabis right for me?" If your doctor is uncomfortable responding, my advice is to seek out a cannabis specialist.

CANNABIS STRAINS AND CONSTITUENTS

Cannabis strains are the topic of many books, conversations between afi-cionados, and street lore. *Cannabis sativa* can be divided into two principal varieties, *sativa* and *indica,* which are well known for their different qualities and growth characteristics.

Indicas are short, broad-leafed plants that mature quickly. Their attri-butes are described as "body stone" and "couch-lock," and people who use indicas report that it makes them lazy and relaxed, making the selection of indicas a good choice for chronic pain and insomnia. The sativas are tall, slender plants that mature slowly. Their attributes are described as "clear-headed," meaning they make one feel alert, euphoric, and functional. Most, if not all, strains are hybrid mixtures of the two.

Without legal access to laboratories and standards, and with only rudi-mentary knowledge of the medicinal value in the various cannabinoids and noncannabinoid components, the goal for cannabis growers in California and elsewhere has been selecting for potency, appearance, and smoking qualities. Tetrahydrocannabinol (THC), which is among the most psycho-active constituents, reportedly accounts for nearly 99 percent of the cannabi-noid fraction, at the expense of the other roughly seventy cannabinoids that occupy the remaining 1 percent. If the cannabinoid fractions are similar in most sativa and indica strains, the differences in their qualities and effects should be found in the scores of terpene and flavonoid molecules.

When patients shop at a cannabis dispensary, they are challenged with selecting a product with ever-changing names and attributes. Given the freedom to analyze and characterize the cannabinoid and terpene fractions of the natural plants, the breeders and patients will have the knowledge to develop the desired strains. For example, the cancer patient may desire a low-THC, high-CBD strain with less psychoactivity and more appetite stimulant and antinausea effects, or one for daytime use and another for bedtime. For other needs, certain cannabis constituents may be best for seizure disorders, psychiatric conditions, or pain control.

CHANGING MEDICAL EDUCATION

As medical education evolves to include the role of the endocannabinoid system in human physiology, pharmacology, and disease, more doctors will gain an understanding of the conditions that are responsive to cannabinoid therapy. At this point, the cannabinoid receptors and the endocannabinoids, with their many regulatory roles, are proving to be very complex and only superficially understood. There are well over one hundred research teams from at least twenty-five nations in hospitals and universities around the world studying the roles and effects of the endogenous and exogenous cannabinoids. In recent years at least ten of the major pharmaceutical companies have revealed their own programs that are researching cannabinoids, and numerous patents have been filed.

CANNABIS SPECIALISTS

Physicians who are considering making cannabis approvals can be reassured that it is their constitutional right to do so. The U.S. Supreme Court's refusal to hear the Ninth Circuit Federal Court decision, *Conant vs. Walter,* meant that the lower court's decision stood. Namely, it is a doctor's right under the First Amendment to have a discussion with his or her patients about the use of cannabis for their medical conditions, and the physician may approve or recommend this medicine in spite of federal laws prohibiting it. That, unfortunately, is not the end of the story. The president of the United States sets priorities for the activities of the Office of National Drug Control Policy, the Justice Department, the Drug Enforcement Administration, Health and Human Services, and the Veterans Administration, and by making various public service announcements. The "Drug War" rages on, despite the waste of resources and the rising tide of dissent against this failed policy.

The pro-cannabis physician must accept that he or she may be targeted by the federal government in a variety of ways. State and federal agents have visited doctors' offices under cover of fictitious names with fake ID cards, records, and feigned symptoms to get a cannabis recommendation. Maintaining high standards in one's practice of medicine is the best and perhaps only defense. The California Medical Board has stated, "A physician who recommends the use of cannabis by a patient should have arrived at that decision in accordance with accepted standards of medical responsibility, that is, history and physical examination of the patient; development of a treatment plan with objectives; provision of informed consent including discussion of side effects; periodic review of the treatment's efficacy and, of critical importance, proper record keeping that supports the decision to recommend the use of cannabis."

Understand that you are establishing not only a medical relationship with your patient, but a legal one as well. You may need to answer to law enforcement, judges, and the courts when you approve cannabis for a patient. Even the most conscientious physicians may be targeted at times. Accept that fact and go about your practice—you'll be nothing less than a hero to your patients.

PRESCRIPTION CANNABINOIDS

Despite the protests of the American Medical Association, the federal government banned the growing of cannabis in 1937, and the pharmaceutical companies stopped making tinctures and salves using whole cannabis extracts. Five decades later the federal government began licensing pharmaceutical companies to market single-molecule cannabis constituents. The first such medicine came out in 1986. It was dronabinol (Marinol brand), a synthetic delta-9-THC. It is now a Schedule III drug, available as an appetite stimulant, an antiemetic agent that controls nausea and vomiting, and a pain medication.

Most of my patients who have tried Marinol prefer the natural product. Marinol is expensive. It is no less psychoactive than cannabis, but apparently less effective in other respects. In 2006 nabilone (Cesamet brand), another synthetic cannabinoid and an analog of Marinol, now on Schedule II, became available for the control of nausea, vomiting, loss of appetite, and pain.

The new medication Sativex is an approximately 50/50 mix of THC and CBD derived from whole-plant extract, including some "minor" cannabinoids and the medicinally active terpene and flavonoid molecules. Manufactured by GW Pharmaceuticals in England (with government approval), it is an oral spray available in Canada and Spain for neuropathic pain and muscle spasticity.

The next product that has come to market in Europe is a research chemical from Sanofi-Aventis. The drug goes by several names, including SR141716A, Rimonabant, and Acomplia. It is a selective cannabinoid (CB1) receptor antagonist, or blocker, that doesn't occur in nature. It is marketed as a drug to treat obesity. It does cause a revulsion to food, but people seem to stop losing weight after the first five to ten pounds. The adverse effects arise from blocking all the CB1 receptors in the brain. In clinical trials of the drug, suicides occurred among people in whom depression had not been a recognized problem. Seizures also occurred in clinical trials. Though it may be available online, Rimonabant should be considered dangerous. To date, the FDA has turned down Sanofi's request to market the drug in the United States.

The development of nonpsychoactive cannabinoid pharmaceuticals is one way to win approval from governments concerned about the mind-altering effect of cannabis. Toward this end, most researchers are looking for single molecules that can be patented. They are turning away from the natural cannabinoids and other natural plant constituents of therapeutic importance because these substances greatly complicate single-molecule drug development, and more importantly, they may not be patentable.

Barbara Costa, an Italian researcher, presented her topic, "Cannabis-based medicine in pain and inflammation. Is it better than pure cannabinoids?" at the IACM Conference on Cannabinoids in Medicine held in Cologne, Germany, on October 5–6, 2007. The title of her paper was "Antihyperalgesic and Antiinflammatory Effects of a Cannabis Extract in Animal Models of Inflammation and Neuropathic Pain." She demonstrated that the whole-plant cannabis extract outperformed individual molecules like THC and CBD in blocking inflammation and neurodegenerative injury in animal studies. She is not alone in encouraging the development of cannabis-based medicines instead of single molecules.

PATTERNS OF CANNABIS USE

People have a personal alliance with the cannabis plant; they tell stories of how their grandmothers and grandfathers used it. Quietly they grow it, share it, and report on the many uses that they have found for it, whether by smoke, vapor, ingestion, salves, or tinctures. Most people deeply resent the federal government's heavy-handed, unscientific denigration of cannabis. Patients often feel that they have no choice but to use the newest pharmaceuticals. They are often fearful of having their cannabis use discovered and are self-critical about their use, even when it is the best medicine that they have ever used.

Most people prefer to smoke cannabis, though an increasing percentage are vaporizing the resins without actually burning the plant. This is done with tools to heat the plant to baking temperatures, 350 to 375 F°. Smoking is preferred for a variety of reasons, including cost-effectiveness, convenience, easy dosage control, rapid onset of action, and—according to some patients—medical effect. Vaporizers are preferred by others for the subtle flavors and the gentler effect on the lungs and airways. Some people use only edible forms of cannabis. A multiple sclerosis clinic in Switzerland reports that its patients simmer cannabis buds in milk and drink it on a regular basis. Other people use cannabis topically, through the skin, and use it this way exclusively.

Frequency of use is highly variable, from once a month to every other hour, depending on one's condition. On average, my patients report using it four to seven days per week, usually after work and in the evening. The dosage of cannabis is easily determined, as users know what state they are looking to achieve. This precise titration is easiest with smoked cannabis, and least so with edible forms. Typically patients use *less* cannabis as their age and experience with controlling their pain increases.

TOLERANCE/DEPENDENCE AND ADDICTION*

Although the "high" is significantly diminished with regular use of cannabis, control of pain, nausea, anorexia, insomnia, and uscle spasm does not seem to diminish with frequent use. Dependence is not a significant problem with cannabis users. If it is available, they prefer it to other pharmaceuticals. If it is unavailable, they get by without withdrawal symptoms or dysfunctional behavior. There are those who admittedly use too much, but no one that I'm treating shows any classical signs of addiction, such as physical and psychological habituation to the use of the medicine, the deprivation of which gives rise to symptoms of distress, abstinence or withdrawal symptoms, and an irresistible compulsion to take the drug again, often in increasing amounts. Though the National Institute of Drug Abuse (NIDA) would have you believe otherwise, cannabis is not addictive, nor does it have a significant withdrawal syndrome.

ADVERSE EFFECTS

Every patient is asked about adverse effects. The quick answer to the question is no, there are no bothersome effects. The sarcastic response is that cannabis is still illegal under federal law, hard to obtain, or too expensive. The long answer sometimes includes an acknowledgment that short-term memory is altered for the first hour or two after use. Therefore, cannabis is unacceptable in many work situations. Mild cough and sputum production or bronchitis is common in heavy smokers and older smokers. Cannabis has bronchodilating and expectorant effects, so the cough is infrequently a complaint. The cough readily resolves with use of a vaporizer or edible forms.

A few patients mention paranoia, though it tends to subside with legalized use or a change of strains. Tiredness and sleepiness are also described, sometimes as a therapeutic value, other times as an adverse effect. These effects may prove to be strain-dependent as well.

---

*For a broader discussion of addiction, please see chapter 14.

PRODUCTION AND DISTRIBUTION

California's Compassionate Use Act of 1996 is a powerful and liberating law. It protects citizens' rights to use physician-approved cannabis without imposing a finite list of conditions or creating a registry of qualified patients.

Some pro-cannabis advocates argue that the California law didn't go far enough to protect the patients from arrest, prosecution, and the loss of employment. It also didn't create a mechanism for the proper distribution of cannabis. Physicians can issue approvals allowing their patients to use cannabis but cannot advise them on how to obtain it. Patients have a right to grow and possess cannabis for their personal medical use, but only a small fraction are able to do so. Medical-cannabis dispensaries have proliferated to meet the need of patients who cannot grow their own. These dispensaries exist in a legal limbo, subject to local zoning laws and raids by the DEA. They are recognized by California law SB 420 if organized as nonprofit cooperatives or collectives. Most dispensaries began paying taxes to the state in 2007.

California today is a crazy quilt in which some cities and counties have taken the "tax and regulate" approach, with ordinances governing when, where, and how dispensaries can operate; others have banned them outright. I'm proud of my community, where law enforcement has accepted the will of the voters. People can grow their plants in their backrooms and backyards without interference from the police.

SO WHAT'S THE PROBLEM?

People often ask, "How can this be?" How can it be that the government prohibits cultivation and use of a beneficial medicinal plant? How can it be that good people are labeled "bad" and imprisoned by the thousands? How can our law enforcement officers raid patients' homes and seize their property? How can children be taken away from their parents by child protective service agencies because cannabis brownies were found in the home? Why is it that young people who are legally using cannabis as medicine are smeared by the press as fakers? How can patients, approved under California law, be fired from their jobs because their employer won't allow the medicinal use of cannabis, even if it does not impair their performance? How can we as a society be unable to have an honest discussion about the "War on Drugs"?

In much of the world, when people are asked how they deal with marijuana, the response is, "It isn't a problem." In America, we have developed institutions throughout our government that have *made* cannabis the problem. The DEA and narcotics task forces are behaving as vigilantes under cover of authority. In many cases the narcotics officers don't know or care about the laws that have allowed the medical use of cannabis. They insist that cannabis is dangerous and that the medical marijuana movement is a sham.

Private-sector institutions also help keep prohibition in place. The pharmaceutical, alcohol, and tobacco industries fund the Partnership for a Drug-Free America and lobby against drug-policy reform, which would cost them countless billions of dollars if cannabis prohibition were relaxed. The prison industry also has a vested interest in ongoing prohibition.

But the American people do not, and it's time the federal government put our interests first.

38

Canadian Compassion Clubs

N. Rielle Capler, M.H.A.

The regulations made in 2001 by Health Canada, even though they are a step in the right direction, are fundamentally unsatisfactory. They do not facilitate access to therapeutic cannabis. They do not consider the experience and expertise available in compassion clubs.

SENATE SPECIAL COMMITTEE ON ILLEGAL DRUGS, 2002

The medical use of cannabis poses a conundrum in Canada, as it does in other countries that take a prohibitionist approach to drug policy. While some governments address this by denying outright the therapeutic value of cannabis (US FDA 2006), the Canadian government reluctantly acknowledges it. Canada is one of only a few countries in which cannabis is legal for medical use. Nevertheless, the vast majority of medical cannabis users in this country still face the possibility of criminal prosecution. Of an estimated one million people living in Canada who use cannabis for medical purposes, about four thousand are currently protected by the law (Canadian Centre on Substance Abuse 2004; Health Canada 2009).

In Canada, patients' rights are being fought for in courtrooms and communities. For more than a decade, patients and their advocates have been challenging laws and engaging in acts of civil disobedience to ensure access to those in need. The result is a mix of three medical cannabis distribution systems: a nationally regulated legal program, self-regulated quasi-legal compassion clubs, and the unregulated illegal black market.

For the last ten years I have worked within the quasi-legal realm, distributing cannabis to thousands of critically and chronically ill people in Canada. I have been involved in cannabis-related research and education and have advocated for patients while critiquing the government program and developing standards for compassion clubs.

From people with backgrounds as diverse as their illnesses, I have heard about the relief cannabis provides from pain, spasms, and nausea. I have witnessed the gratitude of patients able to stop taking addictive and liver-damaging prescription opiates by using cannabis. Many of the people I've served have declared that using cannabis has given them a sense of control over their health, elevated their mood, and improved their quality of life.

They've also expressed outrage at being forced to choose between their liberty and their health because of the laws, and their distress at having to choose between their food and costly medicines. They have told me of their frustration in dealing with a government program that was supposed to remedy this situation but has not. In addition to their illnesses, many are also dealing with the stigma and discrimination that the use of cannabis can engender with employers, landlords, insurance companies, health-care providers, and families.

The following account of the current state of medical cannabis in Canada is informed by my experiences and those of the people I have met.

A CONSTITUTIONAL RIGHT TO LIBERTY, HEALTH, AND CANNABIS

In 1987, Terrance Parker, a Canadian man suffering from epilepsy, won the constitutional right to possess cannabis. In 1997 he found himself back in court fighting for the right to access a legal supply. The Ontario provincial court judge presiding over Parker's case ruled that the sections of the Controlled Drugs and Substances Act (CDSA) prohibiting cannabis possession and cultivation violate the constitutional rights to health and liberty and should be read to exempt people with an approved medical need (*R. vs. Parker* 1997). The federal government decided to appeal this ruling. In the meantime, it began using Section 56 of the CDSA, which gives the minister of health the discretion to grant exemptions for the medical or scientific use of controlled substances, to address the medical use of cannabis (*R. vs. Wakeford* 1998).

In July 2000, the Ontario Court of Appeals ruled in agreement with the provincial court that the laws force people to choose between their liberty and their health, and further found the use of Section 56 was inadequate, since it gave unfettered discretionary power to the minister of health to accept or reject applications. In addition, it recognized that the absence of a legal supply posed a significant problem. As a result, the CDSA, as it applies to cannabis possession and cultivation, was declared unconstitutional and of no force and effect. The declaration of invalidity was suspended for one year to give Parliament time to amend the law (*R. vs. Parker* 2000).

The Canadian government did not appeal the Parker decision to the Supreme Court of Canada. Instead, it announced that it intended to develop a new regulatory approach for Canadians to access cannabis for medical use (Regulatory Impact Analysis Statement 2001).

AN UNCONSTITUTIONAL FEDERAL PROGRAM

On July 4, 2001, Health Canada's Marihuana Medical Access Regulations (MMAR) were published. The stated objective of these regulations is to "provide seriously ill Canadian patients with access to marihuana while it is being researched as a possible medicine" (Medical Marihuana Access Regulations 2001). In practice, however, the government program falls short of its objective. As of June 2009, only 4,029 people had been authorized to possess cannabis for medical use (Health Canada 2009). Funding for research was cut in 2006 (Comeau 2006).

The MMAR sets out a process for the authorization to possess and access a legal supply of cannabis. To be eligible, a person suffering from symptoms associated with a terminal illness, or other specific conditions including multiple sclerosis (MS), spinal cord injury, cancer, HIV/AIDS, arthritis, or epilepsy, must obtain the support of his or her physician to fill out the application form. Those with debilitating symptoms related to other medical conditions require a specialist's confirmation of diagnosis and the specialist's agreement that conventional treatments have failed or are inappropriate.

In the original version of the MMAR, there were two options for legal attainment of cannabis: those who had been issued an Authorization to Possess (AP) could either grow their own supply (with a Personal-Use Production License), or they could designate another person to grow it on their behalf (with a Designated-Person Production License, or DPL). A DPL holder was allowed to supply cannabis to one AP holder, and no more than three DPL holders could combine their efforts in one facility.

✓ In 2003, the highest court in the province of Ontario found the MMAR to be unconstitutional. In addition to other shortcomings, the court found that the government's supply options were inadequate, and that the regulations merely provided an "illusion of access." Instead of striking down the program, the court specified several remedies that the government was required to implement to establish the constitutionality of the regulations. One remedy was to expand the 1:1 ratio of DPLs to APs. This was specifically designed to clear the way for licensing compassion clubs, to which the government had pointed (in defense of its lack of supply options) as "an established part of the black market which has historically provided a safe source of marijuana to those with the medical need for it" and claimed "should continue to serve as the source of supply for those with a medical exemption" (*Hitzig vs. Canada* 2003).

The government did not appeal the decision. Nor did it implement all the court-ordered remedies, leaving the constitutionality of the program in question. Instead, Health Canada amended the regulations to add a third option for access to a legal supply of cannabis (Regulations Amending the MMAR 2003). As of July 2003, AP holders have been able to purchase cannabis from Prairie Plant Systems (PPS), a private company that had previously been contracted to grow cannabis for research purposes deep in the abandoned mineshafts of Flin Flon, Manitoba. Sometimes PPS cannabis is referred to as "mine shwag" due to the place of origin and its poor quality (Moote 2003).

Because of the inadequacy of the PPS supply option, later court cases in Ontario and British Columbia reiterated the earlier finding regarding the constitutionality of the regulations and the required remedy (*Canada vs. Sfetkopoulos* 2008; *R. vs. Beren and Swallow* 2009). In 2009, Health Canada responded with an amendment to the regulations, slightly increasing the allowable ratio of APs to DPLs to 2:1 (Regulations Amending the MMAR 2009). This amendment does not comply with the spirit of the court rulings meant to open new channels to legal distribution, again leaving the constitutionality of the program in question.

CIVILLY DISOBEDIENT
COMMUNITY-BASED DISTRIBUTION

In 1997, predating the government's program, Canada's first nonprofit compassion club opened its doors in Vancouver, British Columbia. Today, there are about a dozen well-established medical cannabis dispensaries across the country providing high-quality medicine to between ten thousand and fifteen thousand patients who have a legitimate diagnosis of a medical condition for which cannabis has therapeutic potential (Thaczuk 2007).

Compassion clubs provide access to diverse strains of high-quality organically grown cannabis and other cannabis-based products such as tinctures and edibles. Clients receive education about the safe and effective use of cannabis and advice regarding strain and product selection. By providing a safe place to access services and engage in social activities, compassion clubs offer a sense of connection and belonging that is an added health benefit for people who risk isolation due to their illnesses and choice of medicine (Reiman 2008). Compassion clubs are at the forefront of peer-reviewed research relevant to their clients and policy-makers alike.

Despite calls for the legal recognition of compassion clubs from the Senate, the courts, and various patient groups, these dispensaries continue to operate without legal sanction or protection. As a consequence, compassion clubs are faced with the challenge of finding landlords willing to rent their premises, laboratories willing to break the law to test products, and staff and cultivators willing to engage in civil disobedience. The possibility of police raids is always present and could result in criminal prosecution and the seizure of valuable supplies of medicine.

While there are regional differences, most municipal governments, law enforcement agencies, and communities tolerate dispensaries that ensure services are strictly for medical purposes. Most dispensaries have not faced police raids, and those that have, have received favorable court outcomes recognizing the need they fulfill and the manner in which they operate (*R. vs. Richardson* 2000; *R. vs. Lucas* 2002). However, if a mandatory minimum bill that was introduced in 2009 passes into law, compassion clubs would be at greater risk, since absolute or conditional sentences could no longer be issued at the discretion of a judge.

To remain open, compassion clubs must skillfully balance the criminal prohibition of cannabis with the personal autonomy of their clients in making important health-care decisions. Where the government has failed to officially recognize and therefore regulate these organizations, compassion clubs have taken the lead in creating self-regulations that ensure they provide a high standard of care and promote an understanding of their practices to the wider community (Capler and Lucas 2006).

BARRIERS TO MEDICAL CANNABIS ACCESS

Patients and their advocates have indicated numerous barriers to accessing cannabis either through legal or compassionate channels (Lucas, Black, and Capler 2004; Canadian AIDS Society 2006; Belle-Isle and Hathaway 2007). The most serious are physician support, quality of medicine, and cost.

Physician Support

Both the MMAR and compassion clubs position health care practitioners as gatekeepers to their programs. Although no doctor has ever faced prosecution for recommending medical cannabis, many report that they are reluctant to be associated with this substance because of its illegality and related stigma. They also cite inadequate knowledge of the therapeutic benefits (Jones and Hathaway 2008).

Initially professional associations, including the Canadian Medical Association (CMA) and some provincial Colleges of Physicians and Surgeons, advised physicians not to participate in the MMAR, and the Canadian Medical Protective Association (CMPA), insurers of the medical profession, warned that physicians could face potential legal difficulties. Health Canada's practice of phoning physicians who prescribe more than five grams a day has also discouraged participation in the program (Comeau 2007). After amendments to the regulations that explicitly place responsibility for risk with the patient, the CMA has expressed limited support, and the CMPA has provided a special liability release form.

Many compassion clubs limit the role of physicians to confirmation of diagnosis, a practice advocated by the Canadian Senate, and some accept confirmation from other licensed health care practitioners familiar with herbal medicine (Senate Special Committee on Illegal Drugs 2002). Patients and their advocates have had to take on the role of providing information to their doctors, as Health Canada does not provide such support.

Quality of Product

The quality of cannabis is directly linked to its effectiveness. If Health Canada follows through on its stated plans to discontinue Personal-Use Production Licenses and Designated-Person Production Licenses, the PPS product will be the sole legal supply of medical cannabis in Canada (Regulatory Impact Analysis Statement 2004).

Only about eight hundred AP holders currently order cannabis from

PPS. Many patients have expressed dissatisfaction with the product, and its return rate has been as high as 30 percent (Beeby 2003; Bueckert 2004). Concerns include lack of strain selection (there is only one strain available), poor quality, low potency, and the use of chemical fertilizers, pesticides, and gamma-irradiation in its production.

The medicine's safety was further questioned after independent lab-test results showed elevated levels of arsenic and heavy metals in the PPS product (Canadians for Safe Access 2005). Health Canada responded by suggesting that these levels were "similar to what one finds in Canadian tobacco and are well within allowable limits." There are, however, no Canadian standards limiting heavy metal content in tobacco (Lucas 2008).

Cost

Health Canada sells cannabis to patients for $5 per gram, a prohibitive price for some patients. In 2006, it ceased supplying medicine to those who were behind on payments and sent collection agencies after them (Beeby 2006; Canadians for Safe Access 2008). In 2009, it implemented a policy requiring payment in advance. By doing this, it effectively cut off one of the only legal sources of medicine to patients who cannot afford it (Beeby 2009).

A report reviewing Health Canada's cultivation contract with PPS revealed that the government is charging patients a 1,500 percent markup. Although it spent more than $10 million over seven years, as of July 2007, Health Canada had distributed cannabis to only 435 AP holders. This is reflective of gross inefficiencies in the government program. For approximately the same yearly cost, Health Canada provided cannabis to seven hundred end-users ($3,889.49 per person), and a compassion club supplied three thousand clients ($739.25 per person). The compassion club cost taxpayers nothing (Capler 2007). Compassion club prices are at or below street prices, and donations of medicine are given to those in need whenever possible.

Some support is available for those accessing cannabis through the government program: cannabis ordered from PPS or paid to a designated producer can be claimed as a medical expense for income tax purposes; and in 2009, Veterans Affairs Canada created a policy to cover the cost of cannabis obtained through Health Canada (Canadian Press 2009). Although helpful, these offers do not go far enough. Patients and their advocates continue to stress the importance of having provincial or private health insurance plans cover the costs of this medicine, as they do other prescription drugs.

CONCLUSION

Some of these people are terminally ill. To suspend our
remedy if they may die in the meantime is, in our view,
inconsistent with fundamental Charter values.

HITZIG VS. CANADA, 2003

The small minority of medical cannabis users who have managed to obtain Health Canada licenses may no longer face criminal prosecution, but they do still face discrimination. For those without licenses, things are even harder, as the MMAR creates the false impression that the only legitimate medical cannabis users are those with licenses.

In 2009, Marilyn Holsten, a nearly blind diabetic double amputee was evicted from her subsidized rental apartment in Vancouver because she was using cannabis to treat her pain. She lost a rental arbitration case, and days before she had to leave her home, she died of a heart attack (Chan 2009). A 2009 ruling from the Quebec Human Rights Commission declaring that medical cannabis users are protected from discrimination under the Charter of Rights and Freedoms may help avoid such tragic situations in the future (Quebec Human Rights Commission 2009).

Despite the rights being won by patients and advocates, the medical use of cannabis will always be a myth under the larger umbrella of cannabis prohibition. Under this legal regime, the rationale for obstructing access to cannabis is that it is not an approved medicine. However, cannabis was an approved medicine in Canada before it was prohibited in 1923, and it was not prohibited as a result of scientific evidence of harm or lack of effectiveness (Senate Special Committee on Illegal Drugs 2002).

Canada is currently a signatory to international drug treaties that strictly control some of the most effective plant medicines, including cannabis. Although these treaties make explicit exceptions for medical use and research, in practice this seems to pertain only to pharmaceutical-grade drugs (Rush 2001). Indeed, it would appear that the MMAR is being used as a stopgap measure until the government can "move the provision of marihuana for medical purposes in Canada toward a more traditional health care model" (Regulations Amending the MMAR 2005).

In the experience of those using medical cannabis, its effectiveness and low level of toxicity cannot be replicated by any available pharmaceutical drug. These patients emphatically insist on their right to whole-plant medicine as an essential health care choice (BC Compassion Club Society 2001).

Prohibiting it, taking it off the approved list of medicines, and making access to a legal supply extremely difficult has not altered the medical efficacy of cannabis. Considering the thousands of years this medicine has been used and the relief it has provided to those who are suffering, it is safe to assume that many people will continue to use cannabis outside the purview of the medical profession and the law if necessary. Only a regulatory framework that recognizes the beneficial uses of this plant will support medical cannabis users in fully exercising their constitutional rights to health and liberty. A public health approach to drug control is one such option that is currently being developed and discussed in Canada (Canadian Public Health Association 2007).

39

Dutch Drug Policy

Mario Lap

RECREATIONAL CANNABIS

Based on a report filed in 1972 by the Baan commission (www.drugtext
.org/library/reports), the Dutch Opium Act on Illicit Drugs of 1976 brought
a clear-cut distinction between drug users and traffickers. At the same time,
a distinction was introduced between illegal drugs with so-called unacceptable health risks (all other illicit drugs) and cannabis products by means of
a de-penalization of the latter. The main goal was to create a separation of
markets, preventing hard drug use and addiction.

A policy was developed permitting the retail trade of cannabis products
in about 1,500 so-called coffee shops under specific conditions through a
system of prosecution guidelines called AHOJ-G: A = no advertisement or
public display of products, etc.; H = no hard drugs (meaning all illegal drugs
but cannabis); O = no nuisance and/or disturbance of public order; J = no
sale to minors (anyone under 18 years of age); G = no wholesale (a maximum
of 5 grams per transaction) and the involvement of the so-called Triangle
Committee (mayor, chief of police, and district attorney.) Although now,
some thirty years later, as cannabis is by far the most commonly used illicit
drug in the Western world, only in the Netherlands can one freely buy cannabis products in these cannabis retail facilities called coffee shops.

The cannabis products sold in these coffee shops are hashish (cannabis product) and marijuana (dried parts of the cannabis plant). Most of the

hashish sold is imported from Morocco, but the vast majority of cannabis products sold in the coffee shops consists of so-called Nederweed.

This Nederweed, marijuana grown in the Netherlands, is produced both on a small scale and on a larger scale in a semiprofessional way. Although the retail trade of hashish and marijuana in the coffee shops is tolerated, no similar systems are applied toward the wholesale trade or production and growing of cannabis in the Netherlands.

In 1994, when Dutch marijuana started to become more dominant on the Dutch market, the Netherlands Institute for Alcohol and Drugs, where I was employed at the time, was concerned that the production of this marijuana would fall into the hands of organized crime. A law was proposed to regulate the Dutch cannabis market (www.drugtext.org/library/articles/lexlap.html). This proposal did not pass Parliament, and the prosecution of Dutch cannabis production has since become a high priority for the Dutch police, with foreseeable results.

Today we may conclude that the intensified judicial attention on the supplying of coffee shops has pushed the coffee shops toward more criminal circles. These judicial interventions disturb the normalized supply patterns and recently even caused undesirable price increases ("The Czar's Reefer Madness," *New York Times,* August 26, 2006). A large number of coffee shops offer resistance to this drift toward a more criminal existence; the proprietors of these coffee shops would prefer a normal legal status with corresponding taxation and contributions, but the current legislation prevents this. A solution for this dilemma would be to extend the guideline system to cannabis production, but although the hypocrisy of the current situation is realized by many parties, such as city mayors, judges, and scientists, the legislators refuse to consider this option, using international treaties, pressure, and politics as an excuse. It almost seems like the Dutch legislators suffer from an amotivational syndrome concerning cannabis.

Now, to put my critical approach to Dutch cannabis policy in the right perspective, I have to emphasize that its consequences and effects are, in my view, superior to those of cannabis policies carried out elsewhere, both in Europe and especially in the United States. Hence my criticism is to be regarded from a Dutch and constructive perspective.

The following data from the Centre for Drug Research (CEDRO, a department of the School of Environmental Sciences at the University of Amsterdam) and the EMCDDA clarifies this position (from "Cannabis: The Changing Picture of Cannabis Use in Europe, 2007, European

Monitoring Centre on Drugs and Drug Addiction," www.emcdda.europa/
eu/publications/online/ar2007/en/cannabis.

Table 39.1 clearly shows that Dutch cannabis use was and is lower than
American cannabis use.

TABLE 39.1. DRUG USE IN THE POPULATION OF TWELVE YEARS AND OVER IN THE UNITED STATES AND THE NETHERLANDS, 1997 AND 2001

1997	Ever used		Used past year		Used past month	
	U.S.	Netherlands	U.S.	Netherlands	U.S.	Netherlands
Alcohol	81.9	90.2	64.1	82.5	51.5	73.3
Tobacco	70.5*	67.9	32.7*	38.1	29.6*	34.3
Cannabis	39.2	15.6	9	4.5	5.1	2.5
Cocaine	10.5	2.1	1.9	0.6	0.7	0.2
Inhalants	5.7	0.5	1.1	0.1	0.4	0.0
Heroin	0.9	0.3	0.3	0.1	not measurable	00

*cigarettes only
Source: *National Household Survey 1997* SAMHSA, Office of Applied Studies, Washington, D.C.
M. Abraham, P. Cohen, M. DeWinter *Licit and illicit drug use in the Netherlands, 1997* CEDRO/
Mets and Schilt.

2001	Ever used		Used past year		Used past month	
	U.S.	Netherlands	U.S.	Netherlands	U.S.	Netherlands
Alcohol	81.7	91.6	63.7	83.8	48.3	75.1
Tobacco	71.4*	66.4	34.8*	34.6	29.5*	30.2
Cannabis	36.9	17.0	9.3	5.0	5.4	3.0
Cocaine	12.3	2.9	1.9	0.9	0.7	0.4
Inhalants	8.1	0.8	0.9	0.2	0.2	0.1
Heroin	1.4	0.4	0.2	0.1	0.1	0.1

*cigarettes only
Source: *National Household Survey on Drug Abuse, 2001* SAMHSA, Office of Applied Studies, Washington, D.C. M. Abraham, H. Kaal, P. Cohen, *Licit and illicit drug use in the Netherlands, 2001* CEDRO/
Mets and Schilt.

TABLE 39.2. EUROPEAN CANNABIS USE

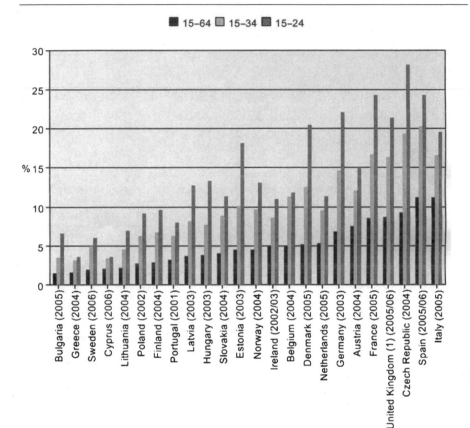

Table 39.2 gives us a picture of European cannabis use, showing Dutch cannabis use was in the mid-range in 2005 and considerably lower than, for example, French cannabis use where French cannabis policy is far more repressive.

Before I move to medicinal cannabis, let me conclude this section on recreational cannabis by briefly discussing two recent issues in the Netherlands and the lack of new realistic prevention efforts.

The Christian Democrat mayor of the city of Maastricht, Gerd Leers, has recently announced the move of a significant number of coffee shops toward the border (Maastricht is a border town of both Belgium and Germany) to decrease the nuisance caused by large numbers of Belgian and French citizens visiting these coffee shops ("Forget Politics, Let's Rap," *The Guardian,* February 28, 2006; Leers: For the Regulation of Cannabis, *ANP,* April 26, 2006; "Belgians Afraid of Maastricht Coffeeshop Policy," *ANP,*

June 1, 2006). He also called for the immediate regulation of production and delivery of cannabis to the Maastricht coffee shops. Whereas he faced opposition for his relocation plans only from Belgian politicians (probably for electoral reasons), his regulatory plans were greeted positively by a majority in Dutch Parliament but were swiftly denied by the minister of justice from the same Christian Democrat party.

As almost everywhere else in the world, drug policy in the Netherlands is rarely based on empirical studies or cost-benefit analyses. Many decisions are based on political opportunism, innuendo, and populism. Bearing this in mind is the only way to understand the recent political decisions concerning coffee shops in the near vicinity of schools ("Coffeeshops in the Vicinity of Schools: A Real or Political Problem?" *TNI*, May 31, 2007).

Not based on any scientific or other data, and without even examining the possible consequences of such proposals for cannabis availability and consumption, or the influence on the main goal of cannabis police—the separation of markets—a decision was made to set minimum distances between coffee shops and schools. This, while no policy whatsoever is in place for what is in my view the main public health problem with cannabis consumption in the Netherlands as well as the rest of Europe.

Cannabis in Europe is mostly consumed in so-called joints. These joints consist of 80 to 90 percent tobacco with some cannabis or hashish mixed in. In fact, many youngsters' first tobacco consumption is by means of these joints. Now at the age of, for example, thirty, most of these youngsters have stopped consuming cannabis but have ended up with a significant tobacco addiction.

Therefore, for many years now, I have suggested a prevention campaign informing young people of the hazards of the above form of cannabis use and of alternative ways of consumption (pure cannabis joints and/or with tobacco replacements). Recent Swiss scientific research has revealed further negative aspects of combined cannabis-tobacco use (*Archives of Pediatric and Adolescent Medicine* 2007, 161 (11): 1–42–1047), but realistic Dutch government prevention efforts concerning such use are nonexistent (Tips for Cannabis Consumers, www.drugtext.org/sub/tips.htm).

MEDICINAL CANNABIS

Thanks to the health minister at that time, Dr. Els Borst, patients in the Netherlands can obtain fully legal medicinal cannabis by prescription from pharmacies since September 1, 2003. This cannabis is produced under control of the Government Bureau of Medicinal Cannabis (BMC) and consists of three varieties of cannabis. Medicinal cannabis is prescribed to a wide variety of patients, such as people suffering from AIDS/HIV; multiple sclerosis and other muscle-related diseases; Tourette's syndrome; rheumatism; and cancer ("The Future of Legal Medicinal Cannabis," quickscan by the Ministry of Health, December 2004).

Recently, Germany, Italy, and Finland have also decided to enable the prescription of such medicinal cannabis and to facilitate such practice on the basis of cannabis imported from and produced by the BMC in the Netherlands ("Dutch Medicinal Marijuana Imported by Germany, Italy, and Finland," *ANP,* August 22, 2009). Additional countries are expected to follow in the near future.

The main problem with medicinal cannabis in the first years was the availability of more varieties of cannabis at a much lower price in the coffee shops, but now more varieties are prescribed, and significant price cuts have been realized; more patients and doctors have realized the advantages of cannabis produced for medicinal purposes, and hence of consistent quality and constant strength (October 13, 2009, De Volkskrant, Cannabis as medicine).

The current Dutch minister of public health, welfare and sport, Ab Klink, has just decided that the production and prescription of medicinal cannabis will be extended for at least another seven years. Further scientific studies are also being facilitated.

40

A Cost-Benefit Analysis of Legalizing Marijuana

Jeffrey Miron, Ph.D.

Government prohibition of marijuana is the subject of enormous debate. Advocates believe prohibition reduces marijuana trafficking and use, thereby discouraging crime, improving productivity, and increasing health. Critics believe prohibition has only modest effects on trafficking and use while causing many problems typically attributed to marijuana itself. In particular, prohibition does not eliminate the marijuana market but merely drives it underground, which has numerous unwanted consequences.

One issue in this debate is the effect of marijuana prohibition on government budgets. Prohibition entails direct enforcement costs. If marijuana were legal, enforcement costs would be zero, and governments could levy taxes on the production and sale of marijuana. Thus, government expenditure would decline and tax revenue would increase. The reduction in expenditure constitutes a net saving in resources as well; that is, these funds would be available for other uses. The increase in tax revenues would be a transfer from drug users and producers to the general public. In attempting to change current policy, advocates of decriminalization or legalization have often emphasized these budgetary impacts as important pieces of their argument.

This essay discusses issues related to the savings in government expenditure and the gains in tax revenue that would result from legalizing marijuana. The first section provides a brief review of existing estimates and discusses some limitations and caveats. The second section discusses the broad range of issues relevant to analyzing legalization versus prohibition and argues that legalization is the better policy even if the budgetary impacts are minor.

THE BUDGETARY IMPACTS OF MARIJUANA LEGALIZATION

In a legalized marijuana regime, all criminal and civil penalties against production, distribution, sale, and possession would cease. Instead, marijuana would be treated like other legal goods subject to standard regulations and taxes. Policy might also impose marijuana-specific regulations and taxes, as occurs now for alcohol and tobacco. These should be moderate enough, however, that marijuana would be produced and distributed in a legal market, not driven underground.

This policy change would affect government budgets in the following ways. First, government would save the resources currently devoted to arresting, prosecuting, and incarcerating marijuana producers and consumers. Second, governments would collect tax revenue on the production and sale of legal marijuana. The tax rates on marijuana might be the same as those applied generally, or they might be higher, as with alcohol and tobacco.

Earlier research (Miron 2006) indicates that marijuana legalization would reduce government expenditures by roughly $8 billion annually. As shown in Table 40.1 below, approximately $5.5 billion of this would come from decreased state and local expenditures and approximately $2.5 billion from decreased federal expenditures. At the state and local levels, the reduced expenditures would consist of $1.8 billion less spent on police, $3.2 less on prosecutions, and $0.5 billion less on incarceration. (At the federal level, a detailed breakdown is not readily available.)

TABLE 40.1. REDUCED GOVERNMENT EXPENDITURE DUE TO MARIJUANA LEGALIZATION, IN BILLIONS OF DOLLARS

	State and local	Federal	Total
Arrests	$1.8		
Prosecutions	$3.2		
Incarcerations	$0.5		
Total	$5.5	$2.5	$8.0

Marijuana legalization would also generate tax revenue of approximately $2.4 billion annually if marijuana were taxed like all other goods, and $6.2 billion annually if marijuana were taxed at rates comparable to those on alcohol and tobacco. (A 2007 study from George Mason University reports that lost revenue from failing to tax a $113 billion business, as well as costs incurred enforcing marijuana laws, cost U.S. taxpayers $41.8 billion yearly.) These budgetary impacts rely on a range of assumptions, but the estimates are most likely biased downward. A few comments about these estimates are in order.

The tax rates on legalized marijuana could be higher than those on most other goods. It is critical, however, that these rates not become so elevated that they drive the marijuana market underground and amount to de facto prohibition. Moreover, high tax rates have many of the same negatives as prohibition, such as penalizing marijuana users who consume responsibly. Thus assuming a legalized regime can generate huge revenues, or justifying legalization by asserting that high taxes will be just as strong a deterrent as prohibition, is not an appealing line of argument. The revenue goals for a legalized marijuana market should be moderate, meaning no more extreme (relative to price) than those for alcohol or tobacco.

A second caveat is that although marijuana is more commonly used than other drugs, prohibition targets other drugs disproportionately relative to marijuana. Thus, at least from the perspective of saving enforcement resources, it is misguided to think only about legalizing marijuana. The same caveat potentially applies if the focus is raising tax revenue, since the demands for some other drugs are plausibly less responsive to price than is marijuana. This means policy can raise substantial revenue from these drugs even if the markets are smaller. Plausibly, the budgetary impacts from these other drugs would be several times larger than those from legalizing marijuana, even though they constitute a much smaller share of the market in terms of users.

An important clarification is that the tax revenues that would accrue to governments from legalization are not as cost-saving in the economic, "opportunity" sense of costs. Instead, these amounts represent transfers from those paying the tax (marijuana producers and users) to the general public. Under prohibition no taxation occurs, but consumers pay higher prices to producers. Thus, the distributional consequence of legalization is to redistribute wealth from people who choose to violate the law—by producing and selling marijuana under prohibition—to the general public. This redistribution is one that most people would endorse, but it does not represent a net increase in resources.

One criticism of legalization proposals that highlight the increase in tax revenues asserts that the underground marijuana industry would remain underground even if legalized, thereby limiting the scope for taxing legalized marijuana. This concern has a grain of truth but is almost certainly irrelevant in practice. Home production of alcohol was widespread during Prohibition, but after repeal most of the demand reverted to being met by commercial suppliers. This makes sense, since large-scale, commercial production is more efficient, and most people seem to prefer purchasing from a reliable, long-term supplier who can maintain quality and consistency. (Most people could grow their own tomatoes, but only a tiny fraction of the population chooses to do so.)

THE BROADER ISSUES RELATED
TO MARIJUANA LEGALIZATION

The budgetary impacts of marijuana legalization are not trivial. A savings of $7.7 billion per year in resources is substantial, and a net improvement in the U.S. government budget of $10–14 billion annually is worth achieving. Compared to the size of the U.S. economy or government, however, these are not enormous amounts. Thus, if prohibition has some nontrivial benefit and few unintended negatives, prohibition advocates could rationally argue that the budgetary benefits do not justify legalization. It is crucial, therefore, to consider the broader range of issues involved. In fact, prohibition has minimal benefits and substantial negative side effects beyond its direct costs.

Prohibition does not eliminate the market for marijuana. Instead, prohibition creates a black market. The key question for analysis of prohibition versus legalization is therefore to what degree marijuana use in this black market is less than what would occur under legalization. To address this issue, consider the effects of prohibition on the demand for and supply of marijuana.

Prohibition affects the demand for marijuana in several ways. The mere existence of prohibition might reduce demand if some consumers exhibit respect for the law. The evidence suggests, however, that "respect for the law" exerts only a mild effect, since violation of weakly enforced laws (speeding, tax evasion, blue laws, sodomy laws) is widespread. The penalties for marijuana purchase or possession might reduce demand by raising the effective price of marijuana use. Again, however, the evidence does not suggest a major impact given that most such penalties are mild and rarely imposed. Potentially countering any tendency for prohibition to reduce demand, prohibition might increase demand because it makes marijuana a "forbidden fruit." Prohibition also affects the supply of marijuana. Because black market marijuana suppliers must operate in secret and attempt to avoid detection by law enforcement, they face increased costs of manufacturing, transporting, and distributing marijuana. Conditional on operating in secret, however, black market suppliers face low marginal costs of evading tax laws and regulatory policies, and this partially offsets the increased costs of operating secretly. Other differences between a black market and a legal market (e.g., differences in advertising incentives or market power) have ambiguous implications for supply costs under prohibition versus legalization.

The bottom line is that prohibition probably reduces marijuana use, since the direct effects on both supply and demand suggest this outcome. Theory does not dictate that prohibition causes a large reduction in marijuana use, however, and the evidence suggests prohibition has at most a moderate impact. Alcohol prohibition in the United States, for example, did not appear to have reduced alcohol consumption dramatically. Comparisons of countries with weakly versus strongly imposed prohibitions find little evidence of higher marijuana consumption in the weak enforcement countries. Thus the evidence does not rule out the possibility that marijuana consumption might increase, say, 25 percent under legalization, but no evidence suggests it would be increased by orders of magnitude.

Whatever the impact of prohibition on marijuana consumption, prohibition has numerous effects beyond any direct costs of enforcement. The main ones are as follows:

Increased crime and corruption. Because participants in illegal markets cannot resolve disputes with nonviolent mechanisms like courts and lawyers, they use guns instead; thus prohibition increases violent crime. By diverting criminal justice resources to prohibition enforcement, prohibition causes reduced deterrence of all kinds of crime. Because participants in a black market must either evade law enforcement authorities or pay them to look the other way, prohibition encourages corruption.

Harm to marijuana users. By raising prices and creating the threat of arrest and other legal sanctions, prohibition reduces the welfare of those who use marijuana illegally. These users also spend more time trying to buy marijuana and must deal with criminals to do so.

Reduced product quality. In a legal market, consumers who purchase faulty goods can punish suppliers by pursuing liability claims, by generating bad publicity, by avoiding repeat purchases, or by complaining to private or government watchdog groups. In a black market, these mechanisms for ensuring product quality are unavailable or less effective. This means product quality is lower and more uncertain in an underground market.

Enriching criminals. In a legal market, the income generated by production and sale of marijuana is subject to taxation, and the tax revenues accrue to the government. In a black market, suppliers capture these revenues as profits. Prohibition thus enriches the segment of society most willing to evade the law.

Restrictions on medicinal uses of marijuana. Because of prohibition, marijuana is even more tightly controlled than morphine or cocaine and cannot be used for medical purposes despite abundant evidence that it alleviates nausea, pain, and muscle spasms, as well as symptoms of glaucoma, epilepsy, multiple sclerosis, AIDS, and migraine headaches, among other ailments.

Compromised civil liberties. Because marijuana "crimes" involve voluntary exchange, enforcement relies on asset seizures, aggressive search tactics, and racial profiling. All these tactics strain accepted notions of civil liberties and generate racial tension.

Respect for the law. All experience to date indicates that, even with substantial enforcement, prohibition fails to deter a great many persons from supplying and consuming marijuana. This fact signals users and nonusers that "laws are for suckers"; prohibition therefore undermines the spirit of voluntary compliance that is essential to law enforcement in a free society.

Most effects of prohibition are unambiguously undesirable. The only possible exception is prohibition's impact in reducing marijuana consumption. According to some people, marijuana use is inherently evil, or promotes socially undesirable behavior, or lowers health and productivity, implying policy-induced reductions in marijuana use might be desirable.

The claim that marijuana is inherently wrong is simply an assertion devoid of any science or reason, however, and no valid evidence supports the claim that marijuana use causes poor health, diminished productivity, or other unwanted behaviors.

An alternative view is that marijuana consumption can generate negative side effects, such as traffic accidents. This view is defensible, but a better approach would be policies that target the negative behavior itself, namely laws against driving under the influence. This is exactly what current policy does regarding alcohol. A total prohibition on marijuana targets millions of otherwise law-abiding citizens whose use does not generate adverse effects for anyone.

Overall, therefore, the reduction in marijuana consumption caused by prohibition is a cost rather than a benefit. That is, preventing responsible people from consuming marijuana makes them worse off, just as preventing responsible people from consuming alcohol would make them worse off. This means virtually all of prohibition's consequences are undesirable, so it is impossible to justify any government expenditure in the attempt to implement this policy.

CONCLUSION

The government expenditure utilized in the attempt to enforce marijuana prohibition is an unambiguous cost of prohibition relative to legalization. It is far from the only cost, however. Prohibition has a host of unintended negative effects that should receive at least as much consideration in evaluations of marijuana policy.

Perhaps most importantly, prohibition reduces the welfare of people who can and do use marijuana with little harm to themselves or others and who believe they receive a benefit—whether recreational or medicinal—from marijuana use. A policy that prohibits marijuana makes no more sense than a policy that prohibits alcohol, ice cream, or driving on the highway. Each of these activities—and millions of others—can generate harm when conducted irresponsibly but also has the potential to benefit the vast majority of users. This is a crucial effect of marijuana legalization that all analyses should recognize.

41

The Marijuana Policy Project

Bruce Mirken

This article was written in August 2007. Please see any and all footnotes for updates since that time, as well as the website www. mpp.org.

The Marijuana Policy Project was founded in 1995 on one simple principle: Marijuana laws ought to make sense, reducing harm rather than increasing it. No drug is harmless, including marijuana, but the current marijuana laws in the United States (and most other countries) cause vastly more harm than they prevent. The Marijuana Policy Project (MPP) advocates for common-sense, harm reduction–based marijuana policies through state and federal lobbying, ballot initiative campaigns, public education, and grant support of local activists.

All policy decisions come down to assessments of risks versus benefits: in this case, the risks and benefits of marijuana use as opposed to its prohibition. While a detailed analysis of these risks and benefits could be—and has been—the subject of entire volumes, it may be useful to recap some essential points.

Few Americans realize that the United States' first national antimarijuana law, the Marijuana Tax Act of 1937, was passed without any sort of rational assessment of the risks and benefits of either marijuana or the proposed new policy. While antimarijuana propaganda of the era was often hysterical and dripping with overt racism, the brief congressional hearings were alarmingly perfunctory, described in one history as "a case study in legislative carelessness"(Bonnie and Whitebread 1970). The "evidence" cited at the hearings, linking marijuana to insanity and criminality, consisted almost entirely of anecdotes taken from newspaper stories (Bonnie and Whitebread 1970).

Since then, numerous expert reviews have considered the evidence regarding marijuana's effects. Government panels in the United States, Canada, Britain, and elsewhere; reviews by scientific bodies such as the Institute of Medicine in the United States and the British government's Advisory Council on the Misuse of Drugs; and numerous independent researchers have produced consistent reports that, while not harmless, the health risks of marijuana use are, for most users, relatively minor and markedly less than those of many drugs that are legal in most countries, including tobacco and alcohol.

For example, the Institute of Medicine (IOM) called dependence on marijuana "relatively rare"—affecting just 9 percent of users, as opposed to 15 percent for alcohol users and 32 percent for tobacco smokers—and "less severe than dependence on other drugs." The IOM panel also found no persuasive evidence that marijuana causes cancer, brain damage, or "amotivational syndrome," or that it causes users to progress to hard drugs (Joy, Benson, and Watson 1999).

In a March 2002 report to Britain's home secretary, the Advisory Council on the Misuse of Drugs noted various health risks associated with marijuana use, most notably a risk of bronchitis and other pulmonary problems associated with smoking. Nevertheless, the council concluded that these risks are relatively small, writing, "The high use of cannabis is not associated with major health problems for the individual or society. The occasional use of cannabis is only rarely associated with significant problems in otherwise healthy individuals" (Advisory Council on the Misuse of Drugs 2002).

So marijuana, especially when smoked, is not without health risks; but when compared with other drugs, including legal substances such as tobacco and alcohol, these risks appear to be fairly small. What, then, are the risks and benefits of attempting to curb marijuana use by criminalizing its production, sale, and possession?

This question can be logically divided into two parts: First, has marijuana prohibition succeeded in curbing marijuana use, and thus the harms associated with such use? Second, has prohibition had other effects on society, good or bad, that must be weighed when considering whether present policies are beneficial?

MPP examined the first question, with an emphasis on use by young people, in a detailed report issued in late 2006 and briefly summarized here. If the idea of banning marijuana was to keep people, especially youths, from using or having ready access to it, then the policy has manifestly failed.

Although marijuana has been used by humans for thousands of years, widespread prohibition did not come about until well into the twentieth century. As stated earlier, in the United States, national marijuana prohibition began with the Marijuana Tax Act of 1937. By nearly all accounts, marijuana use in the United States was rare in the pre-prohibition era, with marijuana virtually unknown across large sections of the United States. For example, according to a 1996 report from the U.S. Department of Health and Human Services' Substance Abuse and Mental Health Services Administration, of individuals born from 1919 to 1929—before the advent of marijuana prohibition—only 1.2 percent had used marijuana even once by the time they reached age thirty-five (Johnson et al. 1996).

The numbers shifted markedly during the prohibition era. For those born from 1941 to 1945, the figure for marijuana use by age thirty-five had jumped to 24.1 percent. For every birth cohort from 1951 forward, more than 50 percent had used marijuana by the time they turned thirty-five (Johnson et al. 1996). Put another way, during the era of marijuana prohibition, use of marijuana by Americans under thirty-five (who have traditionally been the largest proportion of users) increased by more than 4,000 percent.

This is not to say, of course, that prohibition caused use to increase. What is clear, however, is that a policy whose express purpose was to wipe out what was commonly described as a scourge, or even an "assassin of youth," failed utterly in this purpose.

Still, the possibility remains that marijuana prohibition did curb use somewhat, keeping it to lower levels than would have occurred without a ban. A controlled test of this proposition is, for all intents and purposes, impossible, but some clues can be gleaned from what has occurred in various states in the United States and other countries with regard to legal schemes and levels of penalties for marijuana possession. This evidence suggests that criminal penalties have had relatively little impact on use.

For example, in a 2001 report commissioned by the White House, the National Research Council (NRC) concluded, "In summary, existing research seems to indicate that there is little apparent relationship between severity of sanctions prescribed for drug use and prevalence or frequency of use, and that perceived legal risk explains very little in the variance of individual drug use." The bulk of the evidence cited by the NRC in support of this conclusion comes from studies of "the impact of decriminalization on the prevalence of marijuana use among youths and adults" in the United States and Australia (Manski, Pepper, and Petrie 2001).*

Since 1999, the National Survey on Drug Use and Health has published state-level drug-use figures that reinforce these earlier studies, showing marijuana use levels in decriminalized states (California, Colorado, Maine, Massachusetts, Minnesota, Mississippi, Nebraska, Nevada, New York, North Carolina, Ohio, and Oregon) to be virtually indistinguishable from states that still jail those convicted of marijuana possession. For example, in Mississippi, 8.26 percent of those aged twelve and over used marijuana in the past year, while in two neighboring states with much stiffer penalties, Alabama and Louisiana, the rates were 8.76 percent and 9.31 percent, respectively (Wright, Sathe, and Spagnola 2007).

In the Netherlands, where possession and purchase of small amounts of marijuana are effectively legal (technically against the law but permitted under regulation in a policy of official "tolerance"), rates of marijuana use have moved up and down over the years, much as in the United States, but at a consistently lower level. The latest Dutch government figures, from 2001, show that 17 percent of Netherlands residents aged twelve and up have ever used marijuana (van Laar et al. 2006). In contrast, 40.1 percent of Americans aged twelve and up have used marijuana (Substance Abuse and Mental Health Services Administration 2006).

So, if the benefits of prohibition are limited, what of the risks? A policy that does little good might still be justified if it does no harm. Can this be said of marijuana prohibition?

One population is clearly harmed by prohibition: those arrested on marijuana charges—and with U.S. marijuana arrests consistently running over three quarters of a million per year, that's not an insignificant population. In addition to whatever fines or jail sentences are meted out, arrestees are also likely to face legal expenses, disruptions to jobs, families, and educations, and an array of collateral consequences that can include temporary or permanent loss of student loans, the right to vote, driving privileges, access to public

---

*Decriminalization doesn't mean making marijuana legal. What it means varies widely from state to state, and it generally refers to a reduction in penalties for possession of small amounts for personal use—e.g., a fine rather than jail time, a misdemeanor offense rather than a felony. However, in general, in the case of possession of large amounts, it is assumed that it is intended to be sold, and that's still usually a felony.

housing, and many other rights and privileges. (Please see chapter 18 by Richard Glen Boire on collateral consequences of marijuana convictions.)

But a strong case can be made that the rest of society suffers as well, as prohibition forces a large chunk of economic activity into the criminal underground ($35.8 billion worth of economic activity in 2006, according to one estimate, making marijuana America's largest cash crop) (Gettman 2006). This has the effect of exempting a substantial block of business activity from taxation as well as labor and environmental standards. The latter is a growing issue, as pressure from law enforcement has driven more and more marijuana producers to hide clandestine gardens in national parks, forests, and other environmentally sensitive areas not suitable for agriculture. This carries great potential for environmental harm as well as possible risks to hikers, campers, and other innocent frequenters of these wild lands (Breitler 2007).

Beyond that, prohibition means foregoing the controls and restrictions that society has chosen—wisely, most would say—to impose on other psychoactive substances. Consider, for example, the rules imposed on producers and sellers of alcoholic beverages, none of which can be applied to marijuana under prohibition: Producers, distributors, and sellers must be licensed. As a licensing requirement, they are subject to rules covering, among other things, how the product is labeled, including disclosure of the alcohol content; the days, times, and by what means it can be sold; to whom it can be sold; who may be admitted on the premises of alcohol-selling establishments; and where such establishments may be located. While adherence to these rules is imperfect, the vast majority of sellers and producers abide by them, as failure to do so can mean the loss of a lucrative liquor license.

If there is one group that is most profoundly harmed by marijuana prohibition, it is patients suffering from a variety of conditions who might be helped by use of marijuana as medicine. This is a population to which MPP has devoted and will continue to devote much of our attention and resources.

An extensive discussion of the medical marijuana literature is beyond the scope of this chapter, but suffice it to say that recent studies have resoundingly reaffirmed the Institute of Medicine's 1999 conclusion that "nausea, appetite loss, pain and anxiety . . . all can be mitigated by marijuana"(Joy, Benson, and Watson 1999). The continued development and testing of vaporizer technology have removed the last significant objection to medical marijuana, the potential pulmonary risks of smoking (Abrams 2007; Earleywine and Smucker Barnwell 2007).

Fortunately, the medical marijuana front is the area where we've seen the most progress. California passed the first effective medical marijuana law in 1996. As of this writing, August 2007, a total of twelve states have passed laws permitting patients to possess and, in nearly all cases, cultivate a limited amount of marijuana for medical purposes if they meet certain conditions.* MPP played the principal role in drafting and gaining passage of four of the newest such laws, in Hawaii (2000), Montana (2004), Vermont (2004), and Rhode Island (2006).

A particularly encouraging sign is the shift in how medical marijuana laws are being passed. All the medical marijuana laws passed in the 1990s were enacted via ballot initiatives, a difficult and expensive process that is not available in many states. Of the four new laws cited above, three were passed by state legislatures, as was the medical marijuana law enacted in New Mexico in 2007. In a remarkable show of legislative strength, Rhode Island's law was passed via an override of Governor Donald Carcieri's veto in 2006 and made permanent (having been originally passed with a one-year sunset clause) a year later with an even more overwhelming veto override (Henry 2007).

While states are free to exempt medical marijuana patients from arrest under state laws, these state protections do not confer immunity from federal prosecution. The federal Drug Enforcement Administration (DEA) has primarily targeted medical marijuana dispensaries operating openly in some parts of California, depriving patients in some areas of a safe supply of medicine. While individual patients have not been the DEA's primary focus, some patients have been caught up in the raids, which have been routinely denounced by local officials and major newspapers (*Los Angeles Daily News* 2007).

A key MPP goal is to end such federal interference with state medical marijuana laws. MPP, which employs the only full-time marijuana policy lobbyist on Capitol Hill, has worked on several legislative approaches. Most notable among these is the Hinchey-Rohrabacher amendment, a rider to the appropriations bill funding the Department of Justice that would bar the department from using any of its funds to interfere with state medical marijuana laws. While the amendment has not passed in five years of attempts, support keeps inching upward, to a record 165 yes votes (of 218 needed for passage) in 2007, the last time passage was attempted (Richman 2007).

---

*The current number of states is fourteen, plus the District of Columbia, with more pending.

MPP also continues to put considerable energy into increasing the number of medical marijuana states. Not only does this provide substantial immediate protection to patients in those states, it expands the pool of congress members likely to look favorably on federal medical marijuana legislation. In 2008, these efforts are expected to include lobbying drives in Minnesota, Illinois, and New York, and ballot drives in Michigan and Arizona.

While medical marijuana is an urgent priority, MPP continues to work on the larger problem of marijuana prohibition—an irrational and failed policy, but a challenging one to address politically: While the American public overwhelmingly supports legal access to medical marijuana, public opinion surveys show voters sharply divided about how to handle nonmedical marijuana use. For example, a 2005 Gallup Poll found 78 percent in favor of allowing doctors to prescribe marijuana, while a smaller majority, 55 percent, said that possession of a small amount of marijuana should not be treated as a criminal offense. But asked whether "use of marijuana should be made legal," only 36 percent agreed—an increase over previous years, but still well short of a majority (Gallup Poll 2007).

MPP's strategy for ending prohibition has two major prongs, public education and political action. MPP spokespeople appear frequently on television and radio to discuss the folly of prohibition, and MPP op-ed columns discussing the need for new policies have appeared in newspapers all over the country as well as on a variety of websites. Special MPP reports, such as 2006's "Does Prohibition of Marijuana for Adults Curb Use by Adolescents?" stimulate public discussion of the mistaken assumptions underlying prohibition.

Unfortunately, no drug policy reform organization has an advertising budget remotely close to that of the White House Office of National Drug Control Policy, which for a decade has been spending an average of well over $100 million per year on ads largely aimed at demonizing marijuana. By comparison, the combined budgets of all U.S. drug policy reform organizations—not just for advertising, but salaries, rent, telephones, and everything else needed to keep organizations running—hovers somewhere in the neighborhood of $25 million annually. Nevertheless, MPP has run targeted radio and television ads and is presently looking at the potential of new educational campaigns.

On the political front, MPP works with legislators willing to introduce legislation to tax and regulate marijuana in a manner similar to alcohol, and supports state ballot initiatives to do the same. MPP-supported campaigns in Alaska (2004) and Nevada (2006) produced the largest-ever votes (44 percent voting yes) in favor of measures to end marijuana prohibition completely. We are actively looking at prospects for future such measures. In the meantime, a 2008 decriminalization initiative (replacing arrest and jail for possession of a small amount of marijuana with a fine similar to a traffic ticket) is likely in Massachusetts and would represent a significant step forward.

Politicians often fear embracing marijuana policy reform, believing they will be subject to attack for being "soft on drugs." Surprisingly, this even extends at times to reforms with broad public support, such as medical marijuana laws. MPP's lobbyists hear this in private discussions with elected officials and their staff members with disturbing frequency. Overcoming such misconceptions remains one of our biggest challenges.

One way to make statewide reform measures seem less frightening to politicians is to demonstrate support via local ballot measures. MPP's grant program has funded many local campaigns, the vast majority of them successful, for measures calling for an end to marijuana arrests. MPP-supported measures making marijuana arrests the lowest priority for local police or repealing local marijuana penalties have passed in locations all over the country, including Seattle; Denver; the California cities of Oakland, Santa Cruz, Santa Monica, and Santa Barbara; and even in Missoula County, Montana. MPP continues to work with local activists to identify and support campaigns that have a good chance of success, in hope of helping reach the critical mass needed to enact statewide reforms.

MPP's efforts will continue and expand on all these fronts over the next few years. Reforming America's marijuana laws can be likened to assembling a jigsaw puzzle: finding the first few pieces to join together is difficult and time consuming, but the more pieces come together, the clearer the puzzle's pattern becomes, and the easier the job gets. One by one, often with great difficulty, the pieces are coming together. The pattern is becoming clearer. MPP is committed to leading the fight for reform until, like the Berlin Wall, the edifice of marijuana prohibition comes crashing down under the weight of its own futility.

42

The ACLU and Cannabis Drug Policy

An Interview with Graham Boyd, J.D.

Julie Holland, M.D.

JULIE HOLLAND: How has the American Civil Liberties Union (ACLU) been involved in defending civil liberties as they relate to drug policy?

GRAHAM BOYD: While the American Civil Liberties Union has favored the legalization of marijuana for adults for many years, only since 1998 have we had a project specifically dedicated to the litigation of drug policy issues. I started that project in a small office in New Haven, Connecticut, and it has since grown to about twenty people working around the country on a variety civil rights and civil liberties issues related to the "war on drugs." The project, now known as the ACLU Drug Law Reform Project, arose at a particularly interesting crossroads in our nation's drug policy, as states, led by California, began to break from the federal government and allow the use of medical marijuana by qualified patients. This process raised a host of legal questions, and our project really began, first and foremost, working to resolve some of the questions brought up by medical marijuana. Our first case, *Conant vs. McCaffrey,* concerned the federal government's policy of threatening to arrest or to strip the license of any physician who recommended medical marijuana to a patient.

JULIE: This seems to me a freedom of speech issue; I should be able to talk to my patients about whatever I want.

GRAHAM: It is a core First Amendment issue, but it really concerns the federal government's devotion to blocking state medical marijuana laws, which has continued to this day. As soon as the ink was dry on Proposition 215—the first state medical marijuana law, which was passed by a wide margin of California voters in November 1997—the federal government, led by then–"drug czar" Barry McCaffrey, started plotting a response. Essentially, they planned to reverse the outcome of the election—to overturn the will of California voters—and they sought to accomplish this through an official and well-publicized policy of threatening severe punishment of doctors who recommended medical marijuana.

In the course of the litigation, we learned that the drug czar, Barry McCaffrey, had been asked by President Clinton to convene a group of high-ranking officials to formulate a federal response to Proposition 215. While the deliberations of that group weren't publicly known, through our lawsuit we succeeded in uncovering the agendas and minutes and summaries of many of their meetings. One of the first things they considered was filing a lawsuit against California, where the federal government would sue California and claim that Proposition 215 was preempted, or trumped, by federal laws. The lawyers in the Department of Justice recognized, quite correctly, that such a legal claim would most certainly fail. The states are clearly free to decide not to criminalize particular conduct under state law, regardless of whether that conduct remains prohibited under federal law. The federal government can say, We consider it to be a crime, and the state can say, Well, we don't.

So, having realized they couldn't undo Proposition 215 in court, the federal government looked for other means to derail it. And they hit upon this linchpin in the system, which is the doctors. You see, under California law, a patient is permitted to use medical marijuana only if a doctor recommends it. So the federal government figured that if no doctor is willing to recommend marijuana to a patient, then no patient would be authorized to use it, and the system would effectively collapse.

At the time, I was a lawyer in private practice and was hired by the sponsors of Proposition 215 to prepare for its legal defense. So when these threats against the doctors were made, we were ready to go to court. We brought a lawsuit on behalf of Dr. Marcus Conant, a well-known doctor in the HIV/AIDS community, who was featured in the book and movie *And the Band Played On*. He'd been around a long time with a good reputation, and he very much believes that the use of marijuana is medically appropriate for some people. He and a group of other doctors wanted to be represented in a lawsuit against the federal government arguing that they have a right to give honest medical advice to their patients. The case turned into a class action suit on behalf of all the doctors in California, as well as a group of patients with cancer, HIV, and other medical conditions, who wanted to be able to receive honest and accurate medical information from their doctors.

We immediately asked for a court order—a preliminary injunction that would compel the federal government to stop making these threats against doctors, as well as to not follow through on the threats. The judge, rightly, granted our order—a major blow to the strategy of the federal government—which set the stage for Proposition 215 to be effectively implemented.

The Conant litigation eventually reached the Ninth Circuit Court of Appeals—the appellate court for the western United States. We ended up prevailing there in front of a panel that included a mix of liberal, moderate, and conservative judges. They all agreed that the First Amendment strongly protected doctors' right to discuss and recommend marijuana to their patients. But the judges were also disturbed by the heavy-handedness of the federal policy—how it completely lacked compassion. They clearly did not like it, and this was across ideological and political spectrums.

After that, pretty much everyone, myself included, expected the case to go to the Supreme Court. It had all the necessary criteria: it was a court order that had stopped a federal policy, that found an unconstitutional application of the nation's vain, prohibitionist drug policy, and review in the Supreme Court was being sought by the solicitor general, the top government lawyer. But the court ended up not taking the case, which everybody took to mean that a majority of the Supreme Court agreed with the lower courts—in other words, they would have ruled in our favor. The Supreme Court's decision not to take the case was a very powerful signal that the federal government had gone too far by threatening doctors, by threatening medical care, by violating First

Amendment rights in trying to squelch the nation's first medical marijuana law.

There were some really interesting and revelatory moments during the litigation. We ended up being able to take deposition testimony from the highest drug officials in the country—from the head of the DEA, from Barry McCaffrey, the drug czar, from his chief council, who, by the time we deposed her, was the sitting federal judge in Miami. It's quite unusual to have these people placed under oath and subjected to questioning about their drug policies, and from that we gained insight into how the medical marijuana policy was so heavily politically driven, and that it didn't really care about medical facts or patients' well-being. I think at the heart of it was this deep, deep fear about sending the wrong message to children. If children were able to hear that marijuana could be medicine, then they wouldn't believe any of the things that they were told about how dangerous marijuana was, and that, in turn, would cause more children to use marijuana and eventually other drugs.

JULIE: Well, the fear is genuine, but unfounded. Think of something like lithium or chemotherapy that's helping Daddy stay calm or helping Mommy fight her cancer, and obviously it's dangerous for somebody else to have it.

GRAHAM: Absolutely. There are a number of other prescription medications that we allow people to have access to under a doctor's supervision that are the very same substances that are prohibited for what would be called recreational use.

But saying the fear is genuine doesn't mean that we'd agree with it. It's a great illustration of what our nation's drug policies are about. This broad set of scare tactics—that you will go to prison if you use drugs, or you will get terrible diseases if you inject drugs—inflates the fears and harms attached to drug use, believing then that people will just decide not to use drugs. This idea of maximizing the fear and harm associated with drugs as a legitimate tactic in dissuading people from using drugs makes for pretty perverse public policy. Just imagine if the government worked to make cars less impact resistant in an effort to get people to wear their seatbelt or to not speed!

This example seems ludicrous, but it's exactly government's approach to drug use—exacerbate danger to discourage behavior. The policies against syringe exchange and in favor of widespread incarceration are, in some ways, very much akin to a policy that would say you shouldn't allow any discussion of potential medical uses of the drug because it would send the wrong message. Both deny reality and deny what would be best for the individual in order to purportedly further the good of society—though it's clear to anyone paying attention that they harm society as well.

In Conant, the whole sequence of events—the litigation and its outcome, and its high profile—created the political space for other states that wanted to go forward with their own medical marijuana laws. Since then, there has been a steady procession of states enacting such laws, some by popular vote and others by legislative action. We expect that to continue to be a trend for some time to come, until finally the nation as a whole allows for people to use marijuana medically without any legal consequences.

JULIE: So is ACLU involved in these other state battles, or are the Marijuana Policy Project (MPP) and the Drug Policy Alliance (DPA) doing that?

GRAHAM: We've played a role in pushing for these additional laws, but no, the Marijuana Policy Project and the Drug Policy Alliance deserve credit for their leadership in the political process. The ACLU supports these political efforts, but our continuing role has been to defend the political victories that have been gained. Even after Conant, there continue to be recalcitrant public officials who don't like medical marijuana and are trying to reverse it in one fashion or another.

For instance, several governors and attorneys general have asserted that they would not implement the ID card systems called for under some state medical marijuana statutes. The original medical marijuana law in California didn't have any kind of identification cards; it just said if you have a recommendation from a doctor, you are allowed to use marijuana. But subsequent states, and eventually California too, set up systems for getting an ID card. Then, if you're stopped by a police officer, you are able to show the card, and that's the end of the encounter, as opposed to being arrested and charged and then having to prove in court that you're authorized. Several of the states balked at implementing card programs and claimed that federal law prevented them from doing so. Through threat of litigation, we convinced them that they needed to go ahead and issue the IDs.

Another area that we've had to litigate is around grand jury subpoenas. There was a case not too long ago in Washington state and Oregon, in which a federal prosecutor wanted to charge someone who was growing marijuana, some of which he believed was going to patients. So he subpoenaed the federal records of patients that he thought were receiving the marijuana, and he asked for that information from both a doctor and from the Oregon state ID card program. It's not difficult to see how granting law enforcement access to medical marijuana patient records would create a significant chilling effect. We went to court and convinced the judge that this shouldn't be allowed. It has remained a big part of our work to make sure that the relationship between doctors and patients remains protected, that their conversations, their records— everything that happens in a medical context—is treated as a medical issue and not as a law enforcement issue.

JULIE: I was wondering, was the ACLU involved in the Raich case?*

GRAHAM: We were not, and we actually thought from early on that it was better not to pursue a litigation strategy with the Raich case—a strategy that asked the federal courts to create and recognize new individual rights that would protect against federal interference with medical marijuana patients.

It's a really tricky area. Let me just lay out what I see as the two different legal strategies at play here. On the one hand, there now are many states, starting with California, where the people of that state have changed the laws to allow for the medical use of marijuana. That political shift took place at a state level. Federal officials were unhappy with these developments and acted against the popular will and against the political reality of that state by trying to undo these laws—usually through illegal means, by threatening doctors and so forth. By going to court in this posture, you have the political will of the people behind you, and you're taking on an official who is acting against that will and against the law. It's a very strong position to be in.

Contrast that with the situation, like *Raich,* where an individual is challenging federal policy and asserting a right to use medical marijuana.

Gonzales vs. Raich (previously *Ashcroft vs. Raich*), 545 U.S. 1 (2005), was a case in which the United States Supreme Court ruled on June 6, 2005, that under the Commerce Clause of the United States Constitution, which allows the United States Congress "To regulate Commerce . . . among the several States," Congress may ban the use of cannabis even where states approve its use for medicinal purposes.

Although a majority of the people in the United States favor the medical use of marijuana, there isn't a political opening to change the laws at a national level. You can't change the national laws by a popular referendum; it has to be through Congress, and the willingness to do that really hasn't even come close so far. So going to the courts in this posture and asking them to put a halt to enforcement of the federal law and recognize a novel individual right, when there hasn't been any political ability to change that law, and now we're asking the courts to do it . . .

JULIE: It's not likely to happen, and so it's possibly a waste of time.

GRAHAM: Well, it's hard these days. There was a time, I think, when courts were genuinely out in front of what the political system could do, what the legislative system could do. With the dismantling of Jim Crow, for instance, people were asking the courts to go farther than elected officials were willing to go in terms of bringing racial justice to the country. But it's a very different Supreme Court, and, generally, federal courts, than existed in that period, and there's a real reluctance by the courts to do that sort of thing.

So it seems to me the risk of that kind of litigation, such as with *Raich,* is that you're asking something of the courts that I absolutely believe they should do, but it's asking it in a context in which it's hard to imagine that they actually would do it. And that can have some troubling side effects. When the Raich decision came down from the Supreme Court, it simply maintained the status quo and had no bearing on the validity of state medical marijuana laws. But the way both the popular press and the general public interpreted it was that the Supreme Court had sounded the death knell for medical marijuana. In other words, it seemed in a political sense, in a popular sense, that the gains that had already been made at the state levels had been somehow reversed or rolled back.

JULIE: Well, it did feel like a defeat, I think, to most people.

GRAHAM: Granted, sometimes you have to try even when the odds are long, but as we plan litigation strategies for any kind of civil rights or liberties issue, given the current composition and tendencies of the courts, we have to think really carefully about the downside of losing—especially when we have been winning in the political arena. So, for better or worse, the ACLU's strategy has been focused on, and been successful in, defending these political gains from attack by both federal and state officials.

Some of our most recent work regarding medical marijuana has been a case on behalf of the Wo/Men's Alliance for Medical Marijuana (WAMM), a patients' group in Santa Cruz, California, led by Valerie Corral. WAMM is a collective of mostly terminally ill patients who were growing marijuana entirely for their own use. Those who are able to work out in the fields help cultivate the marijuana for the group's own use. There's no money changing hands, no sales. You'd think this wouldn't be at the top of a federal bureaucrat's priority list, but WAMM was, nonetheless, raided by federal drug agents, and in a most disturbing manner.

Federal agents replete with commando gear and assault rifles descended upon the WAMM farm and went so far as to handcuff a patient in her wheelchair as she was trying to explain her situation to them. The raid, appropriately, generated a lot of outrage in the community. The City of Santa Cruz condemned the raid and actually made marijuana available on the steps of City Hall as an act of defiance to the federal government. They ended up filing a lawsuit making many of the same claims that were ultimately rejected in the Raich case. However, they've introduced another, so far successful, claim as well.

This legal claim, which we're now involved in, concerns the ability of particular cities, counties, and states to chart their own course on medical marijuana without undue interference from the federal government. So it's no longer the issue of an individual right to use medical marijuana, which the Supreme Court is unlikely to recognize, as it would mean that any adult anywhere in the United States—be it Alabama or California—has a constitutional right to medical marijuana. Rather, it's about the ability of a city, like Santa Cruz, or a state, like California, to create a separate way of dealing with medical marijuana, and to bar the federal government from deliberately undermining this effort. For the courts to agree with this legal claim, as they have so far, further establishes the legitimacy of state medical marijuana laws and, more importantly, could ultimately bring an end to the federal government's strategic interference with these laws.

JULIE: So it seems there's a huge intersection between civil liberties and drug policy. It makes sense to me that ACLU is to some extent leading the fight against our nation's drug policy.

GRAHAM: The decision to declare a war on drugs, and then escalate it over the last few decades, has had a devastating impact on civil liberties and the lives of countless individuals. Rather than dealing with drug use and abuse as issues of personal choice and public health, we've stuck to an almost purely criminal justice approach, which predetermines the outcomes, and not for the better. For one, it means that we're going to have to build a lot of prisons and empower a lot of police, because, quite simply, a lot of people use drugs, mostly marijuana. So, if it's going to be a war—a war on drugs and a war on people using drugs—then there's going to be a great deal of carnage, and there certainly has been.

While the prison population for crimes other than drugs, like violent crime or property crime, has remained fairly steady through the past 100 to 150 years, incarceration for drug crimes, which essentially didn't exist until relatively recently, has skyrocketed. More than one in 100 adults in the United States is now behind bars, by far the highest rate of incarceration in the world—an inauspicious distinction for a country that purports to be the land of the free.

The boom in building prisons has been fueled by a boom in incarcerating people for drug crimes, and that exacts a huge cost on families, on individuals, on government budgets, on investment in building schools and other public goods. The drug war has also eviscerated the constitutional rights that we take for granted in this country. In recent years, the courts have created what Supreme Court Justice Thurgood Marshall termed a "drug exception" to the Constitution. And that's really true, not just for the Fourth Amendment—the right to be free from unreasonable search and seizure—but in terms of freedom of religion, free speech, the systematic functioning of the courts, and sentencing. You can go through the articles of the Bill of Rights one by one and identify the court decision that most undermined that right over the last generation; and invariably, it's a case that involves drugs.

This outcome is almost unavoidable as a result of our prohibitionist policies, which require that law enforcement be granted, and the courts uphold, the means to enforce laws against consensual crimes—crimes that lack a complaining party. If someone is assaulted, for example, then the victim is going to go to the police and say, I got beat up, and this is the person who did it. But for the vast majority of drug crimes, there isn't a complaining witness. It's a transaction that happens between two willing parties—somebody who's selling and somebody who's buying, and nobody involved wants to be found out by the police. So to enforce the drug laws absent any complaining parties, the police generally have to decide for themselves whom to target for investigation.

This is an obvious invitation for abuse, especially racial stereotyping, which has become a hallmark of the drug war. And it certainly is not that individual police officers are racist. Rather, the system necessitates that investigation and enforcement not be based on actual evidence of wrongdoing, which virtually assures that universal stereotypes, regardless of accuracy, will dictate enforcement patterns. Drug enforcement is also trapped in a readily apparent feedback loop, where law enforcement will continue to devote ever-increasing resources to wherever they focused enforcement initially—in communities of color. Had police focused the drug war in white communities, they also would have uncovered a sizable amount of drug use, which would justify increased enforcement that would, in turn, reveal more drug activity, and so on.

So there are these astonishing racial disparities in drug law enforcement, even though white people use drugs at the same rates as everybody else. In addition to the gross racial disparity seemingly inherent in current drug policy, enforcing laws against consensual crimes requires police to undertake all sorts of unsavory tactics: They have to use informants; they have to do illegal searches; they have to conduct surveillance; they have to bribe people; they have to do all of these kinds of practices that end up generating wrongful convictions and corruption and distrust. The level of distrust right now between many communities and law enforcement reflects how the police have spent so much of their time trying to enforce the drug laws, instead of being responsive to community concerns about safety and quality of life in the community. There are many, many costs to the war on drugs.

JULIE: I want to get your take on forced treatment, in which people go into drug treatment programs to avoid incarceration. One thing I have an issue with is how it's inflating the statistics on cannabis addiction.

GRAHAM: I think the issue of forced treatment is complicated, but the short version is that it's the lesser of two evils. An opportunity to avoid incarceration, even by entering treatment that they don't legitimately need, or treatment that they do need but they're being forced into, I think that is a relative improvement. But at the same time it really is not the right solution. There's a long history in this country of beneficent intervention on behalf of people who the government decides need care—providing asylums and those sorts of things. We're just revisiting that when we talk about the government deciding who is addicted, who needs help, and then saying that the help we're going to offer you is the choice between a prison cell and our version of treatment. And if, at a certain point, you don't manage to become "cured of your medical condition," then you will be punished. Looking at it that way, it's hard to view it as a good thing. But, again, between prison and not-prison, I think not-prison is always better, and I'm sure the many individuals entering treatment for marijuana "addiction" feel the same.

Resources

ADDITIONAL ARTICLES ABOUT MARIJUANA
ARE AVAILABLE AT
THEPOTBOOK.COM.

I owe a debt of gratitude to Philippe Lucas, who helped put me in touch with some of the contributors for this book. His chapter, "Community-Based Research of Medical Cannabis: A Patient-Centered, Public Health Approach," is available on the book's website, ThePotBook.com, as are the following chapters:

Chris Bennet: "Cannabis in the Ancient World"

Richard Glen Boire, J.D.: "Life Sentences: The Collateral Sanctions Associated with Marijuana Offenses"

Jack Cole: "Law Enforcement Against Prohibition"

Deepak Cyril D'Souza, M.D.: "Cannabinoids and Psychosis: Pharmacological Evidence"

Richard Gehr: "Bring Me the Head of Cheech and Chong"

Robert Melamede, Ph.D.: "Endocannabinoids: Marijuana from Within"

Juan Sanchez-Ramos, M.D., and Catherine O'Neill: "Cannabinoids for the Treatment of Movement Disorders"

Soma: "Sacred Cannabis"

Fred Tomaselli: "Stoner in the Studio"

Interview with Carl Olsen, on fighting for his right to use cannabis via the Religious Freedom Restoration Act

Interview with Mr. X., Owner, NYC Pot Delivery Service

Interview with Ms. X, Owner, NoCal Pot Farm

ACLU Drug Law Reform Project

www.aclu.org/drug-law-reform

"The ACLU is our nation's guardian of liberty, working daily in courts, legislatures and communities to defend and preserve the individual rights and liberties that the Constitution and laws of the United States guarantee everyone in this country. [. . .] The ACLU Drug Law Reform Project's goal is to end punitive drug policies that cause the widespread violation of constitutional and human rights, as well as unprecedented levels of incarceration" (from the ACLU website).

Addiction Proof Your Child: A Realistic Approach to Preventing Drug, Alcohol, and Other Dependencies

Stanton Peele (New York: Three Rivers Press, 2007); www.peele.net

Advisory Council on Misuse of Drugs

http://drugs.homeoffice.gov.uk/drugs

The Council is an independent expert body that advises government on drug related issues in the UK. It was established under the Misuse of Drugs Act 1971. The Advisory Council makes recommendations to government on the control of dangerous or otherwise harmful drugs, including classification and scheduling under the Misuse of Drugs Act 1971 and its regulations. It considers any substance which appears to be misused and which is having or appears to be capable of having harmful effects sufficient to cause a social problem. It also carries out in-depth inquiries into aspects of drug use that are causing particular concern in the UK, with the aim of producing considered reports that will be helpful to policy makers and practitioners.

Alliance for Cannabis Therapeutics (ACT)

http://marijuana-as-medicine.org/alliance.htm

The Alliance was the first nonprofit organization dedicated to reforming the laws that prohibit medical access to marijuana. It was founded in 1981 by Robert Randall and Alice O'Leary.

Americans for Safe Access

www.safeaccessnow.org

www.safeaccessnow.net/countyguidelines.htm

Americans for Safe Access is a community-based organization dedicated to the implementation of fair and consistent guidelines in all California counties as a safe harbor from arrest under HS Code 11362.5, the Compassionate Use Act of 1996. Delineated at the URL above is each city's and county's unique medical marijuana laws in California, particularly as they relate to quantities allowed.

Beyond Zero Tolerance: A Reality-Based Approach to Drug Education and School Discipline
Rodney Skager, Ph.D.
www.safety1st.org/images/stories/pdf/bzt.pdf

This booklet offers a comprehensive, cost-effective approach to high school drug education and school discipline focused on helping teenagers by bolstering the student community and educational environment. This unique approach combines honest, reality-based drug education with interactive learning, compassionate assistance, and restorative practices in lieu of exclusionary punishment.

British Columbia Compassion Club Society
www.thecompassionclub.org

The BC Compassion Club is a collectively-run nonprofit natural health center providing safe, high-quality medicinal cannabis and the services of a full wellness center. Since 1997, they have served more than five thousand members with serious or terminal illnesses.

Canadian Addiction Survey 2004, Ottawa, Ontario, Canada
www.ccsa.ca/eng/priorities/research/canadianaddiction/Pages/default.aspx

"The Canadian Addiction Survey (CAS) is one of the most detailed and extensive surveys ever conducted on how Canadians aged 15 years and older use alcohol, cannabis and other drugs, and the impact that use has on their physical, mental and social well-being. This information, when compared with past studies, indicates trends in drug use and harms associated with use" (from the website). The CAS was sponsored by CCSA; Health Canada; the Canadian Executive Council on Addictions (CECA); the Centre for Addictions Research of BC (CAR-BC); and the provinces of Nova Scotia, New Brunswick, and British Columbia.

Canadian AIDS Society
www.cdnaids.ca

Registered as a charity since 1988, the Canadian AIDS Society (CAS) is a national coalition of more than 120 community-based AIDS organizations across Canada. They are dedicated to strengthening the response to HIV/AIDS across all sectors of society and to enriching the lives of people and communities living with HIV/AIDS.

Canadian Centre on Substance Abuse

www.ccsa.ca

The Canadian Centre on Substance Abuse (CCSA) has a legislated mandate to provide national leadership and evidence-informed analysis and advice to mobilize collaborative efforts to reduce alcohol-related and other drug-related harms.

Canadians for Safe Access

http://safeaccess.ca

Canadians for Safe Access (CSA) is a grassroots organization committed to protecting the right of Canadians to safe access to medicinal cannabis.

Cannabis Science

www.cannabisscience.com

Cannabis Science works with world authorities on phytocannabinoid science targeting critical illnesses and adhering to scientific methodologies to develop, produce, and commercialize phytocannabinoid-based pharmaceutical products.

Center for American Progress

www.americanprogress.org

The Center for American Progress (CAP) is dedicated to improving the lives of Americans through progressive ideas and action, addressing 21st-century challenges such as energy, national security, economic growth and opportunity, immigration, education, and health care. It develops new policy ideas, critiques the policy that stems from conservative values, challenges the media to cover the issues that truly matter, and shapes the national debate. Founded in 2003 to provide long-term leadership and support to the progressive movement, CAP is headed by John D. Podesta and based in Washington, D.C.

Common Sense for Drug Policy

www.csdp.org

Common Sense for Drug Policy (CSDP) is a nonprofit organization dedicated to reforming drug policy and expanding harm reduction. CSDP disseminates factual information and comments on existing laws, policies, and practices; provides advice and assistance to individuals and organizations; and facilitates coalition building.

Community Consortium

www.communityconsortium.org

The Community Consortium is an association of Bay Area HIV Health Care Providers, one of the pioneer community-based clinical trials groups, established in 1985. Donald Abrams, M.D., is chairman and principal investigator.

D.A.R.E.
www.DARE.com

Drug Abuse Resistance Education (D.A.R.E) is a police officer–led series of classroom lessons that teaches children from kindergarten through 12th grade how to resist peer pressure and live productive drug- and violence-free lives.

Diagnostic and Statistical Manual of Mental Disorders IV-TR
(Arlington, VA: American Psychiatric Association, 1994)
The Diagnostic and Statistical Manual of Mental Disorders (DSM) is the standard classification of mental disorders used by mental health professionals in the United States. The DSM-V will be published in 2012.

www.drugscience.org
This site provides scientific and other material regarding the medical use of cannabis (marijuana) and its legal status under the laws of the United States.

GW Pharmaceuticals
www.GWPharm.com

"[T]he global leader in prescription cannabinoid medicines," makers of Sativex, sublingual cannabis extract.

Help at Any Cost: How the Troubled-Teen Industry Cons Parents and Hurts Kids
Maia Szalavitz (New York: Riverhead, 2006)
helpatanycost.com

Institute of Medicine
www.iom.edu

"In January 1997, the White House Office of National Drug Control Policy (ONDCP) asked the Institute of Medicine to conduct a review of the scientific evidence to asses the potential health benefits and risks of marijuana and its constituent cannabinoids. That review began in August 1997 and culminated in the report 'Marijuana and Medicine: Assessing the Science Base.'"

International Association for Cannabis as Medicine
www.cannabis-med.org

Founded in March 2000, the aim of the International Association for Cannabis as Medicine (IACM) is to advance knowledge on cannabis, cannabinoids, the endocannabinoid system, and related topics, especially with regard to their therapeutic potential.

Journal of Cannabis Therapeutics
www.cannabis-med.org/membersonly/mo.php

The Journal of Cannabis Therapeutics was published by Haworth Press, Binghamton, New York, and edited by Ethan Russo, M.D., but it ceased publication in 2004.

La Guardia Commission, 1944
www.druglibrary.org/schaffer/library/studies/lag/lagmenu.htm

This was the first in-depth study into the effects of smoking marijuana, prepared by the New York Academy of Medicine on behalf of a commission appointed in 1939 by New York mayor Fiorello La Guardia, who was a strong opponent of the 1937 Marijuana Tax Act.

Law Enforcement Against Prohibition
www.leap.cc

Law Enforcement Againt Prohibition (LEAP) is a Medford, Massachusetts–based group of police officers, judges, prosecutors, prison wardens, and others who want to legalize and regulate all drugs.

Marijuana Myths, Marijuana Facts
John Morgan and Lynn Zimmer (New York: Lindesmith Center, 1997)

Marijuana: What's a Parent to Believe?
Timmen L. Cermak (Center City, MN: Hazeldon Publishing, 2003)

MedicalCannabis.com
This is the website for Patients Out of Time: "A compassionate, science-based eucational forum for the restoration of medical cannabis knowledge."

Multidisciplinary Association for Psychedelic Studies
www.maps.org

The Multidisciplinary Association for Psychedelic Studies (MAPS) mission is 1) to treat conditions for which conventional medicines provide limited relief—such as post-traumatic stress disorder (PTSD), pain, drug dependence, anxiety, and depression associated with end-of-life issues—by developing psychedelics and marijuana into prescription medicines; 2) to cure many thousands of people by building a network of clinics where treatments can be provided; and 3) to educate the public honestly about the risks and benefits of psychedelics and marijuana.

Ethan Nadelmann's NAACP Speech, July 13, 2009
Please go to www.youtube.com and enter "End the Drug War Now" into the search bar.

National Academy of Sciences
www.NationalAcademies.org
The National Academy of Sciences (NAS) is an honorific society of distinguished scholars engaged in scientific and engineering research and dedicated to the furtherance of science and technology and to their use for the general welfare.

National Commission on Marijuana and Drug Abuse, 1972
Created by Public Law 91-513 to study marijuana abuse in the United States.
On March 22, 1972, the Commission's chairman, Raymond P. Shafer, presented a report to Congress and the public entitled "Marijuana, A Signal of Misunderstanding," which favored ending marijuana prohibition and adopting other methods to discourage use.

National Drug Intelligence Center
www.justice.gov/ndic
The mission of the national Drug Intelligence Center (NDIC) is to provide strategic drug-related intelligence, document and computer exploitation support, and training assistance to the drug control, public health, law enforcement, and intelligence communities of the United States in order to reduce the adverse effects of drug trafficking, drug abuse, and other drug-related criminal activity.

National Institute on Drug Addiction
www.drugabuse.gov
The misson of the National Institute on Drug Addiction (NIDA) is to lead the nation in bringing the power of science to bear on drug abuse and addiction.

Nick Snow

www.nicksnow.com

In January 1996, at the age of six, Nick Snow was diagnosed with neuroblastoma, a rare and deadly childhood cancer. He underwent eighty-four months of treatment and finally reached remission in December 2002. Sadly, after more than three years of being cancer-free, he died April 2, 2006, from an infection.

National Organization for the Reform of Marijuana Laws

www.norml.org

The mission of the National Organization for the Reform of Marijuana Laws (NORML) Foundation is to educate the public about the costs of marijuana prohibition and the benefits of alternative policies, to undertake research into various aspects of marijuana and marijuana policy implication, and to provide legal support and assistance to victims of the current laws.

On Drugs

David Lenson (Minneapolis: University of Minnesota Press, 1999)

Patients Out of Time

www.medialcannabis.com

A patient advocacy organization dedicated to educating public health professionals and the public about medical marijuana. Incorporated in 1995, the group is led by medical and nursing professionals and the four remaining participants in the federal government's Investigational New Drug program for cannabis.

Prairie Plant Systems

www.prairieplant.com

Prairie Plant Systems Inc. (PPS) is a biotechnology company with Canadian and U.S. facilities dedicated to the principle of manufacturing pharmaceuticals derived from harvestable plants grown in biosecure GMP production facilities. (GMP refers to the Good Manufacturing Practice Regulations promulgated by the U.S. Food and Drug Administration under the authority of the Federal Food, Drug, and Cosmetic Act.)

Society of Cannabis Clinicians

www.societyofcannabisclinicians.org

The Society of Cannabis Clinicians (SCC) is a project of the California Cannabis Research Medical Group (CCRMG). SCC was formed in autumn

2004 by the member physicians of CCRMG to aid in the promulgation of voluntary standards for clinicians engaged in the recommendation and approval of cannabis under California law (HSC §11362.5).

State of Our Nation's Youth
www.HoratioAlger.com

The 10th State of Our Nation's Youth report was issued in 2008 by the Horatio Alger Association of Distinguished Americans. The report compiles the results of the national survey conducted by Peter D. Hart Research Associates, a comprehensive study of American high school students' opinions, apprehensions, and aspirations.

Safety First Project
www.safety1st.org

Safety First, a project of the Drug Policy Alliance, provides resources for parents, educators, and students who are interested in reality-based approaches to drug education that stress the health, safety, and well-being of young people.

Tourette Syndrome Association
www.tsa-usa.org

The only national voluntary nonprofit membership organization in this field. Its mission is to identify the cause of, find the cure for, and control the effects of Tourette Syndrome.

Understanding Marijuana: A New Look at the Scientific Evidence
Mitch Earleywine (New York: Oxford University Press, 2005)

U.S. National Multiple Sclerosis Society
www.nmss.org

The Society helps people affected by multiple sclerosis (MS) by funding cutting-edge research, driving change through advocacy, facilitating professional education, and providing programs and services that help people with MS and their families move their lives forward.

University of California Center for Medicinal Cannabis Research
www.cmcr.ucsd.edu

The center conducts high-quality scientific studies intended to ascertain the general medical safety and efficacy of cannabis products and examine alternative forms of cannabis administration.

University of Mississippi's Marijuana Potency Project

The project, run by Mahmoud ElSohly, tracks the average potency of seized cannabis according to its percentage of THC.

Vote Hemp

www.votehemp.com

Vote Hemp is a national, single-issue, nonprofit organization dedicated to the acceptance of and free market for industrial hemp, low-THC oilseed, and fiber varieties of cannabis, and to changes in current law to allow U.S. farmers to grow the crop.

Wo/Men's Alliance for Medical Marijuana (WAMM)

www.wamm.org

Founded by Valerie Corral, who used cannabis to manage her seizures, this is a patient collective. Wo/Men's Alliance for Medical Marijuana (WAMM) has emerged as a unique model, a patient self-help alliance, and an alternative to the inflated prices of an illicit black market. A handful of seriously ill patients has grown into a collective membership of more than 250 seriously intentioned citizens.

U.S. Food and Drug Administration

www.fda.gov

The U.S. Food and Drug Administration's (FDA's) mission is to protect consumers and to enhance public health by maximizing compliance of FDA-regulated products and minimizing risk associated with those products.

References

Abel, E. L. "Retrieval of Information after Use of Marijuana." *Nature* 231 (1971): 58.

———. *Marihuana: The First Twelve Thousand Years.* New York: Plenum Press, 1980.

Abi-Dargham, A., J. Rodenhiser, D. Printz, et al. "Increased Baseline Occupancy of D2 Receptors by Dopamine in Schizophrenia." *Proceedings of the National Academy of Sciences USA* 97 (2000): 8104–9.

Abood, M. E., G. Rizvi, N. Sallapudi, et al."Activation of the CB1 Cannabinoid Receptor Protects Cultured Mouse Spinal Neurons against Excitotoxicity." *Neuroscience Letters* 309 (2001): 197–201.

Abrams, D. I. "Medical Marijuana: Tribulations and Trials." *Journal of Psychoactive Drugs* 30 (1998): 163–69.

———. "Marijuana for HIV-related Conditions." *Journal of the San Francisco Medical Society* 79, no. 8 (n.d.): 32–38.

Abrams, D. I., J. F. Hilton, R. J. Leiser, et al. "Short-term Effects of Cannabinoids in Patients with HIV-1 Infection: A Randomized, Placebo-controlled Clinical Trial." *Annals of Internal Medicine* 139 (2003): 258–66.

Abrams, D. I., C. Jay, S. B. Shade, et al. "Cannabis in Painful HIV-associated Sensory Neuropathy: A Randomized Placebo-controlled Trial." *Neurology* 68 (2007): 515–21.

Abrams, D. I., H. P. Vizoso, S. B. Shade, et al. "Vaporization as a Smokeless Cannabis Delivery System: A Pilot Study." *Clinical Pharmacology and Therapeutics* 82 (April 11, 2007): www.nature.com/clpt/journal/vaop/ncurrent/full/6100200a .html. Accessed May 7, 2010.

Addington, J., and D. Addington. "Impact of an Early Psychosis Program on Substance Use." *Psychiatric Rehabilitation Journal* 25 (2001): 60–67.

Adriani, W., A. Caprioli, O. Granstrem, et al. "The Spontaneously Hypertensive-rat as an Animal Model of ADHD: Evidence for Impulsive and Non-impulsive Sub-populations." *Neuroscience Biobehavioral Review* 27 (2003): 639–51.

Advisory Council on the Misuse of Drugs. "The Classification of Cannabis under the Misuse of Drugs Act 1971." London: Home Office Government Printing Office, 2002.

Agarwal N., P. Pacher, I. Tegeder, et al. "Cannabinoids Mediate Analgesia Largely via Peripheral Type 1 Cannabinoid Receptors in Nociceptors." *Nature Neuroscience* 10 (2007): 870–79.

Agurell, S., M. Halldin, J. E. Lindgren, et al. "Pharmacokinetics and Metabolism of Delta-1-tetrahydrocannabinol and Other Cannabinoids with Emphasis on Man." *Pharmacological Reviews* 38 (1986): 21–43.

Aharonovich, E., F. Garawi, A. Bisaga, et al. "Concurrent Cannabis Use during Treatment for Comorbid ADHD and Cocaine Dependence: Effects on Outcome." *American Journal of Drug and Alcohol Abuse* 32 (2006): 629–35.

Akinshola, B. E., A. Chakrabarti, and E. S. Onaivi. "In Vitro and In Vivo Action of Cannabinoids." *Neurochemical Research* 24 (1999): 1233–40.

Akirav, I., and M. Maroun. "The Role of the Medial Prefrontal Cortex-amygdala Circuit in Stress Effects on the Extinction of Fear." *Neural Plasticity* epub 30873 (2007).

Alexander A., P. F. Smith, and R. J. Rosengren. "Cannabinoids in the Treatment of Cancer." *Cancer Letters* 285 (2009): 6–12.

Allen, J. H., G. M. deMoore, R. Heddle, et al. "Cannabinoid Hyperemesis: Cyclical Hyperemesis in Association with Chronic Cannabis Abuse." *Gut* 53 (2004): 1566–70.

Amar, M. B. "Cannabiniods in Medicine: A Review of Their Therapeutic Potential." *Journal of Ethnopharmacology* 105 (2006): 1–25.

American Psychiatric Association. *Diagnostic and Statistical Manual of Mental Disorders,* 4th edition, text revision. Washington, D.C.: American Psychiatric Association, 2000.

Amtmann, D., P. Weydt, K. L. Johnson, et al. "Survey of Cannabis Use in Patients with Amyotrophic Lateral Sclerosis." *American Journal of Hospice and Palliative Medicine* 21 (2004): 95–104.

Andreasson, S., P. Allebeck, A. Engstrom, et al. "Cannabis and Schizophrenia: A Longitudinal Study of Swedish Conscripts." *Lancet* 2 (1987): 1483–86.

Anonymous. "Marijuana Strains, Pictures, and Descriptions" (2007): www. marjuanastrains.com. Accessed December 8, 2007.

Anthony, B., and R. Solomon, eds. *The Black Candle* by Emily Murphy. Toronto, ON.: Coles Publishing, 1973.

Anthony, J. C., L. A. Warner, and R. C. Kessler. "Comparative Epidemiology of Dependence on Tobacco, Alcohol, Controlled Substances and Inhalants: Basic Findings from the National Comorbidity Survey." *Experimental and Clinical Psychopharmacology* 2 (1994): 244–68.

Anthony, J. C., and J. Helzer. "Epidemiology of Drug Dependence." In M. T. Tsuang, M. Tohen, and G. E. Zahner, eds., *Textbook in Psychiatric Epidemiology.* New York: John Wiley and Sons, 1995.

Appelboam, A., and P. J. Oades. "Coma Due to Cannabis Toxicity in an Infant." *European Journal of Emergency Medicine* 13 (2006): 177–79.

Armentano, P. "Crimes of Indiscretion: Marijuana Arrests in the United States." http://norml.org/index.cfm?Group_ID=6411. Accessed April 29, 2010.

Aronow, W. S., and J. C. Cassidy. "Effect of Marihuana and Placebo-marihuana Smoking on Angina Pectoris." *New England Journal of Medicine* 291 (1974): 65–67.

———. "Effect of Smoking Marihuana and of a High-nicotine Cigarette on Angina Pectoris." *Clinical Pharmacology and Therapeutics* 17 (1975): 549–54.

Aronow, W. S., and S. N. Rokaw. "Carboxyhemoglobin Caused by Smoking Nonnicotine Cigarettes: Effects in Angina Pectoris." *Circulation* 44 (1971): 782–88.

Arseneault, L., M. Cannon, J. Witton, et al. "Causal Association between Cannabis and Psychosis: Examination of the Evidence." *British Journal of Psychiatry* 184 (2004): 110–17.

Ashton, C. H., P. B. Moore, P. Gallagher, et al. "Cannabinoids in Bipolar Affective Disorder: A Review and Discussion of Their Therapeutic Potential." *Journal of Psychopharmacology* 19 (2005): 293–300.

Ashton J. C., and M. Glass. "The Cannabinoid CB2 Receptor as a Target for Inflammation-dependent Neurodegeneration." *Current Neuropharmacology* 5 (2007): 73–80.

Associated Press. "Hashish Evidence Is 1,600 Years Old." June 2, 1992.

Austin, G., and R. Skager. "11th Biennial California Student Survey: Drug, Alcohol and Tobacco Use, 2005–2006." Sacramento: California Attorney General's Office (2006): www.safestate.org/documents/CSS_11_Highlights.pdf. Accessed in May 2006; site no longer in operation.

Azorlosa, J. L., S. J. Heishman, M. L. Stitzer, et al. "Marijuana Smoking: Effect of Varying Delta 9-tetrahydrocannabinol Content and Number of Puffs." *Journal of Pharmacology and Experimental Therapeutics* 261 (1992): 114–22.

Bab I., and A. Zimmer. "Cannabinoid Receptors and the Regulation of Bone Mass." *British Journal of Pharmacology* 153 (2008): 182–88.

Bachman, J. G., L. D. Johnston, and P. M. O'Malley. "Explaining the Recent Decline in Cocaine Use among Young Adults: Further Evidence That Perceived Risks and Disapproval Lead to Reduced Drug Use." *Journal of Health and Human Social Behavior* 31 (1990): 173–84.

Bachman, J. G., P. M. O'Malley, L. D. Rodgers, et al. "Changes in Drug Use during the Post-high School Years." Monitoring the Future Occasional Paper No. 35. Ann Arbor, MI: Institute for Social Research, 1992: www.monitoringthefuture.org/pubs.html#papers. Accessed May 7, 2010.

Baker, D., G. Pryce, J. L. Croxford, et al. "Cannabinoids Control Spasticity and Tremor in a Multiple Sclerosis Model." *Nature* 404 (2000): 84–87.

Barber, E. M. *Pre-historic Textiles*. Princeton, NJ: Princeton University Press, 1989.

Barrowclough, C., G. Haddock, N. Tarrier, et al. "Randomized Controlled Trial of Motivational Interviewing, Cognitive Behavior Therapy, and Family Intervention for

Patients with Comorbid Schizophrenia and Substance Use Disorders." *American Journal of Psychiatry* 158 (2001): 1706–13.

Beal, J. E., R. Olson, L. Laubenstein, et al. "Dronabinol as a Treatment for Anorexia Associated with Weight Loss in Patients with AIDS." *Journal of Pain and Symptom Management* 10 (1995): 89–97.

Beal, J. E., R. Olson, L. Lefkowitz, et al. "Long-term Efficacy and Safety of Dronabinol for Acquired Immunodeficiency Syndrome-associated Anorexia." *Journal of Pain and Symptom Management* 14 (1997): 7–14.

Bealle, M. A. 1949. *The Drug Story*. Spanish Fork, UT: The Hornet's Nest, 1949.

Beardsley, P. M., R. L. Balster, and L. S. Harris. "Dependence on Tetrahydrocannabinol in Rhesus Monkeys." *Journal of Pharmacology and Experimental Therapeutics* 239 (1986): 311–19.

Beardsley, P. M., and T. H. Kelly. "Acute Effects of Cannabis on Human Behavior and Central Nervous System Functions." In H. Kalant, W. A. Corrigall, W. Hall, et al., eds., *The Health Effects of Cannabis*. Toronto: Centre for Addiction and Mental Health, 1999.

Becker, H. S. "Becoming a Marihuana User." *American Journal of Sociology* 59 (1953): 235–42.

Bedard, M. Dubois, and B. Weaver. "The Impact of Cannabis on Driving." *Canadian Journal of Public Health* 98 (2007): 6–11.

Beeby, D. "Health Canada Dope Stinks, Patients Say." *Globe and Mail,* September 16, 2003

———. "Ottawa Has Trouble Collecting Marijuana Debt." *Globe and Mail,* February 6, 2006.

———. "Health Canada Wants Cash Up Front for Medical Marijuana." *Canadian Press,* November 1, 2009.

Belle-Isle, L., and A. Hathaway. "Barriers to Access to Medical Cannabis for Canadians Living with HIV/AIDS." *AIDS Care* 19 (2007): 500–506.

Benet, S. "Early Diffusions and Folk Uses of Hemp." In *Cannabis and Culture*. The Hague: Moutan, 1975.

Benetowa, S. [Sula Benet]. 1967. *Tracing One Word Through Different Languages*. N.p., 1936. Republished in Andrews, S., and S. Vinkenoog. *The Book of Grass*. New York: Grove Press, 1967.

Bennett, C., and N. McQueen. *Sex, Drugs, Violence and the Bible*. Gibsons, British Columbia: Forbidden Fruit Publishing, 2001.

Berman, J. S., C. Symonds, and R. Birch. "Efficacy of Two Cannabis Based Medicinal Extracts for Relief of Central Neuropathic Pain from Brachial Plexus Avulsion: Results of a Randomised Controlled Trial." *Pain* 112 (2004): 299–306.

Bersani, G., V. Orlando, G. D. Kotzalidis, et al. "Cannabis and Schizophrenia: Impact on Onset, Course, Psychopathology and Outcomes." *European Archives of Psychiatry and Clinical Neuroscience* 252 (2002): 86–92.

Bicher, H. I., and R. Mechoulam. "Pharmacological Effects of Two Active Constituents of Marijuana." *Archives Internationales de Pharmacodynamie et de Thérapie* 172 (1968): 24–31.

Bilsland, L. G., J. R. Dick, G. Pryce, et al. "Increasing Cannabinoid Levels by Pharmacological and Genetic Manipulation Delay Disease Progression in SOD1 Mice." *FASEB Journal* 20 (2006): 1003–1005.

Blake, D. R., P. Robson, M. Ho, et al. "Preliminary Assessment of the Efficacy, Tolerability and Safety of a Cannabis-based Medicine (Sativex) in the Treatment of Pain Caused by Rheumatoid Arthritis." *Rheumatology* (2006): 50–52.

Blazquez, C., et al. "Inhibition of Tumor Angiogenesis by Cannabinoids." *The Federation of American Societies for Experimental Biology Journal* 17, no. 3 (2003): 529–31.

Block, R. I., R. Farinpour, and K. Braverman. "Acute Effects of Marijuana on Cognition: Relationships to Chronic Effects and Smoking Techniques." *Pharmacology, Biochemistry and Behavior* 43 (1992): 907–17.

Block, R. I., and M. M. Ghoneim. "Effects of Chronic Marijuana Use on Human Cognition." *Psychopharmacology* 110 (1993): 219–28.

Block, R. I., D. S. O'Leary, R. D. Hichwa, et al. "Effects of Frequent Marijuana Use on Memory-related Regional Cerebral Blood Flow." *Pharmacology, Biochemistry, and Behavior* 72 (2002): 237–50.

Bloom, A. S., W. L. Dewey, L. S. Harris, et al. "9-Nor-9B-hydroxyhexahydrocannabinol a Cannabiniod with Potent Antinociceptive Activity: Comparisons with Morphine." *Journal of Phamacology and Experimental Therapies* 200 (1977): 263–70.

Bloom, J. W., W. T. Kaltenborn, P. Paoletti, et al. "Respiratory Effects of Non-tobacco Cigarettes." *British Medical Journal* 295 (1987): 1516–18.

Blows S., R. Q. Ivers, J. Connor, et al. "Marijuana Use and Car Crash Injury." *Addiction* 100 (2004): 605–11.

Bolla, K. I., K. Brown, D. Eldreth, et al. "Dose-related Neurocognitive Effects of Marijuana Use." *Neurology* 59 (2002): 1337–43.

Bolla, K. I., D. A. Eldreth, J. A. Matochik, et al. "Neural Substrates of Faulty Decision-making in Abstinent Marijuana Users." *NeuroImage* 26 (2005): 480–92.

Bonnie, R. J., and C. H. Whitebread II. "The Forbidden Fruit and the Tree of Knowledge: An Inquiry into the Legal History of American Marijuana Prohibition." *Virginia Law Review* 56, no. 6 (1970): www.druglibrary.org/SCHAFFER/library/studies/vlr/vlrtoc.htm. Accessed May 7, 2010.

Bósca, I., and M. Karus. *The Cultivation of Hemp: Botany, Varieties, Cultivation and Harvesting.* Sebastopol, CA: Hemptech, 1998.

Bossong, M. G., B. N. van Berckel, R. Boellaard, et al. "9-Tetrahydrocannabinol Induces Dopamine Release in the Human Striatum." *Neuropsychopharmacology* 34 (2009): 759–66.

Botvin, G., and K. Resnicow. "School-based Prevention Programs: Why Do Effects Decay?" *Preventive Medicine* 22 (1993): 484–90.

Bouaboula, M., B. Bourrie, M. Rinaldi-Carmona, et al. "Stimulation of Cannabinoid Receptor CB1 Induces Krox-24 Expression in Human Astrocytoma Cells." *Journal of Biological Chemistry* 270 (1995): 13973–80.

Bouchard, C. List of approved cultivars. Industrial Hemp Section, Office of Controlled Substances, Drug Strategy and Controlled Substances Programme. Ottawa, Canada, 2007.

Boyce, S. S. *Hemp (Cannabis sativa).* New York: Orange Judd, 1912.

Boyd, N. *High Society: Legal and Illegal Drugs in Canada.* Toronto, ON: Key Porter Books, 1991.

Boydell, J., J. van Os, A. Caspi, et al. "Trends in Cannabis Use prior to First Presentation with Schizophrenia, in South-East London between 1965 and 1999." *Psychological Medicine* 36 (2006): 1441–46.

Brady, C. M., R. DasGupta, C. Dalton, et al. "An Open-label Pilot Study of Cannabis-based Extracts for Bladder Dysfunction in Advanced Multiple Sclerosis." *Multiple Sclerosis* 10 (2004): 425–33.

Brady, C. M., R. DasGupta, O. J. Wiseman, et al. "Acute and Chronic Effects of Cannabis-based Medicinal Extract on Refractory Lower Urinary Tract Dysfunction in Patients with Advanced Multiple Sclerosis: Early Results." *Congress of the IACM* abstracts (2001): 9.

Braitstein, P., T. Kendall, K. Chan, et al. "Mary-Jane and Her Patients: Sociodemographic and Clinical Characteristics of HIV-positive Individuals Using Medical Marijuana and Antiretroviral Agents." *AIDS* 15 (2001): 532–33.

Breitbart, W., M. V. McDonald, B. Rosenfeld, et al. "Pain in Ambulatory AIDS Patients. I: Pain Characteristics and Medical Correlates." *Pain* 68 (1996a): 315–21.

Breitbart, W., B. D. Rosenfeld, S. D. Passik, et al. "The Undertreatment of Pain in Ambulatory AIDS Patients." *Pain* 65 (1996b): 243–49.

Breitler A. "Marijuana Crops Also Bad for Environment." *Stockton Record*, August 6, 2007.

Brewer, D. D., R. F. Catalano, K. Haggerty, et al. "A Meta-analysis of Predictors of Continued Drug Use during and after Treatment for Opiate Addiction." *Addiction* 93 (1998): 73–92.

British Columbia (BC) Compassion Club Society. "Response to Health Canada's Proposed Medical Marijuana Access Regulations" (2001): http://thecompassionclub.org/resources/regs.pdf. Accessed December 17, 2009.

British Medical Association. *Therapeutic Uses of Cannabis.* Edited by D. R. Morgan. Amsterdam: Harwood Academic Publishers, 1997.

Brookmeyer, R., E. Johnson, K. Ziegler-Graham, et al. "Forecasting the Global Burden of Alzheimer's Disease." Johns Hopkins University, Deptartment of Biostatistics Working Papers, Working Paper 130 (2007).

Brown, D. T., ed. *Cannabis: The Genus Cannabis.* Amsterdam: Harwood Academic Publishers, 1998a.

————. *Cannabis: The Genus* Cannabis. Amsterdam: Harwood Academic Publishers, 1998b: 29–54.

Brown, E. R. *Rockefeller Medicine Men: Medicine and Capitalism in America.* Berkeley: University of California Press, 1979.

Brown, J. H., and J. E. Horowitz. "Deviance and Deviants: Why Adolescent Substance Use Prevention Programs Do Not Work." *Evaluation Review* 17 (1993): 529–55.

Budney, A. J., S. T. Higgins, K. J. Radonovich, et al. "Adding Voucher-based Incentives to Coping-skills and Motivational Enhancement Improves Outcomes during Treatment for Marijuana Dependence." *Journal of Consulting and Clinical Psychology* 68 (2000): 1051–61.

Budney, A. J., J. R. Hughes, B. A. Moore, et al. "A Review of the Validity and Significance of the Cannabis Withdrawal Syndrome." *American Journal of Psychiatry* 161 (2004): 1967–77.

Budney, A. J., B. A. Moore, H. L. Rocha, et al. "Clinical Trial of Abstinence-based Vouchers and Cognitive-behavioral Therapy for Cannabis Dependence." *Journal of Consulting and Clinical Psychology* 74 (2006): 307–16.

Budney, A. J., B. A. Moore, R. G. Vandrey, et al. "The Time Course and Significance of Cannabis Withdrawal." *Journal of Abnormal Psychology* 112 (2003): 393–402.

Budney, A. J., P. Novy, and J. R. Hughes. "Marijuana Withdrawal among Adults Seeking Treatment for Marijuana Dependence." *Addiction* 94 (1999): 1311–22.

Bueckert, D. "Nearly a Third of Legal Marijuana Users Reject Pot." *Canadian Press,* April 29, 2004.

Buggy, D. J., L. Toogood, S. Maric, et al. "Lack of Analgesic Efficacy of Oral Delta-9-tetrahydrocannabinol in Postoperative Pain." *Pain* 105 (2003): 169–72.

Byrne, A., R. Hallinan, and A. Wodak. "'Cannabis Hyperemesis' Causation Questioned." *Gut* 55 (2006): 132.

Cadoni, C., A. Pisanu, M. Solinas, et al. "Behavioural Sensitization after Repeated Exposure to Delta-9-tetrahydrocannabinol and Cross-sensitization with Morphine." *Psychopharmacology* 158 (2001): 259–66.

Caffarel, M. M., D. Sarrió, J. Palacios, et al. "Delta-9-tetrahydrocannabinol Inhibits Cell Cycle Progression in Human Breast Cancer Cells through Cdc2 Regulation." *Cancer Research* 66 (2006): 6615–21.

Caldicott, D. G. E., J. Holmes, K. C. Roberts-Thomson, et al. "Keep Off the Grass: Marijuana Use and Acute Cardiovascular Events." *European Journal of Emergency Medicine* 12 (2005): 236–44.

Campbell, V. A. "Tetrahydrocannabinol Induced Apoptosis of Cultured Cortical Neurones Is Associated with Cytochrome C Release and Caspase 3 Activation." *Neuropharmacology* 40 (2001): 702–709.

Canada (Attorney General) *v. Sfetkopoulos,* 2008 FCA 328 (CanLII)—2008-10-27.

Canadian AIDS Society. "Cannabis as Therapy for People with HIV/AIDS: 'Our Right, Our Choice.'" Ottawa, ON: Canadian AIDS Society, 2006.

Canadian AIDS Society. "HIV/AIDS and the Therapeutic Use of Cannabis" (2004):

www.cdnaids.ca/web/position.nsf/pages/cas-pp-0021. Accessed May 6, 2010.

Canadian Centre on Substance Abuse. "Canadian Addiction Survey 2004." Ottawa, ON: Canadian Centre on Substance Abuse, 2004.

Canadians for Safe Access. "Open Letter of Concern for the Health and Safety of Canada's Medicinal Cannabis Community." January 1, 2005: http://safeaccess.ca/research/flinflon/opnltr0105.htm#qandp. Accessed December 17, 2009.

———. 2008. "ATI Request Showing Number of Authorized Users in Debt to Health Canada as of January 31st, 2007" (2008): www.safeaccess.ca/research/flinflon/index.htm. Accessed December 27, 2009.

Canadian Press. "Feds to Pay for Military Veterans Medical Marijuana." May 14, 2009.

Canadian Public Health Association. CPHA Resolution No. 2: Regulation of Psycho-active Substances in Canada. September 17, 2007.

———. Pot and Driving Campaign: www.potanddriving.cpha.ca. Accessed May 3, 2010.

Canadian Senate Special Committee on Illegal Drugs. 2002. *Cannabis: Summary Report: Our Position for a Canadian Public Policy.* (See specifically chapter 15, "Driving Under the Influence.")

Capler, R. "A Review of the Cannabis Cultivation Contract between Health Canada and Prairie Plant Systems" (2007): http://thecompassionclub.org/resources/HC_PPS_Contract_Report_Oct_2007.pdf. Accessed December 17, 2009.

Capler, R., and Lucas, P. "Guidelines for the Community-based Distribution of Medical Cannabis in Canada" (2006): http://thecompassionclub.org/law/reports. Accessed December 17, 2009.

Carracedo, A., M. Gironella, M. Lorente M, et al. "Cannabinoids Induce Apoptosis of Pancreatic Tumor Cells via Endoplasmic Reticulum Stress-related Genes." *Cancer Research* 66 (2006): 6748–55.

Carter, G. T., L. S. Krivckas, P. Weydt, et al. "Drug Therapy for Amyotrophic Lateral Sclerosis: Where Are We Now?" *IDrugs* 6 (2003): 147–53.

Carter, G. T., and R. G. Miller. "Comprehensive Management of Amyotrophic Lateral Sclerosis." *Physical Medicine and Rehabilitation Clinics of North America* 9 (1998): 271–84.

Carter, G. T., and B. S. Rosen. "Marijuana in the Management of Amyotrophic Lateral Sclerosis." *American Journal of Hospice and Palliative Medicine* 18 (2001): 264–70.

Carter, G. T., and V. O. Ugalde. "Medical Marijuana: Emerging Applications for the Management of Neurological Disorders." *Physical Medicine and Rehabilitation Clinics of North America* 15 (2004a): 943–54.

Carter, G. T., and P. Weydt. "Cannabis: Old Medicine with New Promise for Neurological Disorders." *Current Opinion in Investigational Drugs* 3 (2002): 437–40.

Carter, G. T., P. Weydt, M. Kyashna-Tocha, et al. "Medical Marijuana: Rational Guidelines for Dosing." *IDrugs* 7 (2004b): 464–70.

Cary, P. "The Marijuana Detection Window: Determining the Length of Time Cannabinoids Will Remain Detectable in Urine Following Smoking." *Drug Court Review* 5 (2005): 23–58.

CASA Press Release. "National Survey of American Attitudes on Substance Abuse XIII: Teens and Parents." August 14, 2008.

Caspi, A., T. E. Moffitt, M. Cannon, et al. "Moderation of the Effect of Adolescent-onset Cannabis Use on Adult Psychosis by a Functional Polymorphism in the Catechol-O-methyltransferase Gene: Longitudinal Evidence of a Gene X Environment Interaction." *Biological Psychiatry* 57 (2005): 1117–27.

Casswell, S., and D. F. Marks. "Cannabis Induced Impairment of Performance of a Divided Attention Task." *Nature* 241 (1973): 60–61.

Castleman, T. "Hemp Biomass for Energy." CIFAR Conference XIV. June 4, 2001. Cracking the Nut: Bioprocessing Lignocellulose to Renewable Products and Energy. http://fuelandfiber.com/Hemp4NRG/Hemp4NRGRV3.htm.

Centonze D., A. Finazzi-Agro, G. Bernardi, et al. "The Endocannabinoid System in Targeting Inflammatory Neurodegenerative Diseases." *Trends in Pharmacological Sciences* 28 (2007): 180–87.

Cermak, T. *Marijuana: What's a Parent to Believe?* Center City, MN: Hazelden, 2003.

Chadwick, H. *The Early Church.* Harmondsworth, England: Penguin, 1967.

Chan, C. "Sick Woman Evicted for Smoking Pot." *The Province,* May 5, 2009.

Chen, Y, and J. Buck. "Cannabinoids Protect Cells from Oxidative Cell Death: A Receptor Independent Mechanism." *Journal of Pharmacology and Experimental Therapeutics* 293 (2000): 807–12.

Chen, Y., R. M. McCarron, Y. Ohara, et al. "Human Brain Capillary Endothelium-2-arachidonoglycerol (Endocannabinoid) Interacts with Endothelin-1." *Circulation Research* 87 (2000): 323–27.

Chen J., W. Paredes, J. H. Lowinson, et al. "Delta-9-tetrahydrocannabinol Enhances Pre-synaptic Dopamine Efflux in Medial Prefrontal Cortex." *European Journal of Pharmacology* 190 (1990): 259–62.

Chernow, R. *Titan: The Life of John D. Rockefeller, Sr.* New York: Random House, 1998.

Chesher, G., and M. Longo. "Cannabis and Alcohol in Motor Vehicle Accidents." In Grotenhermen, F, and E. Russo. *Cannabis and Cannabinoids: Pharmacology, Toxicology, and Therapeutic Potential.* New York: Haworth Integrative Healing Press, 2002.

Chevaleyre, V., K. A. Takahashi, and P. E. Castillo. "Endocannabinoid-mediated Synaptic Plasticity in the CNS." *Annual Review of Neuroscience* 29 (2006): 37–76.

Chong, M. S., K. Wolff, K. Wise, et al. "Cannabis Use in Patients with Multiple Sclerosis." *Multiple Sclerosis* 12 (2006): 646–51.

Cichewicz, D. L. "Synergistic Interactions between Cannabinoid and Opioid Analgesics." *Life Sciences* 74 (2004): 1317–24.

Clark, W. C., M. N. Janal, P. Zeidenberg, et al. "Effects of Moderate and High Doses of Marihuana on Thermal Pain: A Sensory Decision Theory Analysis." *Journal of Clinical Pharmacology* 21 (1981): 299S–310S.

Clarke, R. C. *Marijuana Botany—An Advanced Study: The Propagation and Breeding of Distinctive Cannabis*, 2nd ed. Berkeley, CA: Ron Publishing, 1993.

Clendinning, J. "Observation on the Medicinal Properties of Cannabis sativa of India." *Medico-Chirurgical Transactions* 26 (1843): 188–210.

Clifford, D .B. "Tetrahydrocannabinol for Tremor in Multiple Sclerosis." *Annals of Neurology* 13 (1983): 669–71.

Coffey, C., J. B. Carlin, L. Degenhardt, et al. "Cannabis Dependence in Young Adults: An Australian Population Study." *Addiction* 97 (2002): 187–94.

Comeau, P. "Cut to Marijuana Research Sends Strong Message." *Canadian Medical Association Journal* 175, no. 12 (2006): doi:10.1503/cmaj.061508.

———. "New Dosage Limits for Medical Marijuana: But Where Is the Science?" *Canadian Medical Association Journal* 177, no. 6 (2007): doi:10.1503/cmaj.071074.

Comer, S. D., E. D. Collins, M. W. Fischman. "Choice between Money and Intranasal Heroin in Morphine-maintained Humans." *Behavioral Pharmacology* 6 (1997):677–690.

Compston, A. "Treatment and Management of Multiple Sclerosis." In *McAlpine's Multiple Sclerosis*. New York: Churchill Livingstone, 1999.

———. "Multiple Sclerosis and Other Demyelinating Diseases." In *Brain's Diseases of the Nervous System*. New York: Oxford University Press, 2001.

Conrad, C. *Hemp: A Lifeline to the Future*. Los Angeles: Creative Xpressions Publications, 1994.

Consroe, P. "Clinical and Experimental Reports of Marijuana and Cannabinoids in Spastic Disorders." *Marijuana and Medicine*. Totowa, NJ: Humana Press, 1999.

Consroe, P., R. Musty, J. Rein, et al. "The Perceived Effects of Smoked Cannabis on Patients with Multiple Sclerosis." *European Neurology* 38 (1997): 44–48.

Copeland, J., and J. C. Maxwell. "Cannabis Treatment Outcomes among Legally Coerced and Non-coerced Adults." *BMC Public Health* 7 (June 14, 2007): www.biomedcentral.com/1471-2458/7/111. Accessed May 7, 2010.

Copeland, J., W. Swift, and V. Rees. "Clinical Profile of Participants in a Brief Intervention Program for Cannabis Use Disorder." *Journal of Substance Abuse Treatment* 20 (2001a): 45–52.

Copeland, J., W. Swift, R. Roffman, et al. "A Randomized Controlled Trial of Brief Cognitive-behavioral Interventions for Cannabis Use Disorder." *Journal of Substance Abuse Treatment* 21 (2001b): 55–64.

Copersino, M. L., S. J. Boyd, D. P. Tashkin, et al. "Cannabis Withdrawal among Non-treatment-seeking Adult Cannabis Users." *American Journal on Addictions* 15 (2006): 8–14.

Croxford, J., and T. Yamamura. "Cannabinoids and the Immune System: Potential for the Treatment of Inflammatory Diseases?" *Journal of Neuroimmunology* 166 (2005): 3–18.

Cunha, J. M., E. A. Carlini, A. E. Pereira, et al. "Chronic Administration of Cannabidiol to Healthy Volunteers and Epileptic Patients." *Pharmacology* 21 (1980): 175–85.

Curran H. V., C. Brignell, S. Fletcher, et al. "Cognitive and Subjective Dose–response Effects of Acute Oral Delta 9-tetrahydrocannabinol (THC) in Infrequent Cannabis Users." *Psychopharmacology* 164 (2002): 61–70.

Dansak, D. A. "Medical Use of Recreational Drugs by AIDS Patients." *Journal of Addictive Diseases* 16 (1997): 25–30.

Darmani, N. A., and J. L. Crim. "Delta-9-tetrahydrocannabinol Differentially Suppresses Emesis versus Enhanced Locomotor Activity Produced by Chemically Diverse Dopamine D2/D3 Receptor Agonists in the Least Shrew (Cryptotis parva)." *Pharmacology Biochemistry and Behavior* 80 (2005): 35–44.

Das, R. *Journey of Awakening: A Meditator's Guidebook*. New York, Bantam Books, 1990.

Das, S. K. "Harmful Health Effects of Cigarette Smoking." *Molecular and Cellular Biochemistry* 253 (2003): 159–65.

Degenhardt, L., W. T. Chiu, N. Sampson, et al. "Toward a Global View of Alcohol, Tobacco, Cannabis, and Cocaine Use: Findings from the WHO World Mental Health Surveys." *PLoS Medicine* 5 (1988): e141.

Dejesus, E., B. M. Rodwick, D. Bowers, et al. "Use of Dronabinol Improves Appetite and Reverses Weight Loss in HIV/AIDS-infected Patients." *Journal of the International Association of Physicians in AIDS Care* 6 (2007): 95–100.

de Jong, B. C., D. Prentiss, W. McFarland, et al. "Marijuana Use and Its Association with Adherence to Antiretroviral Therapy among HIV-infected Persons with Moderate to Severe Nausea." *Journal of Acquired Immune Deficiency Syndrome* 38 (2005): 43–46.

Dell'Osso, L. F. "Suppression of Pendular Nystagmus by Smoking Cannabis in a Patient with Multiple Sclerosis." *Neurology* 54 (2000): 2190–91.

de Meijer, E. P. M., M. Bagatta, A. Carboni, et al. "The Inheritance of Chemical Phenotype in *Cannabis sativa* L." *Genetics* 163 (2003): 335–46.

de Meijer, E. P. M., H. J. van der Kamp, and F .A. van Eeuwijk. "Characterisation of *Cannabis* Accessions with Regard to Cannabinoid Content in Relation to Other Plant Characters." *Euphytica* 62 (1992): 187–200.

Denning, P., J. Little, and A. Glickman. *Over the Influence: The Harm Reduction Guide to Managing Drugs and Alcohol*. New York: Guilford, 2003.

Denson, T. F., and Earleywine, M. "Decreased Depression in Marijana Users." *Addictive Behaviors* 31 (2006): 738–42.

DeSanty, K. P., and M. S. Dar. "Involvement of the Cerebellar Adenosine A(1) Receptor in Cannabinoid Induced Motor Incoordination in the Acute and Tolerant State in Mice." *Brain Research* 905 (2001): 178–87.

Devane, W. A., A. Breuer, T. Sheskin, et al. "A Novel Probe for the Cannabinoid Receptor." *Journal of Medicinal Chemistry* 35 (1992a): 2065–69.

Devane, W. A., F. A. Dysarz III, M. R. Johnson, et al. "Determination and

Characterization of a Cannabinoid Receptor in Rat Brain." *Molecular Pharmacology* 34 (1988): 605–13.

Devane, W. A., L. Hanuš, A. Breuer, et al. "Isolation and Structure of a Brain Constituent That Binds to the Cannabinoid Receptor." *Science* 258 (1992b): 194–249.

De Vries, T. J., and A. N. Schoffelmeer. "Cannabinoid CB1 Receptors Control Conditioned Drug Seeking." *Trends in Pharmacological Sciences* 26 (2005): 420–26.

Deykin, E. Y., J. C. Levy, and V. Wells. "Adolescent Depression, Alcohol, and Drug Abuse." *American Journal of Public Health* 76 (1986): 178–82.

Diaz-Asper, C. M., D. J. Schretlen, and G. D. Pearlson. "How Well Does IQ Predict Neuropsychological Test Performance in Normal Adults?" *Journal of the International Neuropsychological Society* 10 (2003): 82–90.

Di Marzo, V., T. Bisogno, and L. De Petrocellis. "Endocannabinoids: New Targets for Drug Development." *Current Pharmaceutical Design* 6 (2000): 1361–80.

Di Marzo, V., A. Fontana, H. Cadas, et al. "Formation and Inactivation of Endogenous Cannabinoid Anandamide in Central Neurons." *Nature* 372 (1994): 686–91.

Di Marzo, V., and I. Matias. "Endocannabinoid Control of Food Intake and Energy Balance." *Nature Neuroscience* 8 (2005): 585–89.

Dioscorides Pedanius. *De Materia Medica.* Johannesburg, IBIDIS Press, 2000.

Dirikoc, S., S. A. Priola, M. Marella, et al. "Nonpsychoactive Cannabidiol Prevents Prion Accumulation and Protects Neurons against Prion Toxicity." *Journal of Neuroscience* 27 (2007): 9537–44.

Dixon, W. E. "The Pharmacology of *Cannabis Indica.*" *British Medical Journal* 2: 1354–57.

Doblin, R. "The MAPS/California NORML Marijuana Waterpipe/vaporizer Study." *Newsletter of the Multidisciplinary Association for Psychedelic Studies* 5 (1994): 19–22.

Drummer, O., J. Gerostamoulos, H. Batziris, et al. "The Involvement of Drugs in Drivers Killed in Australian Road Traffic Crashes." *Accident, Analysis and Prevention* 36 (2004): 239–48.

D'Souza, D. C., E. Perry, L. MacDougall, et al. "The Psychotomimetic Effects of Intravenous Delta-9-tetrahydrocannabinol in Healthy Individuals: Implications for Psychosis." *Neuropsychopharmacology* 29 (2004): 1558–72.

Duncan, D. F. "Problems Associated with Three Commonly Used Drugs: A Survey of Rural Secondary School Students." *Psychology of Addictive Behavior* 5 (1991): 93–96.

Dunn, M., and R. Davis. "The Perceived Effects of Marijuana on Spinal Cord Injured Males." *Paraplegia* 12 (1974): 175.

Earleywine, M. *Understanding Marijuana: A New Look at the Scientific Evidence.* New York: Oxford University Press, 2005.

———. 2006. "Marijuana Drug Safety." Lecture at the State University of New York, Albany, February 13, 2006.

Earleywine, M., and S. Smucker Barnwell. "Decreased Respiratory Symptoms in

Cannabis Users Who Vaporize." *Harm Reduction Journal* 4 (2007): www .harmreductionjournal.com/content/4/1/11. Accessed April 29, 2010.

Edery, H., Y. Grunfeld, Z. Ben-Zvi, et al. "Structural Requirements for Cannabinoid Activity." *Annals of New York Academy of Sciences* 191 (1971): 40–53.

Eldreth, D. A., J. A. Matochik, J. L. Cadet, et al. "Abnormal Brain Activity in Prefrontal Brain Regions in Abstinent Marijuana Users." *NeuroImage* 3 (2004): 914–20.

Ellis, G. M., M. A. Mann, B. A. Judson, et al. "Excretion Patterns of Cannabinoid Metabolites after Last Use in a Group of Chronic Users." *Clinical Pharmacology and Therapeutics* 38 (1985): 572–78.

Ellis, R. J., W. Toperoff, F. Vaida, et al. "Smoked Medicinal Cannabis for Neuropathic Pain in HIV: A Randomized, Crossover Clinical Trial." *Neuropsychopharmacology* 34 (2009): 672–80.

El-Mallakh, R. F. "Marijuana and Migraine." *Headache* 27 (1987): 442–43.

Elphick, M. R., and M. Egertová. "Cannabinoid Receptor Genetics and Evolution." In *The Cannabinoid Receptors.* Totawa, NJ: Humana Press, 2009.

El-Remessy, A. B., M. Al-Shabrawey, Y. Khalifa, et al. "Neuroprotective and Blood-retinal Barrier-preserving Effects of Cannabidiol in Experimental Diabetes." *American Journal of Pathology* 168 (2006): 235–44.

ElSohly, M. A., J. H. Holley, G. S. Lewis, et al. "Constituents of *Cannabis sativa* L. XXXV. The Potency of Confiscated Marijuana, Hashish, and Hash Oil over a Ten-year Period." *Journal of Forensic Science* 29 (1984): 500–14.

Eshhar, N., S. Striem, and A. Biegon. "HU 211, a Non-psychotropic Cannabinoid, Rescues Cortical Neurones from Excitatory Amino Acid Toxicity in Culture." *Neuroreport* 5 (1993): 237–40.

Esposito, G., A. A. Izzo, M. Di Rosa, et al. "Selective Cannabinoid CB1 Receptor-mediated Inhibition of Inducible Nitric Oxide Synthase Protein Expression in C6 Rat Glioma Cells." *Journal of Neurochemistry* 78 (2001): 835–41.

Eubanks, L. M., C. J. Rogers, A. E. Beuscher, et al. "A Molecular Link between the Active Component of Marijuana and Alzheimer's Disease Pathology." *Molecular Pharmaceutics* 3 (2006): 773–77.

Fan, F., Q. Tao, M. Abood, et al. "Cannabinoid Down-regulation without Alteration of the Inhibitory Effect of CP 55,940 on Adenyl Cyclase in the Cerebellum of CP 55,940-tolerant Mice." *Brain Research* 706 (1996): 13–20.

Fan, P. "Cannabinoid Agonists Inhibit the Activation of 5-HT3 Receptors in Rat Nodose Ganglion Neurons." *Journal of Neurophysiology* 73 (1995): 907–10.

FDA. "FDA Guideline for the Clinical Evaluation of Analgesic Drugs." DHHS Pub. No. 93-3093. Rockville, MD: U.S. Department of Health and Human Services, Public Health Service, Food and Drug Administration, 1992.

Fergusson, D. M., J. M. Boden, and L. J. Horwood. "Cannabis Use and Other Illicit Drug Use: Testing the Cannababis Gateway Hypothesis." *Addiction* 101 (2006): 556–69.

Fernandez-Ruiz, J., M. Gomez, M. Hernandez, et al. "Cannabinoids and Gene Expression during Brain Development." *Neurotoxicity Research* 6 (2004): 389–401.

Ferraro, L., M. C. Tomasini, T. Cassano, et al. "Cannabinoid Receptor Agonist WIN 55, 212-2 Inhibits Rat Cortical Dialysate Gamma Aminobutyric Acid Levels." *Journal of Neuroscience Research* 15 (2001): 298–302.

Fischman, M. W., and R. W. Foltin. "Utility of Subjective-effects Measurements in Assessing Abuse Liability of Drugs in Humans." *British Journal of Addiction* 86 (1991): 760–70.

Fischman, M. W., R. W. Foltin, G. Nestadt, et al. "Effects of Desipramine Maintenance on Cocaine Self-administration by Humans." *Journal of Pharmacology and Experimental Therapeutics* 253 (1990): 760–70.

Fisher, B. A. C., A. Ghuran, V. Vandamalai, et al. "Cardiovascular Complications Induced by Cannabis Smoking: A Case Report and Review of the Literature." *Emergency Medicine Journal* 22 (2005): 679–80.

Fletcher, J. M., J. B. Page, D. J. Francis, et al. "Cognitive Correlates of Long-term Cannabis Use in Costa Rican Men." *Archives of General Psychiatry* 53 (1996): 1051–57.

Flexner, A. *Medical Education in the United States and Canada.* Classics of Medicine Library. Birmingham, AL: Gryphon, 1910.

Fligiel, S. E., M. D. Roth, E. C. Kleerup, et al. "Tracheobronchial histopathology in habitual smokers of cocaine, marijuana, and/or tobacco." *Chest* 112 (1997): 319–26.

Flynn, J., and N. Hanif. "Nabilone for the Management of Intractable Nausea and Vomiting in Terminally Staged AIDS." *Journal of Palliative Care* 8 (1992): 46–47.

Fogarty, A., P. Rawstorne, G. Prestage, et al. "Marijuana as Therapy for People Living with HIV/AIDS: Social and Health Aspects." *AIDS Care* 19 (2007): 295–301.

Ford, D. E., H. T. Vu, C. Hauer, et. al. "Marijuana Use Is Not Associated with Head, Neck or Lung Cancer in Adults Younger than 55 Years: Results of a Case Cohort Study. Paper presented at the National Institute on Drug Abuse Workshop on Clinical Consequences of Marijuana" (August 13–14, 2001): www.nida.nih.gov/MeetSum/marijuanaabstracts.html. Accessed May 7, 2010.

Fox, M. "U.S. Marijuana Even Stronger han Before." Reuters, April 25, 2007.

Fox, P., P. G. Bain, S. Glickman, et al. "The Effect of Cannabis on Tremor in Patients with Multiple Sclerosis." *Neurology* 62 (2004): 1105–1109.

Frich, L. M., and F. M. Borgbjerg. "Pain and Pain Treatment in AIDS Patients: A Longitudinal Study." *Journal of Pain and Symptom Management* 19 (2000): 339–47.

Fried, P. A., and A. M. Smith. "A Literature Review of the Consequences of Prenatal Marihuana Exposure: An Emerging Theme of a Deficiency in Aspects of Executive Function." *Neurotoxicology and Teratology* 23 (2001):1–11.

Fried, P. A., B. Watkinson, and R. Gray. "Neurocognitive Consequences of Marihuana: A Comparison with Pre-drug Performance." *Neurotoxicology and Teratology* 27 (2004): 231–39.

Fried, P. A., D. James, and R. Gray. "Current and Former Marijuana Use: Preliminary Findings of a Longitudinal Study of Effects on IQ in Young Adults." *Canadian Medical Association Journal* 166 (2002): 887–91.

Friedman, H., T. W. Klein, C. Newton, et al. "Marijuana, Receptors and Immunomodulation." *Advances in Experimental Medicine and Biology* 373 (1995): 103–13.

Furler, M. D., T. R. Einarson, M. Millson, et al. "Medicinal and Recreational Marijuana Use by Patients Infected with HIV." *AIDS Patient Care and STDS* 18 (2004): 215–28.

Gabany, S. G., and P. Plummer. "The Marijuana Perception Inventory: The Effects of Substance Abuse Instruction." *Journal of Drug Education* 20 (1990): 235–45.

Gaedcke, F. "Über das Erythroxylin, dargestellt aus den Blättern des in Südamerika cultivirten Strauches Erythroxylon Coca." *Archiv der Pharmazie* 132 (1855): 141–50.

Gaetani, S., F. Oveisi, and D. Piomelli. "Modulation of Meal Pattern in the Rat by the Anorexic Lipid Mediator Oleoylethanolamide." *Neuropsychopharmacology* 28 (2003): 1311–16.

Gallup Poll. "Illegal Drugs." 2005. www.gallup.com/poll/1657/illegal-drugs.aspx.

Galve-Roperh, I, C. Sanchez, M. L. Cortes, et al. "Anti-tumoral Action of Cannabinoids: Involvement of Sustained Ceramide Accumulation and Extracellular Signal-regulated Kinase Activation." *Nature Medicine* 6 (2000): 313–19.

Gaoni, Y., and R. Mechoulam. "Isolation, Structure and Partial Synthesis of an Active Constituent of Hashish." *Journal of the American Chemical Society* 86 (1964): 1646–67.

Garcia de Olalla, P., H. Knobel, A. Carmona, et al. "Impact of Adherence and Highly Active Antiretroviral Therapy on Survival in HIV-infected Patients." *Journal of Acquired Immune Deficiency Syndrome* 30 (2002): 105–10.

Gerdeman, G. L., and D. M. Lovinger. "Emerging Roles for Endocannabinoids in Long-term Synaptic Plasticity." *British Journal of Pharmacology* 140 (2003a): 781–89.

Gerdeman, G. L, J. G. Partridge, C. R. Lupica, et al. "It Could Be Habit Forming: Drugs of Abuse and Striatal Synaptic Plasticity." *Trends in Neurosciences* 26 (2003b): 184–92.

Gerdeman, G. L., J. B. Schechter, and E. D. French. "Inhibition of Stimulus-response (Habit) Learning by Striatal Injection of the CB1 Antagonist Rimonabant." Symposium on the Cannabinoids, International Cannabinoid Research Society, 2006, Burlington, VT.

Gerdeman, G. L. "Endocannabinoids at the Synapse: Retrograde Signaling and Presynaptic Plasticity in the Brain." In A Kofalvi, ed. *Cannabinoids and the Brain.* Boston, MA: Springer, 2008a.

Gerdeman, G. L., and J. Fernandez-Ruiz. "The Endocannabinoid System in the Physiology and Pathology of the Basal Ganglia." In A. Kofalvi, ed. *Cannabinoids and the Brain.* A. Boston, MA: Springer, 2008b.

Gertsch, J., M. Leonti, S. Raduner, et al. "Beta-caryophyllene Is a Dietary Cannabinoid." *Proceedings of the National Academy of Sciences USA* 105 (2008): 9099–104.

Gettman, J. "Marijuana Production in the United States." *Bulletin of Cannabis Reform*

(December 2006): www.drugscience.org/Archive/bcr2/MJCropReport_2006.pdf. Accessed December 1, 2007.

———. "Marijuana Production in the United States" (2006): www.drugscience.org/Archive/bcr2/policy_analysis.html. Accessed April 29, 2010.

Ghalioungui, P. *Magic and Medical Science in Ancient Egypt*. London: Hodder and Stoughton, 1963.

Gieringer, D. "Testimony (to the California Assemby Committee on Public Safety) on the Legalization of Marijuana." *O'Shaughnessy's: The Journal of Cannabis in Clinical Practice* (Winter/Spring 2007).

Gieringer D, J. St. Laurent, and S. Goodrich. "Cannabis Vaporizer Combines Efficient Delivery of THC with Effective Suppression of Pyrolytic Compounds." *Journal of Cannabis Therapeutics* 4 (2004): 7–27.

Gill, E. W., and G. Jones. "Brain Levels of Delta-1-tetrahydrocannabinol and Its Metabolites in Mice: Correlation with Behaviour, and the Effect of the Metabolic Inhibitors SKF 525A and Piperonyl Butoxide." *Biochemical Pharmacology* 21 (1972): 2237–48.

Giuffrida A., L. H. Parsons, T. M. Kerr, et al. "Dopamine Activation of Endogenous Cannabinoid Signaling in Dorsal Striatum." *Nature Neuroscience* 2 (1999): 358–63.

Glass, M., M. Dragunow, and R. L. Faull. "Cannabinoid Receptors in the Human Brain: A Detailed Anatomical and Quantitative Autoradiographic Study in the Fetal, Neonatal and Adult Human Brain." *Neuroscience* 77 (1997): 299–318.

Golub, A., and B. Johnson. "The Shifting Importance of Alcohol and Marijuana as Gateway Substances among Serious Drug Abusers." *Journal of Studies on Alcohol* 55 (1994): 607–14.

Golub, A., and B. D. Johnson. "Variation in Youthful Risks of Progression from Alcohol/tobacco to Marijuana and to Hard Drugs across Generations." *American Journal of Public Health* 91 (2001): 225–32.

Gombos, J. "Drug Testing FAQ: Producing Clean Urine" (1998). The Vaults of Erowid: www.erowid.org/psychoactives/testing/testing_faq.shtml#6. Accessed March 12, 2008.

Goode, E. *Drugs in American Society*, 6th ed. New York: McGraw-Hill, 2004.

Goodyear, K., D. Laws, and J. Turner. "Bilateral Spontaneous Pneumothorax in a Cannabis Smoker." *Journal of the Royal Society of Medicine* 97 (2004): 435–36.

Gorter, R. W., M. Butorac, E. Pulido Cobian, et al. "Medical Use of Cannabis in the Netherlands. *Neurology* 64 (2005): 917–19.

Gracies, J. M., P. Nance, and E. Elovic. "Traditional Pharmacological Treatments for Spasticity. Part II: General and Regional Treatments." *Muscle and Nerve* 20, suppl. 6 (1997): S92–S120.

Graindorge, C. "Les Oignons de Sokar." *Revue d'Egyptologie* 43 (1992).

Grant, I., R. Gonzalez, C. L. Carey, et al. "Non-acute (Residual) Neurocognitive Effects of Cannabis Use: A Meta-analytic Study." *Journal of the International Neuropsychological Society* 9 (2003): 679–89.

Green, G. *The Cannabis Breeder's Bible: The Definitive Guide to Marijuana Genetics, Cannabis Botany and Creating Strains for the Seed Market.* San Francisco: Green Candy Press, 2005.

Green, S. T., D. Nathwani, D. J. Goldberg, et al. "Nabilone as Effective Therapy for Intractable Nausea and Vomiting in AIDS." *British Journal of Clinical Pharmacology* 28 (1989): 494–95.

Greenberg, H. S., A. S. Weiness, and J. E. Pugh. "Short Term Effects of Smoking Marijuana on Balance in Patients with Multiple Sclerosis and Normal Volunteers." *Clinical Pharmacology and Therapeutics* 55 (1994): 324–28.

Greene, L. 2007. "Leo's Story: Looking for Relief, More Time." *Inland Valley Daily Bulletin*, June 18, 2007: www.dailybulletin.com/search/ci_6161392?IADID=Search-www.dailybulletin.com-www.dailybulletin.com. Accessed September 5, 2007.

Greenwald, M. K., and M. L. Stitzer. "Antinociceptive, Subjective and Behavioral Effects of Smoked Marijuana in Humans." *Drug and Alcohol Dependence* 59 (2000): 261–75.

Grey, M. *Drug Crazy.* New York: Random House, 1998.

Grinspoon, L. Quoted in C. Rätsch, C., 2001. *Marijuana Medicine.* Rochester, VT: Healing Arts Press, 2001.

Grinspoon, L., and J. B. Bakalar. *Marihuana, the Forbidden Medicine,* rev. and exp. ed. New Haven: Yale University Press, 1997.

———. "The Use of Cannabis as a Mood Stabilizer in Bipolar Disorder: Anecdotal Evidence and the Need for Clinical Research." *Journal of Psychoactive Drugs* 30 (1998): 171–77.

Grotenhermen, F. "Pharmacokinetics and Pharmacodynamics of Cannabinoids." *Clinical Pharmacokinetics* 42 (2003): 327–60.

———. *Drugs and Driving: Review for the National Treatment Agency, UK.* Nova-Institut (Germany), November, 2007 (2007b).

Grotenhermen, F., G. Leson, G., Berghaus, et al. "Developing Per Se Limits for Driving under Cannabis." *Addiction* 102 (2007a): 1910–17.

Gulland, J. M., and R. Robinson. "The Constitution of Codeine and Thebaine." *Mem Proceedings of the Manchester Literary and Philosophical Society* 69 (1925): 79–86.

Guy, G. W., B. A. Whittle, and P. J. Robson, eds. *The Medicinal Uses of Cannabis and Cannabinoids.* London: Pharmaceutical Press, 2004.

Guzman, M. "Cannabinoids: Potential Anti-cancer Agents." *Nature Reviews Cancer* 3 (2003): 745–55.

Guzman, M., M. J. Duarte, C. Blázquez, et al. "A Pilot Clinical Study of Delta-9-tetrahydrocannabinol in Patients with Recurrent Glioblastoma Multiforme." *British Journal of Cancer* 95 (2006): 197–203.

Guzman, M., C. Sanchez, and I. Galve Roperh. "Control of the Cell Survival/death Decision by Cannabinoids." *Journal of Molecular Medicine* 78 (2001): 613–25.

Hadorn, D. "A Review of Cannabis and Driving Skills." In Guy, G. W., B. A. Whittle, and P. Robson. *The Medicinal Uses of Cannabis and Cannabinoids*. London: Pharmaceutical Press, 2004.

Hall, W., M. Christie, and D. Currow. "Cannabinoids and Cancer: Causation, Remediation, and Palliation." *Lancet Oncology* 6 (2005): 35–42.

Hall, W., R. Room, and S. Bondy. "A Comparative Appraisal of the Health and Psychological Consequences of Alcohol, Cannabis, Nicotine and Opiate Use." In Kalant, H., W. Corrigall, W. Hall, and R. Smart, eds., *The Health Effects of Cannabis*. Toronto: Centre for Addiction and Mental Health, 1999.

Hall, W., and N. Solowij. "Adverse Effects of Cannabis." *Lancet* 352 (1998): 1611–16.

Hall, W., N. Solowij, and J. Lemon. *The Health and Psychological Consequences of Cannabis Use*. National Drug Strategy Monograph Series no. 25. Canberra: Australian Government Publishing Service, 1994.

Hamelink, C., A. Hampson, D. Wink, et al. "Comparison of Cannabidiol, Antioxidants, and Diuretics in Reversing Binge Ethanol-induced Neurotoxicity. *Journal of Pharmacology and Experimental Therapeutics* 314 (2005): 780–88.

Hammond, C., and P. Mahlberg. "Morphogenesis of Capitate Glandular Hairs of *Cannabis sativa* L. (Cannabaceae)." *American Journal of Botany* 65 (1977): 1023–31.

Hampson, A. "Cannabinoids as Neuroprotectants against Ischemia." In F. Grotenhermen and E. Russo, eds., *Cannabis and Cannabinoids: Pharmacology, Toxicology, and Therapeutic Potential*. New York: Haworth Integrative Healing Press, 2002.

Hampson, A., M. Grimaldi, J. Axelrod, et al. "Cannabidiol and (-)Delta9-tetrahydrocannabinol are Neuroprotective Antioxidants." *Proceedings of the National Academy of Sciences USA* 95 (1998): 8268–73.

Hampson, A., M. Grimaldi, M. Lolic, et al. "Neuroprotective Antioxidants from Marijuana." *Annals of the New York Academy of Sciences* 899 (2000): 274–82.

Hill, P. "What Is Neuroprotection?" *Medical News Today*, October 9, 2006: www .medicalnewstoday.com/articles/53700.php. Accesses May 6, 2010.

Haney, M. "The Marijuana Withdrawal Syndrome: Diagnosis and Treatment." *Current Psychiatry Reports* 7 (2005): 360–66.

Haney, M., S. D. Comer, A. S. Ward, et al. "Factors Influencing Marijuana Self-administration by Humans." *Behavioral Pharmacology* 8 (1997): 101–12.

Haney, M., E. W. Gunderson, J. Rabkin, et al. "Dronabinol and Marijuana in HIV-positive Marijuana Smokers: Caloric Intake, Mood, and Sleep." *Journal of Acquired Immune Deficiency Syndromes* 45 (2007): 545–54.

Haney, M., C. L. Hart, S. K. Vosburg, et al. "Marijuana Withdrawal in Humans: Effects of Oral THC or Divalproex." *Neuropsychopharmacology* 29 (2004): 158–70.

Haney, M., C. L. Hart, A. S. Ward, et al. "Nefazodone Decreases Anxiety During Marijuana Withdrawal in Humans." *Psychopharmacology* 165 (2003): 157–65.

Haney, M., A. S. Ward, S. D. Comer, et al. "Abstinence Symptoms Following Smoked Marijuana in Humans." *Psychopharmacology* 141 (1999): 395–404.

Hanrahan, C. "Marijuana." *Encyclopedia of Alternative Medicine,* issue 20010406 (2001): http://findarticles.com/p/articles/mi_g2603. Accessed December 7, 2007.

Hansen, H. H., P. C. Schmid, P. Bittigau, et al. "Anandamide, but Not 2 Arachidonoylglycerol, Accumulates during In Vivo Neurodegeneration." *Journal of Neurochemistry* 78 (2001): 1415–27.

Hanuš, L. O. "Pharmacological and Therapeutic SECRETS of Plant and Brain (Endo) cannabinoids." *Medicinal Research Reviews* 29 (2009): 213–71.

Harcourt, B. E., and J. Ludwig. "Reefer Madness: Broken Windows Policing and Misdemeanor Marijuana Arrests in New York City, 1989–2000." *Criminology and Public Policy* 6:1, 16582. http://papers.ssrn.com/sol13/papers.cfm?abstract_id=948753. Accessed May 21, 2010.

Harris, D., R. T. Jones, and R. Shank, "Self-reported Marijuana Effects and Characteristics of 100 San Francisco Medical Marijuana Club Members." *Journal of Addictive Diseases* 19 (2000): 89–103.

Harris Interactive. CNN/Time Poll. "Marijuana Legalization." October 23–24, 2002.

Hart, C. L. "Increasing Treatment Options for Cannabis Dependence: A Review of Potential Pharmacotherapies." *Drug and Alcohol Dependence* 80 (2005): 147–59.

Hart, C. L., W. van Gorp, M. Haney, et al. "Effects of Acute Smoked Marijuana on Complex Cognitive Performance." *Neuropsychopharmacology* 25 (2001): 757–65.

Hart, C. L., M. Haney, S. K. Vosburg, et al. "Reinforcing Effects of Oral Delta9-THC in Male Marijuana Smokers in a Laboratory Choice Procedure." *Psychopharmacology (Berlin)* 181 (2005): 237–43.

Hart, C. L., M. Haney, A. S. Ward, et al. "Effects of Oral THC Maintenance on Smoked Marijuana Self-administration." *Drug and Alcohol Dependence* 67 (2002b): 301–9.

Hart, C. L., A. B. Ilan, A. Gevins, et al. (under review). "Neurophysiological and Cognitive Effects of Smoked Marijuana in Frequent Users."

Hart, C. L., A. S. Ward, M. Haney, et al. "Comparison of Smoked Marijuana and Oral Delta(9)-tetrahydrocannabinol in Humans." *Psychopharmacology (Berlin)* 164 (2002a): 407–15.

Hashibe, M., D. E. Ford, and Z. Zhang. "Marijuana Smoking and Head and Neck Cancer." *Journal of Clinical Pharmacology* 42 (2002): 103S–7S.

Hashibe, M., H. Morgenstern, Y. Cui, et al. "Marijuana Use and the Risk of Lung and Upper Aerodigestive Tract Cancers: Results of a Population-based Case-control Study." *Cancer Epidemiology Biomarkers and Prevention* 15 (2006): 1829–34.

Hashibe, M., K. Straif, D. P. Tashkin, et al. "Epidemiologic Review of Marijuana Use and Cancer Risk." *Alcohol* 35 (2005): 265–75.

Hashimotodani, Y., T. Ohno-Shosaku, and M. Kano. "Endocannabinoids and Synaptic Function in the CNS." *Neuroscientist* 13 (2007): 127–37.

Hazekamp, A., R. Ruhaak, L. Zuurman, et al. "Evaluation of a Vaporizing Device (Volcano) for the Pulmonary Administration of Tetrahydrocannabinol." *Journal of Pharmaceutical Sciences* 95 (2006): 1308–17.

Health Canada. "Medical Use of Marihuana: Stakeholder Statistics" (2009): www.hc-sc.gc.ca/dhp-mps/marihuana/stat/index-eng.php. Accessed December 16, 2009.

Heard, K., and C. D. Mendoza. "Consequences of Attempts to Mask Urine Drug Screens." *Annals of Emergency Medicine* 50 (2007): 591–92.

Heifets, B. D., and P. E. Castillo. "Endocannabinoid Signaling and Long-term Synaptic Plasticity." *Annual Review of Physiology* 71 (2009): 283–306.

Heishman, S. J., K. Arasteh, and M. L. Stitzer. "Comparative Effects of Alcohol and Marijuana on Mood, Memory, and Performance." *Pharmacology, Biochemistry, and Behavior* 58 (1997): 93–101.

Heishman, S. J., M. L. Stitzer, and J. E. Yingling. "Effects of Tetrahydrocannabinol Content on Marijuana Smoking Behavior, Subjective Reports, and Performance." *Pharmacology, Biochemistry and Behavior* 34 (1989): 173–79.

Henquet, C., A. Rosa, L. Krabbendam, et al. "An Experimental Study of Catechol-O-methyltransferase Val(158)met Moderation of Delta-9-tetrahydrocannabinol-induced Effects on Psychosis and Cognition." *Neuropsychopharmacology* 31 (August 2006).

Henry R. "Rhode Island Budget Problems Dominate Legislative Year." Associated Press, June 22, 2007.

Herkenham, M. "Localization of Cannabinoid Receptors in the Brain and Periphery." In R. G. Pertwee, ed., *Cannabinoid Receptors*. New York: Academic Press, 1995.

Herkenham, M., A. B. Lynn, M. D. Little, et al. "Cannabinoid Receptor Localization in Brain." *Proceedings of the National Academy of Sciences USA* 87 (1990): 1932–36.

Herning, R. I., W. T. Hooker, and R. T. Jones. "Tetrahydrocannabinol Content and Differences in Marijuana Smoking Behaviour." *Psychopharmacology* 11 (1986): 563–83.

Hewitt, D. J., M. McDonald, R. K. Portenoy, et al. "Pain Syndromes and Etiologies in Ambulatory AIDS Patients." *Pain* 70 (1997): 117–23.

Hilario, M. R., E. Clouse, H. H. Yin, et al. "Endocannabinoid Signaling Is Critical for Habit Formation." *Frontiers in Integrative Neuroscience* 1 (2007): 6.

Hill, M. N., and B. B. Gorzalka. "Is There a Role for the Endocannabinoid System in the Etiology and Treatment of Melancholic Depression?" *Behavioural Pharmacology* 16 (2005): 333–52.

———. "The Endocannabinoid System and the Treatment of Mood and Anxiety Disorders." *CNS and Neurologocal Disordorders—Drug Targets* 8 (2009): 451–58.

Hill, M. N., G. E. Miller, W. S. Ho, et al. "Serum Endocannabinoid Content is Altered in Females with Depressive Disorders: A Preliminary Report." *Pharmacopsychiatry* 41 (2008): 48–53.

Hill, S. Y., R. Schwin, D. W. Goodwin, et al. "Marihuana and Pain." *Journal of Phamacology and Experimental Therapeutics* 188 (1974): 415–18.

Hillig, K. W. "Genetic Evidence for Speciation in *Cannabis* (Cannabaceae)." *Genetic Resources and Crop Evolution* 52 (2005):161–80.

Hitzig v. Canada. 2003. ONCA C39532; C39738; C39740.

Hoareau, L., M. Buyse, F. Festy, et al. "Anti-inflammatory Effect of Palmitoylethanolamide on Human Adipocytes." *Obesity* 17 (2009): 431–38.

Hoeffel J. "UC Studies Find Promise in Medical Marijuana." *Los Angeles Times.*

February 18, 2010: www.latimes.com/news/local/la-me-medical-marijuana18-2010feb18,0,1023346.story. Accessed April 13, 2010.

Hohmann, A. G., E. M. Briley, and M. Herkenham. "Pre- and postsynaptic Distribution of Cannabinoid and Mu Opioid Receptors in Rat Spinal Cord." *Brain Research* 822 (1999): 17–25.

Hohmann, A. G., and R. L. Suplita II. "Endocannabinoid Mechanisms of Pain Modulation." *AAPS Journal* 8 (2006): E693–708.

Holland, J. A., L. W. Nelson, P. R. Ravikumar, et al. "Embalming Fluid–soaked Marijuana: New Drug or New Guise for PCP?" *Journal of Psychoactive Drugs* 30 (1998): 215–19.

Hollister, L. E. 1986. "Interactions of Cannabis with Other Drugs in Man." In M. C. Braude and H. M. Ginzburg, eds., *Strategies for Research on the Interactions of Drugs of Abuse.* National Institute on Drug Abuse Research Monograph 68. DHHS Pub. No. (ADM)86-1453. Washington, DC: Supt. of Docs., U.S. Government Print Office, 1986.

———. 1988. "Marijuana and Immunity." *Journal of Psychoactive Drugs* 20 (1988): 3–8.

House of Lords. Select Committee on Science and Technology, Ninth Report. "Cannabis: The Scientific and Medical Evidence." November 11, 1998.

Howlett, A. C., F. Barth, T. I. Bonner, et al. "International Union of Pharmacology. XXVII. Classification of Cannabinoid receptors." *Pharmacological Review* 54 (2002): 161–202.

Huestis, M. A., D. A. Gorelick, S. A. Heishman, et al. "Blockade of Effects of Smoked Marijuana by the CB1-selective Cannabinoid Receptor Antagonist SR 141716." *Archives of General Psychiatry* 58 (2001): 322–28.

Huestis, M. A., J. E. Henningfield, and E. J. Cone. "Blood Cannabinoids: Absorption of THC and Formation of 11-OH-THC and THCCOOH during and after Smoking Marijuana." *Journal of Analytical Toxicology* 16 (1992): 276–82.

Hughes, J. R., S. T. Higgins, and W. K. Bickel. "Nicotine Withdrawal versus Other Drug Withdrawal Syndromes: Similarities and Dissimilarities." *Addiction* 89 (1994): 1461–70.

Hunault, C. C., T. T. Mensinga, K. B. Böcker, et al. "Cognitive and Psychomotor Effects in Males after Smoking a Combination of Tobacco and Cannabis Containing up to 69 Mg Delta-9-tetrahydrocannabinol (THC)." *Psychopharmacology* 204 (2009): 85–94.

Hurd, Y. L., X. Wang, V. Anderson, et al. "Marijuana Impairs Growth in Mid-gestation Fetuses." *Neurotoxicology and Teratology* 27 (2005): 221–29.

Husstedt, I. W., S. Evers, D. Reichelt, et al. "Screening for HIV-associated Distal-symmetric Polyneuropathy in CDC-classification Stages 1, 2, and 3." *Acta Neurologica Scandinavica* 101 (2000): 183–87.

Ilan, A. B., A. Gevins, M. Coleman, et al. "Neurophysiological and Subjective Profile of Marijuana with Varying Concentrations of Cannabinoids." *Behavioural Pharmacology* 16 (2005): 487–96.

Ilan, A. B., M. E. Smith, and A. Gevins. "Effects of Marijuana on Neurophysiological Signals of Working and Episodic Memory." *Psychopharmacology* 176 (2004): 214–22.

Institute of Medicine (IOM), Division of Health Sciences Policy. "Marijuana and Health: Report of a Study by a Committee of the Institute of Medicine, Division of Health Sciences Policy." Washington, D.C.: National Academy Press, 1982.

International Hemp Drugs Commission 1893–94, appendix 3, 246.

Iuvone, T., G. Esposito, R. Esposito, et al. "Neuroprotective Effect of Cannabidiol, a Non-psychoactive Component from Cannabis Sativa, on Beta-amyloid-induced Toxicity in PC12 Cells." *Journal of Neurochemistry* 89 (2004): 134–41.

Iversen L, S. H. Snyder. *The Science of Marijuana.* New York: Oxford University Press, 2000.

Jacobsson, S. O., T. Wallin, and C. J. Fowler. "Inhibition of Rat C6 Glioma Cell Proliferation by Endogenous and Synthetic Cannabinoids: Relative Involvement of Cannabinoid and Vanilloid Receptors." *Journal of Pharmacology and Experimental Therapeutics* 299 (2001): 951–59.

Jager, G., R. S. Kahn, W. Van Den Brink, et al. "Long-term Effects of Frequent Cannabis Use on Working Memory and Attention: An fMRI Study." *Psychopharmacology* 185 (2006): 358–68.

Jain, A. K., J. R. Ryan, F. G. McMahon, et al. "Evaluation of Intramuscular Levonantradol and Placebo in Acute Postoperative Pain." *Journal of Clinical Pharmacology* 21 (1981): 320S–6S.

James, T. "The Baby and the Bathwater." *South African Medical Journal* 84 (1994): 369.

Jankord, R., and J. P. Herman. "Limbic Regulation of Hypothalamo-pituitary-adrenocortical Function during Acute and Chronic Stress." *Annals of the New York Academy of Sciences* 1148 (2008): 64–73.

Jensen, M. P., R. T. Abresch, G. T. Carter, et al. "Chronic Pain in Persons with Neuromuscular Disorders." *Archives of Physical Medicine and Rehabilitation* 86 (2005): 1155–63.

Jiang, H., Li Xiao, You-Xing Zhao, et al. "A New Insight into Cannabis sativa (Cannabaceae) Utilization from 2500-year-old Yanghai Tombs, Xinjiang, China." *Journal of Ethnopharmacology* 108 (2006): 414–22.

Jiang, W., Y. Zhang, L. Xiao, et al. "Cannabinoids Promote Embryonic and Adult Hippocampus Neurogenesis and Produce Anxiolytic and Depressant-like Effects." *Journal of Clinical Investigation* 115 (2005): 3104–16.

Jochimsen, P. R., R. L. Lawton, K. VerSteeg, et al. "Effect of Benzopyranoperidine, a Delta-9-THC Congener, on Pain." *Journal of Clinical Pharmacy and Therapeutics* 24 (1978): 223–27.

Johanson, C. E., and E. H. Uhlenhuth. "Drug Preference and Mood in Humans: d-amphetamine." *Psychopharmacology* 71 (1980): 275–79.

Johnson, D., A. Conradi, and M. McGuigan. "Hashish Ingestion in Toddlers." *Veterinary and Human Toxicology* 33 (1991): 393.

Johnson, R. A., et al. "Trends in the Incidence of Drug Use in the United States, 1919–1992." Substance Abuse and Mental Health Services Administration, U.S. Department of Health and Human Services, 1996.

Johnston, L. D., P. M. O'Malley, J. G. Bachman, et al. "Teen Marijuana Use Tilts Up, While Some Drugs Decline in Use." Ann Arbor: University of Michigan News Service, December 14, 2009.

Johnston, L. D., P. M. O'Malley, J. G. Bachman, et al. "Monitoring the Future National Survey Results on Drug Use, 1975–2008, volume 1: Secondary School Students." NIH Publication No. 09-7402. National Institute on Drug Abuse (2009): http://monitoringthefuture.org/pubs.html. Accessed May 7, 2010.

Jonas, G. The Circuit Riders: Rockefeller Money and the Rise of Modern Science. New York: W. W. Norton, 1989.

Jones, C., and A. Hathaway, "Marijuana Medicine and Canadian Physicians: Challenges to Meaningful Drug Policy Reform." Contemporary Justice Review 11 (2008): 165–75.

Jones, R. T., and N. Benowitz. "The 30-day Trip: Clinical Studies of Cannabis Tolerance and Dependence." In M. C. Braude and S. Szara, eds., Pharmacology of Marihuana, vol. 2. New York: Raven Press, 1976.

Joy, J. E., J. A. Benson, and S. J. Watson, eds. Marijuana and Medicine: Assessing the Science Base. Washington, DC: National Academies Press, 1999.

Joyce, C. R. B., and S. H. Curry, eds. The Botany and Chemistry of Cannabis. London: J. and A. Churchill, 1970.

Kanayama, G., J. Rogowska, H. G. Pope, et al. "Spatial Working Memory in Heavy Cannabis Users: A Functional Magnetic Resonance Imaging Study." Psychopharmacology 176 (2004): 239–47.

Kandel, D. B., ed. "Stages in Adolescent Involvement in Drug Use." Science 190 (1975): 912–14.

———. Stages and Pathways of Drug Involvement: Examining the Gateway Hypothesis. Cambridge, UK: Cambridge University Press, 2002.

Kandel, D. B., M. Davies, D. Karus, et al. "The Consequences in Young Adulthood of Adolescent Drug Involvement." Archives of General Psychiatry 43 (1986): 746–54.

Kandel, D. B., and K. Yamaguchi. "Patterns of Drug Use from Adolescence to Young Adulthood. III: Predictors of Progression." American Journal of Public Health 74 (1984): 673–81.

Kandel, E. R. In Search of Memory: The Emergence of a New Science of Mind. New York: Norton, 2006.

Kann, L., S. A. Kinchen, B. I. Williams, et al. "Youth Risk Surveillance Behavior—United States, 1999." Morbidity and Mortality Weekly Report 29, no. SS-5:1–96 (2000): www.cdc.gov/mmwr/PDF/ss/ss4905.pdf. Accessed May 7. 2010.

Katona, I., and T. F. Freund. "Endocannabinoid Signaling as a Synaptic Circuit Breaker in Neurological Disease." Nature Medicine 14 (2008): 923–30.

Karst, M., K. Salim, S. Burstein, et al. "Analgesic Effect of the Synthetic Cannabinoid CT-3 on Chronic Neuropathic Pain." *Journal of the American Medical Association* 290 (2003): 1757–62.

Kaufman, D. W., J. P. Kelly, L. Rosenberg, et al. "Recent Patterns of Medication Use in the Ambulatory Adult Population of the United States: The Slone Survey." *Journal of the American Medical Association* 287 (2002): 337–44.

Kaufman, M. "Study Finds No Cancer-marijuana Connection." *Washington Post*, May 26, 2006.

Kaufmann I., D. Hauer, V. Huge, et al. "Enhanced Anandamide Plasma Levels in Patients with Complex Regional Pain Symdrome following Traumatic Injury: A Preliminary Report." *European Surgical Research* 43 (2009): 325–29.

Kaymakcalan, S. "Tolerance to and Dependence on Cannabis." *Bulletin on Narcotics* 25 (1973): 39–47.

Kelly, S., and L. F. Donaldson."Peripheral Cannabinoid CB1 Receptors Inhibit Evoked Responses of Nociceptive Neurones In Vivo." *European Journal of Pharmacology* 586 (2008): 160–3.

Kelly, T. H., R. W. Foltin, M. T. Mayr, et al. "Effects of Delta 9-tetrahydrocannabinol and Social Context on Marijuana Self-administration by Humans." *Pharmacology Biochemistry and Behavior* 49 (1994): 763–8.

Kenoyer, C. "Different Medical Marijuana *Cannabis* Strains with Descriptions and photo's [sic.]" (2007): www.onlinepot.org/grow/potstrains.htm. Accessed December 10, 2007.

Khiabani, H. Z. "Relationship between THC Concentration in Blood and Impairment in Apprehended Drivers." *Traffic Injury Prevention* 7 (2006): 111–16.

Killestein, J., E. L. Hoogervorst, M. Reif, et al. "Immunomodulatory Effects of Orally Administered Cannabinoids in Multiple Sclerosis." *Journal of Neuroimmunology* 137 (2003): 140–43.

King, R. S., and M. Mauer. "The War on Marijuana: The Transformation of the War on Drugs in the 1990s." Washington, D.C.: The Sentencing Project, 2005. www.sentencingproject.org/doc/publications/dp_waronmarijuana.pdf. Accessed April 29, 2010.

Kirk, J. M., and H. de Wit. "Responses to Oral Delta9-tetrahydrocannabinol in Frequent and Infrequent Marijuana Users." *Pharmacology Biochemistry and Behavior* 63 (1999): 137–42.

Klein, T. W., C. Newton, and H. Friedman. "Cannabinoid Receptors and Immunity." *Immunology Today* 19 (1998): 373–81.

Kogan, N. M. "Cannabinoids and Cancer." *Mini Reviews in Medicinal Chemistry* 5 (2005): 941–52.

Kofalvi, A., ed. *Cannabinoids and the Brain*. Boston, MA: Springer, 2008.

Korte, F., M. Haag, and U. Claussen. "Tetrahydrocannabinolcarboxylic Acid, a Component of Hashish." *Angewandte Chemie International Edition* 4 (1965): 872.

Kosel, B. W., F. T. Aweeka, N. L. Benowitz, et al. "The Effects of Cannabinoids on the

Pharmacokinetics of Indinavir and Nelfinavir." *AIDS* 16 (2002): 543–50.

Kosersky, D. S., W. L. Dewey, and L. Harris. "Anitpyretic Analgesic and Anti-inflammatory Effects of Delta 9-tetrahydrocannabinol in the Rat." *European Journal of Pharmacology* 24 (1973): 1–7.

Kosier, D. A., K. J. Filipiak, P. Stolarz, et al. "Paroxysmal Atrial Fibrillation Following Marijuana Intoxication: A Two-case Report of Possible Association." *International Journal of Cardiology* 78 (2001): 183–84.

Kouri, E. M., and H. G. Pope. "Abstinence Symptoms during Withdrawal from Chronic Marijuana Use." *Experimental and Clinical Psychopharmacology* 8 (2000): 483–92.

Kouri, E. M., H. G. Pope, and S. E. Lukas. "Changes in Aggressive Behavior during Withdrawal from Long-term Marijuana Use." *Psychopharmacology* 143 (1999): 302–8.

Kreitzer, A. C., and R. C. Malenka. "Endocannabinoid-mediated Rescue of Striatal LTD and Motor Deficits in Parkinson's Disease Models." *Nature* 445 (2007): 643–47.

Krejčí, Z., and F. Šantavý. "Isolace dalšíchch látek z listí indického konopí Cannabis sativa L." *Acta Universitatis Palackianae Olomucensis* 6 (1995): 59–66.

Krivickas, L. S., and G. T. Carter. "Motor Neuron Disease." In J. A. DeLisa, B. M. Gans, and N. E. Walsh, eds. *Physical Medicine and Rehabilitation: Principles and Practice,* 4th ed. Philadelphia: Lippincott, Williams and Wilkins, 2005.

Lane, S. D., D. R. Cherek, O. V. Tcheremissine, et al. "Acute Marijuana Effects on Human Risk Taking." *Neuropsychopharmacology* 30 (2005): 800–809.

Larue, F., A. Fontaine, and S. M. Colleau. "Underestimation and Undertreatment of Pain in HIV Disease: Multicentre Study." *British Medical Journal* 314 (1997): 23–28.

Laumon, B., B. Gadegbeku, J.-L. Martin, et al. "Cannabis Intoxication and Fatal Road Crashes in France: Population Based Case-control Study." *British Medical Journal* 331 (2005): 1371–77.

Lebovits, A. H., M. Lefkowitz, D. McCarthy, et al. "The Prevalence and Management of Pain in Patients with AIDS: A Review of 134 Cases." *Clinical Journal of Pain* 5 (1989): 245–48.

LeDoux, J. *Synaptic Self: How Our Brains Become Who We Are.* New York: Penguin, 2002.

Lehtonen, M., M. Storvik, E. Tupala, et al. "Endogenous Cannabinoids in Post-mortem Brains of Cloninger Type 1 and 2 Alcoholics." *European Neuropsychopharmacology* 20 (2010): 245–52.

Lessem, J. M., C. J. Hopfer, B. C. Haberstick, et al. "Relationship between Adolescent Marijuana Use and Young Adult Illicit Drug Use." *Behavioral Genetics* 36 (2006): 498–506.

Levy, S., S. Van Hook, and J. Knight. "A Review of Internet-based Home Drug-testing Products for Parents." *Pediatrics* 113 (2004): 720–26.

Lewis, H. E. "Cannabis Indica: A Study of its Physiologic Action, Toxic Effects, and Therapeutic Indications." *Merck's Archives of Materia Medica and Its Uses* 2 (1900): 247–51.

Liang, C., M. D. McClean, C. Marsit, et al. "A Population-based Case-control Study of Marijuana Use and Head and Neck Squamous Cell Carcinoma." *Cancer Prevention Research* 2 (2009): 759.

Lichtman, A. H., S. A. Cook, and B. R. Martin. "Investigation of Brain Sites Mediating Cannabinioid-induced Antinociception in Rats: Evidence Supporting Periaquaductal Gray Involvement." *Journal of Pharmacology and Experiemntal Therapeutics* 276 (1996): 585–93.

Ligresti, A., A. S. Moriello, K. Starowicz, et al."Anti-tumor Activity of Plant Cannabinoids with Emphasis on the Effect of Cannabidiol on Human Breast Carcinoma." *Journal of Pharmacology and Experimental Therapeutics* (May 25, 2006): http://jpet.aspetjournals.org/content/318/3/1375.abstract. Accessed May 6, 2010.

Liguori, A. "Marijuana and Driving: Trends, Design Issues, and Future Recommendations." In Mitch Earleywine, ed. *Pot Politics: Marijuana and the Costs of Prohibition*. New York: Oxford University Press, 2007.

Lindstrom, P., U. Lindbolm, and L. Boreus. "Lack of Effect of Cannabinoid in Sustained Neuropathia." *Marihuana International Conference, Melboourne* (1987).

Llewellyn, C. D., K. Linklater, J. Bell, et al. "An Analysis of Risk Factors for Oral Cancer in Young People: A Case-control Study." *Oral Oncology* 40 (2004): 304–13.

Løberg, E., and K. Hugdahl. "Cannabis Use and Cognition in Schizophrenia." *Frontiers in Human Neuroscience* 3 (2009): 53.

Looby, A., M. Earleywine, and D. Gieringer. 2007. "Roadside Sobriety Tests and Attitudes toward a Regulated Cannabis Market." *Harm Reduction Journal* (2007): www.harmreductionjournal.com/content/4/1/4/abstract. Accessed November 24, 2007.

Lopez, H. H., S. M. Goldman, I. I. Liberman, et al. "Cannabis: Accidental Peroral Intoxication." *Journal of the American Medical Association* 227 (1974): 1041–42.

Los Angeles Daily News. "Federal Intervention: It's L.A.'s Business to Regulate Medical Pot, Not Feds.'" July 27, 2007.

Lu, D., V. K. Vemuri, R. I. Duclos, et al. "The Cannabinergic System as a Target for Anti-inflammatory Diseases." *Journal of Neuroimmunology* 166 (2006): 3–18.

Lucas, P. "Regulating Compassion: An Overview of Canada's Federal Medical Cannabis Policy and Practice." *Harm Reduction Journal* 5 (2008): 5.

Lucas, P., H. Black, and R. Capler. "Roadmap to Compassion: The Implementation of a Working Medicinal Cannabis Program in Canada" (2004): CSA, VICS, BCCCS joint publication.

Lundberg, F. *The Rich and the Super-rich*. New York: Bantam, 1968.

Lundqvist, T. "Cognitive Consequences of Cannabis Use: Comparison with Abuse of Stimulants and Heroin with Regard to Attention, Memory and Executive Functions." *Pharmacology, Biochemistry, and Behavior* 81 (2005): 319–30.

Lyman, W. D., J. R. Sonett, C. F. Brosnan, et al. "Delta-9 tetrahydrocannabinol: A Novel Treatment for Experimental Autoimmune Encephalomyelitis." *Journal of Neuroimmunology* 23 (1989): 73–81.

Lynch, M. E., J. Young, and A. J. Clark. "A Case Series of Patients Using Medicinal Marihuana for Management of Chronic Pain under the Canadian Marihuana Medical Access Regulations." *Journal of Pain and Symptom Management* 32 (2006): 497–501.

Lynskey, M. T., A. C. Heath, K. K. Bucholz, et al. "Escalation of Drug Use in Early-onset Cannabis Users vs Co-twin Controls." *Journal of the American Medical Association* 289 (2003): 427–33.

Maccarrone, M. "Endocannabinoids: Friends and Foes of Reproduction." *Progress in Lipid Research* 48 (2009): 344–54.

MacCoun, R., and P. Reuter. "Interpreting Dutch Cannabis Policy: Reasoning by Analogy in the Legalization Debate." *Science* 278 (1997): 47–52.

———. "Evaluating Alternative Cannabis Regimes." *British Journal of Psychiatry* 178 (2001): 123–28.

MacFarlane, B. A. *Drug Offences in Canada,* 2nd ed. Aurora, ON: Law Book Inc., 1986.

Mach, F., and S. Steffens. "The Role of the Endocannabinoid System in Atherosclerosis." *Journal of Neuroendocrinology* 20, suppl. 1 (2008): 53–57.

Mackenzie King, W. L. *The Need for the Suppression of the Opium Traffic in Canada.* Ottawa, ON: S.E. Dawson, 1908.

Mackesy-Amiti, M. E., M. Fendrich, and P. J. Goldstein. "Sequence of Drug Use among Serious Drug Users: Typical vs Atypical Progression." *Drug and Alcohol Dependence* 45 (1997): 185–96.

Mackie, K., and I. Katona. "Get Stoned in GABAergic Synapses." *Nature Neuroscience* 12 (2009): 1081–83.

Mahler, S. V., K. S. Smith, and K. C. Berridge. "Endocannabinoid Hedonic Hotspot for Sensory Pleasure: Anandamide in Nucleus Accumbens Shell Enhances 'Liking' of a Sweet Reward." *Neuropsychopharmacology* 32, no. 11 (November 2007): 2267–78.

Malcher-Lopes, R., S. Di, V. S. Marcheselli, et al. "Opposing Crosstalk between Leptin and Glucocorticoids Rapidly Modulates Synaptic Excitation via Endocannabinoid Release." *Journal of Neuroscience* 26 (2006): 6643–50.

Mangieri, R.A., and D. Piomelli. "Enhancement of Endocannabinoid Signaling and the Pharmacotherapy of Depression." *Pharmacological Research* 56 (2007): 360–66.

Mann, R. *Grass: The Paged Experience.* New York: Autonomedia, 2001.

Mannich, L. *An Ancient Egyptian Herbal.* Austin: University of Texas Press, 1989.

Manski C. F., J. V. Pepper, and C. V. Petrie. *Informing America's Policy on Illegal Drugs: What We Don't Know Keeps Hurting Us.* Washington, D.C.: National Academies Press, 2001.

Marchalant, Y., F. Cerbai, H. M. Brothers, et al. "Cannabinoid Receptor Stimulation Is Anti-inflammatory and Improves Memory in Old Rats." *Neurobiology of Aging* 29 (2008): 1894–901.

Marchalant, Y., S. Rosi, and G. L. Wenk. "Anti-inflammatory Property of the Cannabinoid Agonist WIN-55212-2 in a Rodent Model of Chronic Brain Inflammation." *Neuroscience* 144 (2007): 1516–22.

Marez, C. *Drug Wars: The Political Economy of Narcotics.* Minneapolis: Minneapolis University Press, 2004.

Marijuana Policy Project. "Marijuana Use by Young People: The Impact of State Medical Marijuana Laws" (2008): http://mpp.org/assets/pdfs/general/ TeenUseReport_0608.pdf. Accessed April 27, 2010.

Marijuana Policy Review Panel. "Final Report of the Marijuana Policy Review Panel on the Implementation of Initiative 75." December 4, 2007. http://clerk.ci.seattle .wa.us/~cfpdfs/309070.pdf. Accessed April 29, 2010.

Marijuana Treatment Project Research Group. "Brief Treatments for Cannabis Dependence: Findings from a Randomized Multisite Trial." *Journal of Consulting and Clinical Psychology* 72 (2004): 455–66.

Marquéz L., J. Súarez, M. Inglesias, et al. "Ulcerative Colitis Induces Changes on the Expression of the Endocannabinoid System inb the Human Colonic Tissue." *PLoS One* 4, e6893 (2009).

Marrs, J. *Rule by Secrecy.* New York: Perennial, 2000.

Marshall, C. R. "The Active Principle of Indian Hemp: A Preliminary Communication." *Lancet* 1 (1897): 235–38.

Marsicano, G., S. Goodenough, K. Monory, et al. "CB1 Cannabinoid Receptors and On-demand Defense against Excitotoxicity." *Science* 302 (2003): 84–88.

Marsicano, G., C. T. Wotjak, S. C. Azad, et al. "The Endogenous Cannabinoid System Controls Extinction of Aversive Memories." *Nature* 418 (2002): 530–34.

Martin, C. E., D. F. Duncan, and E. M. Zunich. "Students' Motives for Discontinuing Illicit Drug Taking." *Health Values: Achieving High Level Wellness* 7 (1983): 8–11.

Martin, M. S. *Ethnobotanical Aspects of Cannabis in Southeast Asia, in Cannabis and Culture.* Edited by V. Rubin. Paris: Mouton Publishers, 1975.

Martin, M., C. Ledent, M. Oarmentier, et al. "Involvement of CB1 Cannabinoid Receptors in Emotional Behavior." *Psychopharmacology* 159 (2002): 379–87.

Martin, W. J., S. Patrick, P. O. Coffin, et al. "An Examination of the Central Sites of Action of Cannabinoid-induced Antinociception in the Rat." *Life Sciences* 56 (1995): 2103–9.

Martlatt, A. *Harm Reduction: Pragmatic Strategies for Managing High Risk Behaviors.* New York: Guilford, 2002.

Matthias, P., D. P. Tashkin, J. A. Marques-Magallanes, et al. "Effects of Varying Marijuana Potency on Deposition of Tar and Delta9-THC in the Lung During Smoking." *Pharmacology, Biochemistry and Behavior* 58 (1997): 1145–50.

Mattison, J. B. "Cannabis indica as an Anodyne and Hypnotic." *St. Louis Medical and Surgical Journal* 61 (1891): 265–71.

Mayor's Committee on Marijuana. *The Marijuana Problem in the City of New York: Sociological, Medical and Psychological Studies.* Lancaster, PA: Jacques Cattell Press, 1944.

McCormack, J. P., R. Li, D. Zarowny. "Inadequate Treatment of Pain in Ambulatory HIV Patients." *Clinical Journal of Pain* 9 (1993): 279–83.

McGee, R., S. Williams,, R. Poulton, et al. "A Longitudinal Study of Cannabis Use and Mental Health from Adolescence to Early Adulthood." *Addiction* 95 (2000): 491–503.

McGuigan, M. "Cannabinoids." In N. E. Flomenbaum, L. R. Goldfrank, R. S. Hoffman, et al., eds. *Goldfrank's Toxicological Emergencies,* 8th ed. New York: McGraw Hill, 2006.

McHale, S., and N. Hunt. "Executive Function Deficits in Short-term Abstinent Cannabis Users." *Human Psychopharmacology* 23 (2008): 409–15.

McLaren, J. A., E. Silins, D. Hutchinson, et al. 2009. "Assessing Evidence for a Causal Link between Cannabis and Psychosis: A Review of Cohort Studies." *The International Journal on Drug Policy* (2010): 10–19.

McLeod, A. L., C. J. McKenna, and D. B. Northridge. "Myocardial Infarction Following the Combined Recreational Use of Viagra and Cannabis." *Clinical Cardiology* 25 (2002): 133–34.

McMeens, R. R. *Report on the Ohio State Medical Commission on Cannabis indica.* Sulphur Springs, OH: Ohio State Medical Society, 1860.

McMillan, D. E., L. S. Harris, J. M. Frankenheim, et al. "Delta-9-trans-tetrahydrocannabinol in Pigeons: Tolerance to the Behavioral Effects." *Science* 169 (1970): 501–503.

McPartland, J. M., I. Matias, V. Di Marzo, et al. "Evolutionary Origins of the Endocannabinoid System." *Gene* 370 (2006): 64–74.

McRae, A. L., A. J. Budney, and K. T. Brady. "Treatment of Marijuana Dependence: A Review of the Literature." *Journal of Substance Abuse Treatment* 24 (2003): 369–76.

Mead, G. R. S. 1900. *Fragments of a Faith Forgotten: Some Short Sketches Among the Gnostics of the First Two Centuries.* London: Theosophical Publishing Society, 1900.

Mechoulam, R. "Marihuana Chemistry: Review." *Science* 168 (1970): 1159–66.

———, ed. "Marijuana: Chemistry, Metabolism, Pharmacology and Clinical Effects." In *Cannabinoid Chemistry.* New York: Academic Press, 1973.

———, ed. "The Pharmacohistory of *Cannabis sativa.*" In *Cannabinoids as Therapeutic Agents* (monograph). Boca Raton, FL: CRC Press, 1986.

Mechoulam, R., and I. Bab. "An Endogenous Lipid with Novel Bone Anabolic Activity In Vivo." *Proceedings of the 18th International Cannabinoid Research Society,* June 25–29, 2008.

Mechoulam, R., S. Ben-Shabat, L. Hanuš, et al. "Identification of an Endogenous 2-monoglyceride, Present in Canine Gut, that Binds to Cannabinoid Receptors." *Biochemical Pharmacology* 50 (1995): 83-90.

Mechoulam, R., P. Braun, and Y. Gaoni. "A Stereospecific Synthesis of (-)-Delta-1- and (-)-Delta-6-tetrahydrocannabinols." *Journal of the American Chemical Society* 89 (1967): 4552–54.

Mechoulam, R., and Y. Gaoni. "The Isolation and Structure of Cannabinolic, Cannabidiolic and Cannabigerolic Acids." *Tetrahedron* 21 (1965): 1223–29.

Mechoulam, R., and L. Hanuš. "Cannabidiol: An Overview of Some Chemical and Pharmacological Aspects. Part I: Chemical Aspects." *Chemistry and Physics of Lipids* 121 (2002): 35–43.

Mechoulam, R., and A. H. Lichtman. "Neuroscience: Stout Guards of the Central Nervous System." *Science* 302 (2003): 65–67.

Mechoulam, R., L. A. Parker, and R. Gallily. "Cannabidiol: An Overview of Some Pharmacological Aspects." *Journal of Clinical Pharmacology* 42, suppl. 11 (2002): 11S–19S.

Mechoulam, R., M. Peters, E. Murillo-Rodriguez, et al. "Cannabidiol: Recent Advances." *Chemistry and Biodiversity* 4 (2007): 1678–92.

Mechoulam, R., A. Shani, H. Edery, et al. "Chemical Basis of Hashish Activity." *Science* 169, no. 945 (1970): 611–12.

Mechoulam, R., and E. Shohami E. "HU-211: A Cannabinoid Neuroprotective Agent." In F. Grotenhermen and E. Russo, eds., *Cannabis and Cannabinoids: Pharmacology, Toxicology, and Therapeutic Potential.* New York: Haworth Integrative Healing Press, 2006.

Mechoulam, R., and Y. Shvo. "The Structure of Cannabidiol." *Tetrahedron* 19 (1963): 2073–78.

Medical Marihuana Access Regulations. *Canada Gazette*, part 2, vol. 135, no. 14, July 4, 2001. SOR/2001–227.

"Medical Marijuana in California, 1996–2006. *O'Shaughnessy's: The Journal of Cannabis in Clinical Practice.* (Winter/Spring, 2007): 5.

Mehra, R., B. A. Moore, K Crothers, et al. "The Association between Marijuana Smoking and Lung Cancer: A Systematic Review." *Archives of Internal Medicine* 166 (2006): 1359–67.

Meinck, H. M., P. W. Schonle, and B. Conrad. "Effects of Cannabinoids on Spasticity and Ataxia in Multiple Sclerosis." *Journal of Neurology* 263 (1989): 120–22.

Meissner, Bruno. *Wissenschaft und Bildung: Die Kultur Babyloniens und Assyriens.* Leipzig: Quelle and Meyer, 1925.

Melamede, R. "Cannabis and Tobacco Smoke Are Not Equally Carcinogenic." *Harm Reduction Journal* 2 (2005): 21. www.harmreductionjournal.com/content/2/1/21. Accessed April 29, 2010.

Melges, F. T., J. R. Tinklenberg, L. E. Hollister, et al. "Marihuana and Temporal Disintegration." *Science*, 168 (1970): 1118–20.

Melis, M., G. Pillolla, T. Bisogno, et al. "Protective Activation of the Endocannabinoid System during Ischemia in Dopamine Neurons." *Neurobiology of Disease* 24 (2006):15–27.

Mendoza, M. "US Drug War Has Met None of Its Goals." Associated Press, May 13, 2010.

Menetrey, A., M. Augsburger, B. Favrat, et al. "Assessment of Driving Capability through the Use of Clinical and Psychomotor Tests in Relation to Blood Cannabinoid Levels following Oral Administration of 20 mg Dronabinol or of a Cannabis Decoction Made with 20 and 60 mg Delta-9-THC." *Journal of Analytical Toxicology* 29 (2005): 327–38.

Meyer, R. E., R. C. Pillard, L. M. Shapiro, et al. "Administration of Marijuana to Heavy and Casual Marijuana Users." *The American Journal of Psychiatry* 128 (1971): 198–204.

Mikuriya, T. H. "Cannabis Substitution: An Adjunctive Therapeutic Tool in the Treatment of Alcoholism." *Med Times* 98 (1970): 187–91.

Miller, L. L., and T. L. Cornett. "Marijuana: Dose Effects on Pulse Rate, Subjective Estimates of Intoxication, Free recall, and Recognition Memory." *Pharmacology, Biochemistry, and Behavior* 9 (1978): 573–77.

Milman, G., Y. Maor, Y., S. Abu-Lafi, et al. "N-arachidonoyl L-serine, an Endocannabinoid-like Brain Constituent with Vasodilatory Properties." *Proceedings of the National Academy of Sciences* 103 (2006): 2428–33.

Milstein, S. L., K. MacCannell, G. Karr, et al. "Marijuana-produced Impairments in Coordination: Experienced and Nonexperienced Subjects." *Journal of Nervous and Mental Disease* 161 (1975): 26–31.

Miron, J. A. "Budgetary Implications of Marijuana Prohibition in the United States" (June 2005): www.prohibitioncosts.org/mironreport.html. Accessed April 29, 2010.

———. "The Budgetary Implications of Marijuana Prohibition." In M. Earleywine, ed., *New Directions in Marijuana Policy*. New York: Oxford University Press, 2006.

Mishima, K., K. Hayakawa, T. Abe, et al. "Cannabidiol Prevents Cerebral Infarction via a Serotonergic 5-hydroxytryptamine1a Receptor–dependent Mechanism." *Stroke* 36 (2005): 1071.

Mittal, M. K., T. Florin, J. Perrone, et al. "Toxicity from the Use of Niacin to Beat Urine Drug Screening." *Annals of Emergency Medicine* 50 (2007): 587–90.

Mittleman, M. A., R. A. Lewis, M. Maclure, et al. "Triggering Myocardial Infarction by Marijuana." *Circulation* 103 (2001): 2805–809.

Molina-Holgado, F., A. Lledo, and C. Guaza. "Anandamide Suppresses Nitric Oxide and TNF-alpha Responses to Theiler's Virus or Endotoxin in Astrocytes." *Neuroreport* 8 (1997): 1929–33.

Monory, K., F. Massa, M. Egertova, et al. "The Endocannabinoid System Controls Key Epileptogenic Circuits in the Hippocampus." *Neuron* 51 (2006): 455–66.

Moore, T. H., S. Zammit, A. Lingford-Hughes, et al. "Cannabis Use and Risk of Psychotic or Affective Mental Health Outcomes: A Systematic Review." *Lancet* 370 (2007): 319–28.

Moote, N. "Pot Activist Rejects Health Canada Drug." *Coast Reporter,* September 20, 2003: www.medicalmarihuana.ca/govtpot.html. Accessed December 22, 2007.

Moreau, J. J. *Du hachisch et de l'alienation mentale: Etudes psychologiques.* Paris: Fortin Masson, 1845.

Moreira, F. A., B. Lutz. "The Endocannabinoid System: Emotion, Learning, and Addiction." *Addiction Biology* 13 (2008): 196–212.

Morgan, D. R., ed. "Therapeutic Uses of Cannabis." British Medical Association. Harwood Academic, 1997.

Morley, A. *Vancouver: From Milltown to Metropolis.* Vancouver, British Columbia: Mitchell Press, 1961.

Morley-Forster, P. "Prevalence of Neuropathic Pain and the Need for Treatment." *Pain Research and Management* 11, suppl. A (2006): 5A–10A.

Morral, A. R., D. F. McCaffrey, and S. M. Paddock. "Reassessing the Marijuana Gateway Effect." *Addiction* 97 (2002): 1493–1504.

Mortensen, P. B., C. B. Pedersen, T. Westergaard, et al. "Effects of Family History and Place and Season of Birth on the Risk of Schizophrenia." *New England Journal of Medicine* 340 (1999): 603–608.

Moshman, D. *Adolescent Psychological Development: Rationality, Morality and Identity.* Mahwah, NJ: Lawrence Erlbaum, 1999.

Moussouttas, M. "Cannabis Use and Cerebrovascular Disease." *Neurologist* 10 (2004): 47–53.

Movig, K. L. L., M. P. M. Mathijssen, P. H. A. Nagel, et al. "Psychoactive Substance Use and the Risk of Motor Vehicle Accidents." *Accident Analysis and Prevention* 36 (2004): 631–36.

Müller-Vahl, K. R. "Cannabinoids Reduce Symptoms of Tourette's Syndrome." *Expert Opinions in Pharmacotherapy* 4 (2003a): 1717–25.

Müller-Vahl, et al. "Treatment of Tourette's syndrome with Delta-9-tetrahydrocannabinol. *American Journal of Psychiatry,* 1999; 156:495.

Müller-Vahl, K. R., A. Koblenz, M. Jöbges, et al. "Influence of Treatment of Tourette Syndrome with Delta9-tetrahydrocannabinol (Delta9-THC) on Neuropsychological Performance." *Pharmacopsychiatry* 34 (2001): 19–24.

Müller-Vahl, H. Prevedel, K. Theloe, et al. "Treatment of Tourette Syndrome with Delta-9-tetrahydrocannabinol (Delta 9-THC): No Influence on Neuropsychological Performance." *Neuropsychopharmacology* 28 (2003c): 384–88.

Müller-Vahl, K. R., U. Schneider, A. Koblenz, et al. "Treatment of Tourette's syndrome with Delta-9-tetrahydrocannabinol (THC): A Randomized Crossover Trial." *Pharmacopsychiatry* 35 (2002): 57–61.

Müller-Vahl, K. R., U. Schneider, H. Prevedel, et al. "Delta 9-tetrahydrocannabinol (THC) Is Effective in the Treatment of Tics in Tourette Syndrome: A 6-week Randomized Trial." *Journal of Clinical Psychiatry* 64 (2003b): 459–65.

Munro, S., K. L. Thomas, and M. Abu-Shaar. "Molecular Characterization of a Peripheral Receptor for Cannabinoids." *Nature* 365, no. 6441 (1993): 61–65.

Murray, J. B. "Marijuana's Effects on Human Cognitive Functions, Psychomotor Functions, and Personality." *Journal of General Psychology* 113 (1985): 23–55.

Murray, R. M., P. D. Morrison, C. Henquet, et al. "Cannabis, the Mind and Society: The Hash Realities." *Nature Reviews, Neuroscience* 8 (2007): 885–95.

Mushoff, F., and B. Madea. "Review of Biologic Matrices (Urine, Blood, Hair) as Indicators of Recent or Ongoing Cannabis Use." *Therapeutic Drug Monitor* 2 (2006): 155–63.

Musty, R. E. "Possible Anxiolytic Effects of Cannabidiol." In S. Agurell, W. L. Dewey, and R. E. Willette, eds. *The Cannabinoids: Chemical, Pharmacologic and Therapeutic Aspects.* New York: Academic Press, 1984.

Nagayama, T., A. D. Sinor, R. P. Simon, et al. "Cannabinoids and Neuroprotection in Global and Focal Cerebral Ischemia and in Neuronal Cultures." *Journal of Neuroscience* 19 (1999): 2987–95.

Naef, M., M. Curatolo, S. Petersen-Felix, et al. "The Analgesic Effect of Oral Delta-9-tetrahydrocannabinol (THC), Morphine, and a THC-morphine Combination in Healthy Subjects under Experimental Pain Conditions." *Pain* 105 (2003): 79–88.

National Archive of Criminal Justice Date. FBI Uniform Crime Reporting Resource Guide, 1965–2006. www.icpsr.umich.edu/NACJD/ucr.html. Accessed April 29, 2010.

National Drug Intelligence Center. Marijuana, National Drug Threat Assessment (2007): www.usdoj.gov/ndic/pubs21/21137/marijuana.htm.

National Highway Traffic Safety Administration. Young Drivers, Traffic Safety Facts. DOT HS 810 630 (2005).

National Institute on Drug Abuse (NIDA). Research Report Series: "Marijuana Abuse." NIH Publication no. 05-3859. July 2005.

———. "Marijuana Facts for Teens" (2007): www.mentalhealth.com/book/p45-mari.html. Accessed December 12, 2007.

National Organization for the Reform of Marijuana Laws (NORML). "Principles of Responsible Use" (1996): www.norml.org/index.cfm?Group_ID=3417.

Nelson, R. A. *Hemp and History.* Jean, NV: RexResearch, 1996. [Original manuscript for R. Robinson, ed. *The Great Book of Hemp.* Rochester, VT: Inner Traditions, 1996.] Chapter 1, The early history of hemp; chapter 2, Hemp in America: www.rexresearch.com/hhist/hhicon%7E1.htm. Accessed December 5, 2007.

———. *Hemp and Health.* Jean, NV: RexResearch, 1999. Sections 1–14: www.rexresearch.com/hhusb/hmphlth.htm. Accessed November 27, 2007.

Newcomb, M. D., and P. M. Bentler. *Consequences of Adolescent Drug Use: Impact on the Lives of Young Adults.* Newbury Park, CA: Sage, 1988.

Nicholson, T. "The Primary Prevention of Illicit Drug Problems: An Argument for Decriminalization and Legalization." *Journal of Primary Prevention* 12 (1992): 275–88.

Nicoll, R. A., and B. E. Alger. "The Brain's Own Marijuana." *Scientific American,* December 24, 2004, 69–75.

Nordstrom, B. R., and C. L. Hart. "Assessing Cognitive Fucntioning in Cannabis Users: Cannabis Use History an Important Consideration." *Neuropsychopharmacology* 31 (2006): 2798–99.

Notcutt, W., M. Price, R. Miller, et al. "Initial Experiences with Medicinal Extracts of Cannabis for Chronic Pain: Results from 34 'N of 1' Studies." *Anaesthesia* 59 (2004): 440–52.

Nowlan, R., and S. Cohen. "Tolerance to Marijuana: Heart Rate and Subjective 'High.'" *Clinical Pharmacology and Therapeutics* 22 (1977): 550–56.

Noyes, Jr., R., and D. A. Baram. "Cannabis Analgesia." *Comprehensive Psychiatry* 15 (1974): 531–35.

Noyes, Jr., R., S. F. Brunk, D. A. Avery, et al. "The Analgesic Properties of Delta-9-tetrahydrocannabinol and Codeine." *Clinical Pharmacology and Therapeutics* 18 (1975a): 84–89.

Noyes, Jr., R., S. F. Brunk, D. A. Baram, et al. "Analgesic Effect of Delta-9-tetrahydrocannabinol." *Journal of Clinical Pharmacology* 15 (1975b): 139–43.

Nutt, D., L. A. King, W. Saulsbury, et al. "Development of a Rational Scale to Assess the Harm of Drugs of Potential Misuse." *Lancet* 369 (2007): 1047–53.

Office of Applied Studies. Substance Abuse and Mental Health Services Administration. "Treatment Referral Sources for Adolescent Marijuana Users." *The DASIS Report* (March 29, 2002): www.oas.samhsa.gov/2k2/YouthMJtx/YouthMJtx.htm. Accessed May 7, 2010.

———. Substance Abuse and Mental Health Services Administration. "Differences in Marijuana Admissions Based on Source of Referral: 2002." *The DASIS Report* (June 24, 2005): http://oas.samhsa.gov/2k5/MJreferrals/MJreferrals.htm. Accessed May 7, 2010.

———. Substance Abuse and Mental Health Services Administration. "Results from the 2008 National Survey on Drug Use and Health: National Findings." NSDUH Series H-36, HHS Publication No. SMA 09-4434 (2009): www.oas.samhsa.gov/nsduh/2k8nsduh/2k8Results.pdf. Accessed May 7, 2010.

Okie, S. "Medical Marijuana and the Supreme Court. *New England Journal of Medicine* 353 (2005): 648–51.

Oscapella, E. Quoted in Randy Boswell "Murphy Campaigned Against 'Marijuana Menace.'" *Edmonton Journal* (CN AB), March 5, 2004: www.mapinc.org/newstcl/v04/n392/a05.html. Accessed April 27, 2010.

O'Shaughnessy, W. B. "On the Preparation of the Indian Hemp or Ganjah (*Cannabis indica*): The Effects on the Animal System in Health, and their Utility in the Treatment of Tetanus and Other Convulsive Diseases." *Transactions of the Medical and Physical Society of Bombay* 8 (1842): 421–61.

———. "Emerging Clinical Applications of Cannabis." *O'Shaughnessy's: The Journal of Cannabis in Clinical Practice*. Winter/Spring 2007.

Oviedo, A., J. Glowa, and M. Herkenham. "Chronic Cannabinoid Administration Alters Cannabinoid Receptor Binding in Rat Brain: A Quantitative Autoradiographis Study." *Brain Research* 616 (1993): 293–302.

Pacher, P., S. Batkai, and G. Kunos. "The Endocannabinoid System as an Emerging Target of Pharmacotherapy." *Pharmacological Review* 58 (2006): 389–462.

Page, S. A., M. J. Verhoef, R. A. Stebbins, et al. "Cannabis Use as Described by People with Multiple Sclerosis." *Canadian Journal of Neurological Sciences* 30 (2003): 201–5.

Panacek, E. A., A. J. Singer, B. W. Sherman, et al. "Spontaneous Pneumomediastinum: Clinical and Natural History." *Annals of Emergency Medicine* 21 (1992): 1222–27.

Panikashvili, D., R. Mechoulam, S. M. Beni, et al. "CB1 Cannabinoid Receptors Are Involved in Neuroprotection via NF-κB Inhibition." *Journal of Cerebral Blood Flow and Metabolism* 25 (2005): 477–84.

Panikashvili, D., C. Simeonidou, S. Ben-Shabat, et al. "An Endogenous Cannabinoid (2-AG) Is Neuroprotective after Brain Injury." *Nature* 413 (2001): 527–31.

Papafotiou, K., J. D. Carter, and C. Stough. "An Evaluation of the Sensitivity of the Standardised Field Sobriety Tests (SFSTs) to Detect Impairment Due to Marijuana Intoxication." *Psychopharmacology* 180 (2005): 107–14.

Paton, W. D. M. "Pharmacology of Marijuana." *Annual Review of Pharmacology and Toxicology* 15 (1975): 191–220.

Payne, R. J., and S. N. Brand. "The Toxicity of Intravenously Used Marijuana." *Journal of the American Medical Association* 233 (1975): 351–54.

Peele, S. *Addiction Proof Your Child.* New York: Three River Press, 2007.

Pertwee, R. G. "Pharmacology of Cannabinoid CB1 and CB2 Receptors." *Pharmacology and Therapeutics* 74 (1997): 129–80.

———. "Cannabinoid Receptor Ligands: Clinical and Neuropharmacological Considerations, Relevant to Future Drug Discovery and Development." *Expert Opinion on Investigational Drugs* 9 (2000): 1553–71.

Peter D. Hart Associates. "The State of Our Nation's Youth: 2005–2006." Alexandria, VA: Horatio Alger Association of Distinguished Americans, 2005.

Petro, D. J. "Marijuana as a Therapeutic Agent for Muscle Spasm or Spasticity." *Psychosomatics* 21 (1980): 81–85.

Petro, D. J., and C. Ellenberger. "Treatment of Human Spasticity with Delta-9-tetrahydrocannabinol." *Journal of Clinical Pharmacology* 21 (1981): 413S–416S.

Pfeifer, G. P., M. F. Denissenko, M. Olivier, et al. "Tobacco Smoke Carcinogens, DNA Damage and p53 Mutations in Smoking-associated Cancers." *Oncogene* 21 (2002): 7435–51.

Phan, K. L., M. Angstadt, J. Golden, et al. "Cannabinoid Modulation of Amygdala Reactivity to Social Signals of Threat in Humans." *Journal of Neuroscience* 28 (2008): 2313–19.

Piomelli, D. "The Molecular Logic of Endocannabinoid Signalling." *Nature Reviews Neuroscience* 4 (2003): 873–84.

"Plants and Drugs: Cannabis": www.erowid.org. Accessed June 26, 2007.

Polen, M. R. "Health Care Use by Frequent Marijuana Smokers Who Do Not Smoke Tobacco." *Western Journal of Medicine* 158 (1993): 586–601.

Pope, H. G., A. J. Gruber, J. I. Hudson, et al. "Neuropsychological Performance in Long-term Cannabis Users." *Archives of General Psychiatry* 58 (2001): 909–15.

Pope, H. G., and D. Yurgelun-Todd. "The Residual Cognitive Effects of Heavy Marijuana Use in College Students." *Journal of the American Medical Association* 275 (1996): 521–27.

Potter, D. "Growth and Morphology of Medicinal *Cannabis*." In G .W. Guy, B. A.

Whittle, and P. J. Robson, eds. *The Medicinal Uses of Cannabis and Cannabinoids.* London: Pharmaceutical Press, 2004.

Pryce, G., Z. Ahmed, D. J. Hankey, et al. "Cannabinoids Inhibit Neurodegeneration in Models of Multiple Sclerosis." *Brain* 126 (2003): 2191–202.

Pryce, G., S. J. Jackson, and D. Baker. "Cannabinoids for the Control of Multiple Sclerosis." In A. Kofalvi, ed. *Cannabinoids and the Brain.* Boston, MA: Springer, 2008.

Puffenbarger, R. A., A. C. Boothe, et al. G. A. Cabral. "Cannabinoids Inhibit LPS-inducible Cytokine mRNA Expression in Rat Microglial Cells." *Glia* 29 (2000): 58–69.

Quadrel, M.J., B. Fischhoff, and W. Davis. "Adolescent (In)vulnerability." *American Psychologist* 48 (1993): 102–16.

Quebec Human Rights Commission. "The Medical Use of Marihuana and the Right to Equality." Commission des droits de la personne et des droits de la jeunesse Quebec (2009): Cat. 2.120–12.54.

Quimby, M. W. "Botany of *Cannabis sativa.*" *Archivos de investigación médica* 5, suppl. 1 (1974):127.

R. v. Beren and Swallow. 2009 BCSC 429 (CanLII)—2009-02-02. Supreme Court of British Columbia—British Columbia.

R. v. Lucas. 2002 (July 5), no. 113701C, Victoria Registry (B.C.P.C.).

R. v. Parker. 1997 (December 10), per Judge Sheppard, Toronto Registry (Ont. Prov. Div.).

R. v. Parker. 2000. O.J. no. 2787 (Ont. C.A.).

R. v. Richardson. 2000. (January 26), no. 33558, North Vancouver Registry (B.C.P.C.).

R. v. Wakeford. 1998. O.J. no. 3522 (Ont. Gen. Div.).

Raby, W. N., K. M. Carpenter, J. Rothenberg, et al. "Intermittent Marijuana Use Is Associated with Improved Retention in Naltrexone Treatment for Opiate-dependence." *American Journal on Addictions* 18 (2009): 301–308.

Raft, D., J. Gregg, J. Ghia, et al. "Effects of Intravenous Tetrahydrocannabinol on Experimental and Surgical Pain." *Clinical Pharmacology and Therapeutics* 21 (1977): 26–36.

Ramaekers, J. G., G. Berghaus, M. van Laar, et al. "Dose Related Risk of Motor Vehicle Crashes after Cannabis Use." *Drug and Alcohol Dependence* 73 (2004): 109–19.

Ramaekers, J. G., G. Kauert, E. L. Theunissen, et al. "Neurocognitive Performance during Acute THC Intoxication in Heavy and Occasional Cannabis Users." *Journal of Psychopharmacology* 23 (2009): 266–77.

Ramaekers, J. G., G. Kauert, P. van Ruitenbeek, et al. "High-potency Marijuana Impairs Executive Function and Inhibitory Motor Control." *Neuropsychopharmacology* 31 (2006): 2296–303.

Ramaekers, J. G., M. R. Moeller, P. van Ruitenbeek, et al. "Cognition and Motor Control as a Function of Delta-9-THC Concentration in Serum and Oral Fluid: Limits of Impairment." *Drug and Alcohol Dependence* 85 (2006): 114–22.

Raman, A. "The *Cannabis* Plant: Botany, Cultivation, and Processing for Use." In D. T. Brown, ed. *Cannabis: The Genus Cannabis*. Amsterdam: Harwood Academic Publishers, 1998.

Raman, C., S. D. McAllister, G. Rizvi, et al. "Amyotrophic Lateral Sclerosis: Delayed Disease Progression in Mice by Treatment with a Cannabinoid." *Amyotrophic Lateral Sclerosis and Other Motor Neuron Disorders* 5 (2004): 33–39.

Ramirez, B. G., C. Blázquez, T. Gómez del Pulgar, et al. "Prevention of Alzheimer's Disease Pathology by Cannabinoids." *Journal of Neuroscience* 25 (2005): 1904–13.

Ranalli, P., ed. *Advances in Hemp Research*. Binghamton, NY: Haworth Press, 1999.

RAND Corporation. "RAND Study Casts Doubt on Claims that Marijuana Acts as a 'Gateway' to the Use of Cocaine and Heroin" (December 2, 2002): www.rand.org/news/press.02/gateway.html. Accessed May 7, 2010.

Rätsch, C. *Marijuana Medicine*. Rochester, VT: Healing Arts Press, 2001.

Recht, L. D., R. Salmonsen, R. Rosetti, et al. "Antitumor Effects of Ajulemic Acid (CT3), a Synthetic Non-psychoactive Cannabinoid." *Biochemical Pharmacology* 15 (2001): 755–63.

Regelson, W., J. R. Butler, J. Schulz, et al. "Delta 9-Tetrahydrocannabinol as an Effective Antidepressant and Appetite-stimulating Agent in Advanced Cancer Patients." In M. C. Braude and S. Szara, eds., *Pharmacology of Marihuana*, vol. 2. New York, Raven Press, 1976.

Reggio, P., ed. *The Cannabinoid Receptors*. New York: Humana Press, 2009.

Regulations Amending the Marihuana Medical Access Regulations (MMAR). *Canada Gazette,* part 2, July 4, 2001. SOR/2001–227.

———. *Canada Gazette,* part 2, vol. 137, no. 26, December 17, 2003. SOR/2003–387.

———. *Canada Gazette,* part 2, vol. 139, no. 12, June 29, 2005. SOR/2005–177.

———. *Canada Gazette,* part 2, vol. 143, no. 11, May 27, 2009. SOR/2009–142.

Regulatory Impact Analysis Statement. *Canada Gazette,* part 1, vol. 135, no. 14, April 7, 2001.

———. *Canada Gazette,* part 1, vol. 138, no. 43, October 23, 2004.

Reid, R. D., B. Quinlan, D. L. Riley, et al. "Smoking Cessation: Lessons Learned from Clinical Trial Evidence." *Current Opinion in Cardiology* 22 (2007): 280–85.

Reiman, A. "Self-efficacy, Social Support and Service Integration at Medical Cannabis Facilities in the San Francisco Bay Area of California." *Health and Social Care in the Community* 16 (2008): 31–41.

Reinarman, C. Personal communication, October 2006.

Reinarman, C., P. D. Cohen, and H. L. Kaal. "The Limited Relevance of Drug Policy: Cannabis in Amsterdam and in San Francisco." *American Journal of Public Health* 94 (2004): 836–42.

Reisine, T., and M. J. Brownstein. "Opioid and Cannabinoid Receptors." *Current Opinion in Neurobiology* 4 (1994): 406–12.

Reynolds, C. R. "Are Zero Tolerance Policies Effective in the Schools? An Evidentiary Review and Recommendations." A Report to the American Psychological Association Zero Tolerance Task Force (2006). American Psychological Association: www.apa .org/pubs/info/reports/zero-tolerance.pdf. Accessed May 7, 2010.

Reynolds, J. R. "On Some of the Therapeutic Uses of Indian Hemp." *Archives of Medicine* 2 (1868): 154–60.

———. "Therapeutical Uses and Toxic Effects of Cannabis indica." *Lancet* 1 (1890): 637–38.

Richardson, J., S. Kilo, and K. M. Hargreaves. "Cannabinoids Reduce Hyperalgesia and Inflammation via Interaction with Peripheral CB1 Receptors." *Pain* 75 (1998): 111–19.

Richardson, L. "Dishing Out Dinner as the Anti-drug." *Los Angeles Times*, September 26, 2006.

Richman J. "House Nixes Medical Pot Amendment." *San Jose Mercury News,* July 26, 2007.

Riedel, G., and S. N. Davies. "Cannabinoid Function in Learning, Memory and Plasticity." *Handbook of Experimental Pharmacology* 168 (2005): 445–77.

Robbe, D., S. M. Montgomery, A. Thome, et al. "Cannabinoids Reveal Importance of Spike Timing Coordination in Hippocampal Function." *Nature Neuroscience* 9 (2006): 1526–33.

Roche, E., and P. N. Foster. "Cannabinoid Hyperemesis: Not Just a Problem in Adelaide Hills." *Gut* 54 (2005): 731.

Rog, D. J., T. J. Nurmikko, T. Friede, et al. "Randomized, Controlled Trial of Cannabis-based Medicine in Central Pain in Multiple Sclerosis." *Neurology* 65 (2005): 812–19.

Rolfe, M., C. M. Tang, S. Sabally, et al. "Psychosis and Cannabis Abuse in the Gambia: A Case-control Study." *British Journal of Psychiatry* 163 (1993): 798–801.

Rosenblatt, K. A., J. R. Daling, C. Chen, et al. "Marijuana Use and Risk of Oral Squamous Cell Carcinoma." *Cancer Research* 64, no. 11 (2004): 4049–54.

Rosenfeld, B., W. Breitbart, M. V. McDonald, et al. "Pain in Ambulatory AIDS Patients. II: Impact of Pain on Psychological Functioning and Quality of Life." *Pain* 68 (1996): 323–28.

Rosenthal, E. *Marijuana Growers Handbook*. San Francisco: Quick American Publishing, 1984.

Roth, M. D., A. Arora, S. Barsky, et al. "Airway Inflammation in Young Marijuana and Tobacco Smokers." *American Journal of Respiratory and Critical Care Medicine* 157 (1998): 928–37.

Royal College of Physicians of London, "Cannabis and Cannabis-based Medicines: Potential Benefits and Risks to Health." Report of a Working Party (2005).

Rubino T., N. Realini, C. Castiglioni, et al. "Role in Anxiety Behavior of the Endocannabinoid System in the Prefrontal Cortex." *Cerebral Cortex* 18 (2008): 1292–301.

Ruck, C. "Was There a Whiff of Cannabis about Jesus?" *The Sunday Times,* January 12, 2003.

Rudenko, S. I. 1970. *Frozen Tombs of Siberia.* Berkeley: University of California Press, 1970. Quoted in E. Abel, *Marihuana: The First Twelve Thousand Years.*

Rudolph, K. *Gnosis: The Nature and History of Gnosticism.* San Francisco: HarperSan Francisco, 1987.

Rumpf, G. E., and E. M. Beekman. *The Poison Tree: Selected Writings of Rumphius on the Natural History of the Indies, Library of the Indies.* Amherst: University of Massachusetts Press, 1981.

Rush, B. 2001. "An Anniversary to Regret: 40 Years of Failure of the Single Convention on Narcotic Drugs" (2001): www.ffdlr.org.au/commentary/docs/Single%20 cpnvention.htm. Accessed May 7, 2010.

Rusk, A., and F. Plum. "Neurologic Health and Disorders." In *Textbook of Women's Health.* Philadelphia: Lippincott-Raven, 1998.

Russo, E. "Cannabis for Migraine Treatment: The Once and Future Prescription? An Historical and Scientific Review." *Pain* 76 (1998): 3–8.

———. "Future of Cannabis and Cannabinoids in Therapeutics." *Journal of Cannabis Therapeutics* 3/4 (2003): 163–74.

———. "Clinical Endocannabinoid Deficiency (CECD): Can This Concept Explain Therapeutic Benefits of Cannabis in Migraine, Fibromyalgia, Irritable Bowel Syndrome and Other Treatment-resistant Conditions?" *Neuroendocrinology Letters* 25 (2004): 31–39.

———. "History of *Cannabis* as a Medicine." In G. W. Guy, B. A. Whittle, and P. J. Robson, eds. *The Medicinal Uses of Cannabis and Cannabinoids.* London: Pharmaceutical Press, 2004.

———. "History of Cannabis and Its Preparations in Saga, Science and Sobriquet." *Chemistry and Biodiversity* 4 (2007): 1614–18, 2624–48.

———. "Clinical Cannabis in Ancient Mesopotamia: A Historical Survey with Supporting Scientific Evidence." *Cannabis Culture,* 2007.

Russo, E. B., et al. "Phytochemical and Genetic Analyses of Ancient Cannabis from Central Asia." *Journal of Experimental Botany* 59 (2008): 4171–82.

Russo, E. B., G. W. Guy, and P. J. Robson. "Cannabis, Pain, and Sleep: Lessons from Therapeutic Clinical Trials of Sativex, a Cannabis-based Medicine." *Chemistry and Biodiversity* 4 (2007): 1729–43.

Russo, E. B., H. E. Jiang, X. Li, et al. "Phytochemical and Genetic Analyses of Ancient Cannabis from Central Asia." *Journal of Experimental Botany* 59 (2008): 4171–82.

Safo, P. K., B. F. Cravatt, and W. G. Regehr. "Retrograde Endocannabinoid Signaling in the Cerebellar Cortex." *Cerebellum* 5 (2006): 134–45.

Sanchez, C., M. I. de Ceballos, T. G. del Pulgar, et al. "Inhibition of Glioma Growth In Vivo by Selective Activation of the CB(2) Cannabinoid Receptor." *Cancer Research* 61 (2001): 5784–89.

Sanchez, C., I. Galve-Roperh, C. Canova, et al. "Delta9-tetrahydrocannabinol Induces

Apoptosis in C6 Glioma Cells." *FEBS Letters* 436 (1998): 6–10.

Sarchielli, P., L. A. Pini, F. Coppola, et al. "Endocannabinoids in Chronic Migraine: CSF Findings Suggest a System Failure." *Neuropsychopharmacology* 32 (2007): 1384–90.

Sarfarez, S., V. M. Adhami, D. N. Syed, et al. "Cannabinoids for Cancer Treatment: Progress and Promise." *Cancer Research* 68 (2008): 339–42.

Sasco, A. J., M. B. Secretan, and F. Straif. "Tobacco Smoking and Cancer: A Brief Review of Recent Epidemiological Evidence." *Lung Cancer* 45 (2004): S3–S9.

Schifitto, G., M. P. McDermott, J. McArthur, et al. "Incidence of and Risk Factors for HIV-associated Distal Sensory Polyneuropathy." *Neurology* 58 (2002): 1764–68.

Schindler, F., I. Anghelescu, F. Regen, et al. "Improvement in Refractory Obsessive Compulsive Disorder with Dronabinol." *American Journal of Psychiatry* 165 (2008): 536–37.

Schon, F., P. E. Hart, T. L. Hodgson, et al. "Suppression of Pendular Nystagmus by Smoking Cannabis in a Patient with Multiple Sclerosis." *Neurology* 53 (1999): 2209–10.

Schultes, R. E. "Random Thoughts and Queries on the Botany of *Cannabis*." In C. R. B. Joyce and S. H.Curry, eds. *The Botany and Chemistry of Cannabis.* London: J. and A. Churchill, 1970.

Schultes, R. E., and A. Hoffman. *The Botany and Chemistry of Hallacinogens*, 2nd ed. Springfield, IL: Charles C. Thomas, 1991.

———. *Plants of the Gods: Origins of Hallucinogenic Use.* London: McGraw-Hill, 1979. Reprinted Rochester, VT: Healing Arts Press, 1992.

Schuster, C. R., W. S. Dockens, and J. H. Woods. "Behavioral Variables Affecting the Development of Amphetamine Tolerance." *Psychopharmacologia* 9 (1966): 170–82.

Schurab U., J. Callaway, A. Erkkilä, et al. "Effects of hempseed and flaxseed oils on the profile of serum lipids, serum total and lipoprotein lipid concentrations and haemostatic." *European Journal of Nutrition* 45, vol. 8 (2006): 470–77.

Schwarcz, G., B. Karajgi, and R. McCarthy. "Synthetic Delta-9-tetrahydrocannabinol (Dronabinol) Can Improve the Symptoms of Schizophrenia." *Journal of Clinical Psychopharmacology* 29 (2009): 255–58.

Schwartz, R. H., and R. L. Hawks. "Laboratory Detection of Marijuana Use." *Journal of the American Medical Association* 254 (1985): 788–92.

Schweizer, A., and H. P. Bircher. "Reposition of a Dislocated Shoulder under Use of Cannabis." *Wilderness and Environmental Medicine* 20 (2009): 301–2.

Scragg, R. K. R., E. A. Mitchell, R. K. R. Ford, et al. "Maternal Cannabis Use in the Sudden Death Syndrome." *Acta Paediatrica* 90 (2001): 57–60.

Seligman, K. "Connoisseurs of Cannabis." *San Francisco Chronicle*, April 22, 2007.

Senate Special Committee on Illegal Drugs. "Cannabis: Our Position for a Canadian Public Policy." Ottawa: Senate of Canada, 2002.

Sertürner, F. "Über das Morphium, eine neue salzfähige Grundlage, und die

Mekonsäure, als Hauptbestandtheile des Opiums." *Annals of Physics* 55 (1817): 56–89.

Shedler, J., and J. Block. "Adolescent Drug Use and Psychological Health: A Longitudinal Inquiry." *American Psychologist* 45 (1990): 612–30.

Sherrill, D. L., M. Krzyzanowski, J. W. Bloom, et al. "Respiratory Effects of Nontobacco Cigarettes: A Longitudinal Study in General Population." *International Journal of Epidemiology* 20 (1991): 132–37.

Shoyama, Y., T. Fujita, T. Yamauchi, T., et al. "Cannabichromenic Acid: A Genuine Substance of Cannabichromene." *Chemical and Pharmaceutical Bulletin* 16 (1968): 1157–58.

Sidney, S. C. P. Quesenberry Jr., G. D. Friedman, et al. "Marijuana Use and Cancer Incidence." *Cancer Causes and Control* 8 (1997): 722–28.

Silver, G. *The Dope Chronicles, 1850–1950.* San Francisco: Yellow Press, 1979.

Sim, L. J., D. E. Selley, R. Xiao, et al. "Differences in G-protein Activation by Mu- and Delta-opioid, and Cannabinoid, Receptors in Rat Striatum." *European Journal of Pharmacology* 307 (1996): 97–105.

Singer, E. J., C. Zorilla, B. Fahy-Chandon, et al. "Painful Symptoms Reported by Ambulatory HIV-infected Men in a Longitudinal Study." *Pain* 54 (1993): 15–19.

Singh G. K. "Atrial Fibrillation Associated with Marijuana Use." *Pediatric Cardiology* 21 (2000): 248.

Sinha, D., T. I. Bonner, N. R. Bhat, et al. "Expression of the CB1 Cannabinoid Receptor in Macrophage-like Cells from Brain Tissue: Immunochemical Characterization by Fusion Protein Antibodies." *Journal of Neuroimmunology* 82 (1998): 13–21.

Sinor, A. D., S. M. Irvin, and D. A. Greenberg. "Endocannabinoids Protect Cerebral Cortical Neurons from In Vitro Ischemia in Rats." *Neuroscience Letters* 14 (2000): 157–60.

Skager, R. "Beyond Zero Tolerance: A Reality-based Approach to Drug Education and School Discipline" (2007): www.safety1st.org/iimages/stories/pdf/bzt.pdf. Accessed May 7, 2010.

Skopp, G., and L. Potsche. "Serum Cannabinoid Levels 24 to 48 Hours after Cannabis Smoking." *Archives of Criminology* (Germany) 212 (2003): 83–95.

Sloman, L. *Reefer Madness.* New York: St. Martin's Press, 1979.

Small, E., and A. Cronquist. 1976. "A Practical and Natural Taxonomy for *Cannabis.*" *Taxon* 25 (1976): 405–35.

Small, E., and D. Marcus. "Hemp: A New Crop with New Uses for North America." In J. Janick and A. Whipkey, eds. *Trends in New Crops and New Uses.* Alexandria, VA: ASHS Press, 2002.

———. "Tetrahydrocannabinol Levels in Hemp (Cannabis sativa) Germplasm Resources." *Economic Botany* 57 (2003): 545–58.

Smiley, A. "Marijuana: On-road and Driving-simulator Studies." In Kalant, H., Centre for Addiction and Mental Health, et al., eds. *The Health Effects of Cannabis.*

Toronto, ON: Canadian Centre for Addiction and Mental Health, 1999.

Smink, B. E., K. J. Lusthof, J. J. De Gier, et al. "Drug Use and the Severity of Traffic Accident." *Accident, Analysis and Prevention* 37 (2005): 427–33.

Smit, F., L. Bolier, and P. Cuijpers. "Cannabis Use and the Risk of Later Schizophrenia: A Review." *Addiction* 99 (2004): 425–30.

Snyder, S. H., and S. R. Childers. "Opiate Receptors and Opioid Peptides." *Annual Review of Neuroscience* 2 (1979): 35–64.

Sofia, R. B., S. D. Nalepa, J. J. Harakal, et al. "Anti-edema and Analgesic Properties of D9 Tetrahydrocannabinol." *Journal of Pharmacology and Experimental Therapeutics* 186 (1973): 646–55.

Solowij, N., P. T. Michie, and A. M. Fox. "Differential Impairments of Selective Attention Due to Frequency and Duration of Cannabis Use." *Biological Psychiatry* 37 (1995): 731–39.

Solowij, N., R. S. Stephens, R. A. Roffman, et al. "Cognitive Functioning of Long-term Heavy Cannabis Users Seeking Treatment." *Journal of the American Medical Association* 287 (2002): 1123–31.

Somerset, M., R. Campbell, D. J. Sharp, et al. "What Do People with MS Want and Expect from Health-care Services?" *Health Expectations* 4 (2001): 29–37.

Staquet, M., C. Gantt, and D. Machin. "Effect of a Nitrogen Analog of Tetrahydrocannabinol on Cancer Pain." *Journal of Clinical Pharmacy and Therapeutics* 23 (1978): 397–401.

Starks, M. *Marijuana Chemistry: Genetics, Processing, and Potency,* 2nd ed. Berkeley, CA: Ronin Publishing, 1990.

Stearn, W. T. "The *Cannabis* Plant: Botanical Characteristics." In C. R. B. Joyce and S. H. Curry, eds. *The Botany and Chemistry of* Cannabis. London: J. and A. Churchill, 1970.

Steiner, M. A., K. Wanisch, K. Monory, et al. "Impaired Cannabinoid Receptor Type 1 Signaling Interferes with Stress-coping Behavior in Mice." *Pharmacogenomics Journal* 8 (2008): 196–208.

Stella, N. "Endocannabinoid Signaling in Microglial Cells." *Neuropharmacology* 56 suppl. 1 (2009): 244–53.

Stephens, R. S., T. F. Babor, R. Kadden, et al., and The Marijuana Treatment Project Research Group. "The Marijuana Treatment Project: Rationale, Design, and Participant Characteristics." *Addiction* 97, S1 (2002): 109–24.

Stephens, R. S., R. A. Roffman, and L. Curtin. "Comparison of Extended versus Brief Treatments for Marijuana Use." *Journal of Consulting and Clinical Psychology* 68 (2000): 898–908.

Stephens, R. S., R. A. Roffman, and E. E. Simpson. "Adult Marijuana Users Seeking Treatment." *Journal of Consulting and Clinical Psychology* 61 (1993): 1100–1104.

———. "Treating Adult Marijuana Dependence: A Test of the Relapse Prevention Model." *Journal of Consulting and Clinical Psychology* 62 (1994): 92–99.

Stewart, J., and A. Badiani. "Tolerance and Sensitization to the Behavioral Effects of Drugs." *Behavioral Pharmacology* (1993): 289–312.

Strakowski, S. M., M. P. DelBello, D. E. Fleck, et al. "Effects of Co-occurring Cannabis Use Disorders on the Course of Bipolar Disorder after a First Hospitalization for Mania." *Archives of General Psychiatry* 64 (2007): 57–64.

Strohbeck-Kuehner, P., G. Skopp, and R. Mattern. "Cannabis Improves Symptoms of ADHD." *Cannabinoids* 3 (2008): 1–3.

Students for Sensible Drug Policy. "Harmful Drug Law Hits Home: How Many College Students in Each State Lost Financial Aid Due to Drug Convictions?" (2006): www.ssdp.org/states/ssdp-state-report.pdf. Accessed May 7, 2010.

Subramanian, R. "Motor Vehicle Traffic Crashes as a Leading Cause of Death in the United States, 2003." Traffic Safety Facts, DOT HS 810 568 (2006).

Substance Abuse and Mental Health Services Administration (SAMHSA), "Trends in the Incidence of Drug Use in the United States, 1919–1992." Substance Abuse and Mental Health Services Administration, Office of Applied Studies, Division of Population Surveys, 1998.

———. *Summary of Findings from the 2000 National Household Survey on Drug Abuse.* USDHHS, 2001.

———. National Survey on Drug Use and Health, 2005 (2006).

———. National Survey on Drug Use and Health (2006): www.icpsr.umich.edu/cocoon/SAMHDA/STUDY/21240.xml. Accessed May 2, 2010.

———. Office of Applied Studies. Treatment Episode Data Set (TEDS): 1995–2005. National Admissions to Substance Abuse Treatment Services, DASIS Series: S-37, DHHS Publication No. SMA 07-4234, 2007.

———. *National Household Survey on Drug Use and Health, Data from 2006 Survey.* Ann Arbor, MI: Substance Abuce and Mental Health Data Archive, 2007

———. Office of Applied Studies. Results from the 2007 National Survey on Drug Use and Health: National Findings. NSDUH Series H-34, DHHS Publication No. SMA 08-4343, 2008.

Sugiura, T., S. Kondo, A. Sukagawa, et al. "2-Arachidonoylgylcerol: A Possible Endogenous Cannabinoid Receptor-ligand in Brain." *Biochemical and Biophysical Research Communications* 215 (1995): 89–97.

Swanberg, W. A. *Citizen Hearst.* New York: Bantam Books, 1961.

Sydney, S., C. P. Quesenberry, G. D. Friedman, et al. "Marijuana Use and Cancer Incidence (California, United States)." *Cancer Causes and Control* 8 (1997): 722–28.

Szalavitz, M. *Help at Any Cost: How the Troubled-Teen Industry Cons Parents and Hurts Kids.* New York: Penguin, 2006.

Tan B., D. K. O'Dell, Y. Yu, et al. "Identification of Endogenous Acyl Amino Acids Based on a Targeted Lipidomics Approach." *Journal of Lipid Research* 51 (2010): 112–19.

Tan B., Y. W. YU, M. F. Monn, et al. "Targeted lipidomics approach for endogenous N-acyl amino acids in rat brain tissue." *Journal of Chromatography B* 26 (2009): 2890–4.

Tarter, R. E., M. Vanyukov, L. Kirisci, et al. "Predictors of Marijuana Use in Adolescents before and after Licit Drug Use: Examination of the Gateway Hypothesis." *American Journal of Psychiatry* 163 (2006): 2134–40.

Tashkin, D. P., A. H. Coulson, V. A. Clark, et al. "Respiratory Symptoms and Lung Function in Habitual Heavy Smokers of Marijuana Alone, Smokers of Marijuana and Tobacco, Smokers of Tobacco Alone, and Nonsmokers." *American Review of Respiratory Disease* 135 (1987): 209–16.

Tashkin, D. P., B. J. Shapiro, Y. E. Lee, et al. "Effects of Smoked Marijuana in Experimentally Induced Asthma." *American Review of Respiratory Disease* 112 (1975): 377–86.

Tashkin, D. P., M. S. Simmons, D. L. Sherrill, et al. "Heavy Habitual Marijuana Smoking Does Not Cause an Accelerated Decline in FEV1 with Age." *American Journal of Respiratory and Critical Care Medicine* 155 (1997): 141–48.

Tatarsky, A. *Harm Reduction Psychotherapy: A New Treatment for Drug and Alcohol Problems.* Northvale, NJ: Aronson, 2002.

———. "Harm Reduction Psychotherapy: Extending the Reach of Traditional Substance Use Treatment." *Journal of Substance Abuse Treatment* 25 (2003): 249–56.

Taura, F., S. Morimoto, Y. Shoyama, et al. "First Direct Evidence for the Mechanism of Delta-1-tetrahydrocannabinolic Acid Biosynthesis. *Journal of the American Chemical Society* 117, no. 38 (1995): 9766–67.

Taylor, D. R., D. M. Fergusson, B. J. Milne, L. J. Horwood, et al. "A Longitudinal Study of the Effects of Tobacco and Cannabis Exposure on Lung Function in Young Adults." *Addiction* 97 (2002): 1055–61.

Taylor. D. R., R. Poulton, T. E. Moffitt, et al. "The Respiratory Effects of Cannabis Dependence in Young Adults." *Addiction* 95 (2000): 1669–77.

Taylor, F. M. 1988. "Marijuana As a Potential Respiratory Tract Carcinogen: A Retrospective Analysis of a Community Hospital Population." *Singapore Medical Journal* 81: 1213–16.

Taylor, T. "Supporting Research into the Therapeutic Role of Marijuana." Report published by the American College of Physicians (January 2008).

Teesson, M., M. Lynskey, B. Manor, et al. "The Structure of Cannabis Dependence in the Community." *Drug and Alcohol Dependence* 68 (2002): 255–62.

Terranova, J. P., J. J. Storme, N. Lafon, et al. "Improvement of Memory in Rodents by the Selective CB1 Cannabinoid Receptor Antagonist SR141716." *Psychopharmacology* 126 (1996): 165–72.

Tetrault, J. M., K. Crothers, B. A. Moore, et al. "Effects of Marijuana Smoking on Pulmonary Function and Respiratory Complications: A Systematic Review." *Archives of Internal Medicine* 167 (2007): 221–28.

Texas Police Central. Drug Information: www.texaspolicecentral.com. Accessed June 26, 2007.

Thaczuk, D. 2007. "Cultivating Compassion: The Positive Side." *Canadian AIDS Treatment Information Exchange (CATIE)* 9, no. 1 (Summer 2007).

Thierry, A. M., J. P. Tassin, G. Blanc, et al. "Studies on Mesocortical Dopamine Systems." *Advances in Biochemical Psychopharmacology* 19 (1978): 205–16.

Thomas A., L. A. Stevenson, K. N. Wease, et al. "Evidence that the Plant Cannabinoid Delta-9-tetrahydrocannabivarin Is a Cannabinoid CB_1 and CB_2 Receptor Antagonist." *British Journal of Pharmacology* 146 (2005): 917–26.

Thomas, H. "A Community Survey of Adverse Effects of Cannabis Use." *Drug and Alcohol Dependence* 42 (1996): 201–7.

Thompson, R. C. *The Assyrian Herbal.* London: Luzac, 1924.

Tims, F. M., M. L. Dennis, N. Hamilton, et al. "Characteristics and Problems of 600 Adolescent Cannabis Abusers in Outpatient Treatment." *Addiction* 97 (2002): 46–57.

Tinklenberg, J. R., F. T. Melges, L. E. Hollister, et al. "Marijuana and Immediate Memory." *Nature* 226 (1970): 1171–72.

Tournier, M., F. Sorbara, C. Gindre, et al. "Cannabis Use and Anxiety in Daily Life: A Naturalistic Investigation in a Non-clinical Population." *Psychiatry Research* 118 (2003): 1–8.

Tramer, M. R., D. Carroll, F. A. Campbell, et al. "Cannabinoids for Control of Chemotherapy Induced Nausea and Vomiting: Quantitative Systematic Review." *British Medical Journal* 323 (2001): 16–21.

Ungerleider, J. T., T. Andrysiak, L FGairbanks, et al. "Delta-9 THC in the Treatment of Spasticity Associated with Multiple Sclerosis." *Advances in Alcohol and Substance Abuse* 7 (1987): 39–50.

U.K. Department of Environment, Transport and the Regions, Road Safety Division. "Cannabis and Driving: A Review of the Literature and Commentary" (n.d.): http://webarchive.nationalarchives.gov.uk/+/http://www.dft.gov.uk/pgr/roadsafety/research/rsrr/theme3/cannabisanddrivingareviewoft4764. Accessed April 13, 2010.

UNAIDS. Joint United Nations Programme on HIV/AIDS (2007).

United Nations Office on Drugs and Crime. *World Drug Report 2006,* vol. 1, *Analysis.* Vienna: United Nations, 2006.

United Nations Office for Drug Control and Crime Prevention. *Global Illicit Drug Trends 2002.* New York: UNODCCP, 2002.

U.S. Department of Health and Human Services, Substance and Mental Health Services Association, Office of Applied Studies. "Driving after Drug or Alcohol Use" (1998): www.oas.samhsa.gov/driverrprt/toc.htm. Accessed November 24, 2007.

U.S. Department of Justice, Drug Enforcement Administration. "In the Matter of Marijuana Rescheduling Petition (Docket No. 86-22) Opinion and Recommended Ruling, Findings of Fact, Conclusions of Law and Decision of Administration Law Judge Francis L. Young." (September 6, 1988).

U.S. Department of Transportation, National Highway Traffic Safety Administration. "The Incidence and Role of Drugs in Fatally Injured Drivers: Final Report." DOT HS 808 065 (October 1992): http.trb.org/view.aspx?id=405149. Accessed May 2, 2010.

————. Robbe, H. W. J., and J. F. O'Hanlon, "Marijuana and Actual Driving Performance." DOT HS 808 078 (November 1993): www.druglibrary.org/schaffer/misc/driving/driving.htm. Accessed May 2, 2010.

————. "State of Knowledge of Drug-impaired Driving: Final Report." DOT HS 809 642 (September 2003): www.nhtsa.gov/people/injury/research/StateofKnowledgeDrugs/StateofDrugs. Accessed May 2, 2010.

U.S. Drug Enforcement Administration (DEA). *Drugs of Abuse.* U.S. Department of Justice (2005): www.justice.gov/dea/pubs/abuse/index.htm. Accessed May 7, 2010.

U.S. Food and Drug Administration (FDA). "Inter-agency Advisory Regarding Claims That Smoked Marijuana Is a Medicine" April 20, 2006: www.fda.gov. Accessed December 20, 2007.

U.S. General Accounting Office (GAO). "Drug Use among Youth: No Simple Answers to Guide Prevention." Report to the Chairman, Subcommittee on Children, Family, Drugs, and Alcoholism, Committee on Labor and Human Resources, U.S. Senate. Washington, D.C.: U.S. Government Printing Office (1993): http://archive.gao.gov/t2pbat4/150661.pdf. Accessed May 7, 2010.

U.S. Government Accountability Office. "ONDCP Media Campaign: Contractor's National Evaluation Did Not Find that the Youth Anti-drug Media Campaign Was Effective in Reducing Youth Drug Use." Report to the Subcommittee on Transportation, Treasury, the Judiciary, Housing and Urban Development, and Related Agencies, Committee on Appropriations, U.S. Senate. August 25, 2006.

University of Mississippi Marijuana Potency Monitoring Project. Report 95 (January 9, 2007).

Vadhan, N. P., C. L. Hart, W. G. van Gorp, et al. "Acute Effects of Smoked Marijuana on Decision making, as Assessed by a Modified Gambling Task, in Experienced Marijuana Users." *Journal of Clinical and Experimental Neuropsychology* 29 (2007): 357–64.

Valjent, E., C. Pages, M. Rogard. "Delta 9 Tetrahydrocannabinol Induced MAPK/ERK and Elk 1 Activation In Vivo Depends on Dopaminergic Transmission." *European Journal of Neuroscience* 14 (2001): 342–52.

Van der Elst, W., M. P. van Boxtel, G. J. P van Breukelen, et al. "Rey's Verbal Learning Test: Normative Data for 1855 Healthy Participanst Aged 24–81 years and the Influence of Age, Sex, Education, and Mode of Presentation." *Journal of the International Neuropsychological Society* 11 (2004): 290–302.

Van der Stelt, M., W. B. Veldhuis, P. R. Bar, et al. "Neuroprotection by Delta9-tetrahydrocannabinol, the Main Active Compound in Marijuana, against Ouabain-induced In Vivo Excitotoxicity." *Journal of Neuroscience* 21 (2001): 6475–79.

Vaney, C., M. Heinzel-Gutenbrunner, P. Jobin, et al. "Efficacy, Safety and Tolerability of an Orally Administered Cannabis Extract in the Treatment of Spasticity in Patients with Multiple Sclerosis: A Randomized, Double-blind, Placebo-controlled, Crossover study." *Multiple Sclerosis* 10 (2004): 417–24.

Vandrey, R. G., A. J. Budney, J. R. Hughes, et al. "A Within-subjects Comparison of Withdrawal Symptoms during Abstinence from Cannabis, Tobacco, and Both Substances." *Drug and Alcohol Dependence* 92 (2007): 48–54.

Vandrey, R. G., A. J. Budney, J. L. Kamon, et al. "Cannabis Withdrawal in Adolescent Treatment Seekers." *Drug and Alcohol Dependence* 78 (2005a): 205–10.

Vandrey, R. G., A. J. Budney, B. A. Moore, et al. "A Cross-study Comparison of Cannabis and Tobacco Withdrawal." *American Journal on Addictions* 14 (2005b): 54–63.

van Laar, M. W., A. A. N. Cruts, J. E. E. Verdurmen, et al. *The Netherlands National Drug Monitor Annual Report 2005.* Ultrecht, the Netherlands: Trimbos Institute, 2006.

Velasco, G., A. Carracedo, C. Blazquez, et al. "Cannabinoids and Gliomas." *Molecular Neurobiology* 36 (2007): 60–67.

Verdoux, H., F. Sorbara, C. Gindre, et al. "Clinical Use and Dimensions of Psychosis in a Nonclinical Population of Female Subjects." *Schizophrenia Research* 59 (2003): 77–84.

Verdoux, H., M. Tournier, and A. Cougnard. "Impact of Substance Use on the Onset and Course of Early Psychosis." *Schizophrenia Research* 79 (2005): 69–75.

Viggiano D., L. A. Ruocco, M. Pignatelli, et al. "Prenatal Elevation of Endocannabinoids Corrects the Unbalance between Dopamine Systems and Reduces Activity in Naples High Excitability Rats." *Neuroscience and Behavioral Review* 27 (2003): 129–39.

Vinod, K. Y., and B. L. Hungund. "Role of the Endocannabinoid System in Depression and Suicide." *Trends in Pharmacological Sciences* 27 (2006): 539–45.

Viveros, M.-P., E.-M. Marco, R. Llorente, et al. "Endocannabinoid System and Synaptic Plasticity: Implications for Emotional Responses." *Neural Plasticity* (2007): 5290.

Volfe, Z., A. Dvilansky, and I. Nathan. "Cannabinoids Block Release of Serotonin from Platelets by Plasma from Migraine Patients." *International Journal of Clinical Pharmacology Research* 4 (1985): 243–6.

Volicer, L., M. Stelly, J. Morris, et al. "Effects of Dronabinol on Anorexia and Disturbed Behavior in Patients with Alzheimer's Disease." *International Journal of Geriatric Psychiatry* 12 (1997): 913–19.

Wachtel, S. R., M. A. ElSohly, S. A. Ross, et al. "Comparison of the Subjective Effects of Delta(9)-tetrahydrocannabinol and Marijuana in Humans." *Psychopharmacology (Berlin)* 161 (2002): 331–39.

Wachtel, T. "SaferSanerSchools: Restoring Community in a Disconnected World." International Institute for Restorative Practices (1999): http://fp.enter.net/restorativepractices/SSSRestoringCommunity.pdf. Accessed May 7, 2010.

Wade, D. T., P. M. Makela, H. House, et al. "Long-term Use of a Cannabis-based Medicine in the Treatment of Spasticity and Other Symptoms of Multiple Sclerosis." *Multiple Sclerosis* 12 (2004a): 639–45.

Wade, D. T., P. Makela, P Robson, et al. "Do Cannabis-based Medicinal Extracts Have General or Specific Effects on Symptoms in Multiple Sclerosis? A Double-blind, Randomized, Placebo-controlled Study on 160 Patients." *Multiple Sclerosis* 10 (2004b): 434–41.

Wade, D. T., P. Robson, H. House, et al. "A Preliminary Controlled Study to Determine Whether Whole-plant Cannabis Extracts Can Improve Intractable Neurogenic Symptoms." *Clinical Rehabilitation* 17 (2003): 21–29.

Waksman, Y., Olson, J. M., S. J. Carlisle, et al. "The Central Cannabinoid Receptor (CB1) Mediates Inhibition of Nitric Oxide Production by Rat Microglial Cells." *Journal of Pharmacology and Experimental Therapeutics* 288 (1999): 1357–66.

Walker, J. M., and S. M. Huang. "Cannabinoid Analgesia." *Pharmacology and Therapeutics* 95 (2002): 127–35.

Wallace, M., G. Schulteis, J. H. Atkinson, et al. "Dose-dependent Effects of Smoked Cannabis on Capsaicin-induced Pain and Hyperalgesia in Healthy Volunteers." *Anesthesiology* 107 (2007): 785–96.

Walther, S. R. Malhlberg, U. Eichmann, et al. "Delta-9-tetrahydrocannabinol for Nighttime Agitation in Severe Dementia." *Physcopharmacology* 185 (2006): 524–8.

Walton, R. P. *Marihuana—America's New Drug Problem: A Sociologic Question with Its Basic Explanation Dependent on Biologic and Medical Principles.* Philadelphia: J.P. Lippincott, 1938.

Wang, D., H. Wang, W. Ning, et al. "Loss of Cannabinoid Receptor 1 Accelerates Intestinal Tumor Growth." *Cancer Research* 68 (2008): 6468–76.

Ward, A. S., S. D. Comer, M. Haney, et al. "The Effects of a Monetary Alternative on Marijuana Self-administration." *Behavioral Pharmacolology* 8 (1997): 275–86.

Ware, M. A., C. R. Doyle, R. Woods, et al. "Cannabis Use for Chronic Non-cancer Pain: Results of a Prospective Survey." *Pain* 102 (2003): 211–16.

Ware, M. A., A. Gamsa, J. Persson, et al. "Cannabis for Chronic Pain: Case Series and Implications for Clinicians." *Pain Research and Management* 7 (2002): 95–99.

Ware, M. A., S. Rueda, J. Singer, J., et al. "Cannabis Use by Persons Living with HIV/AIDS: Patterns and Prevalence of Use." *Journal of Cannabis Therapeutics* 3 (2003): 3–15.

Warner, R., D. Taylor, J. Wright, et al. "Substance Use among the Mentally Ill: Prevalence, Reasons for Use, and Effects on Illness." *American Journal of Orthopsychiatry* 64 (1994): 30–39.

Weil, A. T., and D. I. Abrams. *Integrative Oncology.* New York: Oxford University Press, 2008.

Weil, A. T., N. E. Zinberg, and J. M. Nelsen. "Clinical and Psychological Effects of Marihuana in Man. *Science* 162 (1968): 1234–42.

Weiser, M., M. Davidson, and S. Noy. "Comments on Risk for Schizophrenia." *Schizophrenia Research* 79 (2005a): 15–21.

Weiser, M., H. Y. Knobler, S. Noy, et al. "Clinical Characteristics of Adolescents Later Hospitalized for Schizophrenia." *American Journal of Medical Genetics* 114 (2002): 949–55.

Weiser, M., and S. Noy. "Interpreting the Association between Cannabis Use and Increased Risk for Schizophrenia." *Dialogues in Clinical Neuroscience* 7 (2005b): 81–85.

Weiss, L., M. Zeira, S. Reich, et al. "Cannabidiol Lowers Incidence of Diabetes in Non-obese Diabetic Mice." *Autoimmunity* 39 (2006): 143–51.

———. "Cannabidiol Arrests Onset of Autoimmune Diabetes in NOD Mice." *Neuro-pharmacology* 54 (2008): 244–9.

Weiss, M. D., P. Weydt, and G. T. Carter. "A Role for Rational Polypharmacy in the Treatment of Amyotrophic Lateral Sclerosis." *Expert Opinion on Pharmacotherapy* 5 (2004): 735–46.

Welch, S. P., and M. Eads M. "Synergistic Interactions of Endogenous Opioids and Cannabinoid Systems." *Brain Research* 848 (1999): 183–90.

Welch, S. P., and D. L. Stevens. "Antinociceptive Activity of Intrathecally Adminis-tered Cannabinoids Alone and in Combination with Morphine in Mice." *Journal of Pharmacology and Experimental Therapeutics* 262 (1992): 10–18.

Wenger, T., and G. Moldrich. "The Role of Endocannabinoids in the Hypothalamic Regulation of Visceral Function." *Prostaglandins, Leukotrienes and Essential Fatty Acids Journal* 66 (2002): 301–307.

West, D. P. "Hemp and Marijuana: Myths and Realities." North American Industrial Hemp Council, Madison, WI (1998): www.naihc.org/hemp_information/con-tent/hemp.mj.html. Accessed December 7, 2007.

Weydt, P., S. Hong, A. Witting, et al. "Cannabinol Delays Symptom Onset in SOD1 Transgenic Mice without Affecting Survival." *Amyotrophic Lateral Sclerosis and Other Motor Neuron Disorders* 6 (2005): 182–4.

Weydt, P., M. D. Weiss, T. Moller, et al. "Neuroinflammation as a Therapeutic Tar-get in Amyotrophic Lateral Sclerosis." *Current Opinion in Investigational Drugs* 3 (2002): 1720–24.

Whitlow, C. T., A. Liguori, L. B. Livengood, et al. "Long-term Heavy Marihuana Users Make Costly Decisions on a Gambling Task." *Drug and Alcohol Dependence* 76 (2004): 107–111.

Williams, A. F., M. A. Peat, D. J. Crouch, et al. "Drugs in Fatally Injured Young Male Drivers." *Public Health Reports* 1 (1985): 19–26.

Wills, S. "*Cannabis* Use and Abuse by Man: An Historical Perspective." In D. T. Brown, ed., *Cannabis: The Genus Cannabis.* Amsterdam: Harwood Academic Publishers, 1998.

Willstätter, R. "Über die Constitution der Spaltungsproducte von Atropin und Cocaïn." *Berichte der Deutschen Chemischen Gesellschaft* 31 (1898): 1534–53.

Wilson, K. J., A. Doxanakis, and C. K. Fairley. "Predictors for Non-adherence to Anti-retroviral Therapy." *Sex Health* 1 (2004): 251–57.

Wilson, R. I., and R. A. Nicoll. "Endocannabinoid Signaling in the Brain." *Science* 296 (2002): 678–82.

Wilson, W., R. Mathew, T. Turkington, et al. "Brain Morphological Changes and Early Marijuana Use: A Magnetic Resonance and Positron Emission Tomography Study." *Journal of Addictive Diseases* 19 (2000): 1–22.

Winick, C. "Social Behavior, Public Policy, and Nonharmful Drug Use." *The Milbank Quarterly* 69 (1991): 437–59.

Wolf, S. A., S. Tauber, and O. Ullrich. "CNS Immune Surveillance and Neuroinflammation: Endocannabinoids Keep Control." *Current Pharmaceutical Design* 14 (2008): 2266–78.

Woolridge, E., S. Barton, J. Samuel, et al. "Cannabis Use in HIV for Pain and Other Medical Symptoms." *Journal of Pain and Symptom Management* 29 (2005): 358–67.

Wright, D., N. Sathe, and K. Spagnola. State estimates of substance use from the 2005–2006 National Survey on Drug Use and Health. Substance Abuse and Mental Health Services Administration, U.S. Deptartment of Health and Human Services (February 2007).

Wright, K. L., M. Duncan, and K. A. Sharkey. "Cannabinoid CB2 Receptors in the Gastrointestinal Tract: A Regulatory System in States of Inflammation." *British Journal of Pharmacology* 153 (2008): 263–70.

Yee, P. *Saltwater City: An Illustrated History of the Chinese in Vancouver.* Vancouver, British Columbia: Douglas and McIntyre, 2006.

Yin, H. H., and B. J. Knowlton. "The Role of the Basal Ganglia in Habit Formation." *Nature Reviews Neuroscience* 7 (2006): 464–76.

Zachariah, S. B. 1991. "Stroke after Heavy Marijuana Smoking." *Stroke* 22 (1991): 406–409.

Zacny, J. P. "Response to Marijuana as a Function of Potency and Breathhold Duration." *Psychopharmacology* 103 (1991): 223–26.

Zacny, J. P., and L. D. Chait. "Breathhold Duration and Response to Marijuana Smoke." *Pharmacology, Biochemistry and Behavior* 33 (1989): 481–84.

Zajicek, J., P. Fox, H. Sanders, et al. "Cannabinoids for Treatment of Spasticity and Other Symptoms Related to Multiple Sclerosis: Multicentre Randomized Placebo-controlled Trial." *Lancet* 362 (2003): 1517–26.

Zammit, S., P. Allebeck, S. Andreasson, et al. "Self Reported Cannabis Use as a Risk Factor for Schizophrenia in Swedish Conscripts of 1969: Historical Cohort Study." *British Medical Journal* 325 (2002): 1199.

Zeidenberg, P., W. C. Clark. J. Jaffe, et al. "Effect of Oral Administration of Delta-9-tetrahydrocannabinol on Memory, Speech, and Perception of Thermal Stimulation: Results with Four Normal Human Volunteer Subjects." *Comprehensive Psychiatry* 14 (1973): 549–56.

Zimm, A. "Study: Marijuana Halts Growth of Lung Cancer Tumors." *Bloomberg News Wire*, April 18, 2007.

Zimmer, L., and J. P. Morgan. *Marijuana Myths, Marijuana Facts: A Review of the Scientific Evidence.* New York: Lindesmith Center, 1997.

Zuardi, A. W., J. Crippa, S. Dursun, et al. "Cannabidiol Was Ineffective for Manic Episode of Bipolar Affective Disorder." *Journal of Psychopharmacology* 24 (2010): 135–37.

Zuardi, A. W., J. A. Crippa, J. E. Hallak, et al. "Cannabidiol for the Treatment of Psychosis in Parkinson's Disease." *Journal of Psychopharmacology* 23 (2009): 979–83.

Zuardi, A. W., and S. F. Guimaraes. "Cannabidiol as an Anxiolytic and Antipsychotic." In M. L. Mathre, ed., *Cannabis in Medical Practice: A Legal, Historical and Pharmacological Overview of the Therapeutic Use of Marijuana*. Jefferson, NC: McFarland, 1997.

Zuardi, A. W., S. L. Morais, F. S. Guimaraes, et al. "Antipstychotic Effect of Cannabidiol." *Journal of Clinical Psychiatry* 56 (1995): 485–86.

Zuardi A, I. Shirakawa, E. Finkelfarb, et al. "Action of Cannabidiol on the Anxiety and Other Effects Produced by THC in Normal Subjects." *Psychopharmacology* 76 (1982): 245–50.

Contributors

Donald I. Abrams, M.D., is professor of medicine at the University of California, San Francisco. Since 1997, funded by both the National Institutes of Health and the University of California Center for Medicinal Cannabis Research, he has been involved in clinical investigations of smoked and vaporized cannabis in patients with HIV, cancer, and pain. He can be contacted at dabrams@hemeonc.ucsf.edu.

Sunil Aggarwal, M.D., Ph.D., has published several peer-reviewed papers on medicinal cannabis science in international journals of pain management, hospice and palliative medicine, and general medicine, and he has served as a designated external reviewer for the AMA's 2009 report on the use of cannabis for medicinal purposes. He is a resident in physical medicine and rehabilitation at New York University Medical Center. He can be contacted at sunila@uw.edu.

Paul Armentano is deputy director of the National Organization for the Reform of Marijuana Laws (NORML) and the NORML Foundation, a nonprofit foundation established in 1997 to educate the public about marijuana and marijuana policy. He has coordinated lobbying efforts to liberalize successfully so-called zero tolerant drugged driving laws in several states in the United States. He is the author of more than five hundred published papers and magazine articles and was a 2008 recipient of the Project Censored Real News Award for Outstanding Investigative Journalism. He is the coauthor of the book *Marijuana is Safer: So Why Are We Driving People to Drink?* (White River Junction, VT: Chelsea Green Publishing, 2009) and is on the faculty of Oaksterdam University in Oakland. He can be contacted at paul@norml.org.

Lynne Belle-Isle is an epidemiologist by training and is currently a Ph.D. student at the University of Victoria. She has been working as a programs consultant with the Canadian AIDS Society since January 2004. She sat on Health Canada's Stakeholder Advisory Committee on Medical Marihuana. Lynne also works on issues related to harm reduction, drug policy, housing, and community-based research. She can be contacted at LynneB@cdnaids.ca.

Chris Bennet is coauthor of *Green Gold the Tree of Life: Marijuana in Magic and Religion* (Frazier Park, CA, n.p., 1995) and author of *Sex, Drugs, Violence and the Bible* (Gibsons, British Columbia: Forbidden Fruit Publishing, 2001) and *Cannabis and the Soma Solution* (Springfield, OR: Trine Day, 2010). He is the owner of Urban Shaman Entheobotanicals (www.urbanshaman. net) and Forbidden Fruit Publishing (www.forbiddenfruitpublishing.com), and he is also a reverend with the Church of the Universe (www.iamm .com), which recognizes cannabis as the Tree of Life. He can be contacted at freeshiva@hotmail.com.

Richard Glen Boire, J.D., is an attorney and legal scholar whose work centers on subjectivity and the law and the translation of traditional constitutional law into a contemporary, science-based right to freedom of thought. From 1999 through 2004, he was a senior fellow in law and policy at the Center for Cognitive Liberty and Ethics. He can be contacted at www .rgblawgroup.com.

Graham Boyd, J.D., founded the ACLU Drug Law Reform Project in 1998 and was its director until February 2010. In that role, he litigated many of the leading cases around medical marijuana, including the successful effort to protect doctors and patients from federal efforts to shut down the nation's first medical marijuana program. In his current position as a visiting fellow at Stanford Law School's Criminal Justice Center, he is writing articles and a book about drug law reform efforts over the past decade.

Al Byrne, LCDR (retired) is COO and cofounder of Patients Out of Time (medicalcannabis.com.), a pro-cannabis reform group. Before founding the organization with Mary Lynn Mathre, he spent years counseling veterans in Appalachia for the Department of Veterans' Affairs Agent Orange Class Assistance Program. He can be contacted at al@medicalcannabis.com.

N. Rielle Capler is director of Canadians for Safe Access, the Drug Policy Committee, and the BC Civil Liberties Association. She is involved in research, advocacy, and education that supports legal, safe, and effective use of cannabis. She can be contacted at rielle@telus.net, http://safeaccess.ca.

Gregory D. Carter, M.D., is clinical professor of rehabilitation medicine at the University of Washington School of Medicine, Seattle. He is actively involved in research examining the efficacy of cannabis in treating human neuromuscular disease. He can be contacted at gtcarter@u.washington.edu.

Tommy Chong is an actor, comedian, writer, and director. He began his cannabis studies when he was seventeen years old. He found it helped him enjoy the music he was playing (he was a blues guitar player for multiple bands). His cannabis use helped him to quit a four-year cigarette habit. He also found it immensely helpful with writing and directing the Cheech and Chong movies. He can be contacted at tomcheech@yahoo.com.

Cheryl Corcoran, M.D., is assistant professor of clinical psychiatry and director of the Center of Prevention and Evaluation at New York Psychiatric Institute, Columbia University. She is interested in the relationship that may exist between cannabis use and psychosis.

Lyle Craker, Ph.D., is professor in the department of plant and soil sciences and director of the Medicinal Plant Program at the University of Massachusetts. Dr. Craker, author of several research articles, books, and proceedings and editor of the *Journal of Herbs, Spices and Medicinal Plants,* has worked on the physiology and production of medicinal plants for more than thirty years. He can be contacted at craker@pssi.umass.edu.

Danny Danko is senior cultivation editor of *High Times* magazine and a cannabis law reform advocate. He has authored many articles on indoor and outdoor marijuana gardening. He can be contacted at dannydanko @hightimes.com.

Rick Doblin, Ph.D., is founder and executive director of the Multidisciplinary Association for Psychedelic Studies (MAPS, www .maps.org). His dissertation (public policy, Harvard's Kennedy School of Government) was "The Regulation of the Medical Use of Psychedelics and

Marijuana," and his master's thesis (Harvard) focused on the attitudes and experiences of oncologists concerning the medical use of marijuana. He can be contacted at rick@maps.org.

Mitch Earleywine, Ph.D., is professor of psychology at the State University of New York at Albany; author of *Understanding Marijuana* (New York: Oxford University Press, 2002), *Parents' Guide to Marijuana* (New York: High Times Books, 2008), and *Substance Use Problems, Advances in Psychotherapy* (Cambridge, MA: Hogrefe, 2009); and editor of *Pot Politics* (New York:Oxford University Press, 2007) and *Mind-Altering Drugs* (New York: Oxford University Press, 2005). He is also on the advisory board for the National Organization for the Reform of Marijuana Laws (NORML). He can be contacted at mearleywine@albany.edu.

Mahmoud A. ElSohly, Ph.D., is research professor at the school of pharmacy at the University of Mississippi and project director at the National Center for Natural Products Research, a division of the Research Institute of Pharmaceutical Sciences. At the University of Mississippi, he presides over the only federally approved marijuana plantation in the United States. He can be contacted at melsohly@olemiss.edu.

Zoë Gardner is program coordinator of the Medicinal Plant Program at the University of Massachusetts. She is an expert in the botany, cultivation, and processing of medicinal plants and is currently completing her Ph.D. in medicinal plant quality and safety. She can be contacted at zoe@psis.umass .edu. Her website is www.herbnerd.com.

Gregory Gerdeman, Ph.D., is assistant professor of biology at Eckerd College. His research explores the molecular physiology, pharmacology, and evolutionary significance of endocannabinoids and cannabinoid receptors, especially within neural systems. He can be contacted at gerdemgl@eckerd.edu.

Lester Grinspoon, M.D., is professor of psychiatry emeritus at the Harvard Medical School and a well-published author in the field of drugs and drug policy. He is the author of *Marihuana Reconsidered* (Cambridge, MA: Harvard University press, 1971, 1977; American Archives press classic edition, 1994) and *Marijuana, The Forbidden Medicine* (Princeton, NJ: Yale University Press, 1993, 1997), which is now translated into fourteen languages. Dr. Grinspoon currently maintains a medical marijuana website (www.rxmarijuana.com and www.marijuana-uses.com) that chronicles real-life stories of people who have had positive "non-medical" experiences with marijuana. He can be contacted at lester_grinspoon@hms.harvard.edu.

Margaret Haney, Ph.D., is professor of clinical neurobiology at Columbia University. Her interest is to assess empirically the behavioral and neuro-biological effects of cannabis in long-term users. She can be contacted at mh235@columbia.edu.

Lumír Hanuš, Ph.D., is senior scientist at the Institute of Drug Research, School of Pharmacy, Hebrew University in Jerusalem. His research during the last eighteen years has centered on cannabinoids—their chemistry and analysis. He can be contacted at lumir@cc.huji.ac.il.

Carl L. Hart, Ph.D., is associate professor of psychology in both the departments of psychiatry and psychology at Columbia University and director of the Residential Studies and Methamphetamine Research Laboratories at the New York State Psychiatric Institute. A major focus of Dr. Hart's research is to understand complex interactions between drugs of abuse and the neurobiology and environmental factors that mediate human behavior and physiology. He is the author or coauthor of dozens of peer-reviewed scientific articles in the area of neuropsychopharmacology, coauthor of the textbook *Drugs, Society, and Human Behavior* (New York: McGraw-Hill, 2009), and a member of a National Institutes of Health (NIH) review group. He can be contacted at clh42@columbia.edu.

Jeffrey Hergenrather, M.D., is president of the Society of Cannabis Clinicians (SCC), a project of the California Cannabis Research Medical Group, a nonprofit public benefit corporation whose mission includes collecting and reporting data associated with the medical conditions for which cannabis provides relief. SCC physicians meet quarterly to share their findings in the field of cannabinoid medicine. He can be contacted at jeff@trashtalk.net.

Julie Holland, M.D., is assistant clinical professor of psychiatry at New York University School of Medicine. She has a private practice in psychopharmacology in New York City. She is a harm reductionist and drug policy reformer and believes in cognitive liberty and personal freedom with regard to health maintenance. She is editor of *Ecstasy: The Complete Guide: A Comprehensive Look at the Risks and Benefits of MDMA* (Rochester, VT: Park Street Press, 2001) and author of *Weekends at Bellevue: Nine Years on the Nightshift at the Psych ER* (New York: Bantam, 2009). Her websites include DrHolland.com, NaturalMood.com, ThePotBook.com, and WeekendsAtBellevue.com. She can be contacted at taxandregulate@gmail.com.

William J. Holubek, M.D., is an emergency medicine physician and medical toxicologist at Vassar Brothers Medical Center in Poughkeepsie, New York. He has written numerous articles on the use and abuse of medications. He can be contacted at wjh2118@columbia.edu.

Matthew Kirkpatrick is a Ph.D. candidate in the department of psychology at Columbia University and the division on substance abuse at the New York State Psychiatric Institute. His NIDA-funded research focuses on understanding the direct effects of alcohol, marijuana, and methamphetamine on human behavior and physiology. He can be contacted at mk627@columbia.edu.

Mario Lap is director of Drugtext Foundation (www.drugtext.org) and advisor to the Dutch Drug Policy Foundation. He is also director of the Foundation on Drug Policy and Human Rights and he has written widely on the legal basis, philosophy, and rationale of drug prohibition. He can be contacted at mario@lap.nl.

Harry G. Levine, Ph.D., is professor of sociology at Queens College, City University of New York. He has been writing about drug use and policy for many years and is the coauthor of *Crack in America: Demon Drugs and Social Justice* (Berkeley: University of California Press, 1997) and *Marijuana Arrest Crusade: Racial Bias and Police Policy in New York City* (New York: New York Civil Liberties Union, 2008).

Peter Lewis is nonexecutive chairman of the Progressive Corporation (Progressive Insurance Companies). Lewis has long held an unorthodox approach to business. As a retired CEO of Progressive, he has made many donations to various charities and political groups. Since the late 1970s, Mr. Lewis has supported many efforts to reduce or eliminate the penalties for marijuana use.

David Malmo-Levine is an educator, agitator, and the curator of the Herb Museum in Vancouver, BC. He is interested in helping to relegalize cannabis in order to end the drug war, empower farmers and gardeners, and remove red tape around hemp ethanol. He can be contacted at malmolevine@gmail .com, cannabisculture.com, pot.tv.

Caroline Marvin is a Ph.D. candidate in the department of psychology at Columbia University. The aim of her research is to understand better the cognitive effects produced by marijuana and methamphetamine. She can be contacted at cbm2118@columbia.edu.

Mary Lynn Mathre, R.N, C.A.R.N., is president and cofounder of Patients Out of Time (medicalcannabis.com). She is also editor of *Cannabis in Medical Practice: A Legal, Historical and Pharmacologic Overview of the Therapeutic Use of Marijuana* (Jefferson, NC: McFarland and Co, Inc. 1997) and coeditor of *Women and Cannabis: Medicine, Science and Sociology* (New York: Haworth Herbal Press, 2002). She can be contacted at mlmathre@hughes.net.

Raphael Mechoulam, Ph.D., is professor of medicinal chemistry (emeritus) at the Institute of Drug Research, Faculty of Medicine, Hebrew University, in Jerusalem. He is a member of the Israel Academy of Sciences, where he serves as head of the division of natural sciences. His scientific interests are in the chemistry and biological effects of natural products and synthetic drugs. He has published on plant cannabinoids since 1963 and on endocannabinoids since 1992. He can be contacted at mechou@cc.huji.ac.il.

Bruce Mirken, a longtime health journalist, served as director of communications for the Marijuana Policy Project from 2001 through 2009. He became interested in cannabis during the 1990s while covering medical marijuana controversies. He left the Marijuana Policy Project at the end of 2009 as a result of concerns over the organization's governance and is no longer affiliated with the organization in any way. He is now media relations coordinator at the Greenlining Institute in Berkeley, California. He can be contacted at sftroubl@att.net.

Jeffrey A. Miron, Ph.D., is senior lecturer and director of undergraduate studies in the department of economics at Harvard University. He has published more than twenty-five articles in refereed journals and fifty op-eds.

His commentary on economic policy has appeared in dozens of other television, radio, and print media around the world. He currently writes the blog *Libertarianism from A to Z* at jeffreymiron.com.

Ethan Nadelmann, J.D., Ph.D., is founder and executive director of the Drug Policy Alliance, the leading organization in the United States advocating for drug policies grounded in science, compassion, health, and human rights. Described by *Rolling Stone* as "the point man" for drug policy reform efforts, he is widely regarded as the outstanding proponent of drug policy reform both in the United States and abroad. He can be contacted at Enadelmann@drugpolicy.org.

William Notcutt, M.D., F.R.C.A., F.F.P.M.R.C.A., is a consultant in pain medicine at the James Paget University Hospital, Great Yarmouth, UK, and a senior lecturer at the University of East Anglia, Norwich, UK. He has been researching the clinical use of cannabinoids for the last fifteen years and has participated in about eighteen studies. He can be contacted at william.notcutt@jpaget.nhs.uk.

Denis J. Petro, M.D., is a board-certified neurologist in private practice in Pennsylvania. He has also served as a clinical drug researcher. He supports the medicinal use of cannabis and has written widely on the subject. He can be contacted at djpetromd@gmail.com.

Ben Platt, M.D., has a private practice in Vancouver, Washington. He is affiliated with Southwest Washington Medical Center. He has a particular interest in neuromodulation and cancer pain management. Dr. Platt is intrigued by the evolving role of cannabinoids in pain medicine.

Neal Pollack is the author of *Stretch: The Unlikely Making of a Yoga Dude* (New York: Harper Perennial, 2010). He is a card-carrying medical marijuana patient in the state of California. He can be contacted at alternadad@gmail.com.

Michael Pollan is Knight Professor of Science and Environmental Journalism at Berkeley and author of six books, including *The Botany of Desire* (New York: Random House, 2001), which has a chapter on the coevolution of humans and cannabis, and *The Omnivore's Dilemma* (New York: Penguin, 2006).

Marsha Rosenbaum, Ph.D., a National Institute on Drug Abuse–funded researcher and founder of the Safety First Project (www.safety1st.org), is currently director emerita of the San Francisco office of the New York–based Drug Policy Alliance (www.drugpolicy.org). Her interest in marijuana education spans four decades. She can be contacted at mrosenbaum@drugpolicy.org.

Doug Rushkoff is founder of the Institute for Applied Memetics and is the author of *Cyberia: Life in the Trenches of Hyperspace* (San Francisco: HarperSan Francisco, 1994); *Media Virus!: Hidden Agendas in Popular Culture* (New York: Ballantine, 1994); and *Life Inc.* (New York: Random House, 2009). He believes cannabis can save the economy and compensate for America's addiction to stimulants. He can be contacted at http://rushkoff.com.

Allen St. Pierre is executive director of NORML and the NORML Foundation, a nonprofit organization established in 1997 to educate the public about marijuana and marijuana policy. He strongly supports legalization and responsible adult use of marijuana. He can be contacted at director@norml.org www.norml.org.

Jason B. Schechter, Ph.D., is CEO of Cortical Systematics LLC, a scientific consultancy and support firm. He is a classically-trained neuropharmacologist with a focus on the cannabinoids. He can be contacted at jbs@corticalsystematics.net.

Andrew Tatarsky, Ph.D., is a clinical psychologist and psychotherapist in private practice in New York City. He is codirector of Harm Reduction Psychotherapy and Training Associates and is the author of *Harm Reduction Psychotherapy: A New Treatment for Drug and Alcohol Problems* (Lanham, MD: Rowman and Littlefield, 2007). He can be contacted at atatarsky@andrewtatarsky.com.

Ryan Vandrey, Ph.D., is assistant professor at Johns Hopkins University School of Medicine. He conducts controlled human research studies on the behavioral pharmacology of cannabis. The primary focus of his work has been to characterize the consequences of abruptly stopping heavy cannabis use and then applying that knowledge to improve treatment interventions to assist those who have trouble stopping use of cannabis. He can be contacted at rvandrey@jhmi.edu.

Mark Wallace, M.D., is professor of clinical anesthesiology and chair of the division of pain medicine, Department of Anesthesiology, University of California, San Diego. He has received state grants from the California Center for Medicinal Cannabis Research; he has completed one study using experimental pain in healthy volunteers and is conducting a clinical trial on the effects of cannabis on painful diabetic peripheral neuropathy. He can be contacted at mswallace@ucsd.edu.

Mark A. Ware, M.D., is assistant professor of anesthesia and family medicine at McGill University, director of clinical research at the Alan Edwards Pain Management Unit at the McGill University Health Centre, and executive director of the Canadian Consortium for the Investigation of Cannabinoids, a nonprofit organization dedicated to promoting research and education on cannabis and cannabinoids. He teaches pain medicine at McGill University, and his main research interests are in the use of cannabinoids in pain management and the epidemiology of chronic pain. He can be contacted at mark.ware@muhc.mcgill.ca.

Andrew Weil, M.D., is founder and director of the Arizona Center for Integrative Medicine at the University of Arizona, where he is also clinical professor of medicine, professor of public health, and Lovell-Jones Professor of Integrative Rheumatology. He is an internationally known author, lecturer, and expert on integrative, natural, and botanical medicine. He conducted the first controlled human experiments with cannabis in 1968 and has always been interested in the plant and its many uses. He can be contacted at nancy@x9ranch.com.

Jeremy Wolff is an artist who has created photo-collages for the cover of *Newsweek* and whose writing has been featured in *The Wall Street Journal*. He lives in a small town north of New York City. An expanded and updated version of his chapter is online at http://very.com/pot.

Index

Page numbers in *italics* indicate illustrations.

2-AG, *71*, 71–72

Abrams, Donald, 247, 249, 252–60, 262, 405
absorption, 142–43
abstinence, 354
abuse potential, 15–16
acute harms, 224–25
acute pain, 331
ADD/ADHD, 290–91, 419–20, 423–24
addiction, 137–40, 187–95, 229, 292, 352–53, 429. *See also* harm reduction
Addiction Proof Your Child, 360
administration, xix–xxi, 157, 275, 337, 338–40, *339*, 428–29
adolescence, 291–92, 344–45
adulterants, 150–51
aeroponics, 46–47
Aggarwal, Sunil, 295–310
AIDS, xiii, xiv, 249, 252–60, 311–17, 419–20
Alabama, 76
Alaska, xi–xii, 77–78
alcohol, 136, 306–9, 397
Alliance for Cannabis Therapeutics (ACT), 413
Alzheimer's disease (AD), 301–3
ambivalence, 236–37
American Bar Association, xii
American Civil Liberties Union (ACLU), 462–72
American Medical Association (AMA), xii, 401

American Nurses Association (ANA), 399–400
American Psychiatric Association, xii
amyotrophic lateral sclerosis (ALS), 297–99
anandamide, *71*, 71–72, 244–45, 374
Ann Arbor, Michigan, 99
anorexia, 419–20
Anslinger, Harry, 7, 31
anti-inflammatory, 245
anxiety, 180, 184–85, 289–90
appetite, 250, 315
Arizona, 78–79
Arkansas, 79
Armentano, Paul, 196–201
arrests, xxi–xxii, 202–6, 409–10, 457–58
Ashcroft, John, 207
Asiatic Exclusion League, 28–29
asset forfeiture, 382
Assurbanipal, King, 20
awareness/relaxation exercise, 232–34

Bearman, David, 404
beauty, 393
Benet, Sula, 21–22
Bennett, Chris, 17–26
Bevan, Arthur Dean, 30
"Beyond Zero Tolerance", 355–56
Bible, 24–26, 27
biopsies, 156
bipolar disorder, 289
Black Candle, The, 31
bladder dysfunction, 324–25

Bloomberg, Michael, 202–3
Boire, Richard Glen, 219–22
bongs, 158
Borst, Els, 445–46
botany of *Cannabis,* 35–36
    applications, 41–43, *42*
    botanical history of, 37–38
    morphology of, 37–41, *39–41*
    nomenclature, 36–37
    plant constituents and, 65–70
Botany of Desire, The, 8, 377
Bourne, Peter, xii
Boyd, Graham, 462–72
brain, xiii–xiv, 57–61. *See also* cannabinoid
        receptors; neuroprotection
brain injury, 306–9
bronchoscopes, 156
Brown, Prentiss, 32
bubblehash, 50
Buchanan, Mary Beth, 207, 210
Bush, George H. W., xii
Bush, George W., 33
Byrne, Al, 399–415
Byrne Grant Program, 206

California, 80–82, 206, 416–31, 466
California Compassionate Use Act
    (Proposition 215), 253–54, 417, 463–65
Canada, 28–29, 432–40
Canadian Medical Association (CMA), 437
Canadian Medical Protective Association
    (CMPA), 437
cancer, 151–52, 245–46, 247–48, 249,
    329–30, 341, 420–23
cannabidiol (CBD), 65–66, *66,* 244, 246,
    281, 286–87, 290, 296–97
cannabinoid receptors, 53–55, *54*
cannabinoids, 35, 36, 43, 65–70, *66–69,*
    154–55, 159, 162, 183, 420. *See also*
    neuroprotection
cannabis, origin of word, 389–90.
cannabis fingerprint, 269–71, 338
Capler, N. Rielle, 432–40

Carcieri, Donald, 459
cardiovascular toxicity, 146–47
Carter, Gregory T., 295–310
Carter, Jimmy, 2
Cayetano, Ben, 89
Cermak, Timmen, 360
Cheney, Dick, 33
children, 150, 344–46, 349–60
China, 18–19, 37
Chong, Tommy, 207–18
chronic harms, 226–28
chronic pain, 331–33, 336–37, 418–19
cigarettes, 136, 160, 245–46, 397
civil disobedience, 435–36
civil liberties, xxiii–xxiv, 452. *See also*
        American Civil Liberties Union (ACLU)
CMCR, 261–65
cocaine, 64, 194, 379
cognition, 161–70, 327
    effects of cannabis on, 170–77
Colorado, 82–84
Compassionate IND Program, xiii, xix,
    243, 272–74, 279, 396, 407, 413–14
Compassionate Use Act of 1996. *See*
    Proposition 215
compassion clubs, Canadian, 432–40
Comprehensive Drug Abuse and Control
    Act, xxi
Conant, Marcus, 464–65
Connecticut, 84
consciousness, 136
consequences, 356–57
Controlled Drugs and Substances Act
    (CDSA), 433–34
Controlled Substance Act of 1970, 1
convictions, collateral consequences of,
    219–22
Corcoran, Cheryl, 178–86
Corral, Valerie, 469
Corzine, Jon, 108
Costa, Barbara, 428
cost-benefit analysis of legalization, 447–53
Craker, Lyle, 263, 406

Creighton, C., 21
crime, 451
Crohn's colitis, 423–24
cultivation laws. *See* specific states
curiosity, 231
Curtis, Alva, 30
cyclical hyperemesis, 149–50

dangers. *See* risks
Danko, Danny, 44–51
dehabituation, 293–94
Delaware, 84–85
delivery methods, xix–xxi, 157, 275, 337,
    338–40, 339, 428–29
delta-9 THC. *See* THC
dementia, 301–2
depression, 185, 288–89
Devane, William, 70
diabetes, 246, 309
Diagnostic and Statistical Manual (DSM),
    188, 195
dishabituation, 387–94
distribution, 430
District of Columbia, 85–87
Doblin, Rick, 252–53, 257, 261–65, 406–7
Dogoloff, Lee, xii
dosage, 293, 316
Doughton, Robert, 32
Douglas, James, 124
Dreher, Melanie, 401–2
driving, 196–201
dronabinol, 258–59. *See also* Marinol
Drug Enforcement Agency (DEA), xiii,
    xvi–xvii, 242–43, 263–64, 403–7, 459
Drug Policy Alliance (DPA), 405, 466–67
drug testing, 144–45, 266–67, 350, 356,
    358–59, 408
drug treatment, 15, 138, 187, 353, 471–72
drug war, 3, 130–31, 382, 409, 426, 470–71

Earleywine, Mitch, 153–60, 248
economics, 32–34, 447–53, 457–58
education, 10–11, 355–56, 425–26

effects of cannabis, 9–16
    adverse, 429
    dishabituation, 387–94
    individual's history of use and, 13–15
    source of education on, 10–11
Effron, Dan, 63
Egypt, 7
Eliot, Charles, 30
ElSohly, Mahmoud A., 266–81, 406–7
endocannabinoid system, 52–62, 70–72,
    71, 296–97, 336
enforcement of marijuana laws, xxi–xxii.
    See also specific states
epilepsy, 24, 246
euphoria, 15
excretion, 144

fatigue, 325
Federal Bureau of Narcotics, 31
female plants, 46
femininity, 388–89, 392–93
fertilization, 48–49
fiber production, 42
flaxseed oil, 8
Flexner, Abraham, 30
Flexner, Simon, 30
Florida, 87
flowering growth, 47–48
Food and Drug Administration, U.S.
    (FDA), 262–63
Fry, Marian, 345–50

Gaoni, Yehiel, 64–65
gardener's rights, 376–82
gateway hypothesis, 193–95, 353, 367
Gehringer, Dale, 257
genetic selection, 271–72
Georgia, 87–88
Gerdeman, Gregory L., 52–62
Gettman, Jon, 402–3
Ginsberg, Douglas, xii
Giuliani, Rudolph, 202
gliomas, 304–6

goals, 237–38
Gonzales vs. Raich, 466–67
gravity, 390–91
Grinspoon, Lester, xi–xxiv
grow revolution, 44–45
    future of, 50–51
    indica vs. sativa, 45
    indoor vs. outdoor, 48
    males vs. females, 46
    medical marijuana and, 50
    organic vs. chemical fertilization, 48–49
    organic vs. chemical pest control, 49–50
    soil vs. hydroponics, 46–47
    vegetative vs. flowering growth, 47–48
guilt, 346–47

Hand of the Ghost, 20
Haney, Margaret, 187–95
Hanuš, Lumír, 63–72
Harcourt, Bernard, 203
harm reduction, 137, 224, 279, 397–98
Hart, Carl L., 9–16, 161–77
hashish, 43, 50, 142, 441–42
Hawaii, 88–90
headaches, 333–34
Hearst, William Randolph, 31, 32
Hebrew Scriptures, 21–23
Help at Any Cost, 360
hemp, 8, 250–51, 280–81, 381, 389
hemp ethanol, 32
herbalism schools, 31–32
Hergenrather, Jeffrey, 416–31
Herodotus, 19–20
heroin, 194
history, early/ancient
    in China, 18–19
    Mideast, 19–26
    role of, 17–18
history, recent, 27–34
    anti-Asian riots, 28–29
    closing of herbal schools, 30
    first laws against, 30–31
    politics of, 31–33

popularity of cannabis as patent
    medicine, 29
HIV, 311–17. *See also* AIDS
holding smoke, 158–59
Holland, Julie, 1–8, 136–40, 242–46,
    282–94, 344–48, 396–98
    interview with Abrams, Donald, 252–60
    interview with Boyd, Graham, 462–72
    interview with Bryne and Mathre, 399–415
    interview with Chong, Tommy, 207–18
    interview with ElSohly, Mahmoud, 266–81
    interview with Lewis, Peter, 383–86
    interview with Pollan, Michael, 373–82
    interview with Weil, Andrew, 247–51
Holubek, William, 141–52
homegrown, 44–45
Howlett, Allyn, 70
Hua T'o, 18
Huffman, Alice, 132
human rights, 130–31
hydroponics, 46–47

Idaho, 74, 90–91
Illinois, 91–92
immune response, 6
immune system, 316–17
Indiana, 74, 92–93
indica, 45, 271–72, 392, 425
individual's history of use, 13–15
indoor growing, 48
infants, 150
infectious diseases, 228
inflammatory bowel disease, 423–24
inhalation, 12
Institute of Medicine (IOM) Report,
    xix–xxi, 455
interviews. *See* Holland, Julie
intoxication, 150–51
Iowa, 74, 93–94
IQ, 166–67, 182

Jealous, Ben, 132
Jefferson, Thomas, 37

Jenks, Barbara, 413–14
Jenks, Kenny, 413–14
Jesus Christ, 24–26
Joy, Janet, 401–2
"just say no," 354

K2, 286
Kansas, 94
Kentucky, 94–95
King, William Lyon Mackenzie, 28–29,
    30
Kirkpatrick, Matthew G., 9–16
Klink, Ab, 446
Kurgans, 17

Lap, Mario, 441–46
Lawn, John, xvi, 242, 405
laws, cannabis in United States, 30–31,
    73–129. See also specific states
Leary, Timothy, 366
Leers, Gerd, 444–45
legalization, 1, 347–48, 396–98, 447–53
Lenson, David, 379
Leonhart, Michele, 264
Leshner, Alan, 254
Lewis, Peter, 383–86
lighting, 44–45
Louisiana, 95
Ludwig, Jens, 203
lung cancer, 153–55, 353–54
lung function, 155, 228
Lust, Benedict, 30

Maine, 73, 95–97
male plants, 46
Malmo-Levine, David, 27–34
Mannich, Lise, 21
MAPS, 261–65
Marihuana Reconsidered, xii, xiii
Marijuana and the Cannabinoids, 266
Marijuana: A New Look at the Scientific
    Evidence, 351
Marijuana Myths, Marijuana Facts, 351

Marijuana Policy Project (MPP), 158, 405,
    454–61, 466–67
Marijuana Research Institute, 215–16
Marijuana Tax Act, 31–32
Marijuana: What's a Parent to Believe?, 360
Marinol, xiv, xx, xxi, 243–44, 250, 272–
    73, 276, 427–28
Marshall, Thurgood, 470
Marvin, Caroline B., 161–77
Maryland, 97–98
masking techniques, 145, 210–11
Mason, James O., xiii
Massachusetts, 98–99
Mathre, Mary Lynn, 399–415
McCaffrey, Barry, 463–65
McCormick, Todd, 409
McMahon, George, 415
McQueen, Neil, 23
McWilliams, Peter, 409–10
measurements, 75
Mechoulam, Raphael, 63–72, 374–75
medical marijuana, xiv–xxiii, 50, 398
    interview with Andrew Weil, 247–51
    interview with Donald Abrams, 252–60
    interview with Mahmoud ElSohly,
        266–81
    MPP and, 458–60
    obstruction of research, 261–65
    See also California; Canada;
        Netherlands; Patients Out of Time
meditation, 246
Mellon, Andrew, 32
memory, 291, 375. See also cognition
mental health, 178–86, 192–93, 225
Mesopotamia, 20
metabolism, 143–44
metabolites, 196–97
Mexico, 30–31
Michigan, 99–100
Mideastern ancient history, 19–26
migraines, 333–34
Mikuriya, Tod, 421–22
Minnesota, 100–101

Mirken, Bruce, 454–61
Miron, Jeffrey, 75, 447–53
Mississippi, 101–2
Missouri, 102
MMAR (Marihuana Medical Access
    Regulations), 434–35
moderation, 344–46, 356
monopoly, 33
Montana, 103–4
Morgan, John, 154
morphology of *Cannabis,* 37–41, *39–41*
Moses, 27
multiple sclerosis (MS), 299–301, 318–27,
    336, 340–41
Murphy, Emily, 31
muscle relaxants, 244

nabilone, 272–73, 337
Nadelmann, Ethan, 130–33, 405
National Commission on Marijuana and
    Drug Abuse, xi–xii
National Council of Churches, xii
National Institute on Drug Abuse
    (NIDA), xii–xiv, 7–8, 242–43, 253–
    54, 261–62, 267–68, 429
National Institutes of Health, 63
National Organization for the Reform of
    Marijuana Laws (NORML), xvi, 196,
    242, 405
National Research Council (NRC), 456–57
nature, 294, 376–77, 388, 394
nausea, 247, 276, 314–15, 419–20
Nebraska, 104
Netherlands, 2, 3, 178, 441–46, 457
neurological toxicity, 147–48
neuropathic pain, 324, 330–31, 341
neuroprotection, 295–310
neurotransmitters, 184
Nevada, 104–6
New Hampshire, 106
New Jersey, 107–8
New Mexico, 108–10
New York, 110–11

New York (city), 202–6
Niño, Carla, 360
North Carolina, 111
North Dakota, 111
Notcutt, William, 336–41, 412
Nutt, David, 397
nystagmus, 325

Obama, Barack, 264
odor, 393
Ohio, 74, 112
oil industry, 32–34
Oklahoma, 112–13
O'Leary, Alice, 413
On Drugs, 379
Operation Green Merchant, xii
opiates, 408, 419
opiod systems, 293
opium, 28–29
oral administration, 157, 275, 339
oral delta-9-THC, 15–16
Oregon, xi–xii, 74, 113–16
outdoor growing, 48

pain, 244, 247, 312–14, 324, 340–41
pain management, 328–35
paranoia, 193, 369, 429
paraphernalia laws. *See* specific states
parenting, 344–46, 349–60, 361–65
Parker, Terrance, 433
Partnership for a Drug-Free America, 32–33
patent medicines, 29
patents, xviii–xix, 426
Patients Out of Time, 399–415
Peele, Stanton, 360
peer pressure, 349–50
Pennsylvania, 116–17
Pen Ts'ao, 18, 37
Pertwee, Roger, 71
pest control, 48, 49–50
pharmaceuticalization of cannabis, xix–
    xxi, xxii–xxiii
pharmacodynamics, 142–44

pharmacokinetics, 142–44
physicians, as cannabis specialists, 426–27
physician support, 437
Pierre, Allen St., 73–129
Platt, Ben, 328–35
Pollack, Neil, 345–50, 361–65
Pollan, Michael, 8, 373–82
pollination, 41
Posse Comitatus Act, xxiii–xxiv
possession arrests. *See* arrests
postural regulation, 327
potency, 268–69, 272–74, 351–52
pregnancy, 149
prevention strategies, 350
prison, 2–3, 75, 131–32, 384
production, xix, 3, 430
prohibition, xxii, xxiii–xxiv, 27–28, 130–33, 447, 451–53, 456, 458
Proposition 215, 253–54, 417, 430, 463–65
protease inhibitors, 255
pruning, 291–92
psychiatry, cannabinoids and, 282–94
psychomotor performance, 198, 225
psychosis, 179–84, 286–88
psychotherapy, harm reduction, 223–39
PTSD, 264–65, 289–90
Public Health Service, xiii
pulmonary harm, 153–60
pulmonary toxicity, 148–49

quality, 212, 317, 412, 437–38, 451–52
qunabu, 20

race and racism, 7, 28–29, 130–31, 471
    arrest statistics and, 202–6, *204*
    early cannabis laws and, 31
    politics and, 32–33
Raich, Gonzales vs., 466–67
Ramses II, 7
Randall, Bob, 243, 399, 413
Rathbun, Mary, 252
Rätsch, Christian, 29
Reefer Madness, xii, 161

reform, efforts in 1970s, xi–xii. *See also* legalization
relaxation, 246
religion, freedom of, 26
research, 11–16, 63–65, 261–65. *See also* Abrams, Donald
resin, 158–59
respiratory illness, 156–57
Reynolds, John Russel, 284
rheumatoid arthritis, 341, 423
Rhode Island, 117–18
Rice, Condoleezza, 33
Richardson, Bill, 109
Rimonabant, 427–28
riots, 28–29
risks, xii–xiii, 136–37, 140, 316, 454–55, 457–58. *See also* addiction; arrests; cognition; harm reduction; mental health; pulmonary harm; toxicity
rituals of use, 139
Robinson, Robert, 64
Rockefeller Institute, 30
Roosevelt, Franklin D., 31–32
Rosenbaum, Marsha, 349–60
Roth, Geneen, 347
Ruck, Ruck, 22–23
Rudenko, S. I., 20
Rushkoff, Doug, 366–72
Russo, Ethan, 20, 263, 326, 406

sativa, 45, 271–72, 392, 425
Sativex, xxi, 248, 272–73, 276–77, 326, 331, 336–41, 396, 412, 427–28
scare tactics, 351
Schechter, Jason B., 52–62
scheduled drugs
    cannabis as, xvii–xviii, 242, 243–44, 267, 274–75, 278, 396–97, 402, 404–5
    definitions of, xv–xvi
schizophrenia, 181–84, 185–86, 286–88
screens, 393–94
Scythians, 19–20
Seattle, Washington, 74

seeds, 8
self-acceptance, 229–38
self-administration, 15
Sex, Drugs, Violence and the Bible, 23
sex and sexuality, 392–93
sexual dysfunction, 326
Shen-Nung, 18
Sherrat, Andrew, 17
Skager, Rodney, 355–56
skunk, 286
slang terms, 150–51
sleep disturbance, 326
smell, 393
smoking, 12, 245–46, 337, 428
soil, 46–47
South Carolina, 118–19
South Dakota, 74, 119–20
spasticity, 319, 322–24, 340–41, 419
specialists, 426–27
Spice, 286
spices, 22–23
Standard Oil, 31–32
stealth goddess, cannabis as, 366–72
stigma, 229–30
stroke, 306–9
sublingual administration, 339, 411–12
Sullivan, Louis, 414
synaptic plasticity, 57
Szalavitz, Maia, 360

Tashkin, Donald, 422–23
Tatarsky, Andrew, 223–39
tax revenue, 448–50
Tennessee, 120–21
Testimony of Truth, 25
Texas, 121–22
THC, xiii–xiv, 36–37, 43, 53–55, 65–70,
    67–69, 162, 184, 199, 268, 277–78,
    280–81, 296–97, 425
therapeutic ratio, xx–xxi
Thompson, Samuel, 30
tobacco, 140, 151, 153–54, 160, 445
tolerance, 14–15, 164, 189, 429

Tourette's syndrome (TS), 303–4
Tours, Jacques-Joseph Moreau de, 284
toxicity, 145–50, 153–60
transdermal applications, 411–12
tree of life, 33–34
tremor, 326–27

uncontrolled use, 190–92
United Kingdom, 178
United States
    cannabis laws in, 73–129
    cannabis use compared to Netherlands, *443*
    drug use in, 1–3
    See also specific states
Utah, 74, 123

Vandrey, Ryan, 187–95
vaporizers, 157–58, 248, 257, 279–80, 411,
    428
Vasconcellos, John, 261
vegetative growth, 47–48
Vermont, 123–25
Virginia, 125

Wallace, Mark S., 328–35
WAMM (Wo/Men's Alliance for Medical
    Marijuana), 469
Washington, 74, 126–27
Washington, George, 37
water pipes, 158
Weil, Andrew, 247–51, 412
West Virginia, 128
Williams, Montel, 410
Willstätter, Richard, 64
Wisconsin, 128–29
withdrawal, 189–90
Wolff, Jeremy, 387–94
working memory, 375
World Health Organization (WHO), 1–2
Wyoming, 129

Yanghai Tombs, 6, 19
Young, Francis L., xvi–xvii, 242

BOOKS OF RELATED INTEREST

Cannabis and Spirituality
An Explorer's Guide to an Ancient Plant Spirit Ally
Edited by Stephen Gray

Cannabis in Spiritual Practice
The Ecstasy of Shiva, the Calm of Buddha
by Will Johnson

Marijuana Medicine
A World Tour of the Healing and Visionary Powers of Cannabis
by Christian Rätsch

Hemp for Health
The Medicinal and Nutritional Uses of Cannabis Sativa
by Chris Conrad

DMT: The Spirit Molecule
A Doctor's Revolutionary Research into
the Biology of Near-Death and Mystical Experiences
by Rick Strassman, M.D.

The Psychedelic Explorer's Guide
Safe, Therapeutic, and Sacred Journeys
by James Fadiman, Ph.D.

Plants of the Gods
Their Sacred, Healing, and Hallucinogenic Powers
*by Richard Evans Schultes and Albert Hofmann,
and Christian Rätsch*

The Encyclopedia of Psychoactive Plants
Ethnopharmacology and Its Applications
by Christian Rätsch
Foreword by Albert Hofmann

Inner Traditions • Bear & Company
P.O. Box 388
Rochester, VT 05767
1-800-246-8648
www.InnerTraditions.com

Or contact your local bookseller